# The Outpatient Breast Clinic

Alfonso M. Pluchinotta
Editor

# The Outpatient Breast Clinic

## Aiming at Best Practice

Springer

*Editor*
Alfonso M. Pluchinotta
Breast Surgery Department Consultant
Surgeon
Polyclinic Abano Terme
Padova
Italy

ISBN 978-3-319-15906-5 ISBN 978-3-319-15907-2 (eBook)
DOI 10.1007/978-3-319-15907-2

Library of Congress Control Number: 2015938097

Springer Cham Heidelberg New York Dordrecht London


Printed on acid-free paper

Springer International Publishing AG Switzerland is part of Springer Science+Business Media (www.springer.com)

# Foreword

This book is an excellent work by a group of distinguished authors presenting the diagnosis and treatment of benign and malignant diseases of the breast from the point of view of a team of multidisciplinary experts. Indeed, the first chapter – The Breast Clinic – not only discusses basic aspects of breast diseases but portrays the philosophical and intellectual basis of multidisciplinary care. The chapter discusses the importance of the outpatient breast unit and the indications and rationale for referral. Basic but important aspects of clinical care are discussed throughout the book, emphasizing the importance of teamwork, transparency, and respect. Clear and honest communication between clinicians and patients is stressed throughout this work.

Important concepts are discussed with lucidity and intelligence. The approach to the asymptomatic woman, including the high-risk woman, is a practical and useful lesson in clinical care. Chapters on the fundamental evaluation of breast diseases including anatomy, congenital abnormalities, normal physiologic changes, and signs and symptoms of disease are elucidating. Diagnostic procedures, including types of biopsies and tissue diagnosis, with a comprehensive chapter on imaging are discussed in a manner that portrays a systematic approach, yet leaves room for the influence of experience and judgment.

Benign conditions such as breast pain, mastitis, nipple discharge, and proliferative and non-proliferative lesions are discussed in depth. Excellent chapters on non-invasive cancer and the diagnosis of special cancers of the breast will be particularly helpful to clinicians who are not necessarily breast specialists. The authors include a chapter on male breast disease which is often overlooked and misdiagnosed by the clinician. The book ends with an excellent chapter which presents a rational plan for clinical follow-up as well as education for patients.

The book is a practical treatise on the complex subject of diseases of the breast. It is a testament to the importance of the outpatient breast unit and the interaction of the multidisciplinary team and patient. The treatment of breast cancer, although complex, is portrayed in a thoughtful and systematic manner, allowing the reader to comprehend the importance of the different approaches and specialties to the overall management of the patient. Readers of this book – who should include all physicians and non-physicians involved in patient care – will gain further insight and knowledge of their specialty. Physicians who do not routinely treat breast cancer but, of course, will see breast cancer patients in their practice should read this book to gain a rational, scientific, and philosophical approach to their patients. The authors apply guidelines when appropriate, yet do not attempt a one-size-fits-all approach. The authors are to be congratulated for this contribution to breast cancer care.

Armando E. Giuliano
Executive Vice Chair of Surgery for Surgical Oncology
Co-director of the Saul and Joyce Brandman Breast Center
Cedars-Sinai Medical Center
Los Angeles, USA

# Preface

*Every woman is a biography*
*and a life plan within and around her*
amp

*The mind energy generated by the breast unit teamwork.* The development of the breast unit organization has improved the method of treating breast diseases with considerable results, from a medical as well as from a social and cultural point of view. The mind energy generated by the breast unit teamwork allows the specialists involved to deal positively with problems concerning health, modifications of body image, both real and perceived, as well as to implement preventive measures and to promote changes in life style. This is achieved through the construction of a multi-faceted culture that ranges from suitable surgery to one aimed at obtaining cosmetic good results, from predictable risks to targeted therapies, from effective communication to psychology and ethics.

The management of common breast diseases represents a major portion of the dedicated professionals' responsibility, while it only covers a minor share of their training. In fact, the range of clinical cases is so broad that it is difficult to cover in a short time all potential clinical and pathological presentations. Moreover diagnostic and therapeutic work-up is steadily changing, becoming more complex, and making it extremely challenging to keep up with the advancements in biological knowledge and with the applicative results of clinical trials.

This book is an intermediate useful resource which enhances the principles and the practice of the treatment of breast diseases as they turn up in an outpatient clinic. It provides a comprehensive and up-to-date account of the main symptoms, signs, and imaging techniques, and offers guidance on the best practices and optimal management. It also provides some answers to the countless questions that the patient asks herself about the correct interpretation of worrisome symptoms, the outcome of surgery, the use of hormone drugs, and even alternative medicine.

An hand-on peripheral brain useful to trainees working in the breast clinic as well as to established surgeons. It may also be of assistance to other health care professionals involved in the treatment and support of patients with breast cancer, such as gynaecologists, general practitioners, healthcare nurses and psychologists.

If anatomy, physiology and pathology of the breast are the basics, the mastery of a good clinical methodology allows practitioners to choose the shortest route to the ultimate diagnosis. From a logistical point of view, the outpatient clinic represents a crossroad from which several therapeutic possibilities spread out, which today are so complex and particular as to require there to be professionals dedicated to breast diseases in several specialisations: radiologists, pathologists, medical and radiation oncologists, plastic surgeons and other professionals.

It is worth reminding that the breast unit does not only deal with tumours of the breast, but also with benign pathology, frequent and equally alarming, which is improperly considered a less important, little sister of neoplastic pathology. Instead it requires just as specific in-depth knowledge, both to prevent errors in diagnosis and, if possible, to avoid unpleasant consequences with unnecessary or unwarranted surgery.

*A very demanding but fascinating practice*. This book aims at giving priority to suitability, synthesis and established beliefs, the latter founded on evidence-based bibliography and on guidelines that focus on quality objectives, indicating their outcome measures. Many tables, key points, and clinical illustrations reinforce the information in each chapter.

Before starting our journey in the dazing planet of breast diseases, we would like to point out some motivating forces that animated our work.

This textbook is the author's debt to Dr. Guidubaldo Querci della Rovere (named Uccio, 1946–2009), whose personal remarks expressed during a long period of friendship are transmitted in these pages [1]. In the same way, it redirects the experience done with other personal teachers, as Prof. Charles-Marie Gros, who created modern breast discipline starting from all women's complaints, including those of an anthropological and psychological nature. He liked to say "*breast discipline is the most human of sciences for its countless additional meanings, symbolic, social… and even religious*".

If Gros in the 1960s and 1970s brought *women to science*, the rapid progress of breast discipline, especially in its surgical approach, is obliged to the teachings of Prof. Umberto Veronesi, who brought *science to women.* Veronesi definitely placed women at the core of the decision-making process, and exposed the risks of technology by asserting that (*in breast oncology*) *…it is important to separate science from technology. Science responds to the principles of the search for truth, for reproducibility, for universality. Instead, sheer technology lives an amoral life of its own, devoid of intentions and responsibilities.*

We deeply believe all professionals dealing with breast diseases have to follow the basics of the discipline but also the teaching of their masters, of today and from the past. In particular, good surgeons stand out because they know which is the right approach for a specific patient at that particular moment in the evolution of her illness, and so they must also be themselves biologists, imaging experts, clinical oncologists; in conclusion learned doctors, who are also skilled in surgical as well non-surgical subjects.

Outpatient breast clinic practice is complex because it involves many fields of medicine, and treatment and care should take patients' needs and preferences into account, probably more than other practices. For this reason *breast culture is a very demanding but fascinating practice*, difficult however rewarding when effective in solving many of the problems that are encountered along the way. *No greater opportunity or obligation* is given, and open-mindedness is the gratifying outcome. Talking about oncoplastic breast conservation surgery, Prof. Melvin Silverstein writes [2]: *it is a philosophy that requires vision, passion, knowledge of anatomy, and an appreciation and understanding of aesthetics, symmetry and breast function. The oncoplastic surgeon must be constantly thinking 'How can I remove this cancer with large margins of normal tissue while at the same time making the patient look as good or better than she looks now?'*

Doctors who have the hard task to work in the outpatient breast clinic should consider themselves *lifelong students of breast cancer*, as Prof. Sampson Handley liked to define himself. The outpatient clinic is a crucial, strategic place, where we have to apply appropriate directives and acquire different methods that can be customised to suit our patients. At the same time it is a place of training based on the limits of clinical and instrumental tests, but also on the correct consideration of mistakes that are inevitably made, both personal ones to be transformed into learning, and collective ones that will require a change in the course of action. This is what makes medicine an *applied* science and also an art.

*The quality of the relationship between the members of the team and the patient is the ultimate test of medicine as an art.* Modern medicine is apparently built on solid foundations with a robust statistical underpinning and scientific rationale. If in the past medicine was considered more of an art than a science, it can be affirmed that it is now more of a science than an art. Technological advances allow improved outcomes compared with the past, and it is not inconceivable that in the future the cognitive component of medical diagnosis may become partly dispensable.

Nonetheless, other areas of knowledge remain uncertain and demand more complex decision-making procedures that must draw on personal attitudes and experience to reach a balanced solution. Furthermore, certain aspects of medical practice such as communication skills, while being recognized as a valid discipline, are often not translated into practice because of various individual or cultural obstacles.

A 'breast philosophy' animated by 'vision, passion and knowledge' cannot be jailed in detailed guidelines and pathways that should be considered valid for all doctors and patients. In this text we make a large use of guidelines that have undeniable merits, but we do not make the assumption that clinical expertise could be easily packaged and shipped around the world [3].

We are not the only ones who believe that the *one size fits all* approach to patient care is unsatisfactory if not useless. Prof. Barry B. Lowitz writes: *Attempts to reduce medical practice into a fixed set of algorithms that are evidence-based creates* one size fits nobody *programs and can damage optimal care for individual patients. The tools of our art are necessary, but alone do not determine the quality of the art.* Quality care *requires experience, thoroughness, attention to detail, good judgment, and, most of all, caring about the quality of the resulting product* [4]. A resulting product of a medical decision is not solely a physical eradication of the disease. The optimization of the patient's physical ability to function, and/or the psychological comfort of the patient and her significant others are equally important.

Moreover, is it possible to separate knowledge and technology from the individual's distinctive temperament, as is the case for other disciplines? Perhaps, only when patients' clinical concerns can be fulfilled with all the concomitant feelings and contradictions. Who knows? May be such a separation is theoretical rather than practical, given the fact that *man is always something more than what he knows of himself. He is not what he is simply once and for all, but is a process…* (Karl Jasper).

Is technology capable of developing a power of observation? So far, it appears that the opposite has happened, namely that technology has emptied of meaning what is best termed as diagnostic and clinical intuition. This capability was the prerogative of those physicians of the past who, in the absence of sophisticated technical tools, had developed strong powers of observation.

Scientific knowledge is advancing at an ever-increasing pace and the rate of change in methodologies is a potential source of alarm. The prevailing need to define, schematize and prioritize can, in practice, make doctors forget the real purpose and meaning of what they do and lead to a weakening of what could be defined as 'strategic direction'.

Though some capabilities are innate, others such as the power of observation and sense of judgment can be enhanced through learning from inspiring teachers. Modern medicine tends to schematize and this has marginalized the role of those more charismatic individuals entrusted to oversee medical training. New tendencies let medicine be tempted by mass information, which sometimes promotes uniformity and safe (from a forensic viewpoint) mediocrity.

Following this line of thought, Karl Popper comes to mind and the way he reflects on the meaning of honesty in a scientific context when he refers to *intellectual modesty* [*or rather to think about what we don't know*]. To be honest with oneself, while being sensitive and responsive to circumstances, requires the ability to learn from clinical experience.

*The quality of the doctor/patient relationship is the ultimate test of medicine as an art.* This is based on the trust of the patient for the clinician and the maintenance of the rectitude that society has conferred on him. Trust is the only option for a patient without medical knowledge, but it can only flourish within a system where a doctor retains the respect of their patients and behaves in accordance with expectations.

Alfonso M. Pluchinotta

## References


1. Querci Della Rovere G, Pluchinotta A. Personal reflections. In: Querci della Rovere G, Benson JR, Nava M, editors. Oncoplastic and reconstructive surgery of the breast. 2nd ed. London: Taylor & Francis; 2010.
2. Silverstein MJ. Oncoplastic breast conservation surgery. In: Nahabedian MY, editor. Oncoplastic surgery of the breast. Philadelphia: Saunders Elsevier; 2009.
3. Burstein H. Expert opinion vs guideline based care: The St. Gallen study (editorial). Breast. 2013;22:51–2.
4. Lowitz BB, Casciato DA. Principles and definitions. In: Casciato DA, editor. Manual of clinical oncology. Philadelphia: Lippincott William & Wilkins; 2012.

# Acknowledgements

We would like to thank our Teachers who always saw beyond our mistakes not blaming the faults, but showing the right direction. In time we became aware of how much we needed them and how much we are obliged to hand down our experience. We would like to thank all those who reinforced our passion and helped refine our art, above all the nurses to be taken into account as full-fledged cultural mediators. We would like to thank all those patients who, sometimes, turned out to be more useful than any of our books. We thank our families who gently peeked inside our study rooms with an understanding smile.

We would like to thank all those who believed in this book, "Mister Uccio" Querci della Rovere who was its primary inspiration; Prof. Umberto Veronesi for his teachings, always "on women's side"; Prof. Armando E. Giuliano, who like Prof. Veronesi has changed the treatment of breast cancer worldwide, for having encouraged us in this work; Elisa Stefanelli, precious executive secretary; Ilaria Bondi, congenial image-maker of all the illustrations; and all the women who allowed clinical pictures to be taken. And many loved ones who stood by our side, physically and in our memory. In truth, nothing in this book feels concluded, on the contrary, it feels it has opened new paths.

# Contents

# Contributors

**David N. Anderson** Breast Service, Department of Surgery, Memorial Sloan-Kettering Cancer Center (MSKCC), New York, NY, USA

**Giorgio Baratelli** Breast Unit, Hospital "Moriggia-Pelascini", Gravedona, Italy

**Zora Baretta** Division of Oncology, Istituto Oncologico Veneto (IOV), Padova, Italy

**Chiara Boccardo** Division of Breast Surgery, European Institute of Oncology (IEO), Milano, Italy

**Marta Cavalli** Division of Breast Surgery, European Institute of Oncology (IEO), Milano, Italy

**Giuliana Dell'Oste** Department of Radiology, Mammographic Screening, Padova, Italy

**Oreste D. Gentilini** Division of Breast Surgery, European Institute of Oncology (IEO), Milano, Italy

**Cristina Ghiotto** Division of Oncology, Istituto Oncologico Veneto (IOV), Padova, Italy

**Armando E. Giuliano** Samuel Oschin Comprehensive Cancer Institute, Los Angeles, CA, USA

**Barbara Gnocato** Breast Surgery, Policlinic of Abano Terme, Padova, Italy

**Rafaele Grigoletto** Breast Unit, Istituto Oncologico Veneto (IOV), Padova, Italy

**Maria Cristina Leonardi** Division of Radiotherapy, European Institute of Oncology (IEO), Milano, Italy

**Gigliola Lodovichetti** Multicentric Pathological Laboratory, Accredited to Health Local Service USL21, Padova, Italy

**Ornella Lora** Division of Radiotherapy, Istituto Oncologico Veneto (IOV), Padova, Italy

**Giorgio Macellari** Surgical Breast Clinic, Hospital "Guglielmo da Saliceto", Piacenza, Italy

**Alfonso M. Pluchinotta** Breast Surgery, Policlinic of Abano Terme, Padova, Italy

**Virgilio S. Sacchini** Breast Service, Department of Surgery, Memorial Sloan-Kettering Cancer Center (MSKCC), New York, NY, USA

**Gianni Saguatti** Department of Radiology, Mammographic Screening, Hospital "Bellaria", Bologna, Italy

**Silvia Teggi** Department of Radiology, Mammographic Screening, Padova, Italy

**Maria Virginia Thomazini** Division of Breast Surgery, European Institute of Oncology (IEO), Milano, Italy

**Elisabetta Tosi** Department of Radiology, Mammographic Screening, USL16, Padova, Italy

**Vincenzo Vindigni** Plastic Surgery Clinic, University of Padova, Padova, Italy

**Daniela Zuccarello** Unit of Clinical Genetics and Epidemiology, University of Padova, Padova, Italy

# The Breast Clinic

# 1

Giorgio Macellari and Alfonso M. Pluchinotta

## Contents




G. Macellari (✉)
Surgical Breast Clinic, Hospital "Guglielmo da Saliceto", Piacenza, Italy
e-mail: g.macellari@ausl.pc.it

A.M. Pluchinotta
Breast Surgery, Policlinic of Abano Terme, Padova, Italy
e-mail: pluchinotta.alfonso@gmail.com







A.M. Pluchinotta (ed.), *The Outpatient Breast Clinic: Aiming at Best Practice*, DOI 10.1007/978-3-319-15907-2_1

**Abstract**

• Breast cancer (BC) is the leading cause of cancer-related death for women in almost all countries. Even though the majority of the patients seen in an outpatient breast clinic have normal breast or a benign disease, these women need to be reassured. • The landmarks of best practice are three 'triples': diagnostic assessment (clinical, imaging and pathologic), interactive principles (prudence, communication and respect) and essential upholders (multidisciplinary team, evidence-based guidelines and advocacy). Ethics is a tenth, separate but not independent, issue. • Clinicians are responsible for communication, no longer discretionary but routine-bound. They should provide information, at a level that the individual patient can clearly understand, and be able to transmit a strong *sense of efficacy* regarding the patient's treatment. • The optimal treatment for BC can be offered only in a breast unit, the place where dedicated professionals work under the guidance of a multidisciplinary philosophy: in this ideal climate, the mortality can be reduced of about 15–20 %.

*Future Directions*. The best treatment is the one that comes out after a discussion among several people about several options has been carried out. Quality lays on a different level from overdiagnosis to overtreatment, in terms of results, timing and consideration of psychological repercussions. Auditing is the best way to judge quality outcomes and objective measures and should be compulsory in all breast units.

## 1.1 The Strategic Role of the Outpatient Breast Clinic

**Clinical Practice Points**

- An outpatient clinician's job is mainly to be able to recognise and diagnose a real illness, but his/her role doesn't end there. There can be normal conditions which are perceived as illness (e.g. high-risk women) and situations where there has been an illness which are perceived as if the illness was still present (e.g. cancer survivors).
- At the slightest suspect of cancer, some women live the doubt as if it were for certain. The objective, however unwritten, should be getting workup with the least psychological toll on the patient.
- Emotional reactions may have a *domino effect*, and referral to breast clinic should be acted promptly, before the imagination starts to run wild.
- General practitioners (GPs) play a fundamental role in supporting the management of symptomatic breast patients.
- Where a BC is suspected or confirmed, immediate reporting of the referral may affect accuracy and also have detrimental psychological effect. A more useful and constructive second visit should be considered in the management of any cancer detected.

### 1.1.1 Introduction

Breast cancer (BC) is the most common cancer in women in almost all countries, including developing countries. Since 1990, the incidence rate has increased 1.5 % annually. In 2008, the estimated age-adjusted annual incidence of BC in Europe (40 countries) was 88.4/100,000 [1].

The incidence increases and continues to do so with the ageing of the population. There is a steep age gradient, with about 25 % of BCs occurring before age 50 and <5 % before age 35. BC in young women is associated with a positive family history and gene mutation more frequently than in older women. The incidence of BC is highest among women of higher socioeconomic background. Although the incidence of BC is higher in whites, black women are more likely to die from the disease. This disparity may be related both to delay in diagnosis because of restricted access to healthcare and to differing biology of the disease (e.g. higher frequency of negative oestrogen/progesterone receptors and HER2 disease in these populations).

In most Western countries, the mortality rate has decreased in recent years, especially in younger age groups, owing to advances both in early detection and in adjuvant systemic therapy. However, BC is still the leading cause of cancer-related death in women in both developing and developed countries (Fig. 1.1).

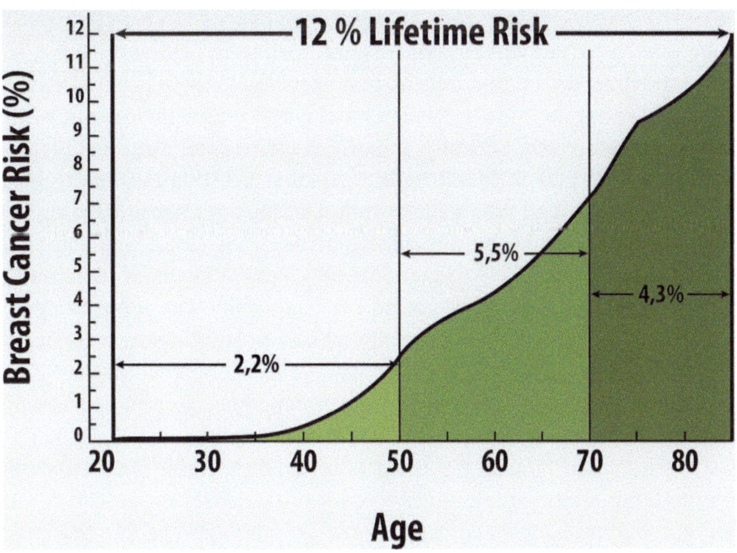


**Fig. 1.1** Percentage of age-related risk for invasive BC based on highest lifetime risk of 12 %. A threefold variation of incidence is observed in all countries of Europe (53–147 cases per 100,000) in different countries, from Belgium (147), Denmark (143), France (137), Iceland (131), the Netherlands (131), the United Kingdom (129) to Ukraine (54) and Moldova (53) [1]

Approximately 5–10 % of BCs are metastatic at diagnosis; of these patients, approximately one-fifth will survive 5 years. Depending on prognostic factors, up to 30 % of node negative and up to 70 % of node-positive BCs will relapse.

The most important risk factors include genetic predisposition, exposure to oestrogens (endogenous and exogenous) and ionising radiation, low parity and history of atypical hyperplasia. The Western-style diet, obesity and consumption of alcohol also contribute to the rising incidence of BC.

BC in males is rare, contributing about 1 % of all BCs. The major risk factors include clinical disorders carrying hormonal imbalances, radiation exposure and, in particular, a positive family history and genetic predisposition as in BRCA2 mutation (see 'Male breast cancer' in Sect. 19.3).

Clinical breast culture and quality of care are fundamental elements, and the outpatient clinic could have a strategic function. Despite the numerous efforts to increase awareness, so many women present late with their BC. There is some evidence that interventions delivered at an individual level can promote cancer awareness in the short term, but insufficient evidence that these might promote early presentation of cancer symptoms. Insisting on awareness is still useful in order to get more long-term results, especially for future generations.

Despite the vast improvement in the last decade in diagnostic procedures, surgical techniques and other systemic therapy offering the prospect of cure or longer life, many patients still experience significant anxiety/depression and sexual dysfunction. The objective, however unwritten, should be getting workup with the least psychological toll on the patient.

Following a diagnosis of BC, a woman finds herself in a new and unfamiliar landscape. This creates different levels of stress that vary from patient to patient and need to be addressed individually with solutions tailored to each woman's needs. Most women will remember the information provided to them in a fragmented way. They will need space and time to process and comprehend their diagnosis, so that they can cope better psychologically with the diagnosis and treatment plan.

Breast clinics are part of breast units, specialised institutions caring for a high volume of BC patients and provided by multidisciplinary teams including at least a surgeon, a radiation oncologist, a medical oncologist, a radiologist and a pathologist – all specialised in BC. Breast clinics may have a strategic function because they are involved in the earlier steps of the *breast journey*. The opportunity to assess and reassure a woman from the beginning avoids worries and concerns and transmits a *sense of efficacy* providing the right care, at the right time, for the right person in the right way. Emotional reactions have a *domino effect*, and it is better to act as soon as possible, before the imagination starts to run wild.

Breast clinics could be also a starting point to start raising breast awareness as well as promoting a more generic health culture (lifestyle, eating habits, mindfulness) that could restore hope and show a 'can-do' attitude. The last few years have seen the growth in the number of breast clinics, breast surgeons and breast nurses. Their roles have expanded to help with the increasing workload regarding BC care. What is not clear is what would be the adequate training for such new individuals. Ideally, before they start making decisions, they should have seen hundreds of

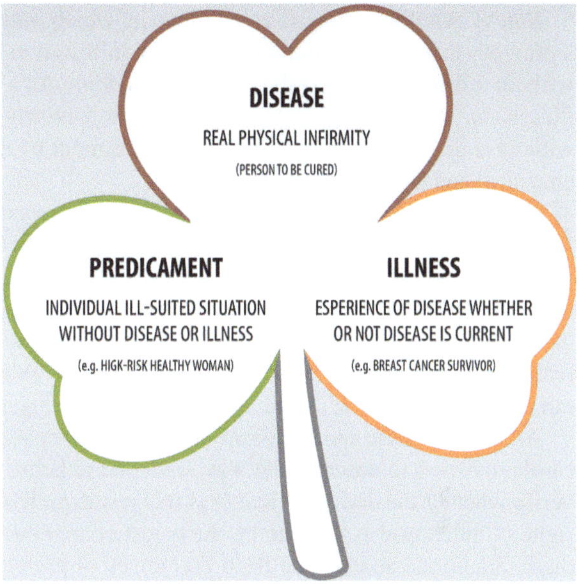


**Fig. 1.2** The woman's *breast journey* includes perception of the risk as a predicament, disease as such, and posttreatment feelings as illness

patients to cover the whole range of common and rare presentations. This is also true for trainees who cover for consultant surgeon in such clinics. Perhaps, the breast surgeons of the future will be less involved in diagnosis and more active surgically, whilst a new figure will come out, that of the outpatient breast clinic doctor.

### 1.1.2 The Woman's *Breast Journey*

By *breast journey* we mean the way a woman becomes aware of having a breast problem. Several distinct conditions related to the seriousness of the disease, the individual's ability to adapt and the prevalence of psychological factors will concur to the development of the woman's perception of the condition on three different levels.

Asymptomatic healthy women, who are at high risk of cancer and ill-suited to that, have a disposition to feel they are in a *predicament*. Women who suffered from the disease, whether or not the disease is current, experience the condition as *illness* [2]. Finally, women who suffer from the actual disease experience it as such. Knowledge of the aspects of predicaments, illness and diseases could help understanding common emotional reactions observed in most women who visit breast clinics (Fig. 1.2).

*Predicament*. A predicament is *a difficult situation*, and it encompasses all of the psychosocial issues which impinge on the individual especially when something interrupts the regularity of their life. As a component of sickness, the predicament is *more personal than the environment*, diffused, multifactorial and has a very unstable structure. Predicaments can be worrisome without disease and sometimes are charged with moral and ethical implications.

*Illness*. An illness, too, is an experience, which may or may not be attributed to a previous disease. An illness is a social manifestation, so that an ill person with or without a disease may exhibit *illness behaviour*. As a component of sickness, the illness can be *overplayed, stoically borne or foolishly denied*. The illness is valid without a discoverable disease, and the treatment of the person with an illness is empirical and palliative.

*Disease*. A disease, lastly, is discernible as physical reality. Diseases are therefore amenable to scientific study and require specific changes in the structure of tissues, even though they are not necessarily organ-specific. The systematic study of a disease leads to a discovery and therefore offers scope for a specific therapy. A disease is real and valid also without illness. It may sound trivial, but a disease is real even if the changes in the body are not severe. A person with a disease should not be judged for being unable to carry out their responsibilities.

Although disease and illness are conceptually separate, the name *disease* is often carelessly used to describe the way someone is being ill, whilst it is important to verify whether the disease is real or if it is just experienced as such. To establish the right attitude towards the patient, the breast clinic consultant must be familiar with these conditions and be free from prejudices or pre-established assumptions. This method should be applied regardless of the psychological evaluation criteria.

### 1.1.3 From Primary Care to Breast Clinic

General practitioners (GPs) play a fundamental role in supporting the management of symptomatic breast patients. They should be facilitated by the specialist in their decision to refer (and to re-refer where necessary) a patient, as it is they who, in turn, will support the patient through the referral process, by providing choices and information and also through any subsequent treatment phases by providing ongoing holistic support [3].

*Presentation of the patient with new breast symptoms*. In the initial consultation, the GP should assess the patient with a view to refer to a symptomatic breast clinic. The GP may find that the patient has normal or benign changes that do not require referral and, at this point, he or she should give reassurance supported by the appropriate literature. All patients should be aware and informed. A good practice is not to wait for their next appointment for clinic or radiological screening if they develop symptoms.

*REFERRAL TO CLINIC* – Patients with the following symptoms or signs should be referred for assessment. In a patient with suspicious symptoms of BC, investigations prior to referral to a breast clinic are not recommended (expert opinion) [4].

Symptoms suggestive of urgent attention are denoted as *U* (*urgent*). Symptoms considered nonurgent but still requiring an appointment within 2 weeks are denoted as *NU* (*not urgent*). Note that family history referrals and cosmetic referrals are excluded from the 2-week wait pathway. That all patients with breast symptoms referred to a specialist should be seen within 2 weeks of referral is a quality indicator (national requirement in UK is 93 %).

*Lump, lumpiness and change in texture* in any woman 30 years and older that persists after next period or presents after menopause (U). The patient's history should always be taken into account. For example, it may be appropriate, in discussion with a specialist, to agree referral within a few days also in patients reporting a lump or other symptom that has been present for several months.

Lump, lumpiness and change in texture at any age:

- Discrete hard lump with fixation +/− skin tethering/dimpling/altered contour (U)
- A lump that enlarges (U)
- A persistent focal area of lumpiness or focal change in breast texture (U)
- Progressive change in breast size with signs of oedema, local pain and reddened skin (U)
- Skin distortion (U)
- Previous history of BC with a new lump or suspicious symptoms (U)

Lump, lumpiness and change in texture under 30 years that do not meet the above criteria (NU). BC in women aged younger than 30 years is rare, but does occur. Benign lumps (e.g. fibroadenoma) are common, however, and a policy of referring these women urgently would not be appropriate; instead, nonurgent referral should be considered (NU).

*Male patients* over 50 years with unilateral firm sub-areolar mass +/− nipple discharge or associated skin changes (U).

*Nipple symptoms*:

- Spontaneous unilateral blood-stained nipple discharge (U)
- Unilateral nipple eczema or nipple change that does not respond to topical treatment (U)
- Recent nipple retraction or distortion (U)

*Breast Pain*. Patient with minor/moderate degree of breast pain with no discrete palpable abnormality that interferes with patient's lifestyle or sleep, when initial treatment fails, and/or with unexplained persistent symptoms (NU).

*Axillary lump* in the absence of clinical breast abnormality, persistent and unexplained (U).

*Personal history of cancer*. Patient with previously histologically confirmed BC, who presents with a further lump or suspicious symptoms, should have an urgent referral, irrespective of age (U).

*High-risk woman*. Request for an assessment by a patient with a strong family history of BC (NU).

*WOMEN MANAGED BY GP* – At least initially, GPs can manage:

- Young women with tender, lumpy breast and older ones with symmetrical nodularity provided that they have no localised abnormality
- Patients with minor and moderate degrees of breast pain who do not have a discrete palpable lesion

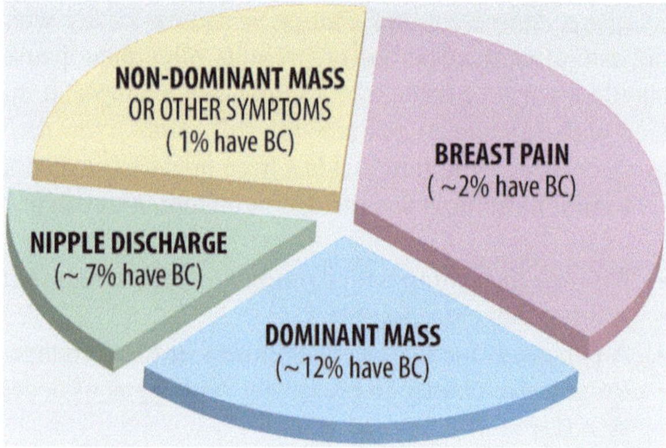


**Fig. 1.3** Approximate incidence of main symptoms observed in a breast clinic

- Women aged under 50 who have nipple discharge, that is, from more than one duct or is intermittent and is not blood-stained or troublesome
- Aspiration of large cysts in patients with a history of multiple breast cysts, even though GPs are not commonly encouraged to do that, because bruising can follow aspiration of a solid mass, making subsequent assessment difficult

*OUTCOME OF REFERRAL* – Most of the patients seen in a breast clinic have normal breasts or a benign disease. Many conditions occur so commonly against the background of breast development, cyclical activity and involution that they are best considered aberrations of this process.

Incidence of symptoms is differently reported in single institutions. Roughly one-third have a dominant mass and one-third painful nondominant mass or lumpiness. Pain alone is referred in about 5 %, nipple discharge in 7 % and nipple retraction in 2–3 %. Rare symptoms are scaling nipple (eczema), infections and axillary lump (Fig. 1.3).

In addition, it can be observed that there are women with a strong family history of BC (see 'High risk woman', Sect. 2.3) or with radiological findings (as calcifications, distortion, non-palpable nodular opacities) (see Sect. 5.1).

Breast pain is common and the majority is related to the chest wall, not the breast itself (see 'Breast pain', Chap. 7). BC is only rarely painful, usually in older women. In young patients presenting solely with breast pain, with no palpable abnormality, there is no evidence to support the use of mammography as a discriminatory investigation for BC.

Bleeding from the nipple too is rarely due to BC. If there is a lump as well, it is more likely to be cancer. Spontaneous, single-duct persistent (>2 per week) or blood-stained nipple discharge requires a definitive diagnosis that may only be obtained by surgical duct excision (see 'Nipple discharge', Chap. 10).

Most benign lumps, some suspicious, usually painless and hard, are irregular in shape. A dominant breast mass can cause dimples to form in the skin of the breast or the nipple to draw in or the breast to change in size. Sometimes the skin looks like an orange peel (*peau d'orange*), due to lymphatic oedema around deepened hair follicles. Breast cysts diagnosed on ultrasound require aspiration only if symptomatic or complex on scan (see Sect. 9.2).

Breast infection requires early antibiotic therapy and sometimes rapid referral to hospital if it does not settle rapidly on antibiotics. Breast abscesses should be assessed by ultrasound and treated by repeated aspiration or mini-incision and drainage (see 'Breast infections', Sect. 8.2).

Gynaecomastia is an increasing problem. The cause should be ascertained and surgery only performed after other options have been exhausted (see 'Gynaecomastia' in Sect. 19.1).

Following a diagnosis of benign disease, reassurance is important, but insufficient, and an explanation of the cause, possible risks and treatment options is required. In any case, breast specialists should convey optimism about getting the control of the situation, because a patient being referred with a breast lump will be naturally concerned.

People of all ages who suspect they have BC may have particular information and support needs. The clinician should discuss these needs with the patient and respond sensitively to them. The patient should receive written and/or verbal information such as regarding accessibility of breast clinic. This information should include waiting times for an appointment and the likely process that will occur during the referral.

Primary healthcare professionals should encourage all patients, including women over 50 years old, to be breast aware in order to minimise delay in the presentation of symptoms. Patients should be reminded of the importance of keeping their appointment.

### 1.1.4 One-Stop Breast Clinic

A one-stop breast clinic has a theoretically considerable advantage to the formation of rapid diagnostic clinics, set up in breast units, where the diagnostic team may work together in a multidisciplinary setting [5]. Women may receive a diagnosis and management plan in the quickest time possible, in the same clinic, or have all the necessary investigations at the same time and return for results within 24–48 h.

In the case of imaging, complex investigations such as MRI, if required, may take longer to organise. In the case of pathological sampling, cytology is the only available method of obtaining an immediate definitive diagnosis, provided that it is executed by an experienced cytopathologist. Core biopsy requires a production time for pathology, and so centres that use core biopsy alone cannot currently offer a one-stop diagnostic service. Core biopsy combined with cytology is increasingly used and easier to interpret, even though partially, in case there is no conclusive result.

One-stop breast assessments are generally more favourable for people without serious disease as they go home without further waiting, knowing they do not have cancer. In fact, some patients do not require all the elements of triple assessment, as those with:

- Resolved symptoms and no clinical abnormality
- Clearly identified benign conditions with no other suspicious features found on clinical and imaging assessment, such as:
- Areas of benign breast change and diffuse nodularity without a dominant mass
- Simple cysts whether aspirated or not
- Breast pain

- Non-bloody nipple discharge
- Gynaecomastia

Regardless of the diagnostic outcome, some patients require a long and unpredictable time to raise questions and concerns. Because the communication cannot be overcharged, closing the case in the same attendance can be counterproductive. Moreover, it is better if these more difficult patients receive information in the presence of a supportive member of their family or a friend.

The main advantages of the one-stop system are the reduction of anxiety and the possibility to provide a certain level of skill and teamwork not otherwise available. In such a service, the benefits are particularly evident for the majority of patients with normal breasts or a benign disease. Patients do like these clinics because they reduce the number of clinic visits and letters, improving administration efficiency, but surprisingly these benefits do not have long-term effects.

Although there have been concerns that immediate reporting may affect accuracy and that there may be a possible detrimental psychological aspect for those with cancer, these are more than offset by the benefits.

It is well recognised that at the time when a patient is given bad news, little other information provided in the consultation is remembered. By concentrating on establishing and delivering a diagnosis at the first visit, it is then possible to have a more useful and constructive second visit to consider the management of any cancer detected. For this reason, as previously recommended, all women with discrete masses or significant signs or symptoms must be referred directly to a specialist breast unit, and not to a basic diagnostic unit.

## 1.2 Landmarks of Breast Practice

**Clinical Practice Points**

- Communication: the issue is not always about it being proper, but more about it being effective; communication is only as good as the message received.
- Guidelines regarding staffing and organisation of breast units have been drawn up worldwide to ensure efficient handling of patients by appropriately experienced staff.
- Guidelines fail their qualitative objectives if related to a 'statistical' patient. Every woman is a person who is fighting a battle you know nothing about. Being respectful is a paramount commitment. Always.
- Multidisciplinary management and care are strongly recommended to avoid an opinionated standard of practice and the risk of over- or undertreat individual cases, as young or elderly or mutation carrying patients.
- Especially for women who want more help with their difficulties, the breast care nurse is an essential support figure and may offer one-to-one counselling or run a support group.
- The role of patients' advocacy is also of crucial importance, particularly for the dissemination of information and knowledge.

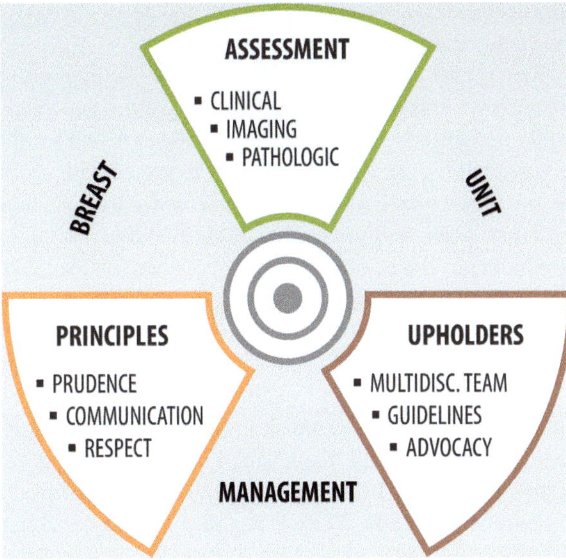


**Fig. 1.4** Landmarks of breast practice. Good practice is comprised of the triple assessment, as well interactive principles and established shields

### 1.2.1 Introduction

In an outpatient breast clinic, the best practice for reaching good results is likely to be founded on three 'triples' landmarks (Fig. 1.4).

- *Triple diagnostic assessment*: clinical, imaging and pathologic
- *Triple interactive principles*: communication, prudence and respect
- *Triple essential upholders*: multidisciplinary team (MDT), evidence-based guidelines and breast care advocacy

Every workup should consider the need to fulfil all these components, which in turn are related to other issues. Outcome measures are never absolute but relative and suffer from the effects of other conditioning elements. For example, imaging is related to the age of the patient, communication is different than plane information and without respect, the slightest annoying thing can become a big concern. Guidelines fail their qualitative objectives if related to a 'statistical' patient.

Changing the view angle of the various elements makes the outpatient practice diversified and inspiring so that personal performance becomes worthwhile. This aspect also entails a lot of obligations but equally delivers its professional and personal rewards.

### 1.2.2 Triple Diagnostic Assessment (TDA)

With triple diagnostic assessment (TDA), the tests used in an individual case will be determined by the presenting symptoms, the clinical findings and the age of the patient. In some circumstances, the clinic assessment should be organised so that all appropriate tests, including imaging and needle biopsy, should be carried out during the same clinic attendance.

The breast imaging facilities should include x-ray mammography and high-frequency ultrasound. Digital mammography is preferred to film screen mammography particularly for women below 50 years and for those with dense breast tissue. Breast imaging facilities should be integrated with, or be within reasonable distance of, the breast clinic for patient convenience and efficient service delivery.

Breast MRI does not form part of the initial imaging assessment of patients in the symptomatic breast clinic. It may, however, be useful in the further investigation of some breast lesions and in the evaluation of patients with confirmed BC. In selected cases, MRI should be carried out according to the local policy agreed by the multidisciplinary team.

The TDA method will enable a diagnosis to be established in the majority of patients, and, in case of breast lumps, diagnostic surgical excision should be rarely required. The delayed diagnosis of cancers after TDA, in women who present with symptoms and are subsequently diagnosed with cancer, is approximately 0.2–0.5 %. Patients in whom the TDA is negative should be advised to seek advice from their GP if they remain concerned or if there is a change in symptoms or signs.

There should be clear administrative links between breast imaging and the breast clinic in order to ensure efficient service delivery, best use of resources, clear and rapid communication for clinic scheduling and exchange of information and results of tests.

*CLINICAL ASSESSMENT* – All patients who attend the symptomatic breast clinic should have a clinical consultation and physical breast examination carried out by a suitably trained member of the multidisciplinary team. This should preferably be a breast surgeon or a gynaecologist, but, in some circumstances, a radiologist, an oncologist or a trained nurse practitioner.

The consultation is aimed at establishing the nature, site and duration of the patient's symptoms and gathering other relevant history, e.g. past history of breast disease or investigation, date of last mammogram, participation in breast screening, family history and history of HRT. It can be helpful to ask the patient to complete a questionnaire at the time of attendance at the clinic.

Minimalist clinically breast-oriented history includes:

- Chief complaint, how long has it been noticed and its characteristics
- Age, pregnancies, presence and regularity of menstrual periods
- Personal history of breast problems and last diagnostic assessment
- Family history of BC in first-degree relatives
- Current taking of hormones and/or other medications
- Living habits: smoking status, alcohol use, change of weight…

The physical examination ('Clinical examination of the breast', Chap. 4) should establish the nature and site of any abnormalities found either on visual inspection or palpation of the breast. In particular, the physical examination should establish whether there is a dominant lump present or an area of textural change. The findings of the clinical examination should be correlated with the area of concern found by the patient or referring doctor.

The physical examination should include an assessment of the axillary and supraclavicular nodes. The results of the physical examination should be recorded clearly using a diagram to indicate the site and extent of any lesions found. It is recommended that the level of *physical assessment* (*P*) should be recorded using the 1–5 scale: P1, normal; P2, benign; P3, uncertain; P4, suspicious; and P5, malignant.

*IMAGING ASSESSMENT* – Appropriate imaging should be carried out by suitably trained members of the multidisciplinary team, i.e. radiologist, radiographer, breast clinician, nurse and surgeon. This should preferably be a radiologist but, in some (rare) circumstances, could be a breast surgeon or a trained nurse practitioner. Ultrasound is the imaging method of choice for the majority of women aged <40 years and during pregnancy and lactation.

X-ray mammography is used in the investigation of women aged ≥40 years with the addition of ultrasound when indicated. X-ray mammography is not indicated for the majority of patients aged <40 years but should be considered in patients aged 35–39 years with clinically suspicious or malignant findings (P4, P5) and in patients with clinically indeterminate lesions (P3) if ultrasound is normal.

If a suspicious abnormality is demonstrated on mammography, it may be helpful to further characterise the mammographic features using magnification or spot compression views. These should be carried out during the clinic as directed by the radiologist or the consultant radiographer in breast imaging.

The level of suspicion for malignancy of ultrasound (U) should be recorded using the U1–U5 classification: U1, normal; U2, benign; U3, indeterminate/probably benign; U4, suspicious of malignancy; and U5, malignant. The level of mammographic suspicion for malignancy should be recorded using the same M1–M5 classification or the BI-RADS categories.

*PATHOLOGICAL ASSESSMENT* – The clinical and imaging workup should be completed before needle sampling (fine needle aspiration cytology or core biopsy) is performed. Breast needle biopsies should be performed under imaging guidance in order to achieve the greatest accuracy and reduce the need for repeat procedures.

Freehand core biopsy may be appropriate for cases of palpable, locally advanced BC and for cases in which the imaging is normal, but there remains a suspicious localised clinical abnormality.

Needle core biopsy is preferred rather than FNA for most solid lesions and for lesions suspicious for cancer because of the higher sensitivity and specificity achieved in most centres and because of the importance of oncological information including tumour type, grade and receptor status obtained with histology. FNA by an experienced cytologist is an acceptable alternative to needle core biopsy in the initial evaluation of symptomatic breast lesions and in patients presenting with a lump in the axilla alone with no known clinical abnormality of the breast.

Biopsy of lesions within or attached to the skin can often be carried out using a 3 or 4 mm punch biopsy needle under local anaesthetic. This is particularly suitable for suspected Paget's disease of the nipple, inflammatory cancer and local recurrences in the skin.

Needle aspiration of clinically obvious cysts in patients with known recurrent cystic disease may be performed following initial clinical assessment. Appropriate imaging with mammography and ultrasound should still be carried out in such cases.

*Conclusions*. The patient should be given their results possibly in the presence of a breast care nurse and any relative/carer/friend of the patient that they wish to have at the consultation. Breast care professionals should previously suggest this solution, especially to emotional patients.

Communicating the diagnosis takes time, and it should be ensured that sufficient time and support is provided for this and that it takes place in an appropriate setting. Sometimes results need to be given by an appropriately trained senior clinician who has experience and training in breaking bad news.

Written information and supportive literature may be appropriate for the patient and their carers or family at this point. The format and language of written information should always be appropriate and easily understood, and information and support should always be tailored to meet the needs of the individual.

GPs should be informed of a diagnosis of cancer within 24 h, and details of test results and care plan should be included in the information. Equally, GPs should be informed if the patient hasn't received a diagnosis of cancer within 10 working days.

Patients with benign/normal results should be given appropriate reassurance and an explanation of their symptoms. Literature to support the results may be useful.

Patients who have an equivocal result or require repeats should have a face-to-face consultation to clearly discuss the need for further tests and possible outcomes, and a simple care plan put together. Clear explanations should be given why further tests may be needed.

Patients who receive a BC diagnosis should have clear routes of referral to specialist, and support services should be in place for any patient identified as needing further support. Around the time of diagnosis, approximately half of all cancer patients experience levels of distress that may adversely affect their quality of life, whilst around one-third report significant levels of anxiety and/or depression.

### 1.2.3 Triple Interactive Principles

*PRUDENCE*. In the practice of medicine, individual values and opinions, even those not strictly belonging to the sphere of science, cannot be underestimated. We need the science of medicine to solve problems at a fundamental level and to advance our knowledge on a solid foundation. At the same time, we need the art of medicine to apply this knowledge to individuals and to society; we need it to be practical and useful. How can we merge these two needs? That is where the word prudence comes in [6].

The art of medicine is comprised of a set of skills. The root word for skill is *techne* in Greek. In Latin, it is *ars* which in English means *art*. The skilful way a clinician practices their profession is the art of medicine. Knowledge is the major requisite, but the skills include the ability to take into account the complexity, uniqueness and unpredictability of the disease in individual patients; the position of the patient within their family and the community; and the values, preferences, fears and expectations of the patient.

Good clinicians will be intuitively considering all these factors at all times, even whilst they are seeing the patient and formulating diagnostic hypothesis and a treatment strategy. This 'reflection-during-action' is the process the practitioner uses when dealing with specific, unique, uncertain and complex situations. This is the art of medicine. Prudence is a big part of it.

Perhaps we should consider the art of medicine as composed of two major parts; one is subjective and 'physician centred' and revolves around the skills of the physician who is using their professional knowledge and experience to make a medical diagnosis and devise a treatment plan. The other component is 'patient and society centred' and defines the factors related to patient's psychology and sociology. The word *prudence* is better suited for the first component and the word *humanities* for the second component.

*COMMUNICATION* – Even though it is established that communication between physicians and patients is a fundamental aspect of care, most physicians have little training in communication. In oncological cases, the aspects of communication most valued by patients are those that help patients and their families feel *guided*, build *trust* and support *hope*. The lack of cross-communication increases the psychological and existential suffering of patients and their loved ones. Communication has been defined an *extraordinary opportunity*, a *key clinician skill*. Moreover, communication opportunities and skills are associated with less burnout and work-related stress [7].

*Behaviours to avoid*. Before even cultivating virtuous behaviours, it is important to avoid harmful ones. Among the several behaviours to avoid include blocking, lecturing, collusion and premature imprudent reassurance.

- *Blocking* occurs when a patient raises a concern but the physician either fails to respond or redirects the conversation. For example, a woman with BC might ask, *How long do you think I have*? To which the doctor responds, *Don't worry about that*. It is important to recognise the mechanisms related to blocking because they are the reasons why the physician typically fails to elicit the range of patient concerns and consequently is unable to address the most important ones.
- *Lecturing* occurs when a physician delivers a large chunk of information without giving the patient a chance to respond or ask questions.
- *Collusion* occurs when patient hesitates to bring up difficult topics and the physician does not ask her directly – a *don't ask, don't tell* situation.
- *Premature (imprudent) reassurance* occurs when physician responds to patient concern with reassurance before exploring and understanding the concern.

*Behaviours to cultivate* are also a number. Some of these are reported below.

- *Ask–tell–ask*. Always ask about the patient's understanding of the issue. *How do you see your health*? Tell the patient in straightforward language what you need to communicate – the bad news, treatment options or other information. Stop short of giving a long lecture or huge amounts of detail. Information should be provided in short, digestible chunks. A useful rule of thumb is not to give more than three pieces of information at a time. Do not use medical jargon. Ask the patient if he or she understood what was said. In few cases and without any pressure, consider asking the patient to restate what was said in his or her own words.

- *Tell me more*. Ask the patient if they need more information or if all their questions are being answered. Ask about how they feel about what has emerged and its meaning.
- *Respond to emotions*. Approaching the person with kindness is key to helping. However, in cases of problematic relationships, covering emotional responses involves naming, understanding, respecting, supporting and exploring the emotional response (NURSE). This acronym also recalls the need for nursing or psychological support.

Communication should be developed in order for the patient to comprehend and agree. Sometimes words can be *as hard as stones*, and each caregiver should therefore calibrate their speech to avoid confusion, anxiety, fear or depression. All staff should possess appropriate communication skills for both communicating with patients and ensuring consistent communication with all health professionals involved in the patient's care.

During the diagnostic process, healthcare professionals should assess patients to ascertain they understand the actual situation and future expectations. The patient should be given clear information that meets their individual needs, at each stage of the diagnostic process, and made aware of the availability of their breast care nurse whose details should be provided to the patient in a timely manner.

For patients who undergo needle biopsy, both written and verbal information should be provided. All patients who undergo needle biopsy should be provided with a definite appointment or other agreed arrangement for communication of the biopsy result, within five working days, so they can arrange to be accompanied by family/friend if they wish.

A discussion between the patient and a clinician who has been involved with the assessment of the patient should occur prior to leaving the clinic. This is to inform the patient of the likely outcome of the biopsy result in light of the clinical examination and imaging findings. If these are thought likely to be malignant, a breast care nurse should be present at that consultation where possible.

Patients who believe they are at high risk of BC may continue to feel distressed following a benign diagnosis, so it is important to accurately, and sometimes again and again, address these (mis)perceptions at the initial consultation.

The results of triple assessment should be discussed at a multidisciplinary meeting for all women who undergo needle biopsy. The results of each element of the TDA should be considered in order to ensure a correct diagnosis and appropriate further management. If there is discordance between the results, further assessment, if necessary including repeat biopsy, should be considered. If surgery is appropriate, the majority of patients do want to be involved in the discussion about which type of surgery they are to receive but do not necessarily wish to choose the treatment.

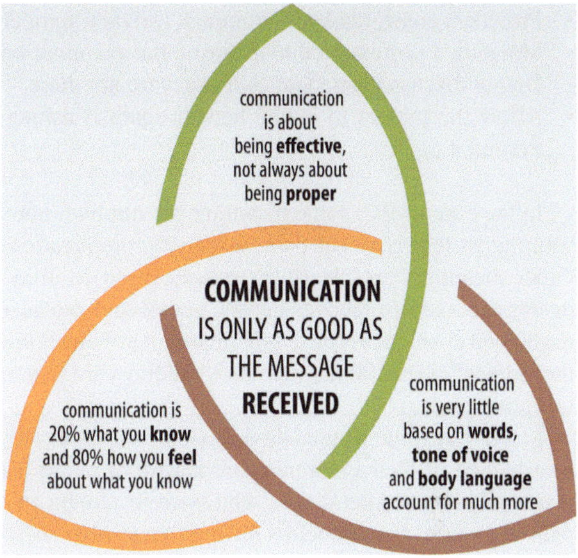


**Fig. 1.5** Some facts about effective communication

It is worthwhile to remember that communication, even if real, has a strong individual component since it is 20 % what the doctor knows and 80 % how they feel about what they know. Moreover, communication is very little based on words; tone of voice and body language account for much more. Finally, effective communication is only as good as the message received (Fig. 1.5).

Different people have different needs for information, and these may change with the stage of treatment. Some women find that gathering information helps them cope with their diagnosis and treatment. Much information is now available to patients, and many resources are directed at trying to prevent or ameliorate psychological stress. Guiding patients to well-established websites and information resource centres might ameliorate anxiety. However, misinformation is as damaging to the psyche as no information at all.

*RESPECT*. At the slightest suspect of cancer, some women live the doubt as if the diagnosis were certain. It is normal for a woman to feel a range of emotions at different times after she learns she has a breast disease. These can include shock, numbness, disbelief, fear and anger. Everybody has different needs and reacts and copes differently.

It is important to show respect but also to tighten a therapeutic alliance founded on transparency, empathy, trust and kindness. Essentials are:

- Treat the patient as a person.
- At the first meeting, introduce yourself and shake hands.
- Then, talk to the patient; do not look at the age on the document or folder.
- Address patient formally (e.g. Mrs. Jones).
- Allow the patient to remain fully clothed during initial interview.

- Provide a comfortable environment (privacy, temperature).
- Maintain a professional tone during the examination.
- Do not discuss the patient as if she were not there.
- Allow the patient to clothe herself again if a long discussion will occur after examination.

In the case of BC, some meanings are implied: not wanting to die of cancer, not wanting to feel physical pain, a fear of complications and a fear of recurrences. Other meanings are clearly expressed: need to allay anxiety; inability to suffer delay; necessity to recover family, sexual and professional position; and desire to have good cosmetic results. Other particular worries are related to children (what do they know?), other family members needing care (e.g. elderly), job concerns, health insurance and so on.

Moreover, some women do not ask for clarifications for many reasons: are afraid or ashamed of their ignorance; are fearful of being pushy, ill-timed; are afraid for wasting health workers' time; and wish to remain in denial because the reality is painful to face. Good doctors *have to try to hear the silent ones*, according to one line by Paul Celan. Everyone praises the silent ones for their reserve, but their inscrutability may conceal deep thinking, a seal of superiority and even a psychological block.

These are some of the reasons why expectations are higher than those the clinicians can understand especially in the course of the first visit. Every woman is a person who is fighting a battle you know nothing about. Being respectful and kind is mandatory. Always.

### 1.2.4 Triple Essential Upholders

*MULTIDISCIPLINARY TEAM* (*MDT*). The complexity that characterises the path of patients with suspected or confirmed BC requires the involvement of a number of specialised figures, the multidisciplinary team (MTD), with special training, working together in a coordinated manner [8].

The patient suffering from BC should be offered prompt access to a group of dedicated operators with a high level of training and, where appropriate, psychiatric services.

- *First level*
  - Radiologist
  - Breast surgeon (oncology surgeon or gynaecologist)
  - Pathologist
  - Breast nurse case manager
- *Second level*
  - Genetic counsellor
  - Nuclear medicine doctor
  - Plastic and reconstructive surgeon

  - Psychologist or psychiatrist
  - Radiation oncologist
  - Medical oncologist
- *Others*, as appropriate, including:
  - Dietician
  - Physical therapist
  - Internal medicine doctor
  - Family medicine doctor

*Multidisciplinary team meeting* (*MDM*). MDT optimises and coordinates patient care in a joint discussion by means of periodical multidisciplinary meetings (MDMs). Many quality indicators underline that the MDT meeting should take place weekly and should be considered a fixed clinical commitment.

All key members of the MDM should be present in person or via video link to ensure full multidisciplinary discussion before the final result is communicated to the patient. The diagnostic MDM must include a pathologist, radiologist or consultant radiographer in breast imaging, surgeon or breast clinician and breast care nurse.

Each MDM should have a MDM coordinator, a lead clinician who should be appointed to ensure that there is good inter-professional communication, that the key personnel required are in attendance and that this attendance is recorded. A record of the meeting, including the attendance, should be kept. Close communication and mutual respect among specialties are required.

*Aims and results*. The purpose of the MDM is to ensure that patients who have undergone full triple assessment receive the correct diagnosis and advice regarding its management. Cases that should be discussed are the following:

- All patients who undergo needle biopsy during assessment should be discussed.
- Patients in whom there is a discrepancy between the clinical findings and imaging should be discussed in order to decide whether further investigation should be undertaken.
- The results of each of the elements of the triple assessment should be discussed to ensure that there is concordance of the results when deciding on the final diagnosis and management (Fig. 1.6).

The outcome for most cases discussed at the MDM will be either a definitive diagnosis of cancer or a benign disease.

The majority of patients with benign disease can be discharged from the clinic. Further review and/or diagnostic intervention may be required following initial assessment for the following:

- Discordance between elements of the triple assessment, e.g. persistent suspicious clinical findings and normal imaging
- Equivocal biopsy results, e.g. B3, B4 core biopsy
- Severe breast pain, where assessment of treatment is required

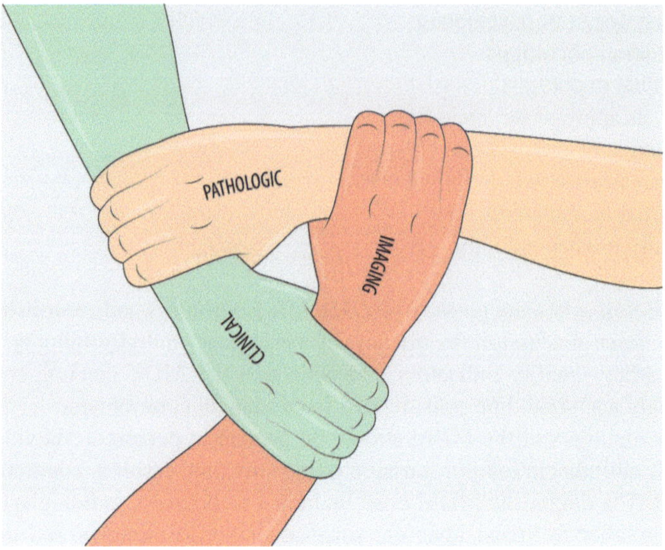


**Fig. 1.6** Triple assessment of a palpable mass. Diagnosis and management are established on the *concordance* of definitive results of the clinical, imaging and pathologic results

- Breast inflammation, infection, cellulitis, abscess
- Nipple discharge if causing significant symptoms, for potential surgical intervention
- Sequelae of traumatic injuries
- Mondor disease

Last, but not least, the MDM is an ideal forum to identify patients who can be offered the opportunity to take part in clinical trials. This is very important for clinical research, and it is estimated that at least 10–15 % of patients could/should enter into controlled clinical trials.

*EVIDENCE-BASED GUIDELINES*. Clinical practice guidelines systematically develop evidence-based statements aiming to assist practitioners in appropriate clinical decision-making, as well as to improve quality of healthcare and outcomes for patients. They also influence national policies for efficient allocation of resources and for better delivery systems.

On the other side, guidelines have inflated public expectations of the effectiveness of treatment beyond measure. For instance, conclusive misdiagnosis of BC is the most common malpractice litigation even if due to intrinsic constitutional factors as dense breast. Equally, even though the current aim of surgery is to produce a result that satisfies the patient's wishes within the limits of technical feasibility, in spite of better and better achievable results, the patient's expectations are increased above the achievable results [8].

There is a lot to say about clinicians sometimes locked into screening, treatment and follow-up protocols with intrinsic limitations, whilst, as everybody knows, medicine encompasses an art and a science. Art is intuition, experience, creativity, respect, empathy and compassion (the patient is *unique*). Science and technology are evidence-based medicine based on the systematic review, meta-analysis and guidelines that lead to standardisation and regulation (the patient is *statistical*).

The indicators do not directly measure the quality. They represent the signals that direct attention to aspects of care intended to be thorough. The indicators are like *the dog pointing the prey*, but is the hunter who interprets the signals and acts at the appropriate time.

Guidelines try to individualise as much as possible the estimation of the risk of BC, as well as to facilitate the clinical decision about providing additional treatment and, ultimately, the most appropriate treatment. Thus, it is important for clinicians not only to be aware of the existence of these tools or 'decision aids' but also to know how they have been developed, how frequently they are revised and if they have been validated [9].

By means of guidelines, we well know the quality of care that we should provide. We have evidence of its usefulness and generally we know what outcomes to expect. Nevertheless, we are far from getting our best performance. Main guidelines working in Europe are listed below.

- *ESMO* (European Society for Medical Oncology)
  Senkus E, Kyriakides S., Penault-Llorca F, et al. Primary BC: ESMO Clinical Practice Guidelines for diagnosis, treatment and follow-up. Ann Oncol, 2013; 24 (Supplement 6): vi7–vi23.
- *EUSOMA* (The European Society of BC Specialists, formerly EUropean SOciety of MAstology)
  (*Quality Indicators*) Rosselli Del Turco M, Ponti A, Bick U, et al. Quality indicators in BC care. Eur J Cancer. 2010; 2344–56.
  (Breast Unit) Wilson ARM, Marotti L, Bianchi S, et al. The requirements of a specialist Breast Centre. Eur J Cancer. 2013; 49:3579–87.
  (*Young Woman*) Cardoso F, Loibl S, Pagani O, et al. The European Society of BC Specialists recommendations for the management of young women with BC. Eur J Cancer, 2012; 48:3355–77.
  (*Elderly Woman*) Biganzoli L, Wildiers H, Oakman C. Management of elderly patients with BC: updated recommendations of the International Society of Geriatric Oncology (SIOG) and European Society of BC Specialists (EUSOMA). Lancet Onc. 2012; 13: 148–60.
  (*Training*) Cataliotti L. Guidelines on the standards for the training of specialised health professionals dealing with BC. Eur J Cancer. 2007; 43, 660–75.
  (*MRI*) Sardanelli F, Boetes C, Borisch B, et al. Magnetic resonance imaging of the breast: Recommendations from the EUSOMA working group. Eur J Cancer. 2010;46:1296–316.
  (*LCIS*) Lakhani SR, Audretsch W, Cleton-Jensen AM, et al, The management of lobular carcinoma in situ (LCIS). Is LCIS the same as ductal carcinoma in situ (DC1S)? Eur J Cancer. 2006;42:2205–11.

(*Diagnosis*) Perry NM, Multidisciplinary aspects of quality assurance in the diagnosis of Breast disease EUSOMA. Eur J Cancer. 2001;37:159–72.
(*Surgery*) Rutgers EJTh, Quality control in the locoregional treatment of BC. (Eusoma group). Eur J Cancer. 2001;37:447–53.
(*Prophylactic mastectomy*) Petit JY, Greco M. Quality control in prophylactic mastectomy for women at high risk of BC. Eur J Cancer. 2002;38:23–6.
(*Endocrine therapy*) Blamey RW. Guideline on endocrine therapy of BC EUSOMA. Eur J Cancer. 202;38:615–34.
(*Alternative Medicine*) Baum M. Role of complementary and alternative medicine in the care of patients with BC: Report of the European Society of Mastology (EUSOMA). Eur J Cancer. 2006;42,1711–4.

- *SIGN* (Scottish Intercollegiate Guidelines Network)
  Treatment of primary BC. A national clinical guideline (sept. 2013). http://www.sign.ac.uk.
- *BASO* (British Association of Surgical Oncology)
  Association of Breast Surgery at BASO, Surgical guidelines for the management of BC, 2009, Eur J Surg Oncol. 2009;35(Suppl.1):1–22.
- *NHS* (National Health Service – Cancer screening programmes)
  NHSBS. Guidelines for Non-Operative Diagnostic Procedures and Reporting in Breast Cancer Screening. http://www.cancerscreening.nhs.uk/breastscreen/publications/nhsbsp50.pdf.
- *NICE* (National Institute for health and Care Excellence)
  NICE Guideline 80, Early and advanced BC: diagnosis and treatment, 2009. In: http://www.nice.org.uk.
- *NCCN* (National Comprehensive Cancer Network)
  NCCN Guidelines. BC (version 1.2014). http:/www.NCCN.org/patients.

*BREAST CANCER ADVOCACY* – Being diagnosed with BC today is an entirely different experience than it was just 30 years ago. Whilst this is partly due to advances in medicine, many significant changes are the result of BC advocacy.

*Women to women movements* arrived in two waves: the first wave, coming in the 1970s, made BC *public* and presented the affirming notion that *It is OK (is a fact) to have BC: you don't have to hide it*. There was a focus on developing less invasive treatments and on giving the patient control over treatment decisions.

The second wave, coming in the 1990s and grounded in political activism, argued that *It is NOT OK to have BC: we have to stop it from happening*. Earlier detection and better treatment were not enough – the goal must be the prevention of BC. A key event during this period was the publication of *Susan Love's Breast Book* in 1990. This wildly successful book was a primary source of information for an entire generation of women diagnosed with BC. For the first time, individuals were truly empowered to understand their diagnosis, their treatment options and what to expect in the future. Nowadays, BC advocates raise funds and lobby for better care, more knowledge and more patient empowerment. Some of them conduct educational campaigns or provide free or low-cost services. Useful websites are listed at the end of this chapter.

*Breast care nurse*. Actually, the main medico-cultural mediator between the patient and the doctor is (and has always been) the nurse. Now more than ever, the importance of a dedicated and specialised breast care nurse (BCN) is well demonstrated in all stages as their work improves the quality of life of patients. All the guidelines suggest that all patients with BC should be assigned to a named breast care nurse specialists in order to:

- Give them emotional support throughout diagnosis, treatment, continuum of care and follow-up
- Encourage patient education at all steps in the process
- Help the doctors in the coordination of care
- Act as an Ariadne's thread to prevent the patient's *pinball bouncing around* feeling

For women who want more help with their difficulties, the breast care nurse may offer one-to-one counselling or run a support group. Some hospitals have a psychologist or a psychiatrist who has a special interest in the emotional needs of women with BC. She, or he, can support the woman also addressing her towards outside organisations that support and inform women with BC. Some are specific to BC and some are aimed at all cancer patients.

The BCN can play a vital role in improving the experience of patients with BC throughout all stages, starting from the referral from the GP until the completion of all treatments. Sure enough, recovery from the emotional upsets of BC can take a year or longer. As well as providing information, BCNs are able to carry out a range of technical and emotional functions, with a coordination role in providing continuity of care throughout the patient pathway whether this involves a benign or a cancer diagnosis.

The BCN works as part of the integrated multidisciplinary team with engagement in appropriate *what if* conversations. The BCN may be required to support and advise patient families and carers. They will have the relevant skills to carry out this role and have undertaken an advanced communication skills course.

## 1.3 Quality Assessment

**Clinical Practice Points**

- Evidence-based practice can be obtained from a number of sources; the most reliable being randomised controlled clinical trials, systematic literature reviews, meta-analyses and observational studies.
- Clinical practice that complies with guidelines is easier to defend, but this principle should not be viewed as absolute.
- Women should be provided with written information at appropriate stages in the diagnostic procedure and informed when results will be issued.
- Delay in diagnosis remains the biggest cause of litigation by breast patients, with missed diagnosis of BC being the most common, and with the highest settlements, in cases involving premenopausal women.
- A clear discharge policy is desirable to prevent clinics being overwhelmed by patients without serious diseases.

**Table 1.1** Levels of evidence (LoE) and Grades of recommendation

| *Levels of evidence (LoE)* | |
|---|---|
| I | Evidence from at least one large, randomised, controlled trial of good methodological quality (low potential for bias) or meta-analyses of well conducted, randomised trials without heterogeneity |
| II | Small, randomised trials or large, randomised trials with a suspicion of bias (lower methodological quality) or meta-analyses of such trials or of trials with demonstrated heterogeneity |
| III | Prospective cohort studies |
| IV | Retrospective cohort studies or case–control studies |
| V | Studies without the control group, case reports, experts' opinions |
| *Grades of recommendation* (may be – or not to be – showed in association with LoE) | |
| A | Strong evidence for efficacy with a substantial clinical benefit, strongly recommended |
| B | Strong or moderate evidence for efficacy but with a limited clinical benefit, generally recommended |
| C | Insufficient evidence for efficacy or benefit that does not outweigh the risk or the disadvantages (adverse events, costs, etc.), optional |
| D | Moderate evidence against the efficacy or for adverse outcomes, generally not recommended |
| E | Strong evidence against the efficacy or for adverse outcomes, never recommended |

Adapted from the Infectious Diseases Society of America-United States Public Health Service Grading System [11] with permission

### 1.3.1 Levels of Evidence

There is evidence that the best practice differs across the countries, also because of the inconsistent availability of certain treatments and procedures. Clinical guidelines help to address the main issue in BC diagnosis and treatment and offer guidance on best practices. Evidence-based practice can be obtained from a number of sources, the most reliable being randomised, controlled clinical trials, systematic literature reviews, meta-analyses and observational studies.

In this textbook, levels of evidence (LoE) with relative grades of recommendation have been applied using the system most referred in many guidelines [10]. For practical purposes, five levels of evidence are considered and, depending on the information available, three grades of recommendations (and two grades of non-recommendation) are addressed (Table 1.1). The recommendation should express the clinical relevance of the procedure. Note that letters (A,B,C…) indicate the *trust* in the entire body of evidence that has been evaluated and that support the recommendation itself; they *not always* reflect the clinical relevance and *are not* a synonym of the importance of the clinical recommendation.

Different but similar criteria of evaluation in some guidelines may lead to minimal changes in few reported LoE within the text. For this reason, it is good to make reference to the quoted source.

### 1.3.2 Times and Ways to Inform

*Delays*. Even in benign conditions, delays at any stage of the diagnostic process may result in anxiety for the woman, which sometimes may be considerable. Targets should be set in terms of working days (w.d.) where delay may arise. Quality assurance in the diagnosis of breast disease is guaranteed by the realisation of the following indicators [11].

- For urgent referral, delay should be 3 days or less.
- Minimum standard for delay between mammography and result: 5 w.d. or less.
- Delay between result of imaging and offered assessment minimum standard: 5 w.d. or less.
- Delay between assessment and issuing of results minimum standard: 5 w.d. or less.
- Delay between decision to operate and date offered for surgery minimum standard: 15 w.d. or less, ideally 7–10 w.d.
- Moreover, 95 % of women should receive full and adequate assessment in three appointments or less.
- 90 % of women with symptoms and signs strongly suggesting the presence of BC should be seen within 2 weeks of referral, and agreed protocols should be in place to facilitate this.

*Information*. Above all, unnecessary distress may be caused not only by delays but also by failure of efficient communication between the diagnostic team and the woman. Failure to reach a definitive diagnosis due to imprecise methods of assessment also results in anxiety.

If possible, the radiologist should be present in the clinic at the time when a woman has her mammogram so that any necessary further investigation (e.g. magnification or spot compression views, ultrasound examination) can be performed without delay. It is also important that full verbal information on the status of her investigations and diagnosis be given to the woman at suitably relevant stages throughout the diagnostic process.

As far as possible, the woman should be informed of the result of her examination before she leaves the clinic and of the need for any necessary further investigation to be performed. The failure of the assessment process to make a definitive diagnosis of either a benign or a malignant condition is an undesirable outcome of assessment and further increases anxiety. For this reason, the use of early recall for a repeat examination at a time shorter than that normally specified for a routine follow-up is to be avoided.

Women must be informed of when to expect results and should be provided with written information at appropriate stages in the diagnostic procedure. However, information regarding the likelihood of malignancy being present should not be given via telephone or letter. Such information should be given verbally to the woman, preferably in the presence of a relative or a nurse counsellor.

### 1.3.3 Ethical and Legal Issues

*Standard of care*. There is no predefined standard of care; on the contrary, a specific standard has to be established for each individual case. One responsibility of the breast specialist is to match the patient's needs with the appropriate measures. The elements used to establish a standard of care are the opinions of peers working in similar circumstances, scientific publications and international, national and local guidelines.

The breast specialist, therefore, is required to display the same behaviours and possess the same skills that are required from the specialists who belong to the same professional community. He or she is required to be up to date with the knowledge and the innovations in their discipline and to possess capacity of judgement and display behaviours respectful of the patient first and foremost as a person rather than a sick person.

*Patient-centred care*. Treatment and care should take into account patients' needs and preferences. Patients with early or locally advanced BC should have the opportunity to make informed decisions about their care and treatment, in partnership with their healthcare professionals. In a few words, doctors should put their patients' interests first.

*Specific ethical issues* are many more than those appear at first sight. Each caregiver facing BC should at least be able to:

- Identify the major sources of medical ethics.
- Manage different approaches to ethical decision-making.
- Respect patient's own right to autonomy.
- Abandon any form of medical paternalism.
- Recognise and solve ethical conflicts
- Give respect and equal treatment to each patient, independently from age, religion, race, class, gender, disease and any personal beliefs or other human rights grounds.
- Resist to any form of sexual attraction.
- Require an interpreter in the case of patients who do not speak their language.
- Keep patient's information confidential and protect any identifiable patient.
- Recognise the principal ethical issues that occur at the end of life.
- Know the main ethical principles relatively to cooperation among colleagues.
- Prevent ethical conflicts among colleagues.
- Know the main principles of research ethics.
- Understand that an even highly competent treatment does not excuse a breach of ethics.

*Consent*. Informed consent should be obtained and documented for most health planned services. For instance, if surgery is indicated, patient should be fully informed of the surgical options available for her specific condition. This includes informed choice among different options, outcome and so on.

*Litigation*. Medicolegal issues are tightly connected with ethical ones. A good breast specialist is not the one who guarantees a good result, but the one who abides by the rules and uses the appropriate means to obtain such result. A negative result is not, in itself, a reason for legal action if the breast specialist is able to demonstrate that they carried out a thorough and sound assessment of the issue and that they have suggested the same solution that the average of other breast specialists would have adopted in that given circumstance.

An evaluation of the clinical judgement is possible only if two (or more) options to solve an issue are available; if the choice made by the breast specialist is accepted by the breast specialists community in that specific moment and in that context, then it is defensible in case it has failed its objective or in case the outcome is unwanted or unpredictable.

Only if the specialist has showed gaps in his/her knowledge, lack of skills, recklessness, negligence or committed omissions in the actions required by the standard of care and only if this resulted in damage to the patient, then they are liable to prosecution.

*Delay in diagnosis.* It remains the biggest cause of litigation by breast patients with missed diagnosis of BC being the most common, and with the highest settlements, in cases involving premenopausal women. Clinical practice that complies with guidelines is easier to defend; nonetheless, guidelines not always take individual context into account. Note the following circumstances.

- BC is less common in younger women, but younger women make up the greater proportion of complainants in failure to diagnose or delayed diagnoses cases.
- False reassurance from a false-negative mammogram or, conversely, unnecessary treatment from a false positive can both result in litigation.
- Incomplete or discordant triple assessment always needs to be properly addressed.
- A benign lump will never become cancerous, but it may grow, resulting in a larger proportion of the breast being removed if it is decided at a later stage to excise the lump.
- If the patient feels a lump that her GP misses, the GP may have been negligent if it emerges that the patient was actually suffering from BC.
- The same where there is no lump, but the patient has other symptoms – for example pain.

More detailed forms of informed consent do not hold down the upward trend of litigation, mainly because the expectations of women are always higher than achievable results. Anyway the concept of negligence can be applied also to the woman who neglects or refuses to adhere to the instructions provided by the breast specialist.

Many litigations are the result of a misunderstanding, and the use of proper terms should always be taken into consideration. Unintentional omissions are considered a logical fallacy; oversight error in judgement and inaccuracies are unforgivable. On the other side, a reflection on the use we make of words could teach us something.

On the other hand, the term *early diagnosis* is, strictly speaking, incorrect and misleading, therefore potentially exposed to medical litigation. The minimum diameter compatible with a clinical diagnosis is, in the best conditions, of about 6 mm, i.e. a tumour that contains over 100 million cells and with a life of more than 27 duplications. A mammogram can detect, always in ideal conditions, cancers of slightly more than 2 mm, i.e. lesions that contain more than 10 million cells and with a life of at least 23 duplications, which therefore have already made 60–70 % of their entire history evolution. Therefore, the term *preclinical* diagnosis should be preferred over the term early diagnosis.

Some results, which are considered *unpredictable*, actually correspond to symptoms insufficiently considered. Other *predictable* results (such as interval tumours in the course of the screening) must be accepted as such. The recurrence of a borderline phyllodes tumour can show a malignant grade, and the recurrence of a pre-invasive cancer may be invasive. The coexistence of lesions at risk (such as atypical hyperplasia) with pre-malignant or invasive lesions is more or less predictable in definitive histology. However less blameworthy, the failure to consider that, as well as how to inform the patient, may still lead to legal consequences.

Defining as *benign* a lesion before all the investigations have been planned or completed may be unwise. For example, in a woman aged >30, it is more prudent to define a typically benign nodule (e.g. fibroadenoma) as *probably benign*. The William Osler's definition of medicine as *a science of uncertainty and an art of probability* still remains valid.

### 1.3.4 Breast Care Training

Last but not least, effective mentoring is very crucial in the training of breast clinicians. In the last decade, the practice of surgery has been changing rapidly at every level, requiring a more complex approach to mentoring young surgeons. Besides clinical and surgical skills, surgical trainees must acquire a broad range of technical, interpersonal, administrative and research skills.

The twenty-first century brings special demands, including changing treatment patterns, increased diversity in trainees and in patient populations, restrictions on how students should be trained, increased concerns about patient's privacy and an ageing population. Besides the classic mentor/mentee relationship, different models of mentoring, including mosaic mentoring and collaborative mentoring, are being used to address these issues. Successful mentoring programs occur in institutions that maintain a culture that actively supports mentoring [12].

In addition to maintaining career satisfaction (use of mentorship's power, engagement in clinical or translational research, time for work-related travels), mentees should maintain personal wellness as regards the relationships (protect time to spend for significant others), attitudes (meaning in work and personal endeavours) and physical and mental well-being.

## References

1. Breast cancer incidence statistics. In http://www.cancerresearchuk.org/cancer-info/cancerstats/types/breast/incidence/uk-breast-cancer-incidence-statistics. Accessed 10 July 2013.

2. Taylor DC. The components of sickness: diseases, illnesses and predicaments. Lancet. 1979;314:1008–10.
3. Willet AM, Michell MJ, Lee MJL, editors. Best practice diagnostic guidelines for patients presenting with breast symptoms. http://www.associationofbreastsurgery.org.uk/media/4585/best_practice_diagnostic_guidelines_for_patients_presenting_with_breast_symptoms.pdf.
4. NICE Guideline 80, Early and advanced breast cancer: diagnosis and treatment, 2009. http://www.nice.org.uk. Accessed 20 July 2013.
5. Dixon MJ. Costs and benefits of a one stop clinic compared with a dedicated breast clinic: randomised controlled trial. Commentary: one stop clinics should not be abandoned. Br Med J. 2002;324:507.
6. Athreya BH. Handbook of clinical skills. Singapore: World Scientific; 2010.
7. Prommer EE. Talking with cancer patients and their families. In: Casciato DA, editor. Manual of clinical oncology. 7th ed. Philadelphia: Lippincott William and Wilkins; 2012.
8. Wilson ARM, Marotti L, Bianchi S, et al. The requirements of a specialist Breast Centre. Eur J Cancer. 2013;49:3579–87.
9. Muñoz M, Estévez LG, Alvarez I, et al. Evaluation of international treatment guidelines and prognostic tests for the treatment of early breast cancer. Cancer Treat Rev. 2008;34:701–9.
10. Dykewicz CA. Summary of the guidelines for preventing opportunistic infections among hematopoietic stem cell transplant recipients. Clin Infect Dis. 2001;33:139–44.
11. Perry NM. Multidisciplinary aspects of quality assurance in the diagnosis of Breast disease EUSOMA. Eur J Cancer. 2001;37:159–72.
12. Singletary SE. Mentoring surgeons for the 21st century. Ann Surg Oncol. 2005;12:848–60.

## Further Reading

Cataliotti L, De Wolf C, Holland R, et al. Guidelines on the standards for the training of specialised health professionals dealing with breast cancer. Eur J Cancer. 2007;43:660–75.

Dixon JM, Thomas J. Symptoms, assessment and guidelines for referral. In: Dixon JM, editor. ABC of breast diseases. 4th ed. Oxford: Wiley-Blackwell; 2012.

ICSI. Evaluation by primary care of patient with symptoms of potential breast disease. www.icsi.org/_asset/v9l91q/DxBrDis.pdf. Accessed 30 Jan 2015.

Julian TB, Venditti CA, Duggal S. Landmark clinical trials influencing surgical management of non-invasive and invasive breast cancer. Breast J. 2015;21:60–6.

Kuerer HM, Pass HA, Simmons R, et al. Multidisciplinary training for breast surgical oncology. In: Kuerer HM, editor. Kuerer's breast surgical oncology. New York: McGraw-Hill; 2010.

Morgan JL, Vijh R. Trends in malpractice litigation in relation to the delivery of breast care in the National Health Service. Breast. 2013;22:964–7.

Perry NM. Multidisciplinary aspects of quality assurance in the diagnosis of breast disease EUSOMA. Eur J Cancer. 2001;37:159–72.

Senkus E. Breast cancer units – improvement in care or expensive "wishful thinking"? Breast. 2014;23:199–200.

Willett AM, Michell MJ, Lee MJR, editors. Best practice diagnostic guidelines for patients presenting with breast symptoms. www.associationofbreastsurgery.org.uk/media/4585/best_practice_diagnostic_guidelines_for_patients_presenting_with_breast_symptoms.pdf. Accessed 30 Jan 2015.

**Websites in Appendix**: *Main Health Professional Websites*, A-1; *Websites Addressed to Patients*, A.2; *BC Coalition for Advocacy*, A.3; *Clinical Trials*, A-4.6.

# The Asymptomatic Woman

# 2

Alfonso M. Pluchinotta, Gianni Saguatti,
and Daniela Zuccarello

## Contents



A.M. Pluchinotta (✉)
Breast Surgery, Policlinic of Abano Terme, Padova, Italy
e-mail: pluchinotta.alfonso@gmail.com

G. Saguatti
Department of Radiology, Mammographic Screening,
Hospital 'Bellaria', Bologna, Italy
e-mail: gianni.saguatti@ausl.bologna.it

D. Zuccarello
Unit of Clinical Genetics and Epidemiology, University of Padova, Padova, Italy
e-mail: daniela.zuccarello@unipd.it



A.M. Pluchinotta (ed.), *The Outpatient Breast Clinic: Aiming at Best Practice*,
DOI 10.1007/978-3-319-15907-2_2

**Abstract**

• Before a woman is a patient, she is a woman with her own biography. • The way a woman looks at her breast is a good indicator of her degree of self-confidence. • Women generally overestimate their risk of developing BC and, as a consequence, overrate the benefits that may be gained from screening or preventive measures. • Although many women with a strong family history do not have an identified genetic mutation, their potential serious risk should be properly considered. • BRCA1 and BRCA2 do not have the same effects, and recent reports show BRCA2 carriers are associated with better survival and therapeutic response than BRCA1 carriers.

*Future Directions*. Every woman faces the risk of developing cancer or she believes she does. Every diagnosis of BC may involve the entire family, while several half-truths and distortions are an obstacle to objectivity. The most challenging element in communication, becoming more and more crucial, is the actual perception and classification of the risk.

## 2.1 Breast Awareness

**Clinical Practice Points**

- There is a lack of evidence for the effectiveness of breast self-examination in reducing cancer mortality. Anyway, clinicians should encourage a form of breast awareness whereby the woman becomes familiar with her own breasts by looking and feeling and reporting promptly any changes.
- Every woman should be reassured and, at the same time, provided with information about her specific risk of suffering from BC. This issue is particularly relevant in discussions about the benefits and harms of screening, preventive measures in gene mutations carriers as well as adjuvant therapy for BC.
- Apart from the fact of being a woman, all things considered, the most significant risk factor for BC is increasing age.
- Major risk factors cannot be changed, while other minor risk factors are related to lifestyle and should suggest preventive measures in healthy habits.

### 2.1.1 Overview

*Perception of risk*. Risk is a poorly understandable and understood concept. Because nothing is risk-free, giving the right perception of the risk is an everyday challenge for the surgeon's communication skills [1]. *Risk* is the measurement of the likelihood that an event will take place, a proportional quantity, but the term carries a negative connotation in spite of being a neutral term. Conversely, odds or probability have a more positive implication even though similar in meaning.

The total effect of a given risk is the product of the risk and the *consequences*. It is known that people tend to pay more attention to negative consequences than positive ones, particularly when the former are seen as gruesome, refractory to treatment and poorly understood. There is an important corollary to the notion that no risk exists in isolation. Conceptually, the proper approach to the assessment of risk would be to sum the product of all possible risks and their consequences. In reality, this is very difficult to do and, as a result, there is often an exaggerated focus on rare, potentially dramatic adverse consequences.

Balance or comparison is another vital principle. The concept of relative or proportionate risk underlies all fields of medicine, and this issue becomes significant also in discussions about the benefits and harms of screening, preventive measures in gene mutation carriers as well as adjuvant therapy for BC.

Explaining the concept of risk is more difficult than it is believed. People have some sense of the total effect of a specific risk and tend not to identify, sum and weigh all hazards and consequences. That without considering that events are constantly changing, the consequences vary with time and circumstances, and also an individual's personal choices change over time.

The best approach is to give a clear explanation of the basic principles and to set individual risks in the context of the other hazards that exist. Thus, when explaining the concept of risk to a patient, there are a number of points worth considering. Firstly it is helpful to set risks in context, by comparing the risk of BC with that of trauma or heart disease. The distinction between risk and consequence should be clarified. Broadly speaking, doubling of a very small risk may be far less worrisome than a 5 % increase in a very large risk. Finally, all interventions, including doing nothing, involve a trade-off of risks.

*Women within the average/mild-risk population.* Incidence of BC and its impression in the media increases the perception of risk. Some women tend to overestimate their own risk of BC, as is usually observed in young women who have experienced relatives (mother, aunt) with BC in postmenopausal age. Every woman should be reassured and, at the same time, provided with information about her specific risk of suffering from BC. Adequate information about genetic counselling and close surveillance programmes should be provided especially to all young women with a strong family history of BC.

To date, the risk factors that have been identified for BC are many, and it is very difficult to assess them thoroughly and establish the real interactions between them. Probably it is the simultaneous presence of risk factors, which by one or other determine a risk only modestly increased, that has an overall multiplicative effect that should be calculated and followed forward in time.

There is a lack of evidence for the effectiveness of breast self-examination (BSE) in reducing BC mortality, and available evidence for its benefit is limited and mostly related to increased breast health awareness. Clinicians should encourage a form of breast awareness whereby the woman becomes familiar with her own breasts by looking and feeling and reporting promptly any changes.

Regular breast self-examination and clinical breast examination should be recommended for all women at average risk over 35–40 years of age. Women also need to be informed about the limitations and risks of breast examination. The ideal time for breast examination is after menstruation. Optimal frequency has not been determined; the usual recommendation is monthly. Regular reminders to perform BSE also promote a culture of screening, according to the recommendations set out by age.

Changes to refer include discomfort or pain, lumps, thickening, uneven areas, nipple changes or discharges or changes in the appearance of the breast, such as the shape or the presence of dimpling of the skin.

*Women with mammographic dense breast.* Density is strongly heritable and decreases with pregnancy, menopause and tamoxifen therapies. At the same time, it is increased by HRT. The ability to detect small tumours is impaired in breast tissue dense on mammogram. Studies found that women with radiologically dense breast tissue (more than 60 % of the breast) had an increased RR=4 of developing BC.

*Women with breast augmentation.* Breast augmentation for cosmetic purposes is more and more common in young women. The presence of breast implants does not represent a risk factor. Several case control and cohort studies have not shown an increased risk for BC due to augmentation mammoplasty and there is no evidence to recommend regular diagnostic surveillance in augmented and non-augmented women at average risk under 40 years of age (LoE III) [2]. Moreover, no evidence exists for recommending periodic MRI in women at average risk with cosmetic breast implants (see 'Magnetic resonance imaging', Sect. 5.3).

To date no studies have investigated screening programmes or imaging surveillance in aesthetically augmented women below 40 years of age who are at average risk. Some data suggest that the presence of implants may lead to a loss of 28–49 % of the breast on mammographic view. The sensitivity of a screening mammography in asymptomatic women is lower in women with breast augmentation in comparison to those without (45 % versus 65 %), while the specificity is slightly higher in women with augmentation.

It was reported that—at time of diagnosis—BCs are more frequently palpable in augmented women than in those without implants (75 % versus 54 %). This observation raises the hypothesis that the presence of breast implants may lead to a delayed diagnosis with all its consequences. Young women planning to have a breast augmentation surgery should be specifically informed about this issue. However, published studies confirmed that prognosis, disease-free time and survival rates are similar between augmented and non-augmented women with BC [2].

*Risk factors.* There is a wide literature about the risk factors for breast tumours, and different levels of risk have been identified based on the importance of the different factors and on the distinction between invariable risk factors and lifestyle-related risk factors. Some of these factors which were considered to be relatively minor, such as alcohol and insulin stimulation, are acquiring more and more importance.

For information regarding the importance of minor factors, it is better to refer to the data of International Agencies (as International Agency for Research on Cancer, AIRC) that evaluates evidence (as sufficient or convincing or probable) on the carcinogenic risk to humans of a large number of exposures [3]. The information is complex because some factors have different impact in pre- or postmenopausal status; moreover, some data are actually controversial, as medical condition or occupational exposure. Our overview considers major and minor risk factors [4].

## 2.1.2 BSC Major Risk Factors

*Gender*. Simply being a woman is the main risk factor. Women to man ratio is about 135:1, with some epidemiological differences depending on ethnicity. Besides anatomical reasons, the explanation is probably because men are exposed to minor quantities of female hormones, which can promote BC cell growth.

*Age*. As age progresses from 35 to 65 years, the risk of developing BC is increased 6-fold. At age 60, about 15–20 in every 1,000 women are expected to develop BC within 5 years. The chance of developing BC is 1:20,000 at 25 years, 1:2,500 at 30, 1:600 at 35, 1:217 at 40, 1:50 at 50 and so on till 1:10 at 80 years.

*Genetic risk factors*. About 5–10 % of all BCs have a genetic inheritance mechanism. All are autosomal dominant and tend to be highly penetrant, and most are bilateral. 50 % of hereditary BC is inherited from the father's side. The best characterised genetic risk factors are represented by germ-line mutations in BRCA1 and BRCA2, so that carriers of these germ-line mutations have a 1.5–4 % per year risk of developing BC. This subject is more largely discussed in the Sect. 2.3.

*Family history*. About 15–20 % of BC patients have a family history of BC. If a mother, sister or daughter has a positive history of BC, the patient's risk is increased 2–4 times (sister more than mother). If two first-degree relatives have BC, the patient's risk is increased 4–6 times and even as high as 50 % if one of the two relatives had bilateral disease before 50 years of age. This subject is more largely discussed in the Sect. 2.3.

*Personal history of BC*. Women with personal history of BC have a 3- to 4-fold increased risk of developing a contralateral BC, with an annual risk of 0.6 % and a cumulative risk increased from 5 % at 10 years to 10 % at 15 years of follow-up (see Sect. 15.1). The lifetime risk of contralateral primary BC is increased by young age at diagnosis of the primary lesion, family history specifically of bilateral BC and presence of DCIS and/or LCIS. These women also have an increased risk of developing ovarian, but also endometrial and colon, carcinomas.

*Ionising radiation*. Radiation therapy is dangerous especially between puberty and before the age of 30 years. Peak incidence of following related cancers has been observed if exposure took place between 15 and 18 years of age. No increased risk of exposure after the age of 40 years has been observed; therefore, mammograms are not dangerous.

Since Hodgkin's disease tends to occur at a younger age, women (but also men) with a previous history of Hodgkin's disease treated with radiation have an increased incidence of BC, especially in medial segments, and more often it is bilateral. For this reason, these patients must undergo screening mammograms beginning at age 35 or 10 years after therapy, whichever comes first.

*Atypical hyperplasia*. Women with atypical hyperplasia have a 4 times higher relative risk of developing BC. Risk is significantly increased if there is a positive family history in first-degree relatives, so that in the presence of a first-degree relative with BC, the risk increases 8–12 times. The cancer risk is bilateral and equally likely to occur in either breast. It is uncertain if the risk remains constant over time, and some studies have observed that the risk may decrease after about 10 years. This subject is more largely discussed in Sect. 9.4 ('Proliferative lesions with atypia').

### 2.1.3 BC Minor Risk Factors

*Menstrual periods*. Uninterrupted menstrual cycling for long periods of time increases risk. Women who have had more menstrual cycles because they started menstruating early (before age 12) and/or went through menopause later (after age 55) have a slightly higher risk of BC. Women who experienced menopause before the age of 45 years are estimated to have one-half the lifetime BC risk of women who experience menopause after the age of 55 years. The increase in risk may be due to a longer lifetime exposure to the hormones oestrogen and progesterone. Decrease in the total number of ovulatory cycles, as in irregularity of menstrual cycles, may be protective.

*Reproductive history*. Having many pregnancies and becoming pregnant at a young age reduces the risk of BC. In this case, the reason for this effect may be that pregnancy reduces a woman's total number of lifetime menstrual cycles. Women who have had no children or who delay childbirth until the age of 30 years have a 2-fold increased risk of developing BC compared with women who have a first child at <20 years of age. It should be noted that there appears to be a transient increased risk of BC after giving birth.

*Breastfeeding*. Some studies suggest that breastfeeding may slightly lower BC risk among premenopausal women, especially if it is continued for 18–24 months, while no reduction in the risk of BC occurred among postmenopausal women with a history of lactation. One explanation for this possible effect may be that breastfeeding reduces a woman's total number of lifetime menstrual cycles (similar to starting menstrual periods at a later age or going through early menopause). Breastfeeding seems to provide a reduction in the risk of ovarian cancer of about 6 % for every 6 months of breastfeeding.

*Hormone use*. Studies have found that women using oral contraceptives have a slightly greater risk of BC than women who have never used them. This risk seems to go back to normal over time once the pills are stopped. Women who stopped using oral contraceptives more than 10 years ago do not appear to have any increased BC risk.

Hormonal replacement therapy (HRT) increases the risk of developing BC of about 1.2–1.4-fold. The longer the duration of HRT, the higher the risk. The increased risk from combined hormone therapy appears to apply only to current and recent users. A woman's BC risk seems to return to that of the general population within 5 years of stopping combined treatment. The use of oestrogen alone after menopause does not appear to increase significantly the risk of developing BC.

Although controversial, at this time there appear to be few strong reasons to use postmenopausal hormone therapy (either combined or oestrogen alone), other than possibly for the short-term relief of menopausal symptoms. Along with the increased risk of BC, combined HT also appears to increase the risk of heart disease, blood clots and strokes. It does lower the risk of colorectal cancer and osteoporosis, but this must be weighed against possible harm, especially since there are other effective ways to prevent and treat osteoporosis.

*Previous history of non-breast cancer*. Women with a personal history mainly of ovarian cancer, but also endometrial, have an increased risk of BC over that of women without such a history. Moreover, an association has been reported among women with melanoma or salivary gland tumours or colon cancer.

### 2.1.4 Main Lifestyle Factors

The main modifiable risk factors are alcohol consumption, leisure physical activity or lack thereof, and body mass index. Some epidemiological studies reports that modifying these factors could reduce the risk in 20 years of around 2 % in menopausal women, of 3–4 % in women with a family history of BC, and up to around 5 % in high-risk women. *Alcohol.*

The use of alcohol is clearly linked to an increased risk of developing BC. The risk increases with the amount of alcohol consumed. Compared with non-drinkers, women who consume 1 alcoholic drink a day have a very small increase in risk. Those who have 2–5 drinks daily have about 1.5 times the risk of women who do not drink alcohol. The effect of alcohol on BC may be enhanced by other factors, such as a low dietary intake of folate that can counteract the effect of alcohol.

*Physical activity.* Evidence is growing that physical activity in the form of exercise reduces BC risk. The main question is how much exercise is needed. In one study from the Women's Health Initiative, as little as 1.25–2.5 h per week of brisk walking reduced a woman's risk by 18 %. Walking 10 h a week reduced the risk a little more.

*Excess weight.* Being overweight or obese after menopause increases BC risk by raising oestrogen levels. As it is well-known, fat tissue produces excess amounts of oestrogen, high levels of which have been associated with the risk of breast and some other cancers. Furthermore, women who are overweight tend to have higher blood insulin levels and insulin-like growth factor-1 (IGF-1), a condition known as hyperinsulinemia or insulin resistance, that have been linked to some cancers, including BC. But the connection between weight and BC risk is complex. For example, the risk appears to be increased for women who gained weight as an adult but may not be increased among those who have been overweight since childhood. Also, excess fat in the waist area may affect risk more than the same amount of fat in the hips and thighs. Researchers believe that fat cells in various parts of the body have subtle differences that may explain this.

*Diet.* The Mediterranean diet (which includes whole grains, fruit, vegetables, nuts and olive oil) may protect against BC. More European studies have revealed that olive oil may be protective against BC by the action of oleic acid that is the main monounsaturated fatty acid of olive oil. Also a diet rich in fish oils seems to be protective, but large randomised studies are needed.

The effect of vitamin intake is questionable. Vitamin A has been shown in some studies to reduce the risk of BC, but this is not proven in large randomised trials. Other antioxidants, such as vitamin C and vitamin E, have not been shown to be protective against BC.

Phytoestrogens (isoflavones derived mainly from soybeans, lignans, black cohosh or *Cimicifuga racemosa*, red clover or *Trifolium pratense*) may act as weak oestrogens, but may also have anti-oestrogenic effects. Their effects vary in different ethnic groups and substantial decrease in BC risk is still controversial.

Finally, more studies have looked for a link between diet and BC risk, but so far the results have been conflicting, as in the amount of fat in the diet and intake of fruits, vegetables and meat. Furthermore, some studies have indicated that diet may play a role, while others found no evidence that diet influences BC risk.

*Chemicals in the environment.* A great deal of research has been reported and more is being done to understand possible environmental influences on BC risk.

Compounds in the environment that have oestrogen-like properties are of special interest. For example, substances found in some plastics, certain cosmetics and personal care products, pesticides (such as DDE) and PCBs (polychlorinated biphenyls) seem to have such properties. These could in theory affect BC risk.

This issue understandably invokes a great deal of public concern, but at this time research does not show a clear link between BC risk and exposure to these substances. Unfortunately, studying such effects in humans is difficult. More research is needed to better define the possible health effects of these and similar substances.

For a long time, studies found no link between cigarette smoking and BC. In recent years more studies have found that long-term heavy smoking is linked to a higher risk of BC in certain groups, such as women who started smoking before they had their first child.

An active focus of research is whether second-hand smoke increases the risk of BC. Both active and second-hand smoke contains chemicals that, in high concentrations, reach the breast tissue and can be found in breast milk. However, the evidence on second-hand smoke and BC risk is controversial, and one possible explanation for this is that tobacco smoke may have different effects on BC risk in smokers and in those who are just exposed to smoke. The 2014 US Surgeon General's report concluded that there is *suggestive but not sufficient* evidence of a link at this point. In any case, this possible link to BC is yet another reason to avoid second hand smoke.

## 2.2 Breast Cancer Screening

**Clinical Practice Points**

- Mammography is the technique of choice that has been shown to be effective on a population basis for a BC screening protocol.
- Screening is targeted at women aged 50–70 years and can be expected to reduce mortality through early detection, allowing more breast-conserving surgeries.
- An increased diagnostic performance is due to independent double reading and computer-aided detection (CAD), while a constant effort is being made to reduce recall rates, false-positive rates and overtreatments.
- Screening is a model of multidisciplinarity since it vouches for the comprehensiveness of the diagnostic pathways in accordance with the main guidelines.

### 2.2.1 BC Screening Strategies

Results from randomised clinical trials show that screening mammography reduces the number of deaths from BC in women between 40 and 74 years of age. The average mortality reduction is estimated to be about 20–25 % with its major impact (mortality reduction of 30 %) in the age group of 49–59 years.

The low incidence of sporadic BC before the age of 40 and the suboptimal performance of diagnostic modalities in these women justify the absence of trials investigating not only the efficacy but also the feasibility of BC screening programmes in women less than 40 years of age. In addition, under the age of 40 years, high recall rates, high rates of additional imaging and low cancer detection rates are commonly recorded. Also the efficacy of a baseline mammogram for women at average risk at the age of 35–40 years to provide a comparison image available for the succeeding screening was tested in the past and failed to show a benefit [2].

Biannual mammography has been shown to have the greatest effect on BC mortality reduction in the age group of 50–69 years, while the effect in women aged 40–49 years is still disputed. Starting from these evidences, many European countries have established national or regional population-based mammography screening programs with the purpose of detecting BCs at a preclinical stage, in order to improve the chance of survival. Guidelines for quality assurance in BC screening and diagnosis recommend standards and describe performance parameters and indicators that should be monitored in any screening programme.

Anyway, there is no consensus about the exact effect of mammography screening on BC mortality reduction, and the estimates reported vary in different countries. In a recent UK review of the randomised, controlled mammography trials, a 20 % relative BC mortality reduction was estimated in women invited to screening in the age group of 50–70 years, although the review stresses the importance of taking into account the risk of overdiagnosis and overtreatment as well as false-positive screening when balancing the benefits and harms of screening. Additionally, screening programs carry the risk of false-negative results and consequently a false feeling of security among patients and doctors.

Actually, although several trials show better cancer-related survival in screened versus non-screened women, a number of important biases may explain that finding.

*Lead-time bias*. Survival time for a cancer found mammographically includes the time between detection and the time when the cancer would have been detected because of clinical symptoms, but this time is not included in the survival time of cancers found because of symptoms.

*Length bias*. Mammography detects a cancer while it is preclinical, and preclinical durations vary. Cancers with longer preclinical durations are, by definition, present during more opportunities for discovery and therefore are more likely to be detected by screening; these cancers tend to be slow growing and to have better prognoses, irrespective of screening.

*Overdiagnosis bias*. It is an extreme form of length bias; screening may find cancers that are very slow growing and would never have become manifest clinically in the woman's lifetime.

*Healthy volunteer bias*. The screened population may be comprised of the most health-conscious women among the general population, even if a variety of factors, including social and economic influences, may restrict women's participation. Because the extent of these biases is never clear in any particular study, most groups rely on randomised controlled trials to assess the benefits of screening. Other prejudices are linked to limited sensitivity and specificity in some group of woman, to the presence of interval cancer and to consistency of equipment.

*Sensitivity*. The sensitivity of mammography is the percentage of BCs detected in a given population, when BC is present. Sensitivity depends on tumour size, eminence and hormone sensitivity, as well as breast tissue density, patient age, timing within the menstrual cycle, overall image quality and interpretive skills of the radiologist. Overall sensitivity is approximately 80 % (range 68 % to >90 %), but is lower in younger women (range 62–76 % in women between 40 and 49 years) and in those with dense breast tissue [4]. The result is that delay in diagnosis of BC is the most common cause of medical malpractice litigation.

*Specificity*. The specificity of mammography is the likelihood of the test being normal when cancer is absent, whereas the false-positive rate is the likelihood of the test being abnormal when cancer is absent. If specificity is low, many false-positive examinations result in unnecessary follow-up examinations and procedures.

*Interval cancers* is a name given to cancers detected/presenting within 12 months after a mammographic screening in which findings are considered normal. The term is a statistical benchmark used in conjunction with other parameters to assess the efficacy of breast imaging programmes and the statistics of mammogram readers. The definition is potentially confusing too because the implication suggests that an imaging error was made and also because interval cancers appear on the statistics of the most recent previous mammogram reader, by convention. The fact is that true-negative interval cancers actually develop in the time period between the last mammogram (read as 'normal') and the one on which the cancer was detected.

Interval cancers might be divided into a number of categories [5].

- *True-negative* interval cancer: no sign of disease may be detected on previous screening mammogram. The lesion is new.
- *Interpreted as benign* interval cancer: a lesion that proves to be malignant showed benign morphological characteristics on the previous mammogram.
- *Retrospectively visible* interval cancer: a now known lesion is seen on the previous screen mammogram. This is an interpretive error on the part of the reader.
- *Single reader* interval cancer: a second reader would have discovered the lesion. Second reads in screening programmes yield up to 10–15 % more cancers.
- *Technical failure* interval cancer: a technically poor image hampered the reader to discover the abnormality. In theory suboptimal images will not be submitted for interpretation and if they are, should not be read.

The review of interval cancers is an integral, essential part of the quality assurance process in any breast imaging programme. It is time-consuming but like pathology review yields benefits for the whole programme. These are cases where careful objective review gives valuable insights and opportunities to learn and improve the whole programme from the image acquisition through to interpretation.

Interval cancer rates are defined parameters in most programmes and the recommended rates vary depending on the country. The rates are higher where the screening interval recommended is longer, i.e. where mammograms are recommended every 3 years as opposed to every year. This value cannot be seen as a stand-alone parameter when assessing the efficacy of a programme or its workers. It is only a single value that needs to be seen in the context of all the other statistical values used in the assessment.

One study on interval cancers reports that interval cancers are more prevalent in women aged 40–49 years. Interval cancers appearing within 12 months of a negative screening mammogram appear to be related to decreased mammographic sensitivity, attributable to greater breast density in 68 % of cases. Those appearing within a 24-month interval appear to be related both to decreased mammographic sensitivity due to greater breast density in 37.6 % and to rapid tumour growth in 30.6 % [4].

Another study found that interval cancers is much more likely to occur in women younger than 50 years and to be of mucinous or lobular histology or to have high histologic grade, high proliferative activity and relatively benign features mammographically and/or to lack calcifications. In the same study, screen-detected cancers: are more likely to have tubular histology; are smaller, low stage and hormone sensitive; and have a major component of ductal carcinoma in situ.

Finally, more studies underline that the most important cancers detected at screening are high-grade DCIS, as most cases of this type will progress to grade 2 or 3 invasive BC within the following 3 years, and grade 2 and 3 invasive BCs under 10 mm in diameter, as at this size these tumours are much less likely to have metastasised [6].

*Equipment.* In the screening, the advent of full-field digital mammography suggests a further positive clinical impact on early detection of BC. Studies comparing the diagnostic performance of full-field digital mammography with screen-film mammography in a corporate screening showed a significantly higher cancer detection rate and positive predictive value for full-field digital mammography, especially in women under the age of 50.

Several new techniques are being tested for screening and diagnostic imaging, such as 3D mammography (breast tomosynthesis), 3D ultrasound, shear wave elastography and contrast-enhanced mammography/spectral mammography. None of them is routinely implemented as yet, but all show promising preliminary results and could increase diagnostic accuracy, especially in women with dense breasts.

### 2.2.2 Benefits and Harms

*Benefits.* As said before, *reduction in mortality* is the first benefit. Breast screening detects BCs and saves lives, with the greatest reduction in mortality seen in women 50–60 years of age.

The *increase in breast-conserving treatments*, due to an increase in the early detection of BC, is another important result. More studies evaluating the quality of life among long survivors of BC demonstrate that body image scores for the breast-conserving surgery group are higher compared to the mastectomy group. Attending for breast screening is associated with short-term anxiety. The overall quality of life is noticeably improved, while the suffering from psychological and physical complaints decreased.

*Harms.* Studies of screening-detected BC have the strongest evidence of overdiagnosis, though estimates of its extent are wide ranging. Up to one-third of all screened women may have unnecessary treatment for the detection of BCs that would not have threatened the lives [7]. Moreover false-positive results in about 1 % of mammograms produce unnecessary anxiety, particularly if further investigations are undertaken.

Other harmful effects are false reassurance due to missed cancer and incorrect diagnosis, pain and discomfort due to mammography and, in general, psychological distress.

*Other concerns*. About 70 % of women participate in screening programs, and there is some evidence that these women have a higher incidence of breast problems than expected. This phenomenon could be explained by the fact that a woman who is reassured by a negative result might ignore changes in her breasts between mammograms. Since approximately 20–30 % of BCs are not detected by mammography, some tumours could, therefore, be missed.

For every BC detected, a substantial number of women will undergo biopsies or surgery for benign breast disease, with attendant morbidity.

Although the total dose of radiation received during mammography is low (<1.5 mGy), it has been suggested that repeated exposure could increase the risk of BC. This risk is, however, low and less perceived.

Small BCs detected by mammography may be biologically different from those detected clinically. Approximately 20 % of cancers detected by mammography are carcinomas in situ, some of which would never progress to invasive disease if left undetected, and the optimal treatment for such tumours is unknown. If these cancers are treated in the same way as invasive cancers, some women may undergo unnecessarily extensive surgery. Conversely, in other women, delaying treatment of an asymptomatic disease may ultimately compromise the chance of cure.

Finally, the optimum interval between mammograms has not been determined and thus, although radiographic screening is the *standard of care* in many places, it still remains controversial.

## 2.3 High-Risk Woman

**Clinical Practice Points**

- Approximately 5–10 % of patients with BC inherit a high-penetrance cancer-predisposing gene. Genes BRCA1 and BRCA2 denote high risk, but account for only a small proportion of cancer. Other rare gene mutations can also lead to inherited BCs but do not increase the risk of BC as much as the BRCA genes.
- In the high-risk woman, genetic counselling and/or psychological testing should precede genetic testing. For many women with a strong family history, no genetic mutation can be identified, though their potential serious risk persists.
- With increasing public awareness of the risk of BC and modern techniques of reconstruction, bilateral prophylactic mastectomy for women at increased risk of developing BC, as well contralateral prophylactic mastectomy for those with unilateral BC (also in seeking a symmetry), is becoming increasingly popular.
- Bilateral risk-reducing mastectomy (RRM) drops the risk of BC in BRCA mutation carriers by over 90 % and can produce profound relief of anxiety, but this major surgery is not an inconsequential decision, and careful consideration should be given to the risks and benefits of such procedures.

### 2.3.1 Breast Cancer Genetics

Cancers occur when an accumulation of genetic mutations in critical genes—those that control the cell growth and division or the repair of damaged DNA—allows cells to grow and divide uncontrollably to form a tumour. In most cases, these genetic changes are acquired during a person's lifetime and are present only in certain cells. These changes, which are called *somatic mutations*, are not inherited. Less commonly, *genetic mutations* inherited from a parent increase the risk of developing cancer. In people with these inherited genetic changes, additional somatic mutations in other genes must occur for cancer to develop.

In addition to specific genetic changes, many individual and environmental factors may influence a person's risk of developing BC. These factors include gender, age, ethnic background, a history of previous BC, certain changes in breast tissue and hormonal factors, as told above.

A history of BC in closely related family members is also an important risk factor, particularly if the cancer occurred at an early age. Some BCs gathered in families are associated with inherited mutations in particular genes, such as BRCA1 or BRCA2, which are the major genes related to hereditary BC. Women who have inherited certain mutations in these genes have a high risk of developing BC, ovarian cancer and also other types of cancer during their lifetimes.

Men with BRCA1 mutations also have an increased risk of developing male BC as well as an increased risk of pancreatic cancer. Mutations in the BRCA2 gene are associated with an increased chance of developing male BC and cancers of prostate and pancreas. Melanoma is also more common among people who have BRCA2 mutations.

Inherited changes in several other genes, including CHEK2 and TP53, have been found to increase the risk of developing BC. Mutations in these genes cause syndromes (as *Li-Fraumeni syndrome*) that greatly increase the chance of developing several types of cancer over a person's lifetime (usually a 70-year interval).

More generally, BC may be sporadic, familial or hereditary with significantly different incidence for both breast and ovarian cancers (Fig. 2.1).

*Sporadic BC (70–75 %)* represents the largest fraction of BC. It appears in individuals of the general population, without a significant familiarity, by the action of somatic mutations, mostly unknown. Few somatic mutations have been identified in the HER2 and TP53 genes associated with some cases of BC.

*Familial*, or family related, *BC (15–20 %)*. In general, family-related cancer is a descriptive term that indicates an aggregation of multiple cases of cancer in the same family (paternal and/or maternal line), without a clear transmission of the disease from one generation to the next or ascertained responsible gene.

However, it is commonly accepted that in some cases the lack of mutation may be due to two main factors: the patient is investigated only in BRCA1 and 2 genes (and not on other susceptibility genes) and international databases of mutation are still extremely poor or plenty of non-informative data.

*Hereditary BC (5–10 %)* is characterised by ascertained (or highly suspected from the analysis of the pedigree) genetic mutations that are transmitted to descendants. Its inherited susceptibility to BC is established on the basis of an

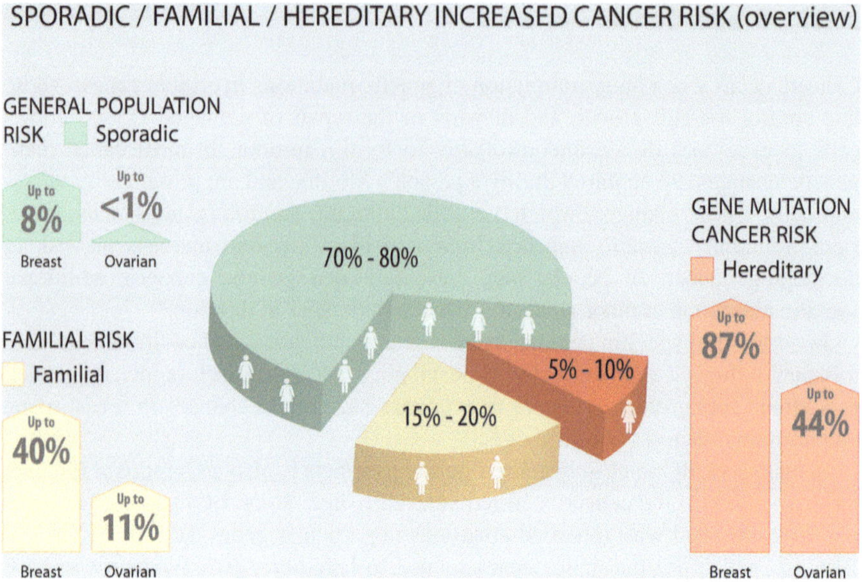


**Fig. 2.1** Incidence of breast and ovarian cancers in women with hereditary (high-risk), familial (moderate-risk) and sporadic (general population) BC [8, mod with permission]

identified germ-line mutation in one allele of a high-penetrance susceptibility gene, such as BRCA1 and BRCA2. Inactivation of the second allele of these tumour suppressor genes would be an early event in the multistep pathway of carcinogenesis.

*Ovarian cancer* (*OC*) too could be involved in the same gene mutations of BC. OC is preferably differentiated only between *sporadic* (*90 %*) and *hereditary* (*10 %*).

Although most cases of BC are not inherited, suspicious hereditary BC should be investigated because the cancer risk depends on the genes involved. This is crucial even if, actually, people inherit an increased risk of cancer, not the disease itself, and not all people who inherit mutations in these genes will develop cancer. In other cases, as in the most family-related BC, the inheritance of BC risk is unclear. However, it can be approximately calculated as a percentage using one of the risk assessment tools, starting from the family tree (pedigree chart).

*FIRST SELECTION*. The presence of an inherited predisposition to BC and/or OC in a family should be suspected on the basis of the following features:

- Incidence significantly higher than expected
- Age of onset younger (<35 years) than sporadic cases
- Increased frequency of bilateral tumours
- Family history of BC in males
- Family history of ovarian cancer
- Association between breast and ovarian cancer in the same patient in the same family

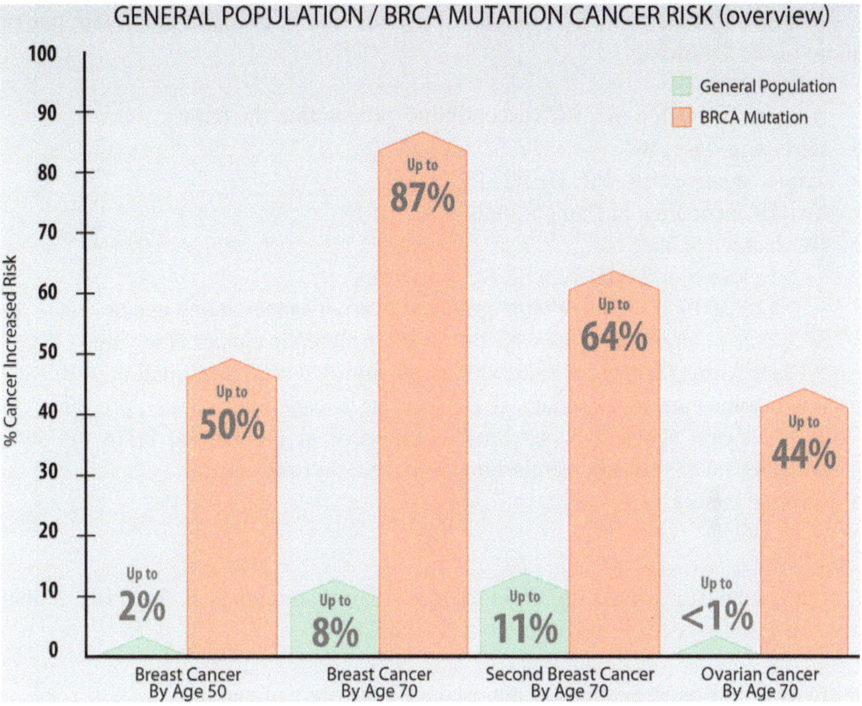


**Fig. 2.2** Incidence of breast and/or ovarian cancer in BRCA mutation carriers and in general population [9, mod with permission]

- BC in a young woman with aggressive phenotype (high-grade DCIS, RE / RPG <10, Ki67 >15, triple negative, HER2 overexpression)

*WOMEN ELIGIBLE FOR GENETIC TESTING* are healthy women as well as women suffering from BC, both with more than 10 % chance of being carriers of mutations in the genes BRCA1/2. Criteria may be different in different countries, but usually all broadly refer to those of the National Comprehensive Cancer Network Guidelines [8, 9] (Fig. 2.2).

*Healthy women* eligible for genetic testing are *unaffected individual* with a family history of one or more of the following:

- A known mutation in a BC susceptibility gene within the family
- ≥2 breast primaries in single individual
- ≥2 individuals with breast primaries on the same side of the family
- ≥1 ovarian cancer primary from the same side of the family
- First- or second-degree relative with BC ≤45 years
- ≥1 family member on the same side of family with a combination of BC and ≥1 of some cancer (especially if early onset) as pancreatic cancer, prostate cancer (Gleason score ≥7), sarcoma, adrenocortical carcinoma, brain tumours, endometrial cancer, leukaemia/lymphoma and thyroid cancer
- Male BC

*Women suffering from BC eligible for genetic testing are individual* with one or more of the following:

- A known mutation in a BC susceptibility gene within the family
- Early-age-onset BC
- Triple negative (ER, PR, HER2) BC
- Two BC primaries in a single individual
- BC at any age and:
  - ≥1 close blood relative with BC ≤50 years or
  - ≥1 close blood relative with epithelial ovarian cancer at any age or
  - ≥2 close blood relatives with BC and/or pancreatic cancer at any age
- ≥1 family member on the same side of the family with a combination of BC and ≥1 of some cancer (especially if early onset) as pancreatic cancer, prostate cancer (Gleason score ≥7), sarcoma, adrenocortical carcinoma, brain tumours, endometrial cancer, leukaemia/lymphoma and thyroid cancer
- Ovarian cancer
- Male BC

Other domestic criteria highlight the age of family members at diagnosis, so that an *average risk* is considered for women who have:

- Only 1 first-degree relative diagnosed after 40 years of age or
- Only 2 first-degree relatives diagnosed after 60 years of age without any other association (i.e. ovarian cancer, male BC, etc.)

In the same way, women likely to be at *moderate risk* are those who have:

- Two first-degree relatives diagnosed between 50 and 59 years of age
- Two second-degree maternal relatives diagnosed before 50 years of age
- One first- or second-degree relative diagnosed between 50 and 59 years of age + 1 familiar first/second-degree relative with ovarian cancer at any age without any other association (i.e. male BC, etc.)

*GENERAL GENETIC TESTING STRATEGIES*. Ideally, genetic testing should begin with a member of the family having the highest probability of having a hereditary condition, typically the member with an early-onset cancer. Doing so increases the likelihood of finding the disease-causing mutation if one can be detected in the family. If the highest risk relative has no detectable mutations, that suggests the disease causing mutation in the family cannot be detected, and therefore, testing other individuals in the family (particularly unaffected individuals) is unlikely to be helpful in the risk assessment. If a mutation has been identified in a blood relative, the consultant can undergo single site testing in order to save on cost.

Testing individuals of Ashkenazi Jewish descent should start with testing of the three common Ashkenazi Jewish founder mutations; reflexing to comprehensive testing can be considered depending on the strength of suspicion for HBOC and whether the individual has any non-Ashkenazi Jewish ancestry.

Testing unaffected patients younger than age 18 years for BRCA1/BRCA2 is not recommended.

### 2.3.2 Genetic Counselling

*Subjects of genetic testing are*:

- *Counsellor*, a specialist in genetic counselling
- *Consultant*, the person who needs the referral and who has never had cancer
- *Proband*, the consultant with BC who is the first subject in a study of a genetic character in a family germ line. The information for the compilation of the family tree is collected starting from the proband. If the consultant is healthy, the proband will be the closest case of tumour in the family tree.

*The Phases of Genetic Counselling*. Firstly a thorough reconstruction of the family history is done by verification of the available data and of the clinical documentation. Practice for collecting clinical data includes some important recommendations:

- Family history can be collected by the specialist in medical genetics.
- History should be accurate and must take into account the maternal line and paternal line; each report must record the age at diagnosis of cancer and age of death and must be verified by examination of the documentation or the type of intervention or therapy.
- In case of doubt (i.e. uncertainty between benign or malignant tumour in a relative) the subject should be considered negative.

If criteria for eligibility to genetic testing subsist, the next steps are a discussion of potential benefits and limitations of the test and then a complete assessment of the case. The patient is allowed a week to decide whether to consent to the test. After that, the test is performed and the patient is recalled for results delivery and, if the mutation is confirmed, details are discussed.

*Pros of genetic testing*. In summary, genetic testing can help to:

- Understand what is the real risk of developing BC or OC
- Implement adequate preventive *custom strategy*
- Participate in programs of intensive surveillance, more close screening than the existing one for the general population
- Provide important information to the consultants' families
- Frame with accuracy the risk of cancer, which may mean, taking, for instance, the case of a negative result of the test on a healthy family, that the consultant has the same risk of contracting BC or OC as the general population, etc.
- Contribute to research

*Cons of genetic testing*. Back to front, the disadvantages are:

- There is currently no preventive strategy of absolute efficacy to prevent the possibility of developing cancer.
- Difficulties may arise in coping with the news of genetic predisposition: anxiety and depression immediately following the notification of the outcome are quite common.
- It is a fact that cannot be changed in the course of life.
- A negative test result could cause a dangerous sense of security, since a negative result does not mean the consultant risk of contracting BC or OC is zero, but that they have the same risk as the general population.

*Reasons why some women wish to undergo the genetic testing* are (in brief):

- Desire to have an explanation why in their own families there have been several cases of cancer.
- Desire to put an end to the uncertainties that create anxiety and worries.
- Knowing the risk of developing cancer can help to better design their lives (marriage, pregnancy).
- Desire to do something useful for their families.
- Feeling of responsibility towards their children.

*Reasons why some women refuse the genetic testing* are:

- Fear of having to live with a risk of cancer, for which there is no decisive preventive intervention
- Embarrassment towards family members
- Sense of guilt towards their children

### 2.3.3 Risk Assessment Tools

Some individuals refuse to do the test for various reasons or because it is expensive. In this case BC risk assessment tools could be exploited to predict individual BC risk [10]. There are a number of models available (Gail, Claus, Tyrer-Cuzick, BRCAPRO and BOADICEA models) to assess both BC risk and the chances of identifying a *BRCA1/2* mutation. Some models perform both tasks, but none are yet totally discriminatory as to which family has a mutation and who will develop BC. Useful in most cases, they do not give a truthful estimate of risk in some women including those:

- With a personal history of invasive BC, ductal carcinoma in situ (DCIS) or lobular carcinoma in situ (LCIS)
- With a strong family history of BC, who may have an inherited gene mutation

The *Gail model* is an accessible interactive computer programme online (http://www.cancer.gov/bcrisktool) that incorporates a number of established risk factors and estimates a woman's risk of developing invasive BC during the next 5-year period and up to age 90 (lifetime risk). A 5-year risk of 1.67 % or higher is considered elevated. This model is not recommended for use with women having a strong family history since it excludes some well-established factors associated with hereditary BC.

The *Claus* model provides a more accurate estimate of risk for women with a family history of BC by taking into account both maternal and paternal histories, including second-degree relatives. The model can also incorporate a family history of ovarian cancer. However, unlike the Gail model, the Claus model does not include many of the other risk factors known to increase risk. It may therefore underestimate the risk in women with exposure to certain environmental, behavioural or reproductive factors.

The *BRCAPRO* is a statistical model, with associated software (http://bcb.dfci.harvard.edu/bayesmendel/software.php), used to estimate the probability of having a BRCA1 or BRCA2 mutation in women whose family histories are suggestive of inherited breast and/or ovarian cancer. It can also be used to estimate BC risk for each individual member of the family. BRCAPRO does not incorporate risk factors that are unrelated to family history.

The *Tyrer-Cuzick* (also called *IBIS*, see http://www.ems-trials.org/riskevaluator/) is a computer-based model that can be used to estimate the probability of carrying a BRCA1 or BRCA2 mutation as well as individual BC risk for the patient and for family members. In addition to factors related to family history, this model incorporates other well-established risk factors when calculating BC risk estimates.

The *BOADICEA* (Breast and Ovarian Analysis of Disease Incidence and Carrier Estimation Algorithm) model (http://www.srl.cam.ac.uk/genepi/boadicea/boadicea_home.html), like the Tyrer-Cuzick, computes the risks of breast and ovarian cancer in women based on their family history. It is also used to calculate the probability that they are carriers of cancer-associated mutations in the BRCA1 or BRCA2 gene. This programme is free and is an example of translational research, where scientific software has been developed into a tool for healthcare professionals. In the United Kingdom, it is recommended as a risk assessment tool in the NICE clinical guidelines and has been incorporated in the guidelines of several countries for the management of familial BC.

### 2.3.4 Pathological Characteristics of Hereditary BC

Eighty per cent of invasive BCs arising in BRCA1 and BRCA2 carriers are invasive ductal carcinomas. A higher frequency of BRCA1 tumours is medullary carcinomas (9 % versus 2 % of sporadic BC), usually poorly differentiated and high grade but with a remarkably favourable prognosis, probably because of low incidence of lymph node metastasis. Notably, 11 % of medullary carcinomas carry BRCA1 germ-line mutations. By contrast, excess of invasive lobular and tubular carcinomas has been reported for BRCA2 relative to BRCA1 tumours [8].

BRCA1 tumours are more frequently high grade compared to sporadic tumours. They have a higher number of mitosis and show a high frequency of necrotic areas, a higher proportion of continuous pushing margins and a considerable lymphocytic infiltration. All these features point towards a more aggressive tumour type. Most

BRCA2 tumours are grade 2/3 with high mitotic rates and have as a common feature continuous pushing margins.

Among sporadic tumours, 70 % are ER positive and 50 % are PR positive, and HER2 overexpression is observed in approximately 15 % of cases. In BRCA1 carriers expression of the hormone receptors is significantly lower from sporadic tumours, even when the ratio is adjusted for the younger age of the BRCA1 patients. A recent study examining pathology data from 4,325 BRCA1 and 2,568 BRCA2 mutation carriers reported that 78 % of tumours arising in BRCA1 carriers were ER negative, while only 23 % of tumours arising in BRCA2 mutation carriers were ER negative. Furthermore, HER2 overexpression was only observed in approximately 10 % of the tumours in mutation carriers. Consequently, 69 % of the BRCA1 tumours were triple negative (i.e. negative ER, PR and HER2; see 'Molecular subtypes', Sect. 13.2), which was true for only 16 % of the BRCA2 tumours. Their prognosis is very poor, not only because these tumours seem to be more aggressive than other BCs but also because endocrine and anti-HER2 therapies are ineffective, leaving chemotherapy as the only treatment option available.

These results suggest that tumours associated with BRCA1 mutations are distinct from those of BRCA2-associated and non-BRCA-associated BCs and that the tumours associated with BRCA2 mutations are similar to the non-BRCA-associated BCs.

On the other hand, as far as the familial non-BRCA1/2 BC is concerned, reports have been shown to comprise a very heterogeneous group of cancers with respect to histopathological characteristics. It has been established that these cancers are often of lower grade compared to sporadic cancers, but with IHC profiles similar to sporadic cancers.

Although only 1 % of all BC develop in men, having a BRCA mutation means an increased risk, particularly for men with BRCA2 (see 'Male breast cancer', Sect. 19.3). BRCA mutations also raise a man's chance of developing cancer of the pancreas and skin and a particularly aggressive form of prostate cancer that develops at an earlier age than men who do not carry a mutation.

### 2.3.5 Current Recommendations/Options

Patients with an established gene mutation, or however significant family history of BC, including patients who did not get tested (because they rejected the option) or with negative/non-diagnostic/uncertain test results should be offered a choice of the most suitable options for primary and secondary prevention. The decision about what to do is a complex process that requires time.

Particularly if the presence of a BRCA1/2 mutation is confirmed, primary or secondary preventive measures may help reduce cancer risk and may either delay the onset of cancer; detect cancer at an earlier, more treatable stage; or even prevent it. While genetic testing and medical society guidelines provide important and useful information, medical management decisions should be made based on consultation between each patient and his or her healthcare provider.

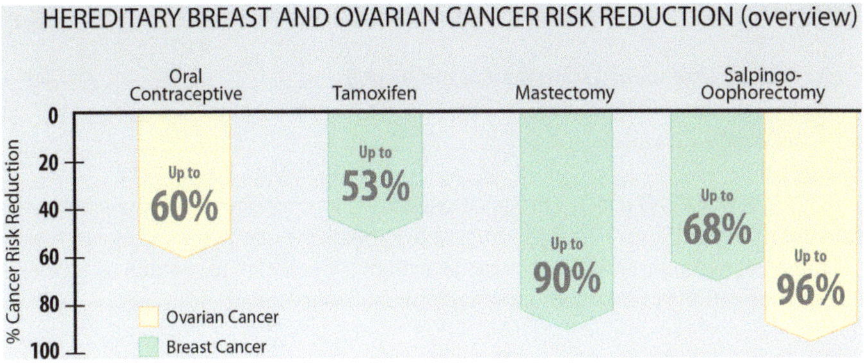


**Fig. 2.3** Overview of strategic measures and expected results in the hereditary breast and ovarian risk reduction [9 mod with permission]

Strategies to reduce the risk include close surveillance, chemoprevention and risk-reducing surgery (Fig. 2.3) [8].

*CLOSE SURVEILLANCE* uses tests to try to detect cancer in its early stages, when it is most treatable. Surveillance does not prevent cancer; however, early detection improves a person's chance of surviving their cancer. Whether close surveillance will lower the death rate from BC in high-risk women is not undisputable. Nevertheless, recommendations for BC screening in the high-risk population differ from recommendations for the general population.

*Close surveillance for breast cancer in mutation carriers*:

- Monthly breast self-exams starting at age 18.
- Annual or semi-annual clinical breast exams starting at age 25.
- Yearly mammography starting at age 25 (ultrasound in case the radiologist recommends it).
- Yearly magnetic resonance imaging (MRI) starting at age 25 or individualised based (usually 10 years before) on earliest case in the family.
- Annual magnetic resonance imaging (MRI) (contrast-enhanced) is the most sensitive exam for women at high risk. MRI lacks ionising radiation and picks up cancers at an earlier stage, but gives more questionable results, and impact on survival is still unknown. Mammography is much less expensive but misses 50 % of cancers in high-risk women in case of dense breast tissue.

MRI is preferable in young women, while mammography may be enough over 50 years of age. Lifetime risk thresholds for including women in surveillance programmes with annual MRI may be determined on the basis of regional or national considerations reflecting an area-specific cumulative risk in the general population, resource availability and practical feasibility.

Further preventive but controversial measures in selected cases are cytology from ductal lavage (DL), or nipple aspirate (NAF), or ductal endoscopy (DE) (see 'Cytological samples', Sect. 6.2).

*Close Surveillance for Ovarian Cancer in Mutation Carriers:*

- Annual or semi-annual transvaginal ultrasound
- Annual or semi-annual blood test for CA125 beginning at age 25
- Annual pelvic exams

*CHEMOPREVENTION* is the use of medication to lower the risk or prevent cancer in healthy people. It uses hormonal drugs able to block the effects of oestrogens, which are responsible for the development and growth of a significant proportion of tumours. Chemoprevention is based on following clinical observations:

- Tamoxifen use has been associated with a reduction of approximately 50% in the risk of a second primary BC in contralateral cancers.
- In previous osteoporosis trials of older postmenopausal women, raloxifene decreased the risk of ER-positive BC by more than 50%. These data have been confirmed by the Study of Tamoxifen and Raloxifene (STAR) trial [11].
- Oral contraceptives, when taken for 6 or more years, have been associated with a reduction of up to 60 % in the risk of ovarian cancer.

Actually, medications should be considered also in women with a strong history of BC and in women who had a breast biopsy that found atypical ductal or lobular hyperplasia or a preinvasive condition such as lobular or ductal carcinoma in situ. The randomised, placebo-controlled BC Prevention Trial demonstrated a 50 % reduction of invasive BC incidence among high-risk healthy women who took tamoxifen. In women with lobular carcinoma in situ (LCIS), the incidence of invasive BC decreased by 56 %, and in cases with atypical hyperplasia, the decrease was 86 % [11]. There were no proven effects in terms of mortality, but an increased risk of developing an endometrial stage I carcinoma has been recognised.

Many past studies of these medications focused on women in the general population or women whose risk for BC was based on risk assessment tools; therefore, the research may not apply to everyone with hereditary cancer risk. Medications for BC chemoprevention are the subject of much ongoing research.

Before choosing the best risk management option, a clear sense of the risk is needed. A healthcare team with expertise in managing high-risk patients should identify the best medication with a clear understanding of the potential benefits and side effects. Drugs known as selective oestrogen receptor modulators (SERMs) act like oestrogen in some tissues, but behave like oestrogen blockers (anti-oestrogens) in others. Two SERMs—tamoxifen, and raloxifene—are approved for BC prevention for high-risk women and, in general, are not recommended as prevention for women at low risk for BC.

*Tamoxifen* acts as an anti-oestrogen in most areas of the body, including the breast. In the uterus, tamoxifen acts like an oestrogen and encourages the growth of the lining of the uterus. For BC risk reduction, tamoxifen is typically taken 5 mg a day (or 10 mg every 2 days) for a total of 5 years. The risk reduction benefit continues for 10 years after the woman stops taking tamoxifen.

Tamoxifen is used to reduce the risk of invasive BC in high-risk women age 35 and older, whether or not they have gone through menopause. Common side effects of tamoxifen include hot flashes, night sweats, vaginal discharge or also dryness. Rarely, taking tamoxifen may cause blood clots, endometrial or uterine cancer, cataracts and stroke. The risk of uterine cancer for premenopausal women taking tamoxifen is very low, compared with those who have undergone menopause.

*Raloxifene* is usually used for prevention and treatment of osteoporosis in postmenopausal women. Like tamoxifen, raloxifene works by blocking oestrogen's effects in the breast and other tissues, but unlike tamoxifen, it does not exert oestrogen-like effects on the uterus.

Common side effects of raloxifene include hot flashes, vaginal dryness or irritation, joint and muscle pain and weight gain. Health risks associated with raloxifene are similar to those associated with tamoxifen.

Both drugs carry an increased risk of blood clots, though the risk may be lower with raloxifene, and raloxifene may be associated with fewer cases of endometrial and uterine cancers than is tamoxifen.

Raloxifene may also be linked to fewer strokes than tamoxifen in women at average risk of heart disease. Although studies indicate raloxifene does not increase the risk of stroke, it can increase the risk of dying from a stroke. Women with a history of current risk factors for stroke or heart disease should discuss with doctors whether raloxifene is an appropriate choice. Raloxifene can cause birth defects and is approved only for postmenopausal women. It should not be taken with the cholesterol-lowering drug cholestyramine (Questran) or with oestrogens.

Tamoxifen reduces BC incidence by 40–50 % and this is maintained in long-term follow-up after cessation of treatment. However, this reduction is almost exclusively a reduction in oestrogen receptor-positive disease and whether this translates into a reduction in cancers related to BRCA1 mutations remains unclear [12]. Trial has shown that raloxifene is nearly as effective as tamoxifen in reducing invasive BC risk and has fewer adverse side effects. However, there are no data available on the efficacy of raloxifene for BC risk reduction among BRCA gene mutation carriers [13].

In conclusion, although tamoxifen may be slightly better than raloxifene at reducing the risk of BC, the risk of blood clots and uterine cancer is higher than with raloxifene, so that it is the medication of choice in patients who have undergone a hysterectomy. Raloxifene may be a preferred option for postmenopausal women who have not undergone a hysterectomy or who have osteoporosis.

*Aromatase inhibitors* (*AIs*) stop the production of oestrogen in postmenopausal women by blocking the enzyme aromatase which turns androgen hormones into small amounts of oestrogens. AIs have been studied and shown to be effective only in postmenopausal women to treat BC and to prevent BC recurrence. Some (few) studies have shown favourable effects in high-risk women, but additional studies are underway to determine whether AIs may reduce the risk of BC in women with genetic mutations.

AIs are not associated with an increased risk of blood clots or uterine cancer, as tamoxifen and raloxifene are, but common side effects of aromatase inhibitors include hot flashes, vaginal dryness, joint and muscle pain, headache and fatigue. Moreover, AIs raise the risk of osteoporosis and so of fractures.

*Retinoids*. In addition to tamoxifen, raloxifene and other selective oestrogen receptor modulators, retinoids are among the most promising agents, given their ability to inhibit mammary carcinogenesis in preclinical models. *Fenretinide*, the synthetic amide of retinoic acid, inhibits cell growth mostly through the induction of apoptosis with mechanisms which may partly involve the retinoid receptors. Because it has a favourable toxicological profile, fenretinide has been extensively investigated in clinical trials.

Results showed a reduction of second breast malignancies in premenopausal women previously treated for BC. In addition, a significant decrease of circulating insulin-like growth factor (IGF-1), a known risk factor for premenopausal BC, was observed after 1 year of fenretinide administration in premenopausal women with BC. Ongoing studies on the validation of the circulating IGF-1 as a surrogate endpoint biomarker of fenretinide activity and on the effectiveness of the combination with low-dose tamoxifen may provide further insight into the future clinical application of fenretinide.

Some studies have evaluated or are evaluating the protective role of the administration of other medications as nonsteroid anti-inflammatory drugs and statins without definitive and unequivocal results.

*RISK-REDUCING MASTECTOMY* (*RRM*). The first study to demonstrate that women with a high risk of BC can significantly reduce their subsequent incidence of the disease with RRM was published in 1999 [14]. This was followed by a Dutch study that confirmed risk reduction in those at highest risk (BRCA1 and BRCA2 carriers). Current evidence would suggest that RRM is associated with an approximately 90–95 % reduction in risk [15].

RRM can be considered in some cases, but only after proper assessment of the case, discussion with the patient about the pros and cons and adequate time to decide without haste and superficiality. The ideal time to propose RRM is between 30 and 50 years. The mean expected rate of BC for cohort of high-risk women is 1 % annually, reflecting a lifetime risk that ranges from 25 to 80 %. To date, although RRM can reduce the risk of BC, it has not been proven to have a survival benefit. It is unlikely there will be randomised trials and hence more cohort studies will be necessary to provide more data to support its use [15].

The decision must be balanced and absorbed after the details related to the reduction of risk and the type of reconstruction have been clarified. The patient must be clearly informed that the risk reduction does not coincide with its own reset. Considering that prophylactic mastectomy reduces the risk of BC by 90–95 % in high-risk patients, for every 100 patients who undergo it—according to data of the literature—5–10 develop the disease anyway. In fact, the whole breast tissue is not always surgically removed: islands of glandular tissue may remain in the flap of skin and subcutaneous tissue, in the retroareolar tissue, in the axillary extension, in the axilla and also (very rarely) in the supraclavicular region or the very cranial portion of the abdominal wall.

RRM is a major surgery with its related risks, generally (bleeding, infections in 10–20 % of cases, seroma, retracting scars or keloids or any form of delayed healing) as well specifically related to mastectomy and to reconstruction (tissue ischaemia/necrosis in case of autologous flap, or of the nipple areola complex if spared). The capsular contracture occurs in 15–20 % of the reconstructions in the absence of radiotherapy and appears even years after and more frequently when the prosthesis is not completely covered by the muscle. A variable degree of durable pain is variously described in one-third of cases.

Any kind of surgery, even if performed with the greatest skill, is unable to return to the same overall situation, in terms of sensitivity and subjective response about body projection. No reconstructive result is guaranteed forever, and the result may change over time, in a totally unpredictable way, often necessitating further operations with a rate of re-interventions reported up to 50 % of cases.

According to EUSOMA [16], RRM gets excellent results in 60 % of cases, with 5 % of the patients not being satisfied with the choice. EUSOMA best practice indicators have excellent results in at least 75 % of cases, minor complications (infection, small area of necrosis) in less than 10 %, asymmetry in less than 20 % and contracture in less than 10 % of cases.

Potential candidates for prophylactic breast surgery are not only women with known BRCA1/2 gene mutation or a significant family history of BC but also patients with BC. The latter should be distinguished in two groups: patients with unilateral BC that is still present subsequently to a recent diagnosis and patients with a previous BC history (and eventual adjuvant treatments) that months/years later decide for a contralateral RRM or for a bilateral one in case of previous breast-conserving surgery.

There are different technical approaches of RRM. The main techniques belong to the so-called conservative mastectomies (subcutaneous, skin-sparing, nipple-sparing, skin-reducing). A sentinel lymph node procedure is recommended.

Having to avoid significant changes in the body projection, RRM is always accompanied by breast reconstruction with expander or sometimes with implants directly, while it is rare to use autologous flaps. In the case where the patient refuses the reconstructive option, this choice must be discouraged and observed only after a multistep decision-making process, accompanied by psychological evaluation and documented in the written informed consent.

Risk-reducing surgery of the breast has some absolute and relative contraindications whether:

- Risk of BC is not high or confirmed.
- Genetic test is unavailable.
- Family history is unreliable.
- Munchausen syndrome (factitious history).
- Risks of surgery outweighing its benefits.

Some contraindications are psychosocial and are related to:

- The choice not being personal, but dictated by family members and/or partner
- Unrealistic expectations of aesthetic results
- Psychiatric disorders

The team should also consider the ability of the patient to understand the procedure and whether she has realistic expectations regarding the possible amount of risk reduction. Finally, they should consider if her choice is motivated by cosmetic rather than oncological reasons. A specialised multidisciplinary team is needed in order to have a complete, detailed, balanced and nonpartisan assessment concerning what to do and how technically to achieve it. The team must include a geneticist, a psychologist and a clinical doctor or, if risk-reducing surgery is considered, a breast surgeon and a reconstructive plastic surgeon for discussion of technical options.

The majority of studies exploring the psychological impact of RRM have found that surgery is associated overall with fairly high levels of satisfaction and reduced anxiety and psychological morbidity among women who undergo this procedure. This is particularly so when there is support from family and friends. A number of studies suggest that provision of presurgical multidisciplinary support appears to have a bearing on outcome, particularly in those who have initial anxiety and negative psychological reactions. These negative effects are usually related to surgical complications and reduce with longer follow-up. A minority of women do express regrets and experience adverse psychosocial events following surgery, including adverse emotional stability, problems in self-esteem, and difficulties in sexual relationships [17].

*Informed consent.* In summary, a patient who wants to start a project of prophylactic surgery, especially if she is not at high genetic risk and has not a positive test for BRCA mutation, should be warned about the possible results. A written informed consent should be comprehensive of all worries such as:

- RRM is a permanent and irreversible act.
- The risk of developing BC is significantly reduced but not reset.
- It is predictable that a psychological benefit linked to the achievement of the risk reduction could be obtained.
- Conversely, a negative impact on the quality of life may be consequent, related to the partial or full loss of sensibility.
- Unsatisfactory effects on the body projection and on the sexual life can happen in some subjects.
- The breast operated can no longer breastfeed.

Women should be given oral and written information regarding their risk and the risks and benefits of mammography and MRI screening or alternative risk-reducing interventions; if these women accept to be screened by MRI, they should be informed about screening intervals and logistics.

*RISK-REDUCING BILATERAL SALPINGO-OOPHORECTOMY (RRSO).* Given that in mutation carriers OC occurs more frequently between 45 and 50 years old, performing the intervention after 35 years to allow a possible pregnancy is recommended [18]. Short-term HRT before age 50 can be considered. For women who have not undergone salpingo-oophorectomy, semi-annual CA-125 and TVUS are recommended, beginning at age 35 or 5 years younger than the earliest age of onset of ovarian cancer in the family. However, no data currently exist to support a benefit of screening for ovarian cancer.

As RRM, BRSO minimises but does not completely eliminate the risk of developing an ovarian cancer, because this may arise from the peritoneum. Moreover, at the time of prophylactic oophorectomy, some occult ovarian neoplasms are incidentally found. In addition to reducing the risk of ovarian cancer, prophylactic salpingo-oophorectomy has also been shown to decrease the risk of BC in women with a BRCA1/2 mutation by 46–56 % [18].

RRSO could be performed between 35 and 40 years, and it results in a 98 % reduction in the risk of ovarian cancer (OC) and 50–70 % of BC. This can be seen from the risk of BC in unaffected women and in the contralateral breast for those with BC. Moreover, a recent study has shown that prophylactic salpingo-oophorectomy not only reduced the risk of breast and ovarian cancer but also lowered all-cause mortality, as well as BC and ovarian cancer-specific mortality.

The RRSO is a risk-reducing procedure that is strongly recommended, much more than the mastectomy, because difficulties in diagnosis of OC, the absence of effective screening measures and poor prognosis. However, there are also some adverse effects among which are decreased libido, early onset of osteoporosis and cardiac problems, all typical of postmenopausal women.

*REPORT OF LEVEL OF EVIDENCE IN HIGH-RISK WOMEN* – According to the recommendation of EUSOMA [2], genetic counselling should be widely available, even if non-mandatory. The proportion of cancer cases referred for genetic counselling should be 5 %, suggested as the minimum standard. Target is not yet applicable.

Annual mammography may be considered for high- risk women starting at age 35 years (LoE III).

Screening mammography should not be performed in high-risk women below 35 years as there is no evidence that the benefits outweigh the risks in this young age group (EPO).

Annual MRI screening should be available starting at age 30. Starting annual screening before age 30 may be discussed, such as in BRCA1 or BRCA2 mutation carriers (starting between age 25 and 29 years) and TP53 mutation carriers (starting at age 20) (LoE IIb).

High-risk breast screening utilising MRI should be conducted only by a nationally/regionally approved and audited service or as part of an ethically approved research study. Periodical audits should be undertaken to ensure that high sensitivity is achieved and that the early recall rate (MR imaging more frequent than annually) is less than 10 % and to monitor detection rate, needle biopsy rate and interval cancers (EPO).

Annual MRI screening should be offered to:

- BRCA1, BRCA2 and TP53 mutation carriers.
- Women at 50 % risk to be carriers of BRCA1, BRCA2 or TP53 mutation (first-degree relatives of mutation carriers) (LoE Ib).
- Women from families not tested or inconclusively tested for BRCA mutation with a 20–30 % lifetime risk or greater (LoE II).
- Women with prior mantle radiotherapy before age 30 (e.g. for Hodgkin's disease), starting 8 years after their treatment (LoE III).

- Women at high risk and who were already diagnosed and treated for BC should be included in screening programmes including MRI (LoE IIb).

If annual MRI is performed, additional screening with breast ultrasound (US) and clinical breast examination (CBE) is not necessary as there is no evidence of any benefit added to MRI (LoE II). They are however recommended in women under 35 years who do not tolerate or have contraindications to MRI or gadolinium-based contrast administration (EPO).

Cases requiring workup after MRI should be initially assessed with conventional imaging, re-evaluation of mammography and targeted US (LoE II). In cases of suspicious findings solely detected by MRI, MRI-guided biopsy localisation should be performed (LoE II).

Risk factors such as prior diagnosis of invasive BC or ductal carcinoma in situ (DCIS), atypical ductal hyperplasia, lobular intraepithelial neoplasia, heterogeneous or dense breasts on mammography, if not associated with other risk factors, do not confer an increased risk justifying the use of screening MRI (LoE III).

## References

1. Baum M, Schipper H. Perception of the risk. In: Baum M, Schipper H, editors. Breast cancer. 3rd ed. Oxford: Health Press; 2005.
2. Cardoso F, Loibl S, Pagani O, et al. The European Society of Breast Cancer Specialists recommendations for the management of young women with breast cancer. Euro J Cancer. 2012;48:3355–77.
3. Cancer Research UK. Breast cancer risk factors. http://www.cancerresearchuk.org/cancer-info/cancerstats/types/breast/riskfactors/breast-cancer-risk-factors.
4. National Cancer Institute. Breast cancer screening. http://www.cancer.gov/cancertopics/pdq/screening/breast/healthprofessional/page4.
5. Radiopaedia. Interval breast cancer. http://radiopaedia.org/articles/interval-breast-cancer.
6. Evans AJ, Pinder SE, Ellis IO, et al. Screen detected ductal carcinoma in situ (DCIS): overdiagnosis or an obligate precursor of invasive disease? J Med Screen. 2001;8:149–51.
7. Foucar E. Addressing overdiagnosis and overtreatment in cancer. Lancet Oncol. 2014;15:306–7.
8. Larsen MJ, Thomassen M, Gerdes AM, Kruse TA. Hereditary breast cancer: clinical, pathological and molecular characteristics. Breast Cancer. 2014;15(8):145–55.
9. BRACAnalisis. http://www.myriad.com/products-services/hereditary-cancers/bracanalysis/. National Comprehensive Cancer Network (MCCN) Guidelines. NCCN Guidelines for Detection, Prevention & Risk Reduction (revised 2011). In: http://www.nccn.org/professionals/physician_gls/f_guidelines.asp.
10. Gareth D, Evans R, Hoell A. Breast cancer risk-assessment models. In: http://breast-cancer-research.com/content/9/5/213.
11. Vogel VG, Costantino JP, Wickerham DL, et al. Update of the National Surgical Adjuvant Breast and Bowel Project Study of Tamoxifen and Raloxifene (STAR) P–2 Trial: preventing breast cancer. Cancer Prevent Res. 2010;3(6):696–706.
12. Cuzick J, Forbes J, Edwards R, et al. First results from the International Breast Cancer Intervention Study (IBIS-I): a randomised prevention trial. Lancet. 2002;360:817–24.
13. Vogel VG. The NSABP Study of Tamoxifen and Raloxifene (STAR) trial. Expert Rev Anticancer Ther. 2009;9:51–60.

14. Hartmann LC, Schaid DJ, Woods JE, et al. Efficacy of bilateral prophylactic mastectomy in women with a family history of breast cancer. N Engl J Med. 1999;340:77–84.
15. Evans DGR, Baildam AD. The genetics of breast cancer, risk-reducing surgery and prevention. In: Dixon JM, editor. Breast surgery. London: Elsevier; 2014.
16. Petit JY, Greco M. Quality control in prophylactic mastectomy for women at high risk of breast cancer. Eur J Cancer. 2002;38:22–6.
17. Frost MH, Schaid DJ, Sellers TA, et al. Long-term satisfaction and psychological and social function following bilateral prophylactic mastectomy. JAMA. 2000;284(3):19–24.
18. Rebbeck TR, Lynch HT, Neuhausen SL, et al. Prophylactic oophorectomy in carriers of BRCA 1 or BRCA2 mutations. N Engl J Med. 2002;346:1616–22.

## Further Reading

American College of Radiology. ACR practice parameter for the performance of screening and diagnostic mammography (Amended 2014). www.acr.org/~/media/ACR/Documents/PGTS/guidelines/Screening_Mammography.pdf.

Balmaña J, Díez O, Rubio IT, Cardoso F On behalf of the ESMO Guidelines Working Group. BRCA in breast cancer: ESMO clinical practice guidelines. Ann Oncol. 2011;22 (Suppl. 6): vi31–4.

Beitsch PD, Whithworth PW. Can breast surgeons provide breast cancer genetic testing? An American Society of Breast Surgeons survey. Ann Surg Oncol. 2014;21:4104–8.

Cuzick J, Sestak I, Bonanni B, et al. Selective oestrogen receptor modulators in prevention of breast cancer: an updated meta-analysis of individual participant data. Lancet. 2013;381:1827–34.

Cuzick J, Sestak I, Forbes JF, et al. Anastrozole for prevention of breast cancer in high-risk post-menopausal women (IBIS-II): an international, double-blind, randomized placebo-controlled trial. Lancet. 2014;383:1041–8.

Domchek SM. Evolution of genetic testing for inherited susceptibility to breast cancer. J Clin Oncol. 2015;33(4):295–6.

Euhus DM, Diaz J. Breast cancer prevention. Breast J. 2015;21:76–81.

Independent UK Panel on Breast Cancer Screening. The benefits and harms of breast cancer screening: an independent review. Lancet. 2012;380:1778–86.

Melchor L, Benitez J. The complex genetic landscape of familial breast cancer. Hum Genet. 2013;132:845–63.

Metcalfe K, Gershman S, Ghadirian P. Contralateral mastectomy and survival after breast cancer in carriers of BRCA1 and BRCA2 mutations: retrospective analysis. BMJ. 2014;348:g226.

Moyer VA on behalf of the U.S. Preventive Services Task Force. Risk assessment, genetic counseling, and genetic testing for BRCA-related cancer in women: U.S. preventive services task force recommendation statement. Ann Intern Med. 2014;160:271–81.

Rich TA, Woodson AH, Litton J, Atun B. Hereditary breast cancer syndromes and genetic testing. J Surg Oncol. 2015;111:66–80.

Visvanathan K, Hurley P, Bantug E, et al. Use of pharmacologic interventions for breast cancer risk reduction: American Society of Clinical Oncology clinical practice guideline. J Clin Oncol. 2013;31:2942–62. Erratum in: J Clin Oncol. 2013;31:4383.

**Websites in Appendix**: *Screening*, A-4.11; *Risk Factors/Genetics*, A-4.19.

# Anatomy, Congenital Aberrations and Physiological Changes

# 3

Alfonso M. Pluchinotta

## Contents



**Abstract**

• The mammary glands have evolved as milk-producing organs to provide appropriate nourishment to the progenies. Breastfeeding provides nourishment and passive immunity to the newborn, promotes postpartum uterine involution, and establishes an important bond between mother and infant. • The breasts are also a distinguishing symbol of femininity in our culture, so that their intrinsic aesthetic value should be always properly considered although not overemphasized. • The mammary gland begins its development early in embryologic life and only culminates in the first postpartum lactation of the adult female. • Some abnormalities of the breast hamper its optimal functioning (e.g. inverted nipple),

A.M. Pluchinotta
Breast Surgery, Policlinic of Abano Terme, Padova, Italy
e-mail: pluchinotta.alfonso@gmail.com





A.M. Pluchinotta (ed.), *The Outpatient Breast Clinic: Aiming at Best Practice*,
DOI 10.1007/978-3-319-15907-2_3

whereas some merely pose a cosmetic problem (e.g. polythelia and congenital asymmetry). Other abnormalities, without any functional deficit, should be considered as deformities (e.g. tuberous breast).

*Future directions.* Congenital breast developmental abnormalities, as well deformities, even though they don't have clinical significance can be extremely psychologically debilitating to the individual. Therefore, it is required to overcome the fatalistic attitude of the past and propose realistic surgical remedies.

## 3.1 Anatomy and Constitutional Patterns of the Breast

**Clinical Practice Points**

- The functional macroscopic structures of the breast are the ductal-lobular segmental units based on the excretory ducts at the nipple. They vary greatly in extent, shape, and functional capability and do not conform (as usually represented) to a regular pyramidal shape radiating from the nipple.
- The functional microscopic structures are the terminal ductal-lobular unit (TDLU) that are the site of origin of milk but also of the most common diseases. The epithelium here consistently shows the highest mitotic rate of any breast epithelium.
- Breast glandular tissue may extend into peripheral or deep structures with substantial clinical implications, so that most mastectomies are successful in removing no more than 90–95 % of breast glandular tissue.
- Ectopic breast tissue, from embryonic inclusion, can be found also in the axillary lymph nodes, even in the sentinel node. Conversely, intramammary lymph nodes can be found, usually in the upper outer quadrant.

### 3.1.1 Anatomy of the Adult Breast

*Location and boundaries.* The adult breast overlies the pectoralis major muscle from the second to the sixth rib in the vertical axis and from the sternal edge to the midaxilla in the horizontal axis. These are the classic descriptions of the boundaries of the breast, but breast tissue can extend beyond these arbitrary boundaries. Ductal tissue can extend as high as the clavicle, beyond the inframammary fold, into the axilla, or beyond the border of the *latissimus dorsi*. Moreover, the fascia overlying the chest wall sometimes harbours breast glandular units. The glands rarely extend beyond this fascia into bands of underlying skeletal muscle. Such extension of breast glandular tissue into these peripheral or deep structures has clinical implications, so that most mastectomies are successful in removing no more than 90 % of breast glandular tissue [1].

The extension of breast tissue from the upper outer quadrant into the axilla is eponymously referred to as the *tail of Spence*. The two breasts may be widely separated on the chest, or partially synthesized at the midline, although ducts do not communicate across the midline of the chest.

*Shape and size* of the breast depend not only upon genetic and racial factors but also upon age, diet, parity and menopausal status of the individual. The breast can appear hemispherical, conical, pendulous, piriform or thinned and flattened; however, typically, the shape of the breast is not spherical, but rather that of a teardrop, more conical in the nulliparous woman and more pendulous in women who have had children. There is a distinct flattening of the superficial contour of the breast superior to the nipple.

The normal mature non-lactating female breast weighs approximately 200 g (±100 g) and fluctuates with the menstrual cycle. The typical lactating breast may weigh more than 500 g. The average adult breast measures 10–12 cm in diameter and 5–7 cm in thickness. The volume of the breast varies greatly among individuals and may vary from left to right. Usually, the right breast is less voluminous and this discrepancy has been correlated to handedness. More than half of women have volume differences greater than 10 % and more than one fourth of women have volume differences greater than 20 %. There is no correlation between breast mass and BC risk because large breasts do not necessarily contain more glandular parenchyma. However, women do not usually tolerate these differences.

*Skin*. The skin of the breast is thin and contains hair follicles, sebaceous glands and eccrine sweat glands. The nipple-areolar complex, centrally located and typically elevated from the surrounding areola, is the focal point of the skin of the breast. It can range from 15 to 60 mm in diameter, and its level in the thorax varies widely but, typically, overlies the fourth intercostal space in younger women and in a non-pendulous breast. Both nipple and areola consist of a keratinizing stratified squamous epithelium with a dense basal melanin deposition and are pink, light brown or darker, depending also upon the general pigmentation of the body. These two structures are somewhat less pigmented in the nulliparous and become increasingly pigmented starting in the second month of pregnancy. The tinctorial change after pregnancy is irreversible.

Within the nipple are multiple sensory nerve endings. Within the dermis are radially arranged smooth muscle fibres that contract with stimulation, hardening and ejecting the nipple. The areola has hair follicles, sebaceous glands and sweat glands. On the areola are the *Montgomery tubercles*, skin elevations formed by openings of the ducts of the *Montgomery glands*, sebaceous gland units usually associated with a lactiferous duct, which are present on the surface of the areola (see Sect. 11.1.3). These 12–20 rounded protuberances become prominent during pregnancy and lactation, reflecting the need for keeping the areola moist during feeding, and regress after menopause. Apocrine and sweat glands are also present in this area. Hair follicles are present at the edge of the areola.

*Fascial layers*. Underneath the skin is the subcutaneous fat, which contributes to the size of the breast and which fluctuates with the amount of total body fat. Fascial tissues, anteriorly the superficial pectoral fascia and posteriorly the deep pectoral fascia, envelop the mammary gland. These two layers of fascia blend with the

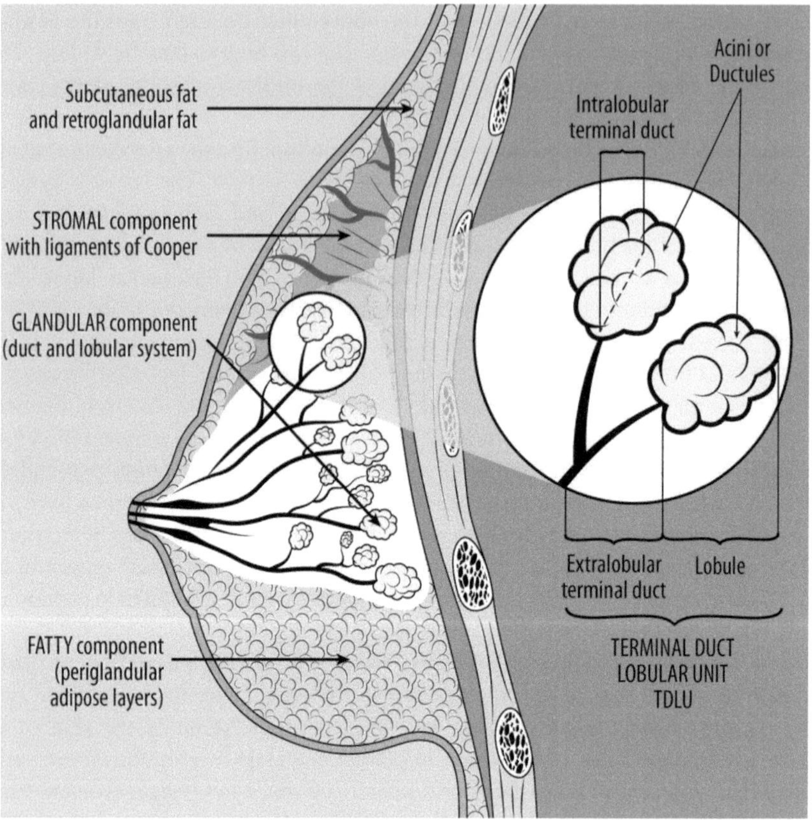


**Fig. 3.1** *On the left*. Basic elements of the breast: (1) glandular component including segmental ducts (and then collecting major ducts) with terminal ductal-lobular units (TDLU); (2) stromal component with Cooper's ligaments of the breast which form fibrosepta in the stroma and provide support for the breast parenchyma; (3) adipose component with subcutaneous fat and adipose tissue distributed around the lobules of the gland which gives its smooth contour and accounts for most of its mass. On average, in premenopausal women, the glandular component varies from 15 to 20 %, while in menopausal woman, it decreases to 2–5 %. *On the right*. Anatomy of terminal ductal-lobular units (TDLUs), a combination of extralobular terminal ducts and lobules. Lobules are composed by intralobular terminal ducts and acini or ductules (for a detail, see Fig. 9.8).

cervical fascia superiorly and with that overlying the abdomen inferiorly. Fibrous bands (*Cooper's ligaments*) connect these two fascial layers and are more numerous in the superior half of the breast and at the lower periphery of the breast, where they maintain the inframammary fold. They are particularly dense, help give the breast its shape, and anchor the gland to the skin. As the breast tissue develops through the layers of the superficial fascia, they remain relatively close to the skin. A retromammary space (or retromammary bursa) filled with loose connective tissue lies between the deep boundary of the breast and the fascia of underlying skeletal muscle and allows the breast some degree of movement over the underlying pectoral fascia (Fig. 3.1).

*Macroscopic functional unit (segment, lobe and lobules).* The fibroglandular tissue of the breast is divided into 12–20 *segments* that converge at the nipple in an unevenly radial arrangement. These segments are not always uniformly distributed around the breast. The upper half of the breast, particularly the upper outer quadrant, tends to contain more glandular tissue than does the remainder of the breast. Each segment contains a *lobe* made of 20–40 lobules, each consisting of more or less 100 alveoli. A 2-mm duct drains each segment into subareolar *lactiferous sinus* (or *ampulla lactifera*) of 5–8 mm in diameter. About 10 major collecting ducts then open at the nipple.

*Microscopic functional unit (TDLU).* The fundamental glandular unit of the breast, and biologically its most actively proliferating part, is the *terminal ductal-lobular unit (TDLU)*. Each of the lobes in the breast contains thousands of TDLUs, which form the functional secretory unit. During pregnancy and lactation, the epithelial cells of the terminal ducts and lobules undergo secretory changes, and the units produce milk, which drains via the branching segmental ducts to their *ampullae* at the surface of the nipple. Hence, the lobules are referred to as acini during pregnancy and lactation.

The TDLU is complex and consists of the extralobular and intralobular terminal ducts and the blindly ending lobules. The epithelial lining of the lobule consists of superficial cells (luminal A) that are involved in milk synthesis. The B cells (basal) have stem cell activity. Except for the terminal portion of the collecting ducts, low-columnar to cuboidal epithelium lines almost the entire duct system of the breast, including the segmental ducts, subsegmental ducts, terminal ducts and acini.

An outer layer of *myoepithelial cells*, which contains contractile fibres, facilitates milk secretion via their contractile property, which is largely under the influence of oxytocin, primarily responsible for the release of milk, a phenomenon called *milk letdown.* The myoepithelial cell layer is generally regarded as being spindle-shaped (see also Fig. 9.5), and it extends from collecting ducts to the tip of the acini.

The *basement membrane*, composed of a relatively attenuated basal lamina, lies immediately outside of the myoepithelial cell layer and divides the glands from the stroma that lies beyond the basement membrane.

The mammary ducts and lobules are embedded within a variable *fibrous and fatty stroma*. The relative portions of glands and fibrous and adipose tissue vary with age and body habitus; however, stromal tissues make up the bulk of the breast in adult non-lactating and non-pregnant women. Adipose tissue is typically present in the *extralobular stroma* and not in the *intralobular stroma* among lobules (at least not until atrophy ensues). The fibrous tissue assists in the mechanical coherence of the gland.

Most disease of the breast arises from the TDLUs, including cysts, which may be the consequence of the unfolding of the terminal ducts and lobular units. Indeed, the only common lesion believed to be strictly of ductal origin may be the larger solitary intraductal papilloma. The sites of origin of common diseases of the breast are represented on Fig. 8.1.

*Superficial lymphatic drainage.* The superficial plexus of lymphatic vessels exists throughout the entire body surface. These vessels are valveless, allowing lymph to flow in any direction, although it does so sluggishly. The subepithelial plexus connects to subdermal lymphatic vessels by vertical lymphatics. The subdermal vessels do have valves. Thus, lymph flows unidirectionally from the superficial to the deep plexus. In the breast, the subepithelial and subdermal plexuses are confluent with the subareolar plexus. Also draining into the subareolar plexus are the fine lymphatics of the lactiferous ducts and the lymphatics of the areola and nipple.

*Deep lymphatic drainage.* From the deep lymphatics, the lymph flow moves centrifugally towards the axillary and internal mammary lymph nodes. About 10 % of the lymph from the breast goes to the intramammary chain, which can come from all quadrants of the breast, not just the inner quadrants. The other 70–90 % of lymph flows to the axillary lymph nodes.

*Boundaries of the axilla.* The axilla is typically thought of as a four-walled pyramid that sits between the upper arm and the chest. The dome-shaped base of the pyramid is the armpit, made of the axillary fascia and the skin. The anterior wall is the pectoralis major and minor muscles. The posterior wall is the subscapularis muscle (and to a lesser extent the teres major and latissimus dorsi muscles and tendons). The medial wall is the serratus anterior muscle. The lateral wall is a thin band of humerus between the insertions of the muscles of the anterior and posterior walls.

*Structures of the axilla.* Coming through the apex of the pyramid are the great vessels and nerves of the upper extremity, enclosed within a layer of fascia, the *axillary sheath*, a dense connective tissue that gradually disappears as the nerves and vessels begin to branch. The axilla is enveloped in fascia. The most significant fascia is the *clavipectoral fascia* that extends from the clavicle towards the floor of the axilla (the *axillary fascia*). The lower portion of the clavipectoral fascia is sometimes called the *suspensory ligament of the axilla* or the *coracoaxillary fascia*.

*Axillary lymph nodes.* The lymph nodes of the axilla are anatomically categorized by several groups (Fig. 3.2): *posterior* or subscapular; *anterior*, laterally to pectoralis; *lateral*, facing the humeral head; *central*; *subclavicular*, posterior to pectoralis minor; *apical*; and *interpectoral* (or *Rotter's nodes*).

Surgically, axillary lymph nodes are categorized in three levels based in their relation to the pectoralis minor muscle: the *level I* lymph nodes are lateral or below the lower border of the pectoralis minor muscle and include the external mammary, axillary vein and scapular lymph node groups, the *level II* lymph nodes are located just beneath the muscle, and the *level III* nodes (or apical) are medial to the medial border of the pectoralis minor.

### 3.1.2 Development of the Breast

The breast undergoes multiple changes throughout life, from intrauterine life to senescence. Although the majority of growth occurs with puberty, the development and differentiation of the breast are truly completed by the end of the first term of pregnancy with the postpartum lactation of the adult female. This is relevant to the

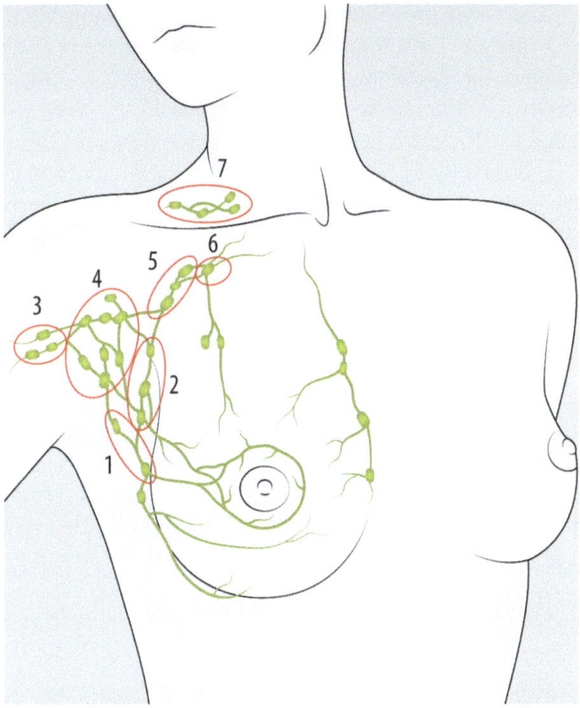


**Fig. 3.2** Lymph drainage and lymph node groups of the axilla and clavicular fossa: *1 posterior* or *subscapular, 2 anterior* or *lateral pectoral, 3 lateral*, facing the humeral head, *4* central, *5 subclavicular*, posterior to pectoralis minor, *6 apical, 7 clavicular* groups. Seventy to ninety percent of the lymphatic drainage from the breast takes place into the axillary nodes. Lymph from three groups of axillary nodes (posterior, anterior and lateral) drains into the main group (central) of nodes that is high in the axilla. All nodes are in continuity with each other, but an arbitrary division in three axillary node levels is considered useful in surgical or pathology reports. *Level I* (low axilla or external nodes) includes *1, 2, 3* and *4* groups. *Level II* (midaxilla) includes subclavicular group, posterior to pectoralis minor. *Level III* (apical axilla) includes an apical group of few nodes superomedial to the pectoralis minor. Intramammary nodes and interpectoral nodes (*Rotter's nodes*) are included in *level I*

development of cancer, because BC risk is somewhat inversely related to the age at which pregnancy first occurs. It is possible that this is secondary to an increased risk of carcinogenesis when the pre-parity, undifferentiated and proliferating mammary epithelium is exposed to carcinogens, as compared to the effect of these same carcinogens on the differentiated breast.

At birth, after the transient secretion stimulated by prolactin production in the neonate, the mammary glands, with their relatively simple architecture, remain quiescent until puberty. During this period, the supporting stromal structures and ducts enlarge in proportion to the increase in body size of the individual, but no lobular development occurs.

*PUBERTY* – The rapid growth that occurs at the onset of puberty is primarily from deposition of fat and development of periductal connective tissue, but elongation and thickening of the ductal system also occur at this stage. Under the influence of gonadotropin-releasing hormone from the hypothalamus, puberty begins in children between 8 and 12–13 years of age. This leads to the release of follicle-stimulating hormone (FSH) and luteinizing hormone (LH) from the pituitary gland, resulting in maturation of the ovarian follicles and the secretion of oestrogens. As puberty begins, the circulating oestrogen causes the ductal epithelium and surrounding stroma to grow. These ducts begin to extend into the superficial pectoral fascia and arborize within the supporting stroma to form collecting ducts and terminal ductal-lobular units. These ultimately form buds that precede further breast lobules. Surrounding the ducts, vascularity increases and connective tissues increase in volume and elasticity, replacing adipose tissue and providing support for the developing ducts.

Ductal growth occurs under the influence of circulating oestrogens, growth hormone and prolactin but is independent of progesterone.

Although there are many ways one can define the stages of breast development from puberty to adulthood, the most commonly used system is the Tanner phases, which is based also on the external appearance of the breast, listed to follow.

- *Tanner I* glandular tissue: areola follows the skin contours of the chest (prepubertal, usually age 10 and younger).
- *Tanner II*: bud forms, with small area of surrounding glandular tissue; areola begins to widen (age 10–11.5).
- *Tanner III*: breast begins to become more elevated and extends beyond the borders of the areola, which continues to widen but remains in contour with surrounding breast (age 11.5–13).
- *Tanner IV*: increased breast size and elevation; areola and papilla form a secondary mound projecting from the contour of the surrounding breast (age 13–15).
- *Tanner V*: breast reaches final adult size; areola returns to contour of the surrounding breast, with a projecting central papilla (age >15).

The development initiated at the onset of puberty is generally complete by age 20 years, but approximately a year or 2 following menarche, the breasts acquire their mature macroscopic structure (Tanner V).

*PREGNANCY* – In the pregnant patient, there is marked growth of the ducts, lobules and alveoli under the influence of luteal and placental sex steroids and prolactin.

In the *first trimester*, during the first 3–4 weeks of pregnancy, under the influence of oestrogen, there is growth and branching of the ducts, as well as increased lobule formation. By the second month, the breasts have enlarged dramatically. The superficial veins dilate and there is increased pigmentation of the nipple-areolar complex. The breasts become tender and the nipples become sore. This can begin just a few weeks after conception.

Oestrogen and progesterone prohibit the hypothalamus from producing prolactin-inhibiting factor (PIF). With this influence gone, prolactin is released and this continues progressively during pregnancy, although increase in prolactin levels is slow during the first trimester.

In the *second trimester* of pregnancy, the effects of progesterone cause the lobular formation to exceed the ductal sprouting. During this time, prolactin levels continue to rise and by the third trimester, blood levels of prolactin are three to five times higher than normal. At this point, the alveoli contain colostrum but no fat. The breast continues to enlarge, but this is not due to epithelial proliferation but rather the filling of the alveoli with colostrum as well as the hypertrophy of myoepithelial cells.

In the *third trimester* of pregnancy, the stroma surrounding the lobules diminishes to make room for the hypertrophied lobules. As pregnancy continues, colostrum composed of desquamated epithelial cells and fluid accumulates. This is released in the immediate postpartum period.

*LACTOGENESIS* – In pregnancy, prolactin is being produced, starting during the eighth week of pregnancy and increasing until birth. During that time, the high levels of oestrogen and progesterone block the prolactin receptors and inhibit milk production. After birth, there is a decline in the serum levels of oestrogen and progesterone over several days. This removes the inhibition on milk production and lactogenesis begins.

*Prolactin* is one of two hormones responsible for milk production, with the other being oxytocin. Prolactin levels were increasing until birth, and after delivery begin to decline. If the mother is not nursing, the prolactin levels will drop slowly in about 14 days. In the nursing mother, prolactin will also drop, but much more slowly, dependent on the time that the infant nurses. Prolactin drives the synthesis and secretion of milk into the alveolar spaces, then the myoepithelial cells contract, and the milk passes through the ductal system and out of the breast.

*Oxytocin* is the second hormone responsible for milk production and delivery. When an infant suckles at the mother's breast, this causes the increase in both prolactin, to stimulate the production, and oxytocin, to increase milk delivery.

During the first few days after delivery, the body does not produce milk but rather a colostrum. This is high in immunoglobulins, which help protect the infant against infections at a time when the infant's own immune system has not fully developed. Colostrum may help decrease the infant's chances of developing asthma and other allergies. When breastfeeding stops, it may take several months for milk production to completely stop. The breasts usually return to their previous size, although they may be smaller after breastfeeding is completed.

Postlactational involution starts on weaning and is initiated by local mechanical factors causing alveolar distension and capillary obstruction. The one-layer secretory alveolar cells regress and reform the two-layered epithelium characteristic of the resting breast. This process is facilitated by cell death and phagocytosis performed by invasion of the alveoli by histiocytes. A lymphocytic infiltrate is also characteristic, but connective tissue regression is limited. The branching alveolar structures become fewer in number but the ductular structure remains mostly intact – this is the fundamental difference between postlactational and postmenopausal involution, where both lobules and ductules are reduced in number.

The ducts become smaller although some secretion remains persistently in the duct lumen in the postlactational breast and can be aspirated or expressed from the nipple in most parous women.

*MENOPAUSE* – During and after menopause, the altered hormonal environment leads to a senescent state, with involution of the glandular component and replacement with connective tissue and fat. The involutive process can be divided into a *preclimacteric* phase starting at about the age of 35 and a postmenopausal phase starting at the time of the menopause, in late 40 and early 50 years of age. The predominant feature is regression of the glandular epithelium and adjacent connective tissue with gradual replacement by fat.

In the *preclimacteric* phase, there is a gradual loss of lobules and infiltration by round cells and the specialized loose connective tissue around the lobules changes into dense collagen. In the *postmenopausal* phase, the typical outline of a lobule is lost and is replaced by dense collagen containing a compressed epithelial remnant. Lobular involution may proceed to formation of microcysts, which may be mistaken for cystic disease microscopically. The essential difference between the two conditions is the preservation of the specialized lobular stroma in the former. The loss of strength of the connective tissue results in an increase in size and sag to the breasts. However, these changes of atrophy are variable and incomplete. Some women in their 60s and 70s still have a lobular appearance similar to a premenopausal state.

Hormone therapy may delay postmenopausal changes in the breast and mimic a more active physiologic or premenopausal state (i.e. cyclic tenderness due to increased nodularity). It would therefore seem logical that fibrocystic changes should resolve with menopause, but this is not always the case. For some women, the breasts can become more tender with menopause, with an increase in nodularity or cysts.

### 3.1.3 Clinical Significance of Constitutional Patterns

Breast density is not an intuitive concept and has little to do with breast size and, in some cases, with age. Though it can be influenced by lifestyle factors, twin studies show that the underlying causes of breast density are mostly inherited. Also, in common practice, constitutional patterns of the breast are similar among first-degree member of family, independently from their body structures.

Higher breast density is more common in some ethnic groups, including white women. It is also more common in younger women, beginning when hormones kick in during puberty and continuing through the childbearing years. Breast density decreases during menopause in a process called breast involution, where the milk glands and ducts atrophy and connective tissue disappears. But in some women, these tissues persist into older age.

The breast composition and relative amount of glandular tissue, connective tissue and fat is well documented in the white (glandular) and black (fat) areas on mammograms. Different methods of estimating the proportion of white area on the mammogram exist and vary from the perception of the radiologist to using a software programme to outline the white area and compare it to the total breast area.

The BI-RADS measuring system involves a radiologist scoring a mammogram in one of four categories according to the extent of contrast within the outline of the breast: x-rays pass easily through fatty tissue, which shows up as darker areas on the image, but are blocked – and thus appear white – by milk ducts, lobes and the web of connective tissue that tethers everything together. Studies have shown that women who have extremely dense breasts have a three- to fivefold increased risk of breast cancer compared with women who have mostly fatty breasts (see Sect. 2.1).

Both in clinical and radiological exam, the major concern is whether dense breasts have a *masking effect*, where the lack of contrast between normal and pathological tissue in dense breasts makes it difficult to identify abnormal clinical densities and radiological opacities (see Sect. 5.1).

Furthermore, from the clinical point of view, the possible extensions of glandular tissue at the periphery of the gland (axillary, subclavian prolongation and extension over normal medial and inferior boundaries) must be taken into account for justifying some unusual clinical manifestations. The pathology of the extended parenchyma or accessory glands is similar to that of the normal mammary gland, with equal possibility of cancerization.

## 3.2 Congenital Breast Deformities

**Clinical Practice Points**

- Congenital malformations of the breast, relating mainly to absence, hypoplasia or ectopia, are sometimes part of wider congenital syndromes, with particular tendency to affect the urinary tract or limb girdles.
- The foetal milk line is not as extensive in humans as in some animals, so most ectopic tissue is found between the axilla and epigastrium.
- Axillary accessory breasts can be subject to all varieties of pathology seen in the breast proper, so axillary masses should be assessed individually, as well as in association with any breast mass.
- Some developmental abnormalities occur so early that are believed to be congenital when they actually are due to abnormal development of the stromal or lobular component.
- Accurate counselling may be necessary to alleviate the sense of deformity and unattractiveness if present. In teenage years, proper timing of surgical intervention is necessary to optimize functional, psychological and aesthetic outcomes.

The mammary malformations are numerous and there are several classifications, most of which descriptive. These malformations generally fall into two categories: the presence of supernumerary breast tissue and the absence or underdevelopment of breast tissue. In a more general framework, which also includes pathological manifestations as altered development, we prefer to distinguish them as follows:

- Deformities regarding the number and location
- Deformities regarding the shape (breast hamartoma and tuberous breast)
- Deformities associated to other congenital anomalies (Poland syndrome)
- Other deformities with not identified causes (asymmetry, synmastia)

Major deformities may cause significant functional, psychological and aesthetic concerns. The affected individual may present for consultation at any age, often early in childhood as a result of parental concern. It is important to be able to counsel the patient and his or her family regarding the nature of the problem, its prognosis for future development, and the appropriate indications, and timing of surgical intervention.

### 3.2.1 Deformities Regarding the Number and the Location

In 1915, Kajava published a classification system for supernumerary breast tissue that remains in use today.

- Class I consists of a complete breast with nipple, areola and glandular tissue.
- Class II consists of nipple and glandular tissue but no areola.
- Class III consists of areola and glandular tissue but no nipple.
- Class IV consists of glandular tissue only.
- Class V consists of nipple and areola but no glandular tissue (pseudomamma).
- Class VI consists of a nipple only (polythelia).
- Class VII consists of an areola only (polythelia areolaris).
- Class VIII consists of a patch of hair only (polythelia pilosa).

The presence of supernumerary breast tissue indicates incomplete involution of the milk line, resulting in the formation of accessory mammary tissue from the redundant clusters of ectopic primordial breast cells. This occurs in 2–6 % of females and 1–3 % of males. Approximately one third of affected individuals have more than one site of supernumerary breast tissue development. Most of this accessory breast tissue has no physiologic significance, but some may enlarge with the onset of puberty, pregnancy, or lactation and can be the site of breast carcinoma.

The extension of the mammary gland towards the armpit is so common that only a few relevant cases we can speak of an anomaly. Sometimes, the accessory glandular tissue is found in a predominantly nodular axillary fat component. In case of real breasts supernumerary, generally, these are highlighted only when breastfeeding following the first or even second pregnancy.

Approximately two out of three cases of accessory breast tissue occur in the thoracic or abdominal portions of the milk line, often just below the inframammary

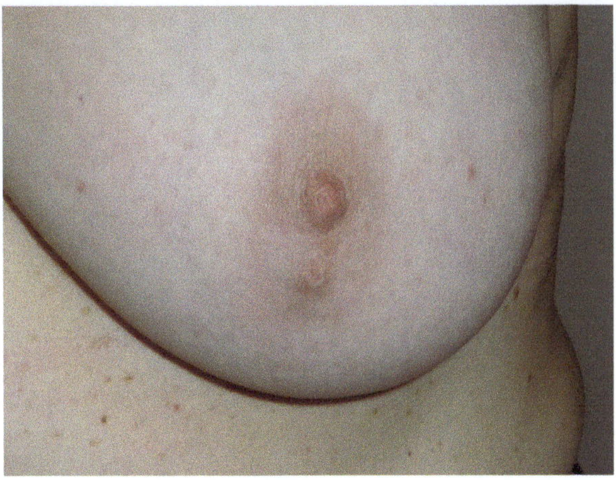

**Fig. 3.3** Supernumerary nipple and areola complex of the left breast

crease and more often on the left side of the body. Another 20 % occurs in the axilla. The remaining locations include anywhere along the milk line or on the buttock, back, face and neck. Supernumerary tissue present in any location other than along the milk line represents a migratory arrest of breast primordium during chest wall development.

*Polythelia*. The most common form of supernumerary breast tissue is polythelia, the presence of more than two nipples on an individual (Fig. 3.3). More than 90 % of supernumerary nipples occur in the inframammary region. This condition is present in 2–5 % of the general population, although many additional patients may go undiagnosed because the nipple is often confused for a nevus or other benign skin lesion because of its diminutive size. Most cases are sporadic, but approximately 6 % are familial and are believed to represent an autosomal dominant trait with variable penetrance.

A correlation exists between renal disease and polythelia. Nephrologic abnormalities such as cysts, duplications or unilateral renal agenesis have been found in approximately 15 % of sporadic cases and twice the amount of familial cases compared to 1–2 % of the general population. Considering the significant incidence of congenital and acquired renal disorders associated to familial polythelia, patients should be aware of the need for regular physical examination and urinalysis. Any abnormality noted should alert the physician to the need for a renal ultrasound.

*Polymastia*, the presence of accessory glandular tissue, is the second most common form of supernumerary breast tissue, occurring in 1–2 % of the female population. Various forms exist, as described by Kajava classes I through IV, but, most commonly, the nipple and areola are absent or rudimentary. The most common location is in the axilla, where they may present as axillary fullness responsive to hormonal cycles of menstruation, pregnancy or lactation. The second most common location is in the inframammary region, similar to polythelia (Fig. 3.4). Most cases are sporadic, but this condition also has been observed as a heritable trait.

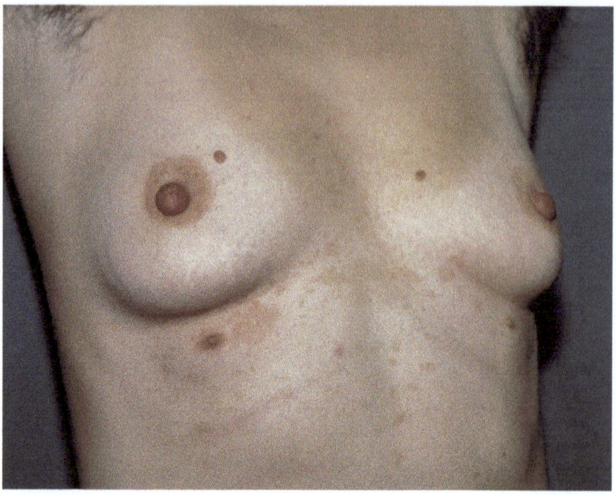

**Fig. 3.4** Supernumerary breast under both breasts

While supernumerary breasts are commonly complete with areolas and nipples, the breasts with areola but no nipple (*polymastia areolaris*) and the breasts with nipple but without areola (*polymastia mamillaris*) are very rare.

The presence of supernumerary tissue can be psychologically disturbing to adolescents. Excision may be recommended prior to puberty or at any age when the condition is recognized and becomes of concern to the individual.

*Amastia, amazia and* marked *hypoplasia*. The absence or marked hypoplasia of breast tissue is less common than the presence of supernumerary tissue. *Amastia*, the complete absence of glandular tissue including nipple and areola, is the most severe form. *Amazia* is a term used when breast tissue is absent but the nipple is present. *Hypoplasia*, the presence of very small rudimentary breasts, is the most common form. These conditions may be unilateral or bilateral and result from partial or complete underdevelopment of the mammary bud. All these conditions of the breast may be associated with scalp defects, ear abnormalities, renal hypoplasia and cataracts in patients with the rare autosomal dominant Finlay-Marks syndrome.

*Athelia*, absence of the nipple and areola in the presence of glandular tissue, is the least common encountered mammary anomaly as an isolated defect, while is usually accompanied by musculoskeletal deformities of the chest wall and ipsilateral upper extremity.

### 3.2.2 Deformities Regarding the Shape

*Hamartoma*. A hamartoma is a non-neoplastic mass characterized by an excess growth of an abnormal mixture of mammary tissues found in an area of the breast (see Sect. 9.3). It is considered a developmental error, called *breast in the breast* meaning that it is a normal tissue in glandular components, but abnormal proportions. Even if the dimensions are varied and can reach 20 cm in diameter so that may change the breast size, the clinical manifestations are mostly negligible.

*Tuberous breasts* are the result of a congenital abnormality of the breasts which can occur in both men and women, one breast or both. The exact cause of this is as

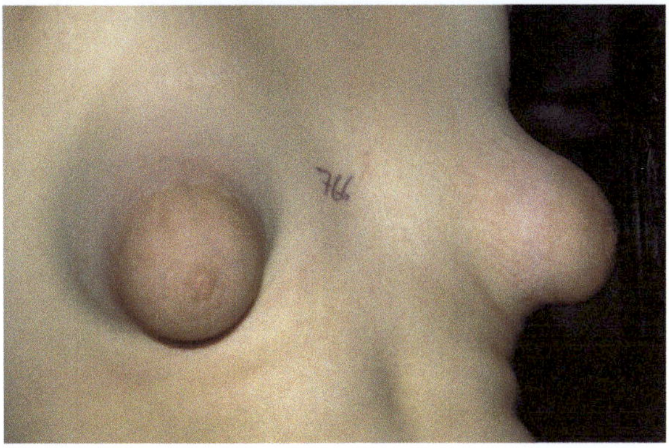

**Fig. 3.5** Tuberous breast in an 18-year-old girl. The breasts are hypoplastic and constricted at the base so that their appearance is conical. The areolar complexes are puffy. More or less herniated with dome-like nipples

yet unclear; however, a recent study suggested a genetic link in a disorder of collagen deposition [2].

In the tuberous breast, the areolar complex is decidedly prominent, separated by a breast cone represented by a narrow cylinder of skin. Narrow in base and sometimes abnormal in position, the breast takes a look reminiscent (in the most poetic figurative interpretation) to tuberose plants, from which for the name of tubular or tuberous breast syndrome. This condition is also known as constricted breasts, snoopy breasts, herniated areolar complexes, conical breast, domen nipple, lower pole hypoplasia and hypoplastic breasts (Fig. 3.5).

Tuberous breasts are not simply small or underdeveloped breasts. The effect of the condition on the appearance of the breast can range from mild to severe, and typical characteristics include enlarged, puffy areola, unusually wide spacing between the breasts, minimal breast tissue, sagging, higher than normal breast fold, and narrow base at the chest wall. The condition can affect the ability of the woman to breastfeed as in some cases the breasts, including the milk glands, have not developed enough to produce breast milk. However, other physical aspects of fertility and pregnancy are not affected by the condition.

When the condition appears psychologically unacceptable, surgery becomes indispensable. Plastic surgery is planned in regard to three main different types:

- Hypoplasia of the inferomedial quadrant with highly developed lateral quadrants (type I)
- Hypoplasia of the lower quadrants with areola downward segment and shortened subareolar skin (sausage or snoopy breast) (type II)
- Hypoplasia of all quadrants with wide reduction of the base and breast parenchyma concentrated below the areola (breast nipple) (type III)

### 3.2.3 Deformities Associated to Other Congenital Anomalies

*Poland syndrome*. Unilateral breast hypoplasia or aplasia is most commonly encountered in Poland syndrome, which includes ipsilateral underdevelopment of the chest muscles, skin and subcutaneous tissues, bones and upper extremities (Fig. 3.6).

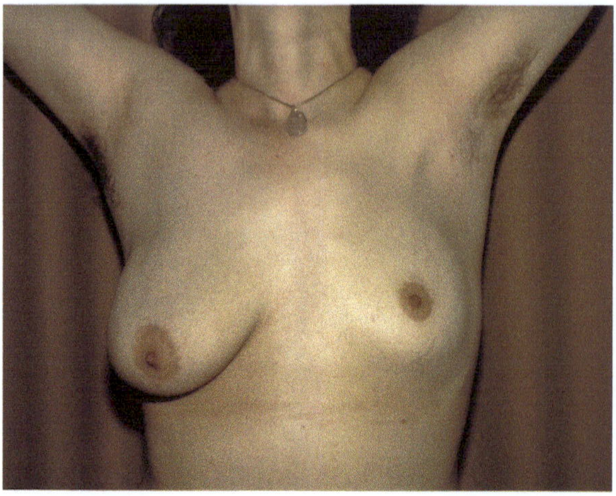

**Fig. 3.6** Unilateral underdevelopment of left breast and pectoralis muscles (Poland syndrome)

The skin of the area is hypoplastic with a thinned subcutaneous layer, and the axillary hair may be absent. The ipsilateral nipple is often smaller and higher in both male and female patients [3].

The absence of the sternal head of the pectoralis major muscle is considered the minimal expression of this syndrome, but the involvement of adjacent muscles includes the pectoralis minor, serratus, latissimus dorsi and external oblique. Skeletal deformities may involve absence of portions of the ribs or costal cartilages anteriorly. The upper extremity also may be hypoplastic so that arm, forearm and fingers may be shortened and complete or incomplete syndactyly can also be found.

Poland syndrome is uncommon but not rare in less severe cases. While plastic surgeons encounter more female patients than male patients with this deformity (because the female patients seek out treatment of breast asymmetry), no gender predilection is exhibited. Many men remain undiagnosed unless they seek attention for the treatment of associated hand anomalies. Because Poland syndrome is underreported and infrequently diagnosed, the exact incidence is difficult to determine. In one review, the incidence of Poland syndrome was estimated at 1 in 30,000. The right side is affected twice as often as the left.

Most Poland syndrome cases arise sporadically. However, several reports exist of family members and twins with the same diagnosis, suggesting some degree of genetic transmission. Poland syndrome has been associated with other syndromes, and haematopoietic malignancies, including leukaemia and non-Hodgkin lymphoma, have been described in patients with Poland syndrome.

### 3.2.4 Other Deformities with No Identified Causes

Some developmental abnormalities occur so early that they are believed to be congenital when they actually are not. They are partly due to factors identified as a pathological development of the stromal (juvenile hypertrophy) or lobular (giant fibroadenoma) component. For instance, breast hypertrophy, which conforms to the ANDI concept, can be loosely categorized as normal (the larger end of the normal spectrum), aberration (when breast weight is sufficient to cause physical symptoms as well as embarrassment), and disease (the rapid, and extreme enlargement of gigantomastia, requiring urgent intervention), as discussed in Chap. 9. Finally, other deformities are due to not identified causes as a distinct asymmetry, a marked hypertrophy or a synmastia.

*BREAST ASYMMETRY* – Breast size asymmetry is the difference of form, position or volume of the breast. It affects more than half of all young women. Typically, the asymmetry is more noticeable during puberty, and up to 25 % of women have a persistent visible breast asymmetry in mature age.

The exact cause of asymmetric breasts is unknown, but possible contributors include hormonal changes or occasionally an underlying medical or skeletal condition, as scoliosis and deformities in the chest wall. Acquired mammary hypoplasia has been reported in patients who have received breast radiation in infancy or childhood, most frequently for the treatment of cutaneous haemangioma. Other iatrogenic causes include previous thoracotomy or excision of both benign and malignant breast tumours during childhood leading to impaired breast development. Burns to the anterior chest can lead to failure of complete mammary expansion from injury to the breast bud.

Generally, slight differences in a woman's breasts are of no concern. If the differences are greater than one bra cup size, however, they may cause some psychological distress, particularly during adolescence, when a young woman's body and mind are already changing so rapidly. An augmentation or reduction surgical procedure may be performed, if the person with the asymmetry wishes to make the breasts more symmetric after development/puberty is complete.

*BREAST HYPERTROPHY* – Breast hypertrophy refers to inappropriate and excessive growth of the breast. Usually, it occurs in both breasts, and when only one breast is affected, the result can produce a minor size variation to an extremely large breast asymmetry.

Many definitions of breast hypertrophy are in use and all are somewhat arbitrary, since an excessive tissue can often be regarded only from an aesthetic viewpoint and not from a medical one. It is known the size of the breasts is not related to their functionality, and therefore, in almost all women, breast tissue is excessive from a functional viewpoint. The line between normal 'big' breasts and a medical condition is an individual one, unless growth is *progressive* and there are ulcerations or other disease-related observations present.

There are varying definitions of what is considered to be excessive breast tissue. The plainest definition of breast hypertrophy is a breast weight that exceeds approximately 3 % of the total body weight. Other definitions define *macromastia* as excessive tissue of over 1.5 kg (3.3 lb) up to 2.5 kg (5.5 lb) and *gigantomastia* where excessive tissue is more than 2.5 kg.

Clinically relevant breast hypertrophy usually occurs in adolescence (see Sect. 3.3) and in pregnancy (see Sect. 3.4). It can be also occasionally observed in adult women without any obvious cause (*idiopathic or constitutional breast hypertrophy*) or related to a pharmacological setting (*iatrogenic breast hypertrophy*). The underlying cause of the rapidly growing breast connective tissue, resulting in gigantic proportions, is thought to be a heightened sensitivity to female hormones, or an abnormally elevated level of circulating hormones, or both.

Extremely large breasts are a source of considerable concern. Some women try to hide or mask their breasts with special clothing, although finding large bra sizes and styles that fit is challenging. Ill-fitting bras with narrow straps can cause chronic irritation, redness and indentations in the shoulders. Skin rashes and intertrigo under the breasts are common, particularly during warm weather. Heavy breasts may cause headaches, neck pain, upper and lower back pain and numbness or tingling in the fingers. Women with this condition may be also subject to psychological problems due to unwanted attention and/or harassment, so that among sufferers depression is common.

Medical treatment has not proven consistently effective. Medical regimens have included tamoxifen, progesterone, bromocriptine, gonadotropin-releasing hormone agonist and testosterone.

In general, breast reduction is not clinically indicated unless at least 1.8 kg (4 lb) of tissue per breast needs to be removed. Actually, in the majority of cases of breast hypertrophy, surgery, even if strictly unnecessary, depends on body weight and severe impediment of the posture. Surgical therapy includes reduction mammoplasty. In some severe cases, a bilateral mastectomy is indicated. A good option is a Goldilocks mastectomy, a completely autologous breast mound created by preserving and de-epithelializing residual mastectomy flap tissue.

*Iatrogenic macromastia* is the excessive growth of breast tissue related to medications. Two drugs that have been most often related to macromastia are penicillamine (mainly used in rheumatoid arthritis) and indinavir (an antiretroviral medication used for the treatment of human immunodeficiency virus infection). Use of cyclosporine, marijuana and cimetidine may also lead to unilateral or bilateral breast enlargement.

*Synmastia* is defined as a confluence of the breast tissue of both breasts across the midline anterior to the sternum. Synmastia can either be a congenital anomaly or iatrogenic. Congenital synmastia is a rare condition with few published cases. Iatrogenic synmastia may occur following breast augmentation. It can be surgically corrected by a plastic surgeon.

## 3.3 Breast Findings in Childhood and Adolescence

**Clinical Practice Points**

- In early puberty, the breast buds are often temporarily asymmetrical.
- Usually, asymmetry becomes less noticeable with age.
- Nipple inversion is common, but self-correcting changes often occur during pregnancy and lactation, allowing breastfeeding.

*NEONATAL BREAST HYPERTROPHY* related to stimulation from maternal hormones can occur in both male and female neonates during the first few weeks of life; it is sometimes associated with a thin milky nipple discharge (*witch's milk*). Neonatal breast hypertrophy usually resolves spontaneously within 2 weeks in boys and several months in girls. However, it may persist if the breast tissue is stimulated (e.g. by attempting to express the milky discharge). Breast abscesses may also occur (see Sect. 8.3).

*PREMATURE THELARCHE* is defined as breast development in females aged 6 months to 9 years, before puberty. Physical examination for this entity should carefully seek out other signs of puberty, such as development of pubic hair, thickening of the vaginal mucosa, and accelerated bone growth. If no other signs of puberty are present, the patient and family should be reassured that this is a benign finding. If other signs of puberty are evident, precocious puberty should be entertained as a diagnosis.

*PREPUBERTAL ASYMMETRICAL DEVELOPMENT OF THE NIPPLE BUD.* The breast buds are often asymmetrical at first and this is much the commonest swelling of the early part of adolescence. Recognition is vital, because ill-advised biopsy will lead to amastia.

*PREPUBERTAL BREAST MASTITIS.* In prepubertal and early pubertal teenagers (11–15 years), discrete superficial cystic masses may occur, but rarely, in sub- or para-areolar location, due to an important oestrogenic stimulation of major ducts. An engorgement of bloody secretions may occur yielding a painful cyst, usually noninfected, but only occasionally. Sometimes, a short but profuse pouring out of a bloody, or dark and brown as chocolate, discharge causes an immediate relief of pain due to the engorgement of retroareolar ducts.

Cold is best for acute onset, numbing painful area and decreasing inflammation due to the acute swelling. Heat pads tend to work best for soothing and easing reabsorption. Usually, symptoms disappear in 2–4 weeks. If infectious mastitis is ruled out, non-specific therapy is advisable.

*PREPUBERTAL BREAST ABSCESS.* In prepubertal girl, infectious abscesses may be rarely observed that manifest as a tender and erythematous mass. The most common organism causing breast abscesses in this age population is *Staphylococcus aureus*. Less common causes include gram-negative enteric organisms (e.g. *Escherichia coli*, *Salmonella*), while anaerobes and methicillin-resistant *Staphylococcus aureus* are more common in community-acquired infections.

Treatment involves antibiotics, needle aspiration or surgical drainage. The literature suggests that drainage alone, without adjunctive antibiotics, may be equally effective, while no definitive antibiotic recommendation regarding breast abscesses in particular is recognized. The decision for surgical drainage should be carefully made because future breast deformation may occur [4].

*PRECOCIOUS PUBERTY* is breast development accompanied by other signs of puberty. Early onset of puberty is more common in girls than in boys and is predominantly mediated by premature activation of the hypothalamic-pituitary-gonadal axis. Hypothalamic hamartomas, trauma or central nervous system lesions may cause central precocious puberty; however, aetiology is most commonly idiopathic.

*ASYMMETRY*. Breast asymmetry may develop as thelarche ensues. In this condition, one breast may develop before or more rapidly than the other. The physical examination findings usually include homogenous enlargement of onc breast with no discrete masses or discharge. Accompanying breast tenderness may be present if the breast bud is starting to develop. If a mass is excluded, by either physical examination or ultrasonography, the patient and parents can be reassured that the asymmetry will become less noticeable with age.

*JUVENILE BREAST HYPERTROPHY*. When breast hypertrophy occurs in young women during puberty, the medical condition is known as *juvenile breast hypertrophy* or *juvenile macromastia* or *juvenile gigantomastia. Juvenile breast hypertrophy* is the postpubertal continuation of unilateral or bilateral breast development in which the gland undergoes massive enlargement (≤2–4 kg each). Breast hypertrophy can be loosely categorized as normal (the larger end of the normal spectrum), as a plane aberration (when breast weight is sufficient to cause physical symptoms as well as embarrassment), and very rarely as a disease (the rapid and extreme enlargement of gigantomastia).

Histologically, the breast tissue shows mainly increase in stromal tissue with pseudoangiomatous stromal hyperplasia (PASH) and may also show some degree of epithelial hyperplasia. Along with the excessive breast size, other symptoms include red, itchy lesions and pain in the breasts. A diagnosis is made when an adolescent's breasts grow rapidly and achieve great weight usually just before or soon after her first menstrual period.

The breasts undergo a massive increase in size over several months. Some adolescent females experience breast growth at a steady rate for several years, after which the breasts, as well as the nipples, rapidly develop exceeding normal growth. Others experience minimal or negligible breast growth until their breasts suddenly grow very rapidly in a short period of time, reaching three or more cup sizes within a few weeks. This may cause considerable physical discomfort.

When hypertrophy occurs in adolescence, non-invasive treatments, including pharmaceutical treatment, hormone therapy and steroid use, are not usually recommended due to known and unknown side effects. Once a girl's breast growth rate has stabilized, breast reduction may be an appropriate choice. In some rare instances, after aggressive or surgical treatment, the breast may continue to grow or regrow; nevertheless, mastectomy may be recommended as a last resort.

*GYNAECOMASTIA* – Lumps in the male breast in adolescence are less common and all due to gynaecomastia. Unlike girls, there is a marked peak incidence at the age of 13 or 14. Inflammatory masses in HIV-positive males have been reported (see Sect. 19.1).

*BREAST MASSES IN ADOLESCENCE* (Table 3.1). Concern has been expressed that fibroadenoma in this age group must be removed because of the possibility of cancer [5]. Cancer in adolescence is exceedingly rare and a review of case reports show that a mistaken diagnosis of fibroadenoma has usually been made because of the age group, not because of typical physical signs of fibroadenoma. Thus, masses with rapid growth, recent nipple retraction, surrounding tissue and lymph node involvement have been diagnosed as fibroadenoma. The risk of cancer can, for

**Table 3.1** Summary of breast masses found during adolescence (10–20 years)

| | Breast mass | Frequency of presentation |
|---|---|---|
| *Male* | Gynaecomastia | Common |
| | Inflammatory mass | Rare |
| *Female* | Premenarchal development of breast bud | Common |
| | Fibroadenoma | Common |
| | Cyst | Rare |
| | Giant fibroadenoma | Rare |
| | Phyllodes tumour | Rare |
| | Adenocarcinoma | Very rare |
| | Metastatic tumour | Very rare |
| Nipple and areola | Retention cysts | Uncommon |
| | Inversion | Uncommon |
| | Molluscum contagiosum | Rare |
| | Leiomyoma | Rare |
| Other conditions | Duct papilloma | Rare |
| | Subareolar mastitis | Uncommon |
| | Subareolar abscess | Very rare |
| | Juvenile hypertrophy | Uncommon |
| | Nipple discharge from Montgomery's tubercle | Rare |

practical purposes, be ignored in an adolescent with a lump showing the typical features of the common fibroadenoma. If anything, there is a very rare risk of metastatic tumour in the breast and, in this age group, the commonest is rhabdomyosarcoma.

## 3.4 Breast Findings Associated with Pregnancy

**Clinical Practice Points**

- Pregnant women may develop any of the breast lesions seen in the population at large but also are disposed to certain pathologic entities unique to the puerperium: lactating adenoma, galactocele, gigantomastia and benign bloody nipple discharge.
- An initial thorough breast examination should be part of the first prenatal visit. This establishes a baseline for comparison should changes be detected later.
- In treatments during pregnancy, two patients – not one – must be considered.
- Management of a new breast mass in pregnancy should maximize diagnostic accuracy and minimize the chances of missing breast cancer. *Watchful waiting*, when a breast mass is discovered, is no more appropriate than in a non-pregnant patient.

During pregnancy, the size and weight of the breasts approximately double as glandular elements proliferate under hormonal stimulation. Both lobular growth and alveolar growth occur. The histology reflects preparation for lactation, with an excess of glandular elements over stroma, in contrast to resting breast tissue, where stroma predominates. Mammary blood flow doubles too [6].

Small amounts of colostrum are produced prior to delivery. After delivery, placental and ovarian hormonal inhibition of lactation is released, and prolactin stimulates galactopoiesis. The mechanical stimulus of suckling allows lactation to continue virtually indefinitely. When nursing is stopped, milk stagnates and lactation ceases within 48 h. Involution of the breasts follows.

Benign lesions that are commonly found in women in general (i.e. fibroadenoma, breast hamartoma and axillary breast tissue) can occasionally enlarge significantly during pregnancy, due to proliferation in response to hormonal stimulation, usually retrieving their original size after childbirth. For this reason, in many cases, it is not necessary to remove simple fibroadenomas before delivery fearing an increasing in their size.

*LACTATING ADENOMA* – Despite the name, lactating adenomas are more common during pregnancy than during lactation. Lactating adenomas are discrete, round, well-demarcated masses unique to pregnancy. Differentiation among other benign lesions (fibroadenomas and hamartomas) that enlarge during pregnancy and lactation may be difficult but clinically irrelevant. Moreover, fibroadenomas and hamartomas together with lactating adenoma in many series are equivalent to each other.

Lactating adenomas typically present as painless, often rather sizable, palpable masses. The most common location is the breast periphery, often in the upper outer quadrant where the bulk of breast tissue is distributed. The histology is characteristic since lobulated masses of acini or lobules are densely packed together with little intervening stroma. The basement membrane is intact. Despite abundant proliferative changes, there are no atypia.

The major task is to differentiate these benign masses from breast cancer. Diagnostic fine-needle aspiration cytology (FNAC) or core biopsy is an acceptable method of diagnosis, provided the cytopathologist is informed of the stage of pregnancy and knowledgeable about the changes seen in these lesions.

*GESTATIONAL HYPERTROPHY* is a rare disease, occurring in 1 out of every 30,000–100,000 pregnancies. Most commonly occurs at the onset of first pregnancy, between the 16th and 20th week of gestation, and may recur in subsequent pregnancies. If normal, resting weight of the breast (200–300 g) typically doubles to 400/600 g; in gigantomastia, weights of 4,000–7,000 g per breast have been recorded. The resulting hypertrophy is not only grotesquely deforming but also may preclude ambulation or progress to skin ulceration, infection or massive bleeding from dilated subcutaneous veins; these complications may be life threatening.

The aetiology is unknown, but the disease is believed to represent an abnormal end-organ (breast) response to the normal rise in progesterone level as pregnancy progresses. This hypertrophy can occur in any pregnancy, not necessarily the first, but the presence of the condition in one pregnancy essentially guarantees its recurrence in subsequent gestations. There is no racial predilection. It is unnecessary and inadvisable to biopsy the breast tissue when gigantomastia is identified because of the risk of bleeding and infection. Biopsy is recommended only when a discrete, suspicious region of abnormality is detected.

Treatment is bromocriptine, which may arrest continued growth of the breasts. Other hormonal interventions have been used with variable success. Sometimes, early delivery and urgent breast surgery are required when life-threatening complications occur, including haemorrhage, infarction, secondary infection or even hyperparathyroidism. Some involution may occur after delivery. Breastfeeding is not advised, because the hypertrophy may continue to increase. Reduction mammoplasty is generally necessary, because the breasts do not revert to normal size even after involution occurs.

*BLOODY NIPPLE DISCHARGE* – During the third trimester of pregnancy, proliferative changes within the ducts of the breasts may lead to bloody discharge from the nipple. This occurs when proliferative spurs of epithelium that extend into the ducts are traumatized, resulting in bleeding. Breastfeeding is not contraindicated, and the bleeding often ceases with the onset of nursing. Cytology of the discharge is apt to be misleading, as proliferative changes are atypical due to pregnancy and may be mistaken for neoplastic alterations. Mammography is usually contraindicated during pregnancy and not useful in case of nipple discharge. Mammography and biopsy are required only if the bloody discharge persists more than 2 months after delivery, localizes to one duct, or is associated with a palpable mass.

*OTHER BREAST MASSES* – The goal in evaluating new breast masses during pregnancy is appropriate diagnosis and confident exclusion of cancer by the least invasive but most reliable means possible.

*Breast infarcts*. Infarcts may occur in fibroadenomas, hamartomas, lactating adenomas or even in regions of hypertrophic breast tissue. The aetiology is believed to be vascular insufficiency related to significantly increased metabolic demands. A pre-existing mass may suddenly increase in size, or a new mass may appear where none was previously palpable. The mass may be ill-defined or even feel tethered to adjacent breast tissue. Sometimes, tenderness, skin fixation or other skin changes may be noted. The rapid increase in size and physical characteristics of the mass may raise concern that the mass may be malignant.

Differentiating these lesions from cancer is more difficult than with lactating adenomas. FNAC is unlikely to be helpful, because it may show only necrotic tissue with some of the proliferative changes noted previously. Generally, a core biopsy is required. Frozen section may be misleading, especially to the inexperienced pathologist, as the histologic picture of extensive central necrosis with an outer zone of proliferation suggests carcinoma.

## 3.5 Breastfeeding and Related Issues

**Clinical Practice Points**

- Several *perceived* barriers to breastfeeding are still influential, so that promotional campaigns are needed.
- The longer women breastfeed, the longer protective factors for woman and child last and the greater the benefits.
- The most appropriate way to breastfeeding should be learned even before the birth.

- Keeping the breast empty of milk promotes healing by helping to drain the culture medium that is facilitating growth of organisms.
- Treatments for benign problems during puerperium should be tailored to allow a woman to continue breastfeeding if she so desires.

As it is known, breastfeeding promotes mother-infant bonding, promotes uterine involution, is economical for the family and the society, and gives a better cognitive development in children, lower incidence of premenopausal breast cancer, lower incidence of premenopausal ovarian cancer, and lower incidence of maternal osteoporosis.

Moreover, breastfeeding brings undeniable health benefits compared to formula feeding, which has a relative illness risk varying from 2 to 6–8 times for diseases as allergies, eczema, urinary tract infections, inflammatory bowel disease, diabetes type 1, gastroenteritis, otitis media and meningitis.

Nevertheless, *perceived* barriers to breastfeeding are loss of freedom, embarrassment, jealousy (paternal and sibling), difficulty returning to work or school, physical discomfort, weaning, lack of confidence (afraid that baby is starving), and perception that formula is equal to breast milk.

The WHO recommends exclusive breastfeeding for the first 6 months of life, after which infants should receive nutritionally adequate and safe complementary foods while breastfeeding may continue up to 2 years of age or beyond. Only for those few health situations where infants cannot, or should not, be breastfed, the choices of the best alternative are, in order, expressed breast milk from an infant's own mother, breast milk from a healthy wet-nurse or a human milk bank, or a breast milk substitute fed with a cup.

Same recommendations come from the National Health Service that point out that any amount of breastfeeding has a positive effect. The longer women breastfeed, the longer the protection lasts and the greater the benefits. The medical and paramedical staff should encourage breastfeeding for its benefits for both the child and the mother, and this beyond some possible difficulties, and in compliance with the will of the woman.

The most appropriate way to breastfeeding should be learned even before the birth. Medical providers should encourage patients to take breastfeeding classes while pregnant so that a proper breastfeeding technique can be learned before delivery. Providers should be sensitive to the impact of negative psychological and physical debilitation subsequent to childbirth when breastfeeding is not successful for missing or insufficient lactation.

Breastfeeding is contraindicated in women with HIV and HTLV infection, with active TB and other specific diseases and with a history of illicit drug abuse. Certain medications are contraindicated during breastfeeding. Breastfeeding women should consult their medical provider before using new medications or supplements. Smoking should be avoided during lactation, and alcohol should be used with caution.

Lactation amenorrhea may not be adequate contraception for lactating women. Other methods should be considered.

Some studies suggest that breastfeeding may slightly lower breast cancer risk, especially if it is continued for 18–24 months. But this has been a difficult area to study, especially in countries where breastfeeding for this long is uncommon. One explanation for this possible effect may be that breastfeeding reduces a woman's total number of lifetime menstrual cycles (similar to starting menstrual periods at a later age or going through early menopause).

*Breastfeeding during cancer treatment.* Most doctors recommend that women who have just had babies and are about to be treated for breast cancer should stop (or not start) breastfeeding. If surgery is planned, stopping breastfeeding will help reduce blood flow to the breasts, make them smaller and help with the operation. It also helps reduce the risk of infection in the breast. Many chemo, hormone and targeted therapy drugs can enter breast milk and be passed on to the baby. Breastfeeding isn't recommended if the mother is getting chemo, hormone or targeted therapy. There is, however, no contraindication in breastfeeding for patients who have had only radiation therapy.

*INFECTION* – Breastfeeding-related disorders are mainly infections (see Sect. 8.2). Nasopharyngeal organisms from the infant are the usual source of breast infections. Terminal ducts emptying into the nipple serve as a portal of entry. Sometimes, cracked or fissured nipples facilitate colonization of the nipple with organisms. An important risk factor is milk stasis. Milk is an excellent culture medium; hence, breast infections are particularly apt to occur when the milk is allowed to stagnate within the breast.

In some cases, milk leucocyte counts and cultures guide antibiotic therapy selection and help in gauging the severity of the infection and progress of treatment. Even when frank abscess formation occurs, serial aspirations may be a useful alternative to surgical drainage in selected cases, as discussed in (Sect. 8.2).

*GALACTOCELE* – Another common problem in breastfeeding is galactocele as a result of ductal obstruction. Galactoceles can occur during lactation but more commonly are noted after cessation of lactation, when the milk is allowed to stagnate within the breast. These smooth, mobile, often tender masses are localized collections of milk. There is no known relationship between galactoceles and the large cysts often seen in fibrocystic changes. Aspiration is both diagnostic and curative, yielding fluid milk when performed during lactation or soon after cessation and yielding more thickened, cheesy material from older lesions aspirated at a time remote from lactation. Several aspirations may be required. Ice packs and good mechanical support of the breast with a well-fitting brassiere are helpful.

Mammography is rarely indicated, as aspiration is both highly diagnostic and in most cases curative. The characteristic mammographic appearance may show layering of fat density over water density. Older lesions containing thickened material may demonstrate a mixed water-fat density similar to that seen in mammary hamartoma. Surgery is rarely required.

## References

1. Sabel MS. Anatomy and physiology of the breast. In: Sabel MS, editor. Essentials of breast surgery. Philadelphia: Mosby; 2009.
2. Klinger M, Caviggioli F, Klinger F, et al. Tuberous breast: morphological study and overview of a borderline entity. Can J Plast Surg. 2011;19:42–4.
3. Moir CR, Johnson CH. Poland's syndrome. Semin Pediatr Surg. 2008;17:161–6.
4. Foxcroft LM, Evans EB, Hirst C, Hicks BJ. Presentation and diagnosis of adolescent breast disease. Breast. 2001;10:399–404.
5. Banikarim C, De Silva NK. Breast disorders in children and adolescents: an overview. http://www.uptodate.com. Accessed 01 July 2014.
6. Scott-Conner CE. Diagnosing and managing breast disease during pregnancy and lactation. http://www.medscape.com/viewarticle/719249_1#showall. Accessed 30 June 2014.

## Further Reading

Conde DM. Treatment approach for breast abscess in nonlactating adolescents. Int J Gynaecol Obstet. 2015;128:72–3.

De Silva NK, Brandt ML. Disorders of the breast in children and adolescents. Part 1: disorders of growth and infections of the breast. J Pediatr Adolesc Gynecol. 2006;19:345–9. Part 2: breast masses. J Pediatr Adolesc Gynecol. 2006;19:415–8.

Kolker AR, Collins MS. Tuberous breast deformity: classification and treatment strategy for improving consistency in aesthetic correction. Plast Reconstr Surg. 2015;135:73–86.

Warren R, Degnim AC. Uncommon benign breast abnormalities in adolescents. Semin Plast Surg. 2013;27:26–8.

**Websites in Appendix**: *Mastitis*, A-4.3.

# Clinical Examination of the Breast

# 4

Giorgio Macellari and Alfonso M. Pluchinotta

## Contents



**Abstract**

• Clinical examination of the breast is the weakest test of the "triple diagnostic assessment", but may be decisive to solve many common symptoms as breast pain, inflammatory changes, acute enlargement of cysts, and many more. • The basic goal of clinical breast examination is to identify a palpable dominant mass, which by definition is a three-dimensional distinct mass that is different from the remainder of the breast tissue and from the tissue of the other breast (not symmetrical). • A dominant breast mass should be definitively diagnosed in a timely manner (old or already recorded, newly or firstly discovered, changing over time, etc.). • Even though a dominant mass in a woman under the age of 40 is most likely benign, a new dominant mass in a postmenopausal woman is most likely malignant.

G. Macellari (✉)
Surgical Breast Clinic, Hospital "Guglielmo da Saliceto", Piacenza, Italy
e-mail: g.macellari@ausl.pc.it

A.M. Pluchinotta
Breast Surgery, Policlinic of Abano Terme, Padova, Italy
e-mail: pluchinotta.alfonso@gmail.com



A.M. Pluchinotta (ed.), *The Outpatient Breast Clinic: Aiming at Best Practice*,
DOI 10.1007/978-3-319-15907-2_4

*Future directions*. The breast surgical oncologist must be highly trained in the differential diagnosis of benign breast entity, appreciate absolute and relative risk, understand genetic counselling and testing, be able to keep up with technological advances in the field, have a keen understanding of molecular diagnostic, and much more. In order to gain breast clinical experience, it is crucial to find many mentors early and lavishly utilize their support.

## 4.1 Introduction

**Clinical Practice Points**

- Consider the reasons of the patient and do not hide her doubt, if motivated, even if you could not found apparent changes.
- Accuracy of CBE is directly related to the time spent on the examination, which should be no less than 3 min per breast.
- A standard sequence should be followed to exclude normal structures and differentiate normal nodularity from a dominant mass. Ultrasound and core biopsy should normally be available at the first visit.
- In CBE it is important whichever symptom is dominant and/or unique. However, the finding may be subtle even for clinical experts.
- Through the CBE, the doctor could take the opportunity to provide the patient with education about breast awareness and breast self-examination.
- Filling in medical records and letter of resignation is mandatory for the follow-up.

Clinical breast examination (CBE) is an important skill for every physician to master. Many practitioners acknowledge receiving inadequate training on this procedure and admit CBE is not their strong point.

CBE is the weakest test of the triple diagnostic assessment, which comprises assessment by the specialist, imaging, and tissue sampling. Nonetheless, it may be decisive to solve many common symptoms as localized pain, inflammatory changes, and acute enlargement of cysts with pain of sudden onset. Moreover, the patient is strongly relying on CBE for a comprehensive evaluation, especially in case of lump or visual change discovered by the patient herself. Prior to discussing technical skills, a few considerations need to be made.

*Benign and malignant symptoms run in parallel*. Normal breast tissue in women is often somewhat nodular, and the physical examination with benign symptoms runs parallel to the examination done in order to avoid missing cancer. There is no reason to be neither optimistic nor fatalistic.

*In CBE it is important whichever symptom is dominant and/or unique*. The first goal of the physical examination is to determine whether a dominant and/or unique mass, thickening, or asymmetry is present. This is particularly important in younger women, whose breasts are more likely to be generally nodular than older women's breasts.

*The finding may be subtle even for clinical experts.* On physical examination, the palpable breast mass can be obvious or subtle; the density soft, firm, or hard; mobile or fixed to the chest wall or skin; and painful, tender, or non-tender. Moreover, the mass may have well-defined or non-discrete margins and be associated with clinical findings including skin changes or nipple discharge. However, the physical examination findings cannot always distinguish between a benign mass and a malignancy.

As to be expected, CBE sensitivity increases with larger tumour size, while obese (for the size of the breast) and younger women (for the density) receive less benefit from CBE. Nevertheless, a small number of BC undetected with conventional mammography may be found with CBE. Mammography may more accurately diagnose a BC when a lump can be felt, so that CBE is the only way to discover interval cancer.

*Suspicious symptoms should not be influenced by the phase of the menstrual cycle.* For premenopausal women, the optimum time for all breast examinations (palpation, mammography, ultrasound, MRI) is at the end of the first half of the menstrual cycle, corresponding to days 7–12 of the cycle. Nevertheless, the evaluation of a clinically suspicious mass should not be influenced by the phase of the menstrual cycle.

*A right clinical diagnosis may be not sufficiently reassuring.* Studies that have examined the usefulness of the physical examination for diagnosing benign versus malignant breast masses have found that clinicians can often make the right diagnosis, but not to a degree that is sufficiently reassuring to the clinician or patient. Also if sensibility for palpable masses may be high, roughly about 90 %, specificity in women over 30 years drops to 70 %. Actually, no single detection method is one hundred percent accurate, but a carefully performed CBE, in combination with other diagnostic procedures, will improve the chances for earlier detection of BC and maximize the patient's options for effective treatment.

*Accuracy is related to time.* Many clinicians report frustration with the lack of time given to complete a comprehensive exam. However, the accuracy of CBE is directly related to the time spent on the examination, which should be no less than (approximately) 3 min per breast.

*Be respectful of different cultural and modesty issues* in your patient population. To lower anxiety, it is important to explain with few words the rationale for each part of the exam to the patient.

## 4.2 History

A thorough history should begin with a review of the patient's concerns or symptoms and include risk factors, such as a personal and/or family history of breast or ovarian cancer and reproductive history. A thorough risk assessment is part of the evaluation of women with breast complaints, and significant negative as well as positive findings should be documented in the medical record. Some questions can give the opportunity to provide patient education throughout the exam. This will help to establish a rapport with the patient and lead to improve patient understanding and compliance.

For masses identified by the patient, subjective information about how and when the mass was first noted, if it is painful, and how it has changed over time should be recorded. Essentially, the history of presenting symptoms includes:

*Any change* in the general appearance of the breast, such as an increase or decrease in size, or a change in symmetry. New or persistent skin changes, including new nipple inversion (see Sect. 11.1.1).

*Nipple discharge*. If nipple discharge is present, whether it is bilateral, unilateral, or from one specific duct. Other important information include the timing, colour, frequency, and spontaneity of the discharge (see Sect. 10.1).

*Pain*. The characteristics of any breast pain, the relationship of symptoms to menstrual cycles (cyclic or non-cyclic), the location within the breast (or both breasts), the duration, and whether it is aggravated or alleviated by any activities or medications (see Chap. 7).

*Mass*. The presence of a breast mass and its evolution, including how it was first noted (accidentally, by breast self-examination, clinical breast examination, or mammogram), how long it has been present, and whether it has changed in size. The precise location of any breast mass (see Sect. 4.6).

*Cyclical modifications*. Whether a mass waxes and wanes during the menstrual cycle. Benign cysts may be more prominent premenstrually and regress in size during the follicular phase.

## 4.3 Physical Examination

The breast examination includes the neck, chest wall, both breasts, and axillae and is part of a complete physical examination. As told before, CBE is best performed when hormonal stimulation of the breasts is minimized, which is usually the second week after the onset of menses in premenopausal women. The timing of the breast examination is not important in postmenopausal women.

*INSPECTION*—Breast experts agree that visual inspection of the breasts is an important component of CBE. The patient should be examined in both the upright and supine positions. The patient must be disrobed from the waist up, allowing the examiner to visualize and inspect the breasts.

The breast examination is started with the patient in a seated position with her arms relaxed. The patient is then asked to raise her arms over her head so the lower part of the breasts can be inspected (Fig. 4.1). Lesions fixed to underlying tissue may present as dimpling when the arms are raised slowly overhead (Figs. 4.2 and 4.3). Point out to the patient that, if she notices skin changes as described, it is important to make an appointment right away.

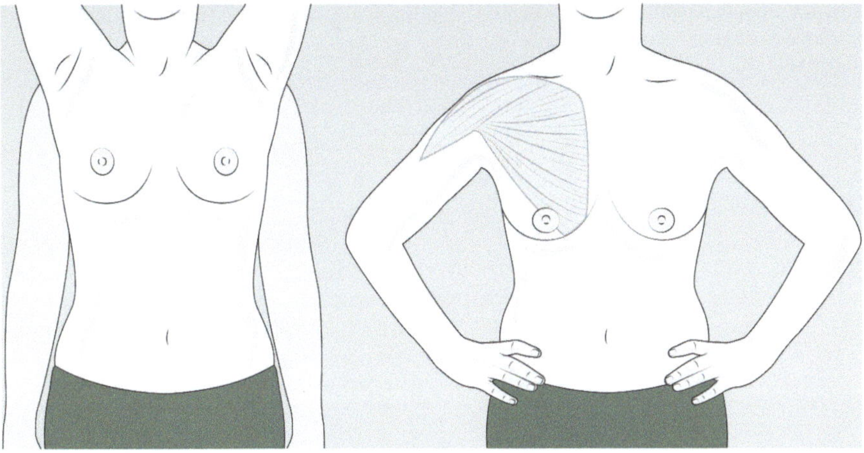

**Fig. 4.1** Inspection of the breast. *Left*: static study of the profile and the surface of the skin (arms raised and lowered). *Right*: dynamic study, since contraction of the pectoralis muscles may accentuate clinical signs

**Fig. 4.2** Minimal skin BC retraction (dimpling) noticeable when raising the ipsilateral arm

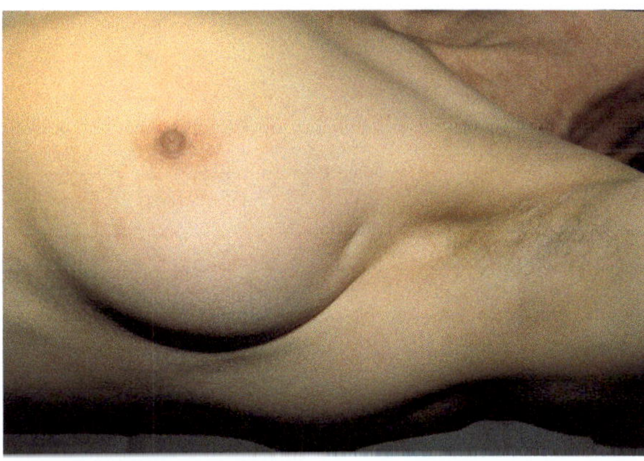

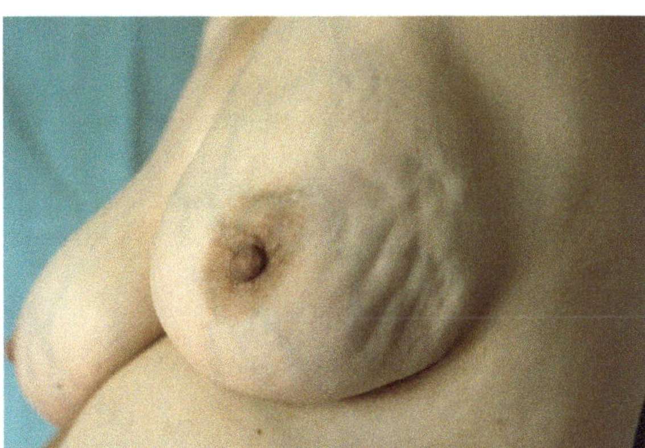

**Fig. 4.3** Large retraction of the skin noticeable only when raising the ipsilateral arm

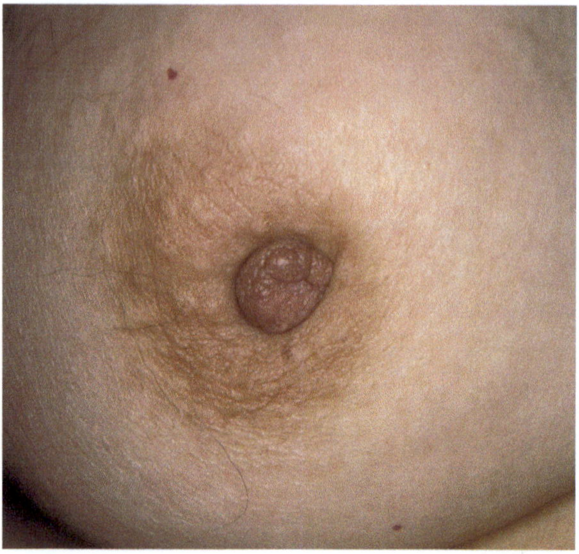

**Fig. 4.4** Nipple partially retracted as a symptom of an underlying BC

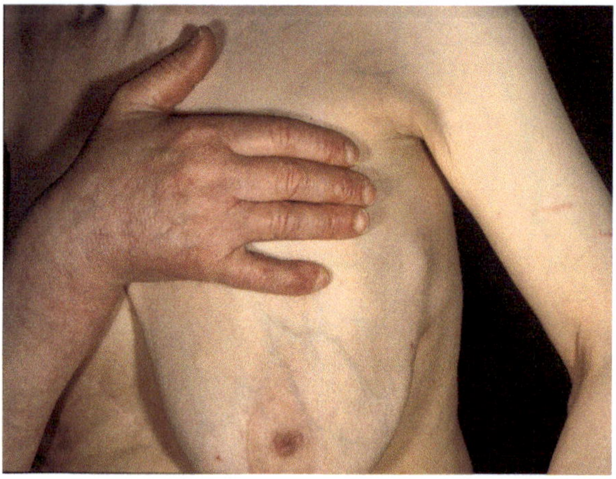

**Fig. 4.5** Very peripheral nodule (enlarging mass or extra-mammary thoraco-lateral lymph node?) of the left breast

Finally, the patient should put her hands on her hips and press in to contract the pectoral muscles so that any other areas of retraction can be visualized. Inspection of the breast includes detection of asymmetry, bulging areas, skin changes (dimpling or retraction, oedema, presence of dermatological lesions), and position of the nipple (inversion or retraction, as in Fig. 4.4). Inspection should include peripheral areas (Fig. 4.5).

*PALPATION*—A bimanual examination of the breasts should be performed while the patient is still in the sitting position, supporting the breast gently with one hand and examining the breast with the other hand (Fig. 4.6). The examination is completed with the patient's arms raised above her head. This allows the examiner to flatten the breast tissue against the patient's chest (Fig. 4.7).

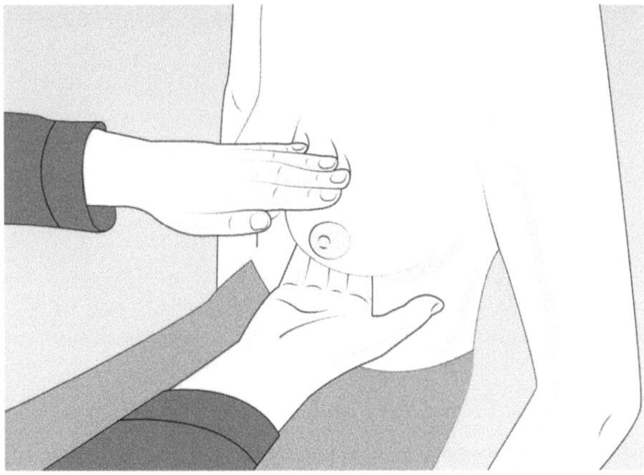

**Fig. 4.6** Bimanual palpation in the sitting position to examine the deep and posterior layers of the breast tissue

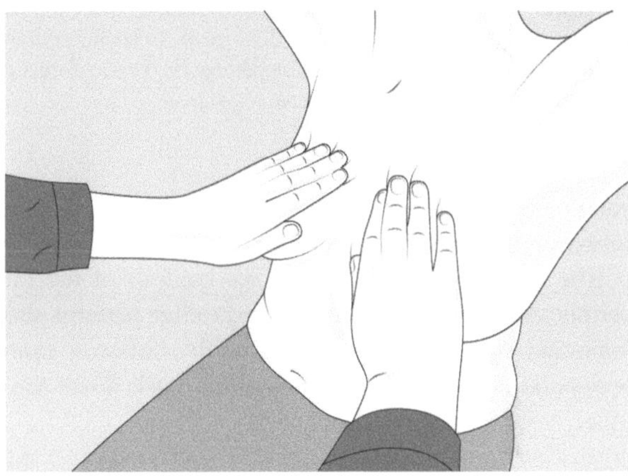

**Fig. 4.7** Bimanual palpation in the sitting position to flatten the breast against the chest wall and check glandular symmetry

In general, to examine the breast, use the pads rather than the less sensitive tips of the three middle fingers, with the hand slightly bowed (Fig. 4.8). Move the pads together as a single unit in a circular or radial way.

Though many patients and some clinicians think of the breast only as the circular mound, breast tissue actually extends from the midaxillary line to the lateral edge of the sternum and from the clavicle to infra-mammary ridge. Covering the entire perimeter is essential in order to avoid missing peripheral areas, where a disease may occur, sometimes undetectable even on mammogram.

Use a consistent pattern that will cover all of the breast tissue within the borders of the perimeter. Begin the vertical strip pattern in the upper outer quadrant. Keep the pads perpendicular to the midaxillary line throughout the exam. Palpate up and down in overlapping strips, being sure to palpate each strip passed the infra-mammary ridge and up to the clavicle. To avoid missing an area, don't lift your fingers from the skin. Be sure to include the nipple and sub-areolar area. Squeezing the nipple to illicit discharge is no longer a part of the screening CBE because only

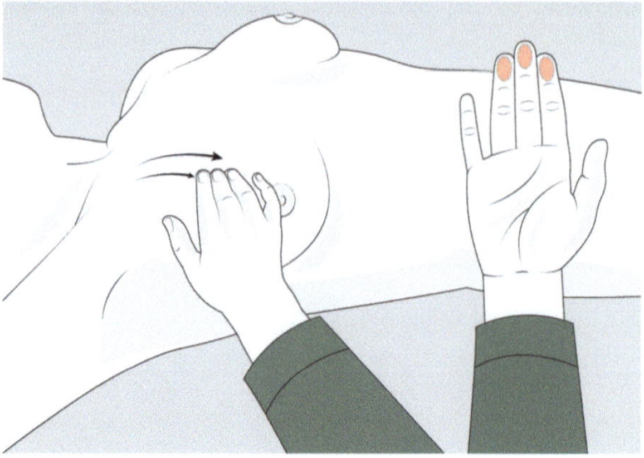

**Fig. 4.8** Palpation with the finger's pads starting from the clavicle towards the infra-mammary ridge. The pads of the second, third, and fourth fingers are the most sensitive. The pads of the fingers are rotated in concentric small *(dime-size)* circles for effective palpation of the breast. Do not pinch the breast tissue to avoid a false perception. Do not forget peripheral extension (axillary tail, subclavicular and parasternal regions)

unilateral spontaneous discharge has any diagnostic significance for breast cancer. However, discharge should be investigated if reported by the patient.

The circular pattern follows the contour of the mound and tends to miss the peripheral areas, and also radial and wedge patterns show some limitations. What is important is that all the surface of the breast is examined, without missing any peripheral areas. With each palpation, push down through the entire depth of the tissue in three sequential manners:

- *Light*: barely moving the surface of the skin
- *Medium*: to the midlevel of the tissue
- *Deep*: to the chest wall or ribs

Come back up through the tissue and slide to the next palpation. Using three levels of pressure will help detect asymmetric thickenings or masses that can occur at different depths in the breast tissue (Fig. 4.9). Keeping the hand bowed assures the use of pads which minimizes discomfort with depression. Repeating a mantra in your head of *light, medium, and deep* will help you to establish a rhythm. Be sure to elicit feedback from your patient regarding comfort level.

Palpation should include the careful application of pressure to the retroareolar region, including the lactiferous sinuses in that area, to check for abnormal discharge (Fig. 4.10). The patient herself is better able to apply concentric pressure to the retroareolar region than is a doctor seated in front of her. Thus, if questionable discharge is noted, the patient should compress the breast herself. If she has noticed the discharge at home, she has usually trained herself over a period of weeks to know exactly where she must push to elicit the discharge.

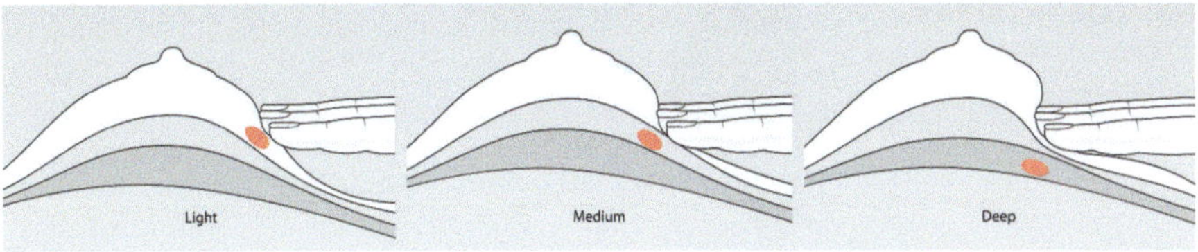


**Fig. 4.9** Varying degrees of pressure are used (*light*, *medium*, *deep*) so that a small mobile mass is not pushed away by the palpating fingers

**Fig. 4.10** Palpation of the retroareolar region. The structure of the nipple and areola complex (NAC) is different from the dominant breast tissue. The major duct area beneath the nipple is less dense and the hand detects as a hollow which is not easy to explore. Small masses may be missed or not easily detectable, unless using a technique that permits to flatten the area to the chest wall

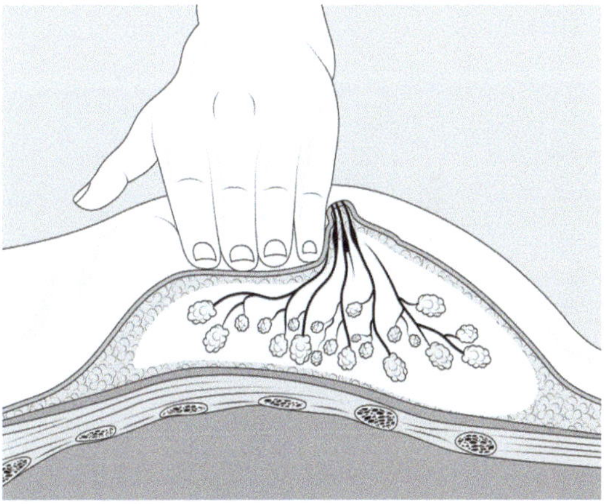

Finally, a dimple indentation underneath the breast, if present, may be elicited by a lateral pressure, as shown in Fig. 4.11.

*The Cahan position.* In the supine position sometimes the distribution of the breast tissue over the chest may be critical to a good exam. To this end, one hand could stabilize the breast whenever the other hand is used to perform the examination. An optimal position can be also accomplished with the Cahan position. Ask the patient to roll onto her hip and shoulder, opposite to the breast you are examining. Her knees should be pulled into a foetal position with her arm at her side. Place a folded towel under her lower lumbar spine for support. Have the patient roll her shoulder back towards you. Raise her arm and place the back of her hand on her forehead. It is this twisting motion that optimally pulls the breast tissue flat (Fig. 4.12).

The Cahan position offers these advantages: it spreads the breast tissue evenly, it raises the midaxillary line and upper outer quadrant for easier access and clinician comfort, and it provides support for the lower back for patient comfort. The Cahan position can be used with all patients, but is especially beneficial for those with large or pendulous breasts where stabilizing the lateral quadrants of the breast tissue is more challenging.

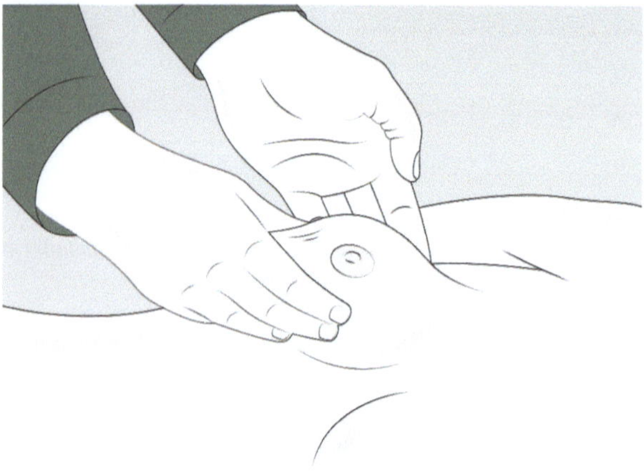

**Fig. 4.11** Search for a dimple indentation underneath the breast elicited by a lateral pressure

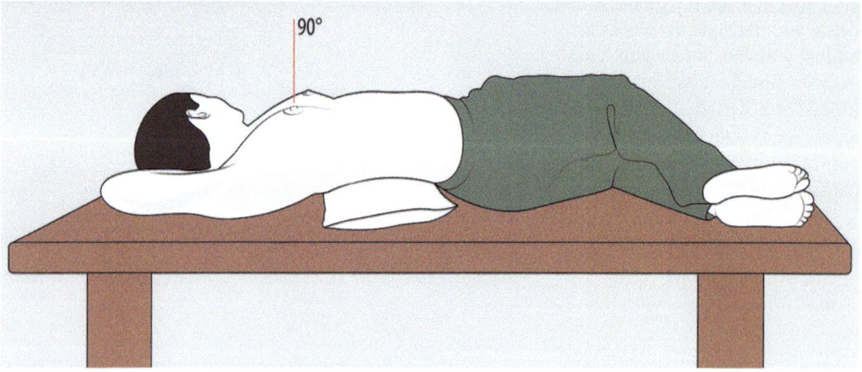


**Fig. 4.12** The Cahan position, a twisting motion that optimally pulls the breast tissue flat and positioned at 90°. The Cahan position provides a steadiness of lateral quadrants of large and pendulous breast

The entire breast must be examined, including the breast tissue that comprises the axillary tail of Spence, which extends laterally towards the axilla. To be sure that all breast tissue is included in the examination, it is best to cover a rectangular area bordered by the clavicle superiorly, the midsternum medially, the midaxillary line laterally, and the lower rib cage inferiorly.

If the pain is the main concern for the patient, pressing on the underlying chest wall to identify any area of localized tenderness may reveal if the pain arises from the breast or from the chest wall (see Sect. 7.1).

*REGIONAL LYMPHONODES EXAMINATION*—The optimal position for the examination of both the clavicular and the axillary lymph nodes is a sitting position, which allows the best access of the deepest nodes. Some clinicians prefer the lymph node exam to be the first physical contact with the patient, since the exam can be done with the gown on, reaching through the arm hole and the neck hole. In their opinion this will maintain the patient's modesty and comfort.

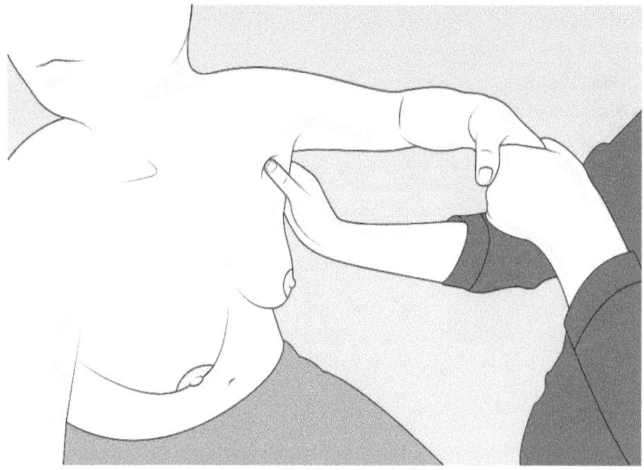

**Fig. 4.13** Palpation of the axillary nodes. Instruct the patient to drop the shoulder and take a deep breath to facilitate relaxation. Support the patient's arm and elbow with the non-examining hand to maintain optimal relaxation. Start palpating the central nodes deep in the apex of the axilla. Proceeding down the midaxillary chest wall, lift the tissue with the examining hand and gently move the pads of the fingers medially and along the border of the pectoral muscle and the pectoral node chain

Regional lymph nodes are examined with attention to the cervical, supraclavicular, infraclavicular, and axillary nodal basins. It is important to note the presence of any palpable nodes and their characteristics, whether they are soft and mobile or firm, hard, tender, fixed, or matted.

The best examination of the axillary nodes requires that the patient relax her shoulders and allow the examiner to support her arm while the axilla is palpated (Fig. 4.13). To facilitate relaxation, have the patient take a deep breath, exhale, and drop her shoulders. The palpation pattern of the axilla should resemble a diamond. First, palpate deep in the midaxilla. Then, rotate your palm anteriorly to palpate deep under the pectoralis muscle. Rotate posteriorly to palpate deep under the subscapular muscles. Finally, rotate your palm towards the ceiling to palpate under the humeral head [1]. Use the pads of the three middle fingers to avoid causing pain to the patient.

Because the clavicular nodes spiral around the clavicle, it is important to palpate above and below the clavicle (Fig. 4.14).

At last, if you palpate something of concern, note it to yourself. Complete the entire screening exam before returning to the abnormal finding to distinguish and document the characteristics. Lingering too long in one spot without explanation can cause patient anxiety.

*What must not be done or missed:*

- Underestimating the inspection
- Examining only one breast or examining the two breasts at the same time
- Grasping the gland
- Not repeating the palpation at least twice

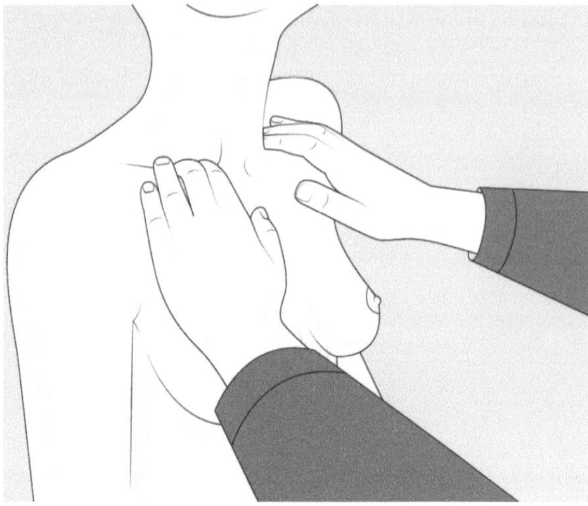

**Fig. 4.14** Palpation of the supraclavicular and infraclavicular nodes. Using firm pressure in small circular movements, palpate above and below the clavicle by applying a spiral movement

- Not checking for the presence of secretions reported by the patient
- Not checking the status of regional lymph nodes

## 4.4 Diagnosis

A breast mass is a nodule or growth of tissue that represents an aggregation of coherent material. A breast mass may be benign or malignant. A benign mass may be solid or cystic, whereas a malignant mass is typically solid. A cystic mass with solid components (complex cyst) can also be malignant.

The clinical presentation of a palpable breast mass is variable [2]. Some masses are detected on a patient's self-breast examination while others are found on a routine CBE. Some masses may be associated with pain and/or nipple discharge (blood, green, white, yellow). Trauma to the breast (e.g. car accident with seat belt, direct injury from a hard object) may result in a breast mass due to the development of fat necrosis or a hematoma. In addition, trauma may be the precipitating event to detection of an existing benign or malignant mass. Any mass after a trauma that fails to resolve within few weeks will require a complete evaluation.

Any lump in the breast obviously causes a lot of anxiety, but by no means all lumps are breast cancer. In any women presenting with a breast lump, it is important to try to differentiate those that are benign from those that may be malignant. Commonly the following features may be found on examination:

- A benign mass is usually mobile and smooth, has regular borders, and is solid or cystic in consistency.
- A malignant mass is usually firm in consistency, has irregular borders, and may be fixed to the skin or the underlying tissue. There may also be skin changes or nipple retraction.

**Table 4.1** Different levels of complexity in clinical diagnosis of breast masses

| | |
|---|---|
| Easy | Cancer with clear symptoms |
| | Simple fibroadenoma, solid, round or lobulated, mobile (can be rolled), solitary or multiple, usually in young women |
| | Simple cysts, solitary or multiple, fluid filled, fluctuating or tense, discrete and compressible, found in pre- and perimenopausal women |
| | Galactocele, a milk retention cyst common in women who are breast-feeding |
| | Symmetrical nodularity |
| | Sheer mastodynia, cyclical or persistent, bilateral or unilateral |
| | Most cases of nipple discharge |
| Difficult | Pseudotumoral inflammation as periductal mastitis |
| | Asymmetrical mastosis |
| | Expansive tumours |
| Hard | Fat necrosis, without a proven previous trauma |
| | Non-nodular invasive lobular carcinoma |
| | Deceitful inflammatory BC |
| Impossible | Occult cancer, as such |
| | Most of non-invasive BCs |

The spectrum of the difficulties likely to be encountered in the diagnosis is very broad. Differentiation is often still not easy and to err on the side of safety is wise. The differential diagnosis of a palpable breast mass includes benign and malignant lesions. Palpable breast masses are very common in women, and most palpable masses are benign. Approximately 90 % or more of palpable breast masses in women in their 20s to early 50s are benign; however, excluding BC is a crucial step in the assessment of a breast mass in a woman of any age. Different levels of complexity in clinical diagnosis of breast masses are listed in Table 4.1.

## 4.5 Special Conditions

Men, women who are breast-feeding, and women with implants, disabilities, or mastectomy scars should receive regular CBE. Some adaptations of the technique are needed for each situation.

*FAKE BREAST LUMPS* may occur, usually during the first examination. Their rapid detection is crucial to ease psychological reactions.

*Prominent fat lobules* are often easily palpable and one may become more prominent than usual. This is seen most frequently along the inferior margin of the breast or over the axillary tail, usually due to pressure from a brassiere. The superficial nature of the lesion, its site, soft smooth consistency, and softness to a needle point will usually allow confident diagnosis.

*Prominent rib* is not uncommon for a patient, usually young. It appears like normal breast tissue over a normal prominent rib. Sometimes the rib is asymmetrical—more often it is identical to the opposite side and it is difficult to know why the patient has suddenly become aware of the rib. Only occasionally, radiology of the rib cage is necessary before reassuring the patient.

*Intramammary lymph nodes* are seen in 5 % of mammographic studies. They are usually confined to the axillary tail of the breast and impalpable since they are small and embedded in the breast stroma. Sometimes they may enlarge sufficiently to be palpable. Intramammary lymph nodes are usually less than 1 cm in diameter, slightly elongated and a characteristic appearance on mammography: a circumscribed oval opacity with a central or peripheral lucency that represents fat within the hilum. The majority of lesions have a lower density at the centre than at the periphery, and sometimes a hilar notch may be seen. Ultrasound shows a hypoechoic area with a similar shape described on mammography. Lymphocytes are found on cytology. It is usually possible to make a diagnosis and avoid surgery.

*External mammary lymph nodes* may be detected along the lateral border of the breast, especially in young, tall, and skinny women. Nodes lie along the lower border of the pectoralis minor, in association with the lateral thoracic vessels. Their mobility is typically lateral, not vertical, as they are joined to vertical lymphatic vessel.

*Extrusion of breast implant.* Breast implants in women with augmentation mammoplasty may provoke changes that adversely affect the clinical examination and the diagnosis. Irregularities or diverticulae of the capsule or implant may present as a palpable lump due to prominent peripheral partial extrusion of prosthesis. More rarely, the capsule that inevitably forms around an implant may become calcified and mimic some hard lumps, which are firm and feel like bone.

*RECURRENT BREAST LUMP* following biopsy. Many breast lumps, such as fibroadenoma and cysts as well proliferative lesion and carcinoma in situ, show a tendency to be multiple over a period of time. However, a new lump may be reassessed in the same way as the original lump. A different situation arises when a lump appears in the region of a previous biopsy. It must also be reassessed completely but a number of additional factors need consideration:

- A recurrent fibroadenoma may represent inadequate removal of the stalk or involvement of adjacent lobules, so that excision biopsy rather than enucleation is indicated.
- A recurrent cyst is common and requires no treatment other than re-aspiration provided the rules governing aspiration are adhered to.
- The breast parenchyma may fail to heal following a biopsy, leaving a palpable dip with prominent edge in the breast tissue, frequently mistaken for a new mass.
- Finally, a recurrent lump following biopsy of nodularity may be due to pathology that was missed at the initial biopsy (usually detected after a short interval) or to progression of the original lesion or to a new lesion.

Such a lump must be carefully reassessed with a view to avoiding biopsy, if not necessary, or to repeat biopsy in case of missed lesions or proliferative lesions where atypiae were originally found.

## 4.6 Documentation

Document all aspects of the exam carefully, preferably on a standardized form with a diagram of the breast. Thorough documentation will help assure continuity of care, facilitate referral for mammography or to another specialist, and is a vital risk management strategy.

The location of the mass as well as any abnormality found on examination should be accurately documented as shape, texture, and mobility. The size of any mass should be measured in centimetres and its location, mobility, and consistency recorded. It is helpful to record the location of any abnormality by documenting both the position on the breast and the distance in cm from the areola. In this manner, the precise location can be easily identified on subsequent follow-up examinations, by the initial examiner as well as other practitioners. The "clock system" can be used for documentation, comparing the breast to a clock and using the location on the clock to indicate the location of a lesion (Fig. 4.15).

The entire examination should be clearly and completely documented in detail, including significant negatives, even if it is completely normal.

*A plan of action* is an essential component of the CBE. In most case a triple diagnostic assessment is required. Be sure to specify whether you are ordering screening or diagnostic imaging. A diagnostic mammogram should be scheduled as soon as

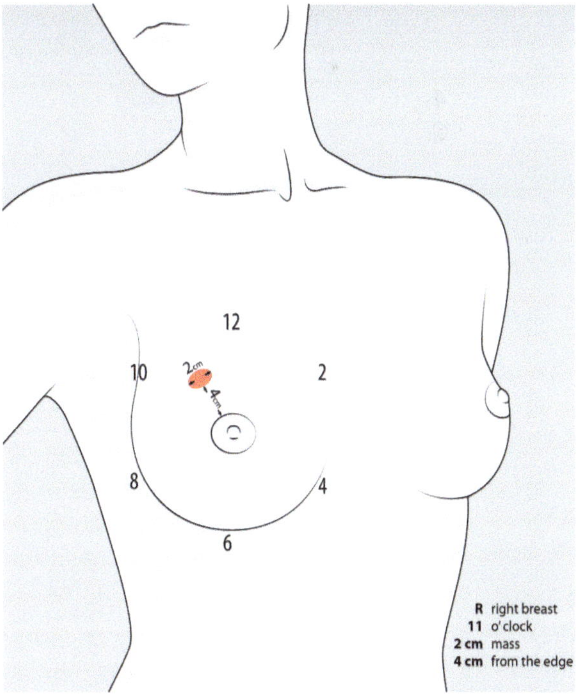


**Fig. 4.15** The precise location and measured size of a mass can be effectively described using the arms of a clock. The mass in this illustration should be recorded as follows: right breast, dominant 2-cm mass at 11 o'clock, 4 cm from the areolar border

possible. If your patient has an abnormal clinical finding or abnormal imaging result, further referral and follow-up are critical. If your CBE has been systematic, normal mammogram never trumps your abnormal finding.

## References

1. California Department of health services. Clinical breast examination: proficiency and risk management. 2005. https://qap.sdsu.edu/resources/tools/pdf/lymphnode.pdf. Accessed 14 July 2014.
2. Klein S. Evaluation of palpable breast masses. Am Fam Phys. 2005;71:1731–8.

## Further Reading

Hindle WH. Breast examination. In: Hindle WH, editor. Breast care, a clinical guidebook for women's primary health care providers. New York: Springer; 1999.

Nelson AL. Controversies regarding mammography, breast self-examination, and clinical breast examination. Obstet Gynecol Clin North Am. 2013;40:413–27.

Schwab FD, Huang DJ, Schmid SM, Schotzau A, Guth U. Self-detection and clinical breast examination: comparison of the two "classical" physical examination methods for the diagnosis of breast cancer. Breast. 2015;24:90–2.

**Websites in Appendix**: *Breast Self-Examination*, A-4.5

# Imaging in Breast-Related Diseases

# 5

Gianni Saguatti and Elisabetta Tosi

## Contents




G. Saguatti (✉)
Department of Radiology, Mammographic Screening, Bellaria Hospital, Bologna, Italy
e-mail: gianni.saguatti@ausl.bologna.it

E. Tosi
Department of Radiology, Mammographic Screening, USL16, Padova, Italy
e-mail: elisabetta.tosi@sanita.padova.it







A.M. Pluchinotta (ed.), *The Outpatient Breast Clinic: Aiming at Best Practice*,
DOI 10.1007/978-3-319-15907-2_5

**Abstract**

• Currently mammography, ultrasound and magnetic resonance are the best radiological imaging modalities for both diagnosis and local staging of breast cancer. To date, there is no evidence on the utility of other emerging diagnostic tools. • The results of imaging are very different if performed as screening procedures in asymptomatic women or as diagnostic procedure in a symptomatic patient. • Mammography is the best technique for a panoramic image; ultrasound is an essential component for localised symptoms and for guided tissue sampling. • Mammography is the technique of choice for a BC screening protocol, but MRI is the technique of choice for very young women at high risk.

*Future directions*. Emerging technologies in breast imaging have resulted in an explosion of areas of investigation: the newer versions of digital mammography including tomosynthesis and digital subtraction mammography, the latest individualised screening strategies that stratify patients with different tools especially for women at high risk and the wide-ranging use of imaging to monitor and adjust efficacy of neoadjuvant regimens in the course of therapy.

## 5.1 Mammography

**Clinical Practice Points**

- Mammography is very accurate when there is a lump in the breast that can be felt (diagnostic/clinical mammography), but much less accurate when the lesion cannot be felt (screening mammography).
- In screening mammography, the use of a double reading by two independent radiologists reduces the rate of human error by 15 %. Sometimes a third reader is used to arbitrate on disagreements.
- Mammography should be performed for all palpable lesions which cannot be characterised as definitively benign.
- There are no absolute mammographic criteria that distinguish malignant from benign lesions. A negative mammogram does not rule out BC.
- Radiological breast density is an important factor in relation to BC risk. Comparison with previous mammograms whenever possible, additional views, spot compression and magnification views may be appropriate.

### 5.1.1 Overview

Mammography is the best radiological imaging modality to identify and characterise palpable and non-palpable, clinically occult lesions. Locating the lesion and establishing its extension are also important as well as identifying multiple (multifocal/multicentric) lesions. Mammography is also able to detect the majority of bilateral synchronous cancers, found in 1–3 % of cases.

- *Screening mammography* is addressed to asymptomatic women and includes an interpretation of the results. In order to reduce the rate of human error for about 15 %, a double reading by two independent radiologists is currently used. It is also expected that a third reader may arbitrate the disagreement. Screening mammography allows to detect tumours that cannot be clinically felt and can find microcalcifications that may, or may not, indicate the presence of BC.

At the present time, mammography is the diagnostic tool of choice for screening for early BC. The sensitivity of mammography in women over the age of 50 has been estimated to be around 85 % (range 70 to >90 %), while it was reported to be lower (range 60–75 %) in women between 40 and 49 years. The advent of full-field digital mammography (FFDM) is giving a further positive clinical impact on early detection of BC in younger women. Moreover, with FFDM *Picture Archiving and Communication System* (*PACS*) technology provides economical storage of and convenient access to images from multiple modalities [1]. Screening mammography concepts are discussed in Sect. 2.2.

*Diagnostic* (or better *clinical*) *mammography* is employed in symptomatic women in order to obtain radiological imaging in the presence of symptoms as definite nodules, indiscrete mass or skin changes. Diagnostic mammography may also be used to better evaluate changes found during standard screening mammography or when screening mammography is difficult to obtain because of special circumstances, such as the presence of breast implants. In such circumstances, additional mammograms are required.

Diagnostic mammography is above all a personalised in-depth analysis, much more than the health measure endorsed by screening mammography. In this way mammography can accurately diagnose over 95 % of cases when there is 'something that can be clinically detected', but only 50 % of cases when the disease cannot be felt.

*Candidates* for diagnostic mammography are all symptomatic patients, even when diagnosis is established. Pregnant women too should have a mammogram when a highly suspicious finding is discovered. Women less than 20 (or maybe 30) years old, instead, should not have a mammogram, because the data regarding the risk itself are inconsistent, even if the risk of a single mammogram at a young age is still low

*Radiation-induced BC*. Few data are available for exposure to low doses, as those used in modern mammography. Extrapolation from existing data suggests two excess BC deaths might result from exposing 1 million women aged >45 years to MGD of 1 mGy. Since in one million women 1500 BC cases are expected with a reduced mortality by about 40 %, with 300 lives saved, the risk/benefit ratio is 300:2.

### 5.1.2 Techniques

*Screen-film mammography* (*SFM*). Screen-film mammography is still the single most common tool for screening and diagnostic detection of BC. However, it has some limitations: contrast resolution may be not ideal, spatial resolution is limited (but in some cases better than digital), and film degradation occurs over the years.

*Computed radiography* (CR) uses very similar equipment to conventional radiography except that, instead of using a film, an imaging plate made of photostimulable phosphor is used. After x-ray exposure, the imaging plate is run through a special laser scanner, or CR reader, that reads and digitises the image. The digital image can then be viewed and enhanced using software that has functions very similar to other conventional digital image-processing software, such as contrast, brightness, filtration and zoom. However, quality of CR, as compared to FFDG, is lower in terms of contrast and spatial resolution.

*Full-field digital mammography* (*FFDM*). Digital mammography has more potential advantages, because it gives images that can be processed in different ways like any digital image (improve contrast, magnify specific areas, etc.). Moreover FFDM mammography allows the use of computer-aided detection and diagnosis software and can be sent to be interpreted or consulted at a different place (teleradiology). Moreover FFDM reduces patient radiation dose.

Comparing SFM and FFDM, the cancer detection rate theoretically is the same, but FFDM used for screening has a lower recall rate and higher positive biopsy rate. Although this difference is not significant, a higher cancer detection rate and positive predictive value for FFDM is observed mainly in women under the age of 50.

*Digital breast tomosynthesis* (*DBT*) and spiral *computed tomography* (*CT*) are other radiological procedures for the study of the breast, briefly illustrated in Sect. 5.4.

### 5.1.3 Findings

*The normal mammogram.* The normal mammographic image is the combination of various structural elements:

- Nodular opacities, corresponding to lobules
- Linear opacities corresponding to ducts, to support connective tissue and vessels
- Homogeneous opacity, corresponding to fibrous tissue
- Radiolucent areas, corresponding to adipose tissue

The combination of these different opacities and transparencies originates five types of mammogram (four in other classifications).

- *Type 1* is the most common in premenopausal women, and the different components will appear represented in a uniform manner (about 25 % each).
- *Types 2–3*, the most characteristic of menopause, are the outcome of processes of involution, with more common prevalence of fatty tissue. Type 3 is distinguished by a greater evidence of the retroareolar ducts and fibrosis.
- *Type 4* is characterised by a preponderance of nodular opacities (at least 50 %), while the other components are equally represented.
- *Type 5* is characterised by extensive fibrosis (at least 80 %), while the other three components are poorly represented. Types 4 and 5, configuring breasts clinically and radiographically 'dense', can be seen in all age groups.

It is important to consider that some therapies may alter the pattern by increasing parenchymal density, as in hormone replacement therapy (HRT), or reducing it, as

**Table 5.1** Findings suggesting benign disorders for well-defined radiological lesions

| Radiolucent lesions | High-density lesions |
|---|---|
| Lipoma | Phyllodes tumour |
| Cyst lipoid | Cyst |
| Galactocele | Abscess |
| Mixed density lesions | Hematoma |
| Fibroadenolipoma | Lymphadenopathy |
| Galactocele | Atheroma |
| Intramammary lymph node | A differential diagnosis may be required with |
| Hematoma | Carcinoma (medullary, solid) |
| Low-density lesions | Atheroma |
| Fibroadenoma | Sarcoma |
| Cyst | Metastasis in breast |
| Giant fibroadenoma | |
| Phyllodes tumour | |
| Mucinous carcinoma | |
| Papillary carcinoma | |
| Abscess | |
| Cavernous haemangioma | |

Note that same lesion may have different patterns

in therapies with selective oestrogen-receptor modulators (SERM), such as tamoxifen and raloxifene.

*Limits*. The errors of diagnostic mammography depend on technical or human factors and are more common in young women with dense or striking fibrocystic dysplasia. Mammography could have a false-negative rate up to 20–30 %. Reasons for false-negative results are as follows:

- *Mass hidden* within dense breast tissue, as the most common reason
- *Technical errors* due to flaws of technology or the inherent limitations of the equipment, inadequate compression and improper placement that does not include all of the breast, so excluding peripheral lesions, as in the submammary crease and in parasternal and subclavicular location, and missed retroglandular lesions because of the inability to pull the breast forward enough
- *Human error*, as inattention for small lesions as infiltrating lobular carcinoma presents with an uneven opacity.

For one or more of these reasons, negative mammogram in the setting of a palpable breast mass requires additional procedures to rule out malignancy. In any case mammography can be used to exclude BC, and an US guided biopsy should be performed for all palpable lesions, which cannot be characterised as definitively benign.

*FINDINGS SUGGESTING BENIGN DISORDERS* are mainly radiological opacities with well-defined margins, listed as related to their density in Table 5.1. Defined borders are characteristic of benign lesions (Fig. 5.1); nevertheless, some

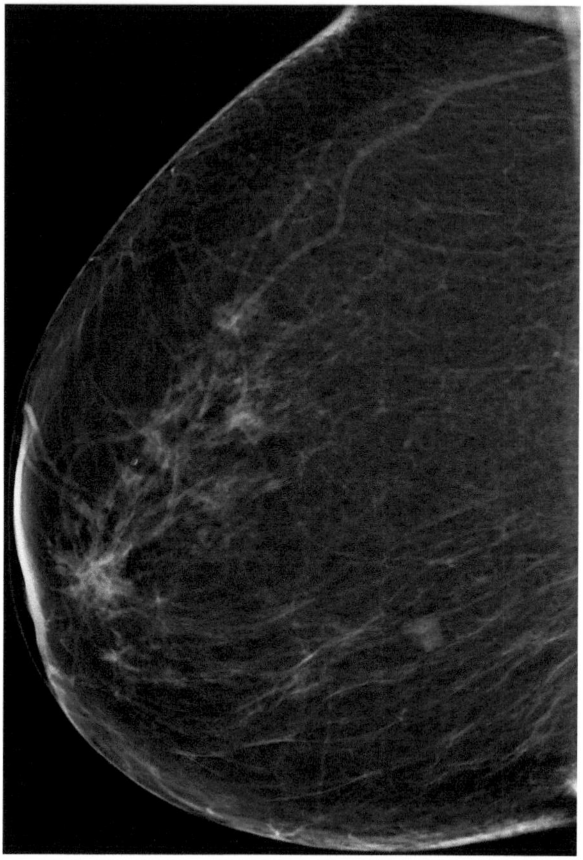

**Fig. 5.1** Probably benign mass with mostly circumscribed margins. A core-needle biopsy (CNB) should be performed to exclude malignancy. In the case of negative result, follow-up should be planned to establish the long-term stability

well-defined high-density opacities could be misinterpreted as benign while are corresponding to fast-growing tumours as medullary or solid BC [2].

*FINDINGS SUGGESTING MALIGNANT DISORDERS.* Findings suggesting malignant disorders are listed in Table 5.2. Ill-defined borders, spicules and distortion are the main characteristics of a malignant mass (Fig. 5.2). Well-defined but lobulated borders are an intermediate feature, shared between benign and malignant lesions.

Spicules represent fibrous reaction to the growth of the mass that usually is dense in the centre. Histologically, the tumour may or may not extend along the spicules. Spiculated abnormality should be considered also to be associated to postsurgical or radial scar (benign) and area of fat necrosis. Apparently normal asymmetric breast tissue could be suspicious also without evidence of architectural distortion, even though it can be found in 3 % of healthy women.

Small malignant findings (Fig. 5.3), if surrounded by connective tissue and without calcifications, are mammographically detectable only when they are located

**Table 5.2** Findings suggesting malignant disorders

| Main findings |
|---|
| Solid mass with ill-defined borders |
| Irregular or spiculated mass |
| Architectural distortion |
| Less common findings |
| Enlarging solid, well-circumscribed mass |
| Developing density compared with previous films |
| Focal asymmetric density |
| Skin thickening |
| Nipple retraction |
| Enlarged and dense axillary lymph nodes |
| *Spiculated abnormality* should be considered with: |
| Postsurgical or radial scar (benign) |
| Area of fat necrosis |
| *Apparently normal asymmetric breast tissue* with or without evidence of architectural distortion (constitutional in 3 % of healthy women) |
| Some typical semiological findings |
| *Infiltrating ductal carcinoma*: high attenuation mass with spiculated margins and focal distortion |
| *Infiltrating lobular carcinoma*: focal distortion with inhomogeneous density |
| *Ductal carcinoma in situ*: cluster of pleomorphic microcalcifications |
| *Pure mucinous carcinoma*: circumscribed opacity with distinct margins |
| *Medullary carcinoma*: lobulated opacity circumscribed oval or round |
| *Inflammatory carcinoma*: diffuse thickening of trabecular density diffusely increased |
| *Metastases* from extramammary primitiveness: round opacity with distinct margins |

at the edge of the breast parenchyma or cause parenchymal asymmetry and/or skin/nipple retraction. Also calcifying diffuse malignancies could be missed by the radiologist, unless additional mammograms or ultrasound are performed.

*CALCIFICATION*. Calcifications are another characteristic of cancer. Calcifying neoplasms, unlike non-calcifying cancers, are radiographically detectable at a relatively early stage, long before they are manifested clinically and also long before they exhibit malignant features at ultrasound or MRI. These relatively slow-growing lesions are definitely in the domain of mammography, and because of this, mammography is still essential for the early detection of BC. The most important elements in the analysis of calcifications are morphology and distribution, but also appearance of calcifications over time.

*Morphology*. Rounds, rings, needles and parallel lines are morphological features of benign lesions, due mainly to sediments of calcium to the bottom of cysts, to the calcified fibrous tissue or to vascular calcifications that have distinctive parallel track appearance. Large calcifications (popcorn-like) in a mass more likely correspond to a benign lesion such as an involuting fibroadenoma or papilloma.

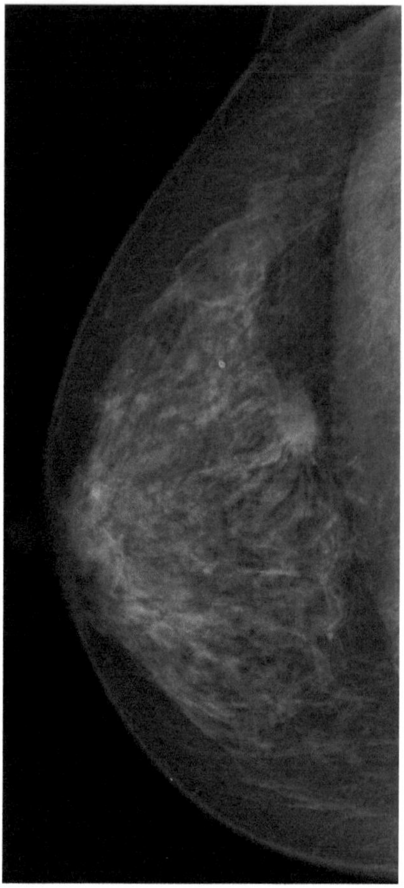

**Fig. 5.2** Mammogram of a typical BC: irregular, dense, spiculated mass lesion, more conspicuous on post-compression view and associated with architectural distortion. No suspicious microcalcifications are noted

Calcifications associated with malignancy are <0.5 mm in diameter and vary in size and shape. Most typical calcification associated to intraductal carcinoma are pleomorphic, linear and branch-shaped (as expression of casting duct) and/or granular (Fig. 5.4).

*Distribution* of benign calcification is in large round areas, while malignant ones have a clustered, linear or segmental distribution. A synopsis of diagnostic features of calcification is shown in Table 5.3. Note that the presence of typical benign calcification does not exclude coexistent malignancy and each area of calcification within a breast should be judged separately.

*Appearance over time.* Intraductal neoplasia (or intraductal component of an infiltrating BC) should be suspected whenever a new microcalcification cluster appears within a short period of time. If the nature of clustered microcalcifications remains uncertain, it is better to recommend a core-needle or vacuum biopsy under digital stereotactic guidance than the usual short-term follow-up.

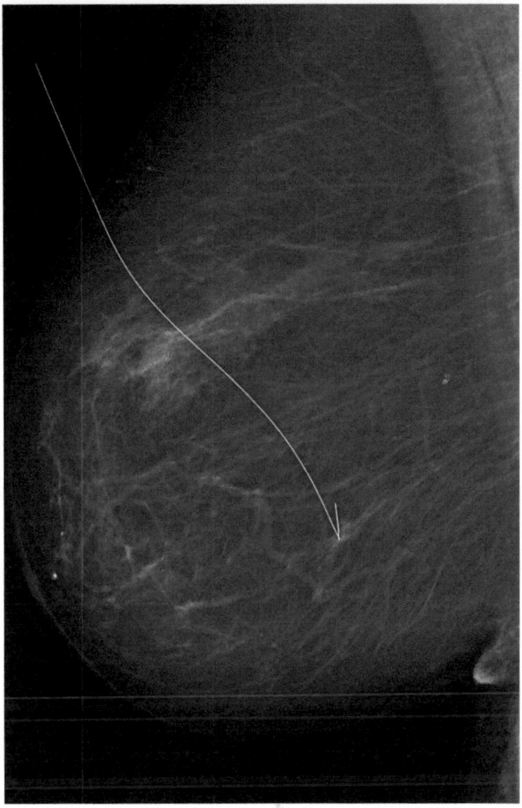

**Fig. 5.3** A typical clinically occult BC detected on a screening mammogram. A small mass with ill-defined irregular margins. The spot compression magnification provides improved resolution and shows a margin which is clearly spiculated with microcalcifications that may not have been visible on the standard image. Mandatory surgical biopsy requires a hook-wire preoperative localisation, as shown in the mammogram

The biopsy can be done quickly on an outpatient basis, is well tolerated and can provide a definitive diagnosis. It also relieves patient anxiety by eliminating the waiting time for future follow-ups. Moreover, follow-ups are often unrewarding because benign adenosis and particularly low-grade in situ carcinomas calcify very slowly over a period of years or even decades and the calcifications may regress or disappear completely on progression to an invasive neoplasm. Short-term follow-up tends to increase more than allay the patient's (and doctor's) level of uncertainty.

### 5.1.4 Mammography in Special Situations

*Calcifications.* Unilateral magnification mammogram (magnification compression views) is the primary technique for further investigation of calcifications. Geometrically magnified images can provide better image quality and, therefore, more accurate diagnosis than electronically zoomed images.

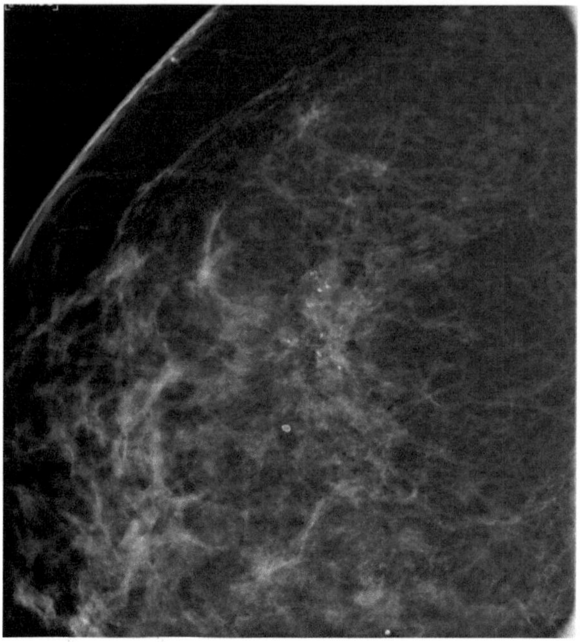

**Fig. 5.4** Area of pleomorphic microcalcifications (magnified view), partly distributed within linear branching arrays. A classic high-grade intraductal carcinoma with calcified necrotic tumour debris within the duct

**Table 5.3** Diagnostic features of radiological calcifications

| Feature | Benign | Malignant |
|---|---|---|
| Distribution | Single, areas or diffuse | Clustered (>5 in a small area) |
| Cluster shapes | Round | Linear, triangular, rhomboid |
| Form | Rounds, popcorn, rings, needles, tea cups, parallel lines | Casting (linear and branching), granular, pleomorphic |
| Size | Uniform | Variable |
| Density | Uniform | Variable within and between calcifications |

*Tissue sampling*. It is always advisable to obtain the mammogram prior to any microinvasive procedure. After core-needle biopsy, it is recommended to wait 2 weeks or more so that tissue changes (as hematoma) can resolve.

*Surgery*. Being sure to acquire mammograms prior to surgery is essential. After surgery mammography to determine need for re-excision should wait 2–3 weeks for oedema to resolve. Focal skin thickening and retraction at surgical site together with variable amount of distortion and/or mass at the tumour bed jeopardises the results.

*Radiation therapy*. After radiation therapy, oedema is usually distributed in the gravity-affected portions of the breast, mostly periareolar and inferiorly. Coarse trabecular changes and early calcifications of fat necrosis may be indistinguishable from malignancy. Infrequent oil cysts are observed.

*Follow-up*. To evaluate for new mass/calcifications, a new baseline mammogram 6 months after radiation therapy should be obtained. Lumpectomy site should always be followed up with magnification, and presence of calcifications or unusual distortions take close-up views every 6 months for the first 3 years after surgery. However, except in justified cases, short-interval mammography after conservative breast surgery adds little benefit and dramatically increases material and psychological costs.

## 5.2 Ultrasound Scanning

**Clinical Practice Points**

- Ultrasound scanning (US) is a diagnostic rather than a screening procedure, more targeted for the study of localised breast lesion than for an overall view.
- Since US is less affected by breast density, it shows a better diagnostic performance than mammography in symptomatic young patients and in women with radiographically dense breasts.
- US is the most operator-dependent of all imaging modalities.
- US guided localisation and sampling is a first-choice diagnostic tool in most cases.
- US may not replace mammography in women older than 40 years, but may equally give an important contribution to diagnosis.

### 5.2.1 Overview

Besides mammography, ultrasound is the technique of choice for further investigation of focal symptomatic breast problems at all ages. Under 35 years of age, when the risk of BC is very low, it is usually the only staging technique required. Over 35 years of age it should be used in association with mammography.

Ultrasound is less sensitive than mammography for the early signs of BC and is therefore not used for screening. However, ultrasound does increase detection of small BC in women who have a dense background pattern on mammography. Moreover, ultrasound is the technique of first choice in the guidance of biopsy of both palpable and non-palpable breast if visible on scanning. The characteristic and main indications of breast ultrasound are shown in Table 5.4.

Ultrasound is an easy performing aid in differential diagnosis between cystic and solid nodules, as well as in differentiation between benign and malignant nodules.

*CYST*. Sonographic features of a simple cyst include well-circumscribed shape, smooth walls with sharp anterior and posterior borders and anechoic signal with posterior acoustic enhancement. Cysts may display calcifications in their periphery and do not increase in size in postmenopausal women, unless they use HRT.

All cysts that do not meet strict criteria are, by default, classified as *complex* cysts. The vast majority of complex cysts fall within the broad spectrum of

**Table 5.4** Ultrasound scanning advantages and diagnostic features

| |
|---|
| The best method to differentiate solid vs. cystic lesions which have: |
| Circumscribed margins |
| Sharp anterior and posterior walls |
| No internal echoes |
| Posterior enhancement |
| The best method to guide tissue sampling by FNA and CNB |
| Easy performing aid: |
| In benign-malignant differentiation of solid nodules |
| In determining BC: |
| Skin invasion |
| Superficial fascia involvement |
| Muscle invasion |
| Findings suspicious for malignancy |
| *Solid hypoechoic non-oval area* with taller (antiparallel or perpendicular to the skin) than wider (parallel to the skin) span that may denote fast growth and invasion of tissue |
| *Irregular margins* |
| *Acoustic shadowing*, associated with malignancy in about 60 % of cases |
| *Anterior echogenic rim*, sometimes corresponding to desmoplastic reaction caused by invasion |
| *Multiple lobulations* (>4 lobules) |
| *Abnormal vascularity* found in Doppler ultrasound |
| *Inside calcifications*, although poorly characterised |

fibrocystic change. For these reasons, the majority of complex breast cysts are not worrisome and do not need to be aspirated or biopsied [3]. With the improved resolution of current high-resolution equipment, a large percentage of breast cysts appear *complex* or *dirty*. This is because there is real stuff within most breast cysts, due to fibrocystic change. With older equipment these internal cells and debris were not visible, and the cysts appeared simple. Internal contents within breast cysts are part of the spectrum of fibrocystic change and include protein globs, cellular debris, cholesterol crystals, foam cells and apocrine cells, floating and papillary.

*FINDINGS SUGGESTING BENIGN DISORDERS*. Benign characteristics of solid nodules are as follows:

- Well-circumscribed, slightly hyperechoic homogeneous structure
- Wider than deep morphology with major axis parallel to the plane of the skin
- Regular gently curving smooth polilobular (<3) margins
- Thin echogenic pseudocapsule in a wider than deep nodule that probably represents normal compressed tissue consistent with a non-infiltrative process

Lesion contour and shape are considered to be the main features that allow in differentiating benign and malignant lesions, the former with high sensitivity and the latter with high specificity. When one aspect does not agree with other findings, tissue sampling (FNA or CNB) is mandatory (Fig. 5.5).

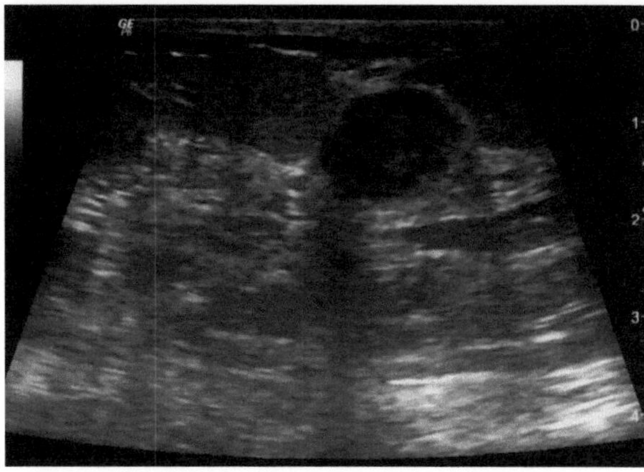

**Fig. 5.5** Ultrasound scan of one lesion with prevailing, but not all, features of benignity: relatively uniform hypoechoic mass, quite delimited margins, transverse diameter wider than taller, posterior acoustic enhancement and no calcifications. According to age, a core-needle biopsy (CNB) should be performed to exclude malignancy

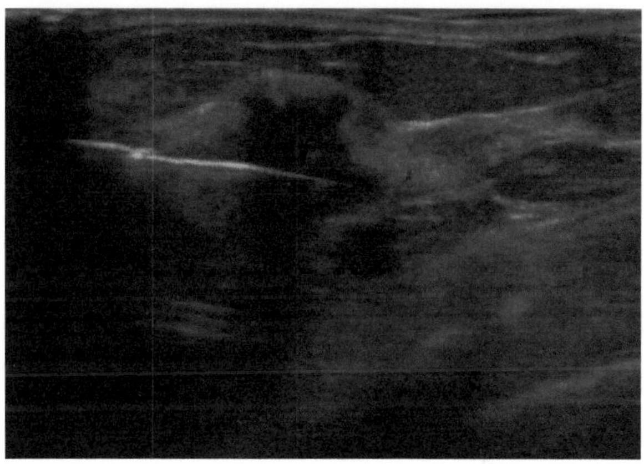

**Fig. 5.6** Ultrasound scan of a typical BC: significantly hypoechoic mass, with irregular and angular margins, taller than wider with a vertical axis and a tree shape, thick echogenic capsule and posterior shadowing. A CNB is the best procedure to get a reliable diagnosis. As shown in the US image, the needle is positioned in the centre of the lesion under US guidance

Among solid nodules, the appearance of intraparenchymal lymph nodes, small, round or kidney-shaped, homogeneous to the periphery with echogenic hilum is typical.

*FINDINGS SUGGESTING MALIGNANT DISORDERS*. Malignant characteristics (with positive predictive values) include the following (Fig.5.6):

- Sonographic spiculation (90 %), that is, alternate hypo-/hyperechoic lines radiating perpendicularly from surface of nodules
- Taller than wide morphology (80 %), except in certain solid expansive G3 breast cancer
- Micro- or small lobulations (75 %), 1–2 mm on the surface, with risk of malignancy related to numbers
- *Thick* hyperechoic halo (75 %)
- Markedly hypoechoic nodule (70 %)
- Sonographic posterior acoustic shadowing (50 %)
- Branching pattern (30 %), that is, multiple projections from the nodule within or around ducts extending away from the nipple, usually seen in larger tumours
- Punctate calcifications (25 %) which usually do not shadow
- Heterogeneous echotexture
- Ill-defined margins

The study of the blood supply with Power Doppler (associated with vocal fremitus) is another element that helps distinguish malignant from benign lesions. In cancer, vibrations are conducted along tumour infiltration into centre; hence, colour pixels run into the centre of the tumour and fill it in. Focal and considerable vascularity with multiple poles is generally related to malignancy, while the absence of vascularisation or the presence of a single pole is suggestive of benign lesions. These are all situations that require pathological sampling.

*Potential pitfalls* in breast ultrasound practice are as follows:

- Not correlating ultrasound with mammogram images. The operator must know where the lesion is located in the breast and its likely nature.
- Reviewing static images of breast pathology without watching them in real time. This is a very significant potential pitfall for the misdiagnosis of breast pathology.

### 5.2.2 Ultrasound in Special Situations

With the high resolution of the newest apparatus, US should be considered even working up on microcalcifications. In cases they are visible on US so that it is possible to supply a tissue diagnosis, US may spare the patient the inconvenience of a stereotactic biopsy.

In the presence of breast implants, breast US gives a good evaluation about the integrity of prosthesis and of fibrous capsule in case of rupture or fluid collections.

If malignancy is diagnosed, bilateral US of the breast and axilla should be performed for loco-regional staging of the disease. In advanced disease US could help in determining superficial fascia involvement, depth and distance and potential muscle invasion.

After surgery US could represent the first imaging modality after clinical examination in patients treated by mastectomy. US of the axillary and supraclavicular region is also useful in the identification of nodal recurrence in both symptomatic and asymptomatic patients.

Finally, second-look US after breast MRI could yield a positive finding, but only in about 50 % of cases.

## 5.3 Magnetic Resonance Imaging

**Clinical Practice Points**

- Although the sensitivity of magnetic resonance imaging (MRI) in the detection of BC is high, its specificity varies with the quality of images obtained. Cyclical changes can critically affect the sensitivity of MRI, while high breast density has been shown to negligibly affect MRI sensitivity.

- MRI has been evaluated as a screening adjunct given its improved sensitivity in specific subgroups of women and is recommended for screening in high-risk populations.
- Significant controversy exists regarding the appropriate use of MRI in patients with breast cancer, particularly as part of the preoperative staging workup. MRI is frequently obtained to exclude the presence of multicentric disease or an occult contralateral BC with the presumed benefit of improving patient selection for breast conservation as well as decreasing ipsilateral breast tumour.
- Despite the lack of clear evidence of its effectiveness in many clinical settings, inappropriate use is common, in most cases leading to an unnecessary number of biopsies. The appropriate use, levels of evidence and grades of recommendations of the MRI of the breast in all main conditions are outlined in the recent guidelines.

### 5.3.1 Overview

Modern strategies for BC detection are founded on triple assessment (mammography, ultrasound and clinical breast examination). However, in a significant minority of patients, breast malignancy could not be adequately assessed (or excluded) with conventional imaging. This is an uncommon occurrence as in:

- Palpable or indeterminate lesion without a focal imaging correlate
- Potential understaging in suspicious multiple or bilateral BC
- Distant or axillary BC metastasis, with no breast lesion found on conventional imaging
- Invasive lobular carcinoma because of its higher incidence of multifocality
- Detection of chest wall invasion and detection of recurrent BC in postsurgical scars and irradiated breast
- Monitoring of the response to neoadjuvant chemotherapy
- Detection of internal mammary lymph node involvement, if suspected

In each of these conditions MRI has been shown to be a sensitive and effective method of detecting, diagnosing and staging BC, even when conventional imaging results have been negative. The use of MRI may change the clinical management in these situations if unexpected abnormalities are detected.

The efficacy of MRI in breast imaging has undergone much advancement in the last years. It shows promise in many areas, including staging of BCs and determination of tumour size and spread, and is a valuable screening tool for high-risk women [4]. It may also be of value in those patients whose breasts are too dense for mammography, because high breast density has been shown to negligibly affect MRI sensitivity. However, because of the cost in addition to high sensitivity with poor specificity which may lead to an unnecessary number of biopsies, it is unlikely to be used for general screening.

**Table 5.5** Characteristics and main clinical indication of MRI

| Main characteristics |
| --- |
| Highly sensitive |
| Poorly specific |
| Leads to an unnecessary number of biopsies |
| Does not visualise calcifications |
| May be useful in detecting internal mammary lymph node involvement |
| Findings suspicious for malignancy: |
| Spicules |
| Ring enhancement |
| Irregular margins |
| Coalescent clump (DCIS) |
| Linear clump (infiltrating carcinoma) |
| Main clinical indications |
| *MRI screening* in high risk women with a genetic mutation or family history with >25 % lifetime risk |
| *MRI screening* in high risk women with personal of radiation to chest or mediastinum |
| *Discordant findings* in physical examination, mammogram and ultrasound |
| *Occult BC* (axillary lymph node involvement with BC, without mammographic or US abnormality) |
| *Lobular carcinoma* (not seen in about 20 % of cases by ultrasound and mammogram) also useful in determining the extent of disease |
| *Extent of known malignancy* in multiple or bilateral cancer |
| *Residual tumour after lumpectomy* with positive margins |
| *Recurrence after surgery* vs. scar, since MRI reflects tumour vascularity |
| *Monitoring of the response* to neoadjuvant therapy |
| *Implant integrity* or with suspicious imaging findings |

In a number of situations, MRI is essentially contraindicated, usually because of the following physical constraints that prevent adequate patient positioning: patient's inability to lay prone, marked kyphosis or kypho-scoliosis, marked obesity, extremely large breasts and severe claustrophobia.

Another contraindication is the inability to use gadolinium-based contrast media in a patient, as in cases of allergy or pregnancy. Relative contraindications are essentially based on the high sensitivity, but limited specificity, of the technique. MRI may not be useful in cancer-phobic patients or for the assessment of mammographically detected microcalcifications.

*Timing* may be a substantial factor in MRI procedure. In young and premenopausal women the ideal time for MRI of the breast is approximately between day 5 and 15 of the menstrual cycle, because the luteal phase of the menstrual cycle with the associated increase in oestrogen and progesterone leads to the stroma being oedematous with development of the lobules. This increases enhancement being maximal 7 days before menstruation.

In addition, the use of hormone therapy in postmenopausal women may lead to enhancement that may be either focal or diffuse. In such cases, it may be necessary to repeat the MRI examination 2 or 3 months after stopping hormone therapy to obtain optimal results.

*REPORTS*. The characteristic and main indications of MRI are shown in Table 5.5. In MRI the lesions are roughly described by morphologic analysis, patterns of enhancement and dynamic analysis [5].

*Morphologic analysis*. The lesion may be described as round, oval, lobulated, irregular or stellate. The margins of the lesion may be described as smooth, scalloped, irregular or spiculated. Margins that are smooth are associated with a 95 % negative predictive value for carcinoma, so they are probably benign. Also lobulated margins have a 90 % negative predictive value for carcinoma. In reverse, irregular margins are associated with an 80 % positive predictive value for malignancy, and spiculated margins are associated with a 90 % positive predictive value for malignancy.

*Pattern of enhancement*. The pattern of enhancement may be described as homogenous, heterogeneous, rim pattern, enhancing internal separations or non-enhancing internal separations. In addition, one may have foci of enhancement without any mass or space-occupying lesion. This may or may not represent an area of malignancy. Linear enhancement may suggest DCIS. Non-enhancing masses as well as masses with non-enhancing septations can also be present, but these tend to be benign lesions.

*Dynamic analysis*. The last of the interpretation is the enhancement intensity versus time curve, with malignant tumours tending to have fast enhancement with fast washout and with benign lesions tending to have a gradual increase in enhancement.

*ADVANTAGES OF MRI*. If early rapid enhancement due to neo-vascularity were unique to malignant tissues, MRI would be the standard in clinical practice today. Unfortunately, such enhancement is not specific, and several benign conditions may enhance in a fashion similar to cancer. Conversely, a small percentage of malignancies either enhance identically to benign breast parenchyma, or, rarely, they do not enhance at all.

Apart from this, the numerous advantages of MRI over conventional breast imaging for the detection of malignancy have become apparent with increasing clinical experience. These advantages include the following:

- No ionising radiation
- All imaging planes possible with a good spatial resolution
- Capability of imaging the entire breast volume and chest wall
- Greater than 90 % sensitivity to invasive carcinoma
- Detection of occult, multifocal or residual malignancies
- Accurate size estimation for invasive carcinoma

*DISADVANTAGES OF MRI*. In practice, the main disadvantages of MRI are the high equipment costs, with a long learning curve for interpretation, and the non-standard technique. In the assessment of diagnosis, the main limitations are false-positive enhancement in some benign tissues (limited specificity), variable enhancement of in situ carcinoma and an incidence of slowly or poorly enhancing invasive carcinomas of about 5 %.

*Incidental abnormalities.* The increasing use of MRI has inevitably been accompanied by incidental enhancing abnormalities, which typically were not detected on earlier, conventional images. These apparent lesions may represent normal or dysplastic tissues, cyclic hormonal changes, benign tumours or even unexpected malignant foci. If the enhancement rate, intensity or pattern is suspicious, the nature of such foci must be clarified so that a cancer is not missed.

*STRATEGIES OF MRI.* Strategies against incidental enhancing abnormalities are commonly used to diagnose these lesions such as MRI-guided second-look ultrasound, repeat MRI examination at another suitable time or MRI-guided needle biopsy.

*MRI-guided second-look ultrasound.* High-resolution US of the suspect region of the breast should be the first method used, because it is rapid and can be performed (possibly by the same radiologist) immediately after the MR examination. MRI is used to guide the examination to determine the size, shape and position of the suspect lesion. Using this technique, malignancies previously missed with routine US are found, particularly in cases with multifocal or occult malignancies. Sometimes, such lesions are subtle. They may even appear benign on sonograms, being confidently detected only because the operator was aware of the existence of the lesion.

*Repeat MRI.* In premenopausal patients, cyclic hormonal enhancement is a common cause of false-positive focal or multifocal enhancement, characteristic of hormonally influenced, benign tissue. If a repeat examination shows a persistent abnormality with suspicious features that cannot be localised with US, the choice is to either continue to observe the lesion or to perform breast biopsy to achieve a definitive diagnosis. The decision should be based on the level of suspicion of the MRI findings; the options should be presented to and discussed with the patient.

*MRI-guided Biopsy.* MRI-guided needle biopsy or hook-wire localisation for surgical biopsy is an inevitable consequence of MRI showing lesions that are occult with all other forms of breast imaging. Techniques range from simple freehand techniques, which remain useful for hook-wire localisation, to complex, robotic, automated systems, which are intended primarily for vacuum-assisted biopsy with large-bore needles.

*Impact in surgical treatment.* Because breast MRI has greater sensitivity in cancer detection than mammography and US do, the increased use of MRI could lead to an increased rate of mastectomy also in women with early stage BC. In most cases there is no evidence that MRI-induced changes from breast conservation to more radical surgery improve surgical care or prognosis. Emerging data even indicate that MRI does not reduce or increases re-excision rates.

These findings are due in part to a non-standard technique that allows different results in different centres. In part they are due to the evidence that occult pathology, found only microscopically (and perhaps on MRI), is more responding to adjuvant treatment, while gross pathology (the only one detected by mammography or ultrasound) is less responsive to treatment and leads more easily to a recurrence (see Sect. 15.1).

### 5.3.2 MRI in Special Situations

Special conditions could require an MRI assessment because of the equivocal or suspicious findings on conventional imaging following treatments that change the normal architecture of breast tissue.

*Core-Needle Biopsy (CNB) changes on MRI Scans*. Since normal tissues do not significantly alter their enhancement after a small sampling, in case of inconclusive result with CNB, MRI should be performed especially in the first 2 weeks.

*Hematoma and seroma* seen shortly after surgery appear as fluid-filled, not enhancing, smoothly bounded cavities. Seromas are hyperintense, and hematomas may be hyperintense or hypointense, depending on the age and oxygenation state of the blood products. This reactive postsurgical enhancement decreases over time. A delay of at least 4–5 weeks after surgery is needed to achieve a reasonable specificity, in about 75 % of cases, for the detection of residual tumour.

*Fat necrosis* appears as an ovoid focus with irregular stellate granulation tissue, which may be intensely enhancing after the administration of contrast material. This necrosis resembles a contracted hematoma or seroma. While this occasionally mimics a recurrent tumour, the typical lesion is usually readily diagnosable by its shape and enhancement pattern.

*Postoperative scarring*. Scar tissue generally appears as a low-signal-intensity, linear irregularity with variable enhancement, which largely depends on the interval since treatment. In the first few months after surgery, the borders of the surgical cavity may have strong enhancement, particularly if haemorrhage or fat necrosis has occurred.

This reactive enhancement gradually subsides. At 6 months after surgery without radiation therapy, most images show slow, minimal or no enhancement, while the appearance of abnormal enhancement raises the suspicion of a recurrent malignancy.

Some patients may nevertheless benefit from MRI soon after surgery if the presence of residual disease is strongly suspected. Although diffuse parenchymal enhancement is of little diagnostic value, the demonstration of typically malignant enhancement in a focal lesion should prompt a re-excision.

*Post-radiation therapy*. In the first 9–12 months after radiation therapy, a diffuse increase in capillary permeability occurs. This change initially causes marked parenchymal enhancement that later becomes patchy. In most women, this enhancement gradually declines after 18 months because of fibrosis. As a result, normal tissues have minimal enhancement, and any enhancing lesion on this background is suggestive of a recurrent tumour, which may appear nodular with carcinoma recurrence or may appear linear with DCIS.

*Post-chemotherapy*. As mentioned above, MRI is useful to assess responses to neoadjuvant chemotherapy. However, more clinical-to-MRI discrepancies need to be pointed out. MRI tends to underestimate a tumour when decreased in vasculature and permeability, leading to poor altered patterns of enhancements. After surgery, occult pathological foci may or may not be found. On the contrary a good tumour response with necrosis and fibrosis may occur with only a slight reduction in the clinical size of the tumour.

*Post-implant MRI*. According to EUSOMA guidelines [6], MRI is not recommended as a screening tool for implant rupture in asymptomatic women with breast implants. In patients with symptoms suggestive for implant rupture (pain, asymmetry, change in shape, etc.), after conventional imaging, non-contrast MRI is recommended to confirm or exclude rupture.

In patients with implants and signs/symptoms of parenchymal disease (e.g. breast lump), when conventional imaging is not diagnostic, non-contrast MRI and dynamic contrast-enhanced MRI are indicated to exclude implant rupture and to evaluate the breast gland parenchyma.

In symptomatic patients that have undergone breast augmentation with direct polyacrylamide gel injection, non-contrast MRI and dynamic contrast-enhanced MRI are indicated. In patients with tissue expanders, the MR compatibility should be evaluated because various breast tissue expanders have magnetic ports to allow for a more accurate detection of the injection site. These devices are substantially attracted to the static magnetic fields of MR systems and, therefore, may be uncomfortable and in some cases contraindicated for patients undergoing MR procedures. Breast tissue expanders with magnetic ports produce relatively large artefacts on MR images, and, as such, assessment of the breast using MR imaging is problematic.

In view of this possibility, it is recommended that patients with tissue expanders who require MRI should be identified prior to MRI so that the radiologist is aware of the potential problems related to the generation of artefacts and the patient is carefully advised about localised symptoms in the region of their expanders during the scan.

### 5.3.3 MRI Guidelines

A recent paper by the EUSOMA working group [6] outlines appropriate use, levels of evidence (LoE), expert panel opinions (EPO), and grades of recommendations of the MRI of the breast in all main conditions. A selection of main topics is shown below.

*Staging before treatment planning*. Acceptable indications to preoperative MRI with potential advantages are for:

- Patients newly diagnosed with an invasive lobular cancer (LoE 2a)
- Patients at high risk for BC (LoE 2b)
- Patients under 60 years of age with discrepancy in size >1 cm between XRM and US with expected impact on treatment decision (LoE 2b)
- Patients eligible for PBI on the basis of CBE and conventional imaging (LoE 3b)

*Screening of high-risk women*. Women with a family history suspicious for inherited predisposition to BC should have their risk assessed by an appropriately trained professional group (genetic counselling). If found at high risk (20–30 % or greater), they should be given written information on their risk and on risks and benefits of XRM and MRI screening and alternative risk-reducing interventions; if they accept to be screened with MRI, they should be informed on how often and where their screening will take place together with relevant contacts (EPO). Lifetime risk thresholds for including women in surveillance programmes with annual MRI may be selected on the basis of regional or national considerations due to area-specific cumulative risk in the general population, availability of resources or practical feasibility (EPO).

High-risk breast screening including MRI should be conducted only at a nationally/regionally approved and audited service or as part of an ethically approved research study. Periodical audit should be undertaken to ensure that high sensitivity is achieved and recall rate (MR imaging more frequently than annual) is less than 10 % and to monitor detection rate, needle biopsy rate and interval cancers (EPO).

Annual MRI screening should be available to be done starting from the age of 30. Starting annual screening before age 30 may be discussed for mutation carriers of BRCA1 or BRCA2 (starting from 25 to 29) and TP53 (starting from 20) (LoE 2b). Annual MRI screening should be offered to:

- BRCA1, BRCA2 and TP53 mutation carriers
- Women at 50 % risk for BRCA1, BRCA2 or TP53 mutation that runs in their family (first-degree relatives of mutation carriers)
- Women from families not tested or inconclusively tested for BRCA mutation with a 20–30 % lifetime risk or greater (LoE 2)
- Women who have had previous mantle radiotherapy before age 30 (e.g. for Hodgkin disease), starting 8 years after their treatment (LoE 3)

Women at high risk who have been already diagnosed and treated for BC should be included in screening programmes including MRI (LoE 2b). Definition of upper age limits for non-enrolling women or discontinuing annual MRI is not possible on the basis of current evidence (EPO).

Women of any age undergoing prophylactic mastectomy should have an MRI examination within 3 months before surgery to screen for occult BC (EPO).

Screening XRM should not be performed in high-risk women below 35 years as there is no evidence that the benefits outweigh the risks at this young age (EPO). In TP53 mutation carriers of any age annual XRM can be avoided based on discussion on risks and benefits from radiation exposure (EPO). Annual XRM may be considered for high-risk women from age 35 (LoE 2–3).

If annual MRI is performed, whole breast XRM and US are not necessary as there is no evidence of any additional benefit to MRI (LoE 2). They are recommended in women under 35 who do not tolerate or have contraindication to MRI or to gadolinium-based contrast material administration (EPO).

Cases requiring workup after MRI should be initially assessed with conventional imaging, re-evaluation of XRM and targeted US (LoE 2). In cases of only MRI-detected suspicious findings, MR-guided biopsy/localisation should be performed (LoE 1).

Risk factors such as previous diagnosis of breast invasive cancer or DCIS, atypical ductal hyperplasia, lobular intraepithelial neoplasia and heterogeneous or dense breasts on XRM, when not associated with other risk factors, do not confer an increased risk that justifies the use of MRI screening (EPO).

*Evaluation of response to neoadjuvant therapy*. MRI does not have a role in the assessment of treatment options in patients with inoperable BC at presentation (EPO). Pretreatment breast MRI should be performed in patients with large potentially operable BC before the first course of NAC, at the condition that performing MRI does not significantly postpone NAC initiation (LoE 1). Post-NAC breast MRI should preferably be performed 2 weeks after the last NAC cycle and within 2 weeks before surgery (EPO); treatment delay due to preoperative MRI should not be larger than 1 month.

Variations between pre- and post-NAC should be based on concomitant evaluation of both pre- and post-NAC MRI examinations; even very low enhancement located at the primary tumour site should be considered as a sign for residual disease (LoE 1). Measurement of residual disease after NAC should be performed according to RECIST or WHO criteria; multifocal or multicentric disease should be evaluated by summing the largest diameter of the visible tumours (EPO).

The ultimate surgical decision should be based on the relative volume of residual tumour compared to that of the affected breast and decided by a multidisciplinary team (EPO). In poor responders to NAC, MRI generally confirms the results of clinical and conventional imaging evaluations and may, therefore, not be mandatory (EPO).

*Occult primary breast cancer*. Breast MRI is indicated in the presence of localised metastatic disease (typically, axillary lymphadenopathy) and negative CBE and conventional imaging (LoE 1b). Breast MRI is not indicated when extensive metastatic disease exists and/or prognosis is poor, where knowledge of the site of the primary tumour is unlikely to influence the treatment options or the likely outcome (EPO). If MRI of the breast is negative, surgical treatment of the breast may be avoided (LoE 2b) and therapy planning should be decided by a multidisciplinary team (EPO).

*BC recurrence*. The previous diagnosis of breast invasive cancer or DCIS does not confer an increased risk that justifies the use of annual MRI screening. If conventional imaging shows a high likelihood of recurrence and needle biopsy can be performed, MRI should not be used as an alternative to needle biopsy (EPO).

In the presence of inconclusive findings on conventional imaging for differential diagnosis between scar and recurrence and when needle biopsy cannot be performed or is judged to be probably inconclusive, MRI is indicated (LoE lb).

*Nipple discharge*. There is insufficient evidence of benefit to recommend the routine use of MRI in the clinical context of suspicious nipple discharge (EPO). In countries where ductography is considered the routine test for suspicious nipple discharge, non-contrast T2-weighted and contrast-enhanced MRI can be considered if ductography fails for technical reasons or the patient refuses the procedure (LoE 3b).

*Equivocal findings at conventional imaging*. MRI should not be used as an alternative to needle biopsy when needle biopsy can be performed (LoE la). MRI-guided needle biopsy should be considered for cases with abnormal imaging but inconclusive findings on conventional imaging where it is not possible to perform or define a site for needle biopsy (EPO).

MRI should not be used for differential diagnosis of inflammatory BCs from acute mastitis before treatment (LoE 1b). If after treatment of a presumed mastitis doubts remain about the presence of an underlying BC, MRI can be considered (LoE 2b).

*Male breast cancer*. MRI should not be used for routine diagnosis of BC in men (EPO).

## 5.4 Other Radiological Procedures for Breast Disease

### 5.4.1 Digital Breast Tomosynthesis

*Digital breast tomosynthesis* (*DBT*), or *3D mammography*, is a method of creating three-dimensional images of the breast using x-rays. Unlike current FFDM, in which two x-ray images of the breast are obtained from different projections, tomosynthesis is performed by taking a series of low-dose exposures (usually 9–15) at different angles across the breast from one projection. From these images and using mathematical methods of back projection reconstruction, a series of 1-mm slices are created in order to show the tissue structure in three dimensions. The ability of tomosynthesis to image the breast three-dimensionally may help to overcome some of the shortcomings of standard mammography caused by overlapping dense tissue.

*Potential advantages*. Mammography is limited in ability to differentiate potential lesions from overlying and underlying tissue structures, which may necessitate recall visits for supplementary views in addition to the standard two-plane views. DBT is an innovation in breast imaging in which sequential tomographic images through the breast are reconstructed from a limited number of 2D images acquired at multiple angles over a short scan [7].

Potential clinical benefits include improved lesion characterisation, improved lesion size assessment at detection, reduced recalls for further imaging and fewer biopsies, increasing not only sensitivity of FFDM but specificity too. For lesions that require biopsy, DBT may also offer accurate localisation. However, although a number of papers have been published, and the DBT-guided biopsy system is already available, the advantages of DBT over other imaging modalities remain to be proven in randomised clinical trials.

*Radiation doses*. The radiation dose for 2D plus 3D with 1 and 2 views is greater than that for the standard 2D, a major potential drawback of 3D imaging, as it exposes all patients who undergo it to additional radiation.

*Indications*. More research is needed to determine the best methods of incorporating 3D tomographic imaging into daily practice. Not all patients benefit equally, and identifying which patient populations receive the greatest benefit is important. Additionally, standards for imaging protocol variations and post-processing algorithms need to be established.

### 5.4.2 Computed Tomography

*Spiral CT* is useful for elucidating problems in the diagnosis of breast lesions, especially when a more thorough staging is needed. Its advantages are the speed of the method, comfort for the patient, absence of movement artefacts, easy standardisation and wide applicability.

*Dynamic contrast-enhanced CT* of the breast has been found to be effective for the detection of intraductal extension of breast carcinoma and is thought (but controversial) to be useful in the preoperative assessment of BCs in selected cases. The lesions appear attenuating compared with fatty background, and they show early enhancement on arterial phase on dynamic contrast-enhanced CT.

*Three-dimensional (3D) helical CT* can provide good information about the spread of BC and could be an alternative to 3D MRI for preoperative examination of BC. In vitro high-resolution helical CT can depict the internal structure of small nodes. Morphologic changes detected on helical CT help distinguish benign from malignant nodes. Tumours appear as dense lesions on CT and usually show early contrast enhancement similar to that seen with dynamic MRI. CT is less sensitive than mammography for detecting microcalcifications when it is the sole manifestation of early cancer.

### 5.4.3 Positron Emission Mammography (PEM)

Positron emission mammography (PEM) is a breast-dedicated high-resolution technology of the positron emission tomography (PET), used to visualise the metabolism of the breast. PET scanning is a nuclear medicine technique that images the flow of a radiotracer F-18 fluorodeoxyglucose (F-18 FDG) that enters into the metabolic pathways of glucose. While anatomic imaging allows visualisation of body structures, PET molecular imaging allows visualisation of molecular flow and metabolic processes within the body [8].

The primary benefit of PET imaging is, in theory, based on detection of an abnormal metabolism before anatomic changes can be seen. In addition, dense breast tissue or scarring may cause anatomic techniques (mammography, ultrasonography) to be indeterminate. In such cases, knowing whether an anatomic structure is glucose hypermetabolic can be critical in the determination of proper medical management.

Whole-body PET cameras are typically combined with a CT scanner to allow acquisition of anatomic and molecular information from a single procedure. These hybrid PET/CT cameras are donut-shaped. While PET/CT cameras are useful for whole-body imaging, breast-specific PET imaging, known as positron emission mammography (PEM), requires the PET camera to be configured like a mammography machine. Current PEM cameras utilise two small movable flat detectors that are pressed directly against the breast.

The camera technology utilised by PEM has been shown to be more sensitive than whole-body PET/CT imaging in the detection of breast tumours. PEM is a relatively new technology, and the clinical indications are evolving rapidly. PEM is particularly useful when other imaging scan results are indeterminate. It has a useful complementary role to mammography, ultrasonography and MRI.

In theory PEM can assist in pre-surgical planning in BC, monitoring response to therapy and evaluating for tumour recurrence. In some cases, it may be useful in BC staging and in helping guide breast biopsies.

## References


1. Pisano ED, Gatsonsis C, Hendrick E, et al. Diagnostic performance of digital versus film mammography for breast cancer screening. N Engl J Med. 2005;353:1773–83.
2. Dongola N. Mammography in breast cancer. http://emedicine.medscape.com/article/346529-overview#showall. Accessed 30 Jan 2015.
3. Thrush S, Dixon JM. The role of imaging in breast diagnosis including screening and excision of impalpable lesions. In: Dixon JM, editor. Breast surgery. 5th ed. London: Elsevier; 2014.
4. Kuhl CK, Schrading S, Leutner CC, et al. Mammography, breast ultrasound, and magnetic resonance imaging for surveillance of women at high familial risk for breast cancer. J Clin Oncol. 2005;23:8469–76.
5. Shah SH, et al. Current role of magnetic resonance imaging in breast imaging: a primer for the primary care physician. http://www.medscape.com/viewarticle/518406_7.
6. Sardanelli F, Boetes C, Borisch B, et al. Magnetic resonance imaging of the breast: recommendations from the EUSOMA working group. Eur J Cancer. 2010;46:1296–316.
7. Lin J. 3D mammography. http://emedicine.medscape.com/article/1970908-overview#showall. Accessed 30 Jan 2015.
8. Eston TF. Breast positron emission tomography. http://emedicine.medscape.com/article/2109054-overview#showall. Accessed 30 Jan 2015.


## Further Reading


American College of Radiology. ACR practice parameter for the performance of screening and diagnostic mammography (Amended 2014). www.acr.org/~/media/ACR/Documents/PGTS/guidelines/Screening_Mammography.pdf.

Ciatto S, Houssami N, Bernardi D, et al. Integration of 3D digital mammography with tomosynthesis for population breast-cancer screening (STORM): a prospective comparison study. Lancet Oncol. 2013;14:583–9.

Houssami N, Ciatto S, Macaskill P, et al. Accuracy and surgical impact of magnetic resonance imaging in breast cancer staging: systematic review and meta-analysis in detection of multifocal and multicentric cancer. J Clin Oncol. 2008;26:3248–58.

Koomen M, Pisano ED, Kuzmiak C, Pavic D, McLelland R. Future directions in breast imaging. J Clin Oncol. 2005;23:1674–7.

Saslow D, Boetes C, Burke W, et al. American Cancer Society guidelines for breast screening with MRI as an adjunct to mammography. CA Cancer J Clin. 2007;57:75–89.

Torjesen I. How much is too much breast screening? BMJ. 2015;350:h139.

Warner E, Hill K, Causer P, et al. Prospective study of breast cancer incidence in women with a BRCA1 or BRCA2 mutation under surveillance with and without magnetic resonance imaging. J Clin Oncol. 2011;29:1664–9.


**Websites in Appendix**: *Imaging*, A-4.11.

# Breast Tissue Diagnosis

# 6

Gianni Saguatti, Giuliana Dell'Oste, and Silvia Teggi

## Contents




G. Saguatti (✉)
Department of Radiology, Mammographic Screening,
Hospital "Bellaria", Bologna, Italy
e-mail: gianni.saguatti@ausl.bologna.it

G. Dell'Oste • S. Teggi
Department of Radiology, Mammographic Screening, Padova USL16, Italy







A.M. Pluchinotta (ed.), *The Outpatient Breast Clinic: Aiming at Best Practice*,
DOI 10.1007/978-3-319-15907-2_6

**Abstract**

• Nonoperative diagnosis should become the norm in breast disease assessment. The aim of sampling procedures should be to fulfil the "triple diagnostic assessment" and achieve as near as possible 100 % nonoperative diagnosis of breast problems. • Automated core needle biopsy (CNB) is the sampling technique of first choice, to prefer over fine needle aspiration (FNA) because of fewer inadequate samples. In most cases, CNB accomplishes the same results of an open incisional biopsy. • Ultrasound guidance, if feasible, is the technique of first choice for biopsy of both palpable and impalpable breast lesions; it is less costly, easy to perform and more accurate than free-hand or other image-guided techniques. • Management of high-risk lesions remains controversial. The likelihood of atypical ductal hyperplasia or radial scar in association with BC is related to the size of the lesion and the age of the patient.

*Future directions*. Percutaneous image-guided biopsies are increasingly an alternative to surgical biopsy for the histological assessment of breast lesions. Moreover, in BC and in some borderline lesions, core needle samples are becoming larger in order to provide a complete set of prognostic factors to guide the decision-making process and to enable new strategies of treatment.

## 6.1 Choice of Sampling Procedure

**Clinical Practice Points**

- Aiming to a nonoperative diagnosis should become the norm in breast disease assessment.
- Histology is better than cytology in breast masses, so that core needle biopsy should be preferred to fine needle aspiration in most cases.
- There is a great individual variability in outcome within each sampling method. Ultrasound guidance, if feasible, is the technique of first choice also in palpable lesions.
- Few but well-identified conditions require a conclusive surgical diagnosis.

### 6.1.1 Overview

*Sampling techniques* may include fine needle aspiration cytology, core biopsy or vacuum-assisted biopsy techniques, the use of which will depend upon the local radiological and cytological expertise and audit of results obtained [1]. Very occasionally, there may remain a significant discordance between suspicious radiological features and benign sampling. Where no reasonable pathological correlation can be made, re-running with another modality or open surgical excision is advisable.

*Fine needle aspiration (FNA)* is particularly useful in the evaluation of cystic lesions detected by ultrasonography. Aspiration of a benign cystic lesion should result in the collapse of the cavity. Persistence of the mass or rapid recurrence following aspiration is a general indication for further workup.

**Table 6.1** Indications, advantages and disadvantages of fine needle aspiration (FNA)

| Major indications | Advantages | Disadvantages |
|---|---|---|
| Lesions characterised by a liquid component and/or necrosis features (complicated cysts, some papillary lesions)<br>Anyway established diagnosis (benign or malignant)<br>Localisation of the lesion in some challenging areas as axilla, close proximity to the chest wall or breast implants | Cheap<br>High sensitivity<br>Provides diagnosis in most common instances<br>Can be referred immediately | Operator dependent<br>Needs experienced cytopathologist<br>Painful<br>Cannot differentiate invasive from in situ cancer<br>Variable percentage of C1 (inadequate or insufficient)<br>Few, but possible, false positives |

**Table 6.2** Indications, advantages and disadvantages of core needle biopsy (CNB)

| Major indications | Advantages | Disadvantages |
|---|---|---|
| Findings highly suggestive or suspicious for malignancy (BIRADS 4/5) or assessed as probably benign (BIRADS 3, C1 and C3 cytological class)<br>Multicentric lesions in order to plan timing and way of treatment<br>Results not correlated with the clinical and imaging findings | Easy to perform<br>High sensitivity, more high specificity with close to zero false-positive rate<br>Provides a definitive histological diagnosis<br>Facilitates in the planning of multimodal treatments for women with BC or who refuse surgery or when surgery can be avoided (very old women) | Operator dependent<br>Cannot easily be reported immediately<br>Uncomfortable but less painful than FNA<br>Bruising and swelling |

Concerning solid lesions, although core biopsy can get a more proper and definitive diagnosis in most cases, FNA should be preferred in solid, easy accessible lumps, easily established as benign (fibroadenoma in young women) or malignant (scirrhous cancer), and in lesions characterised by a liquid component and/or necrosis features (complicated cysts, some papillomatous lesions) or localised in some challenging areas as the axilla, close proximity to the chest wall or breast implants (Table 6.1).

*Core needle biopsy (CNB)* provides increased sensitivity and specificity compared to fine needle aspiration cytology. Sensitivity and specificity are related to the size of the needle. CNB using a 14- or 16-gauge needle is widely accepted to be sensitive (90 %) and specific (98 %) in diagnosing breast masses, compared with 60 and 86 %, respectively, for FNA. In any case, CNB is recommended in most doubtful cases and mandatory for lesions as architectural distortion and microcalcifications.

Diagnosing lesions with needle biopsy has several advantages. For benign lesions, establishing a definitive diagnosis obviates unnecessary surgical excision or protracted follow-up, both of which are costly in psychosocial and resource terms. A definitive diagnosis of cancer allows the patient to make an informed choice and to obtain counselling before surgery (Table 6.2).

*Vacuum-assisted biopsy (VAB)* is a more complex and expensive percutaneous needle biopsy technique. It should be reserved for large sampling as needed in some clusters of microcalcifications or in some radiological areas with architectural distortion. The procedure is accurate as when a tissue sample is removed surgically.

**Table 6.3** Indications, advantages and disadvantages of vacuum-assisted biopsy (VAB)

| Major indications | Advantages | Disadvantages |
|---|---|---|
| Clusters of indeterminate microcalcifications<br>An architectural distortion in the structure of the breast tissue<br>An area of diffuse non-specific abnormality<br>Failed 'conventional' core biopsy<br>Some papillary and mucocele-like lesions | An excellent way to evaluate microcalcifications<br>Generally, the procedure is not painful and the results are as accurate as when a tissue sample is removed surgically | Because device removes larger pieces of tissue, there is a risk (less than 1 %) of bleeding and forming a hematoma, at the biopsy site<br>An occasional significant patient's discomfort can be readily controlled by pain medication |

The core needles are of a large calibre and are mounted onto a spring-loaded device that allows small cylinders of tissue to be cut and collected within the notch of the needle. Technically, the best core biopsy samples are obtained by using 8- or 11-gauge needles. The optimal number of passes required varies according to the mammographic appearances of the lesions being sampled, with fewer passes required for solid lesions compared with microcalcifications. Several investigators have shown that a minimum of 5–6 passes is required when sampling microcalcifications to minimise sampling error. In case it is performed for microcalcifications, a wide-bore needle should be preferred; moreover, a specimen radiography of the cores should be obtained to demonstrate the presence of calcifications.

VAB may be an alternative to open surgery for additional tissue biopsy in patients with microcalcifications or borderline breast lesions. Compared with open surgical biopsy, needle biopsy is cheaper, it causes less trauma and disfigurement, no breast defect remains, and unlike with surgery, it does not distort the breast tissue making it difficult to read in future mammograms (Table 6.3.)

Undoubtedly, VAB is advantageous in increasing the preoperative diagnostic accuracy of impalpable breast lesions and even in reducing the overall costs of diagnosis compared with surgical excision. Even so, each new and incremental development has increased the cost of the procedure; it is therefore prudent to use a biopsy technique with full knowledge and awareness of the individual strengths and weaknesses of not only the individual capability, but also the expertise available in one's institution.

According to all-purpose available expertise, masses may be successfully sampled with FNA or core biopsy under ultrasound guidance, whereas stereotactic vacuum biopsy of small clusters of indeterminate microcalcifications may be more appropriate as a modality of choice compared with FNA or core biopsy. Used in this manner, image-guided percutaneous needle biopsy can be used effectively to ensure that most palpable and impalpable breast lesions are diagnosed with accuracy and certainty.

*Open surgical biopsy.* Some large lesions which are predominantly architectural distortion should be subject to excision biopsy, following preoperative diagnostic workup. That is due to a significant risk of associated malignancy which may not be demonstrated even under ideal sampling conditions. Also, lesions that are proven with atypical ductal hyperplasia (ADH) or radial scar (RS) should be subject to excision due to the risk of associated malignancy (Table 6.4).

**Table 6.4** Indications, advantages and disadvantages of open surgical biopsy

| Major indications | Advantages | Disadvantages |
|---|---|---|
| Clinical suspicion of malignancy not otherwise confirmed by sampling, especially when a mastectomy or axillary clearance is planned<br>Large benign lesions, i.e. benign phyllodes tumours or large fibroadenoma<br>Diagnosis of atypical hyperplasia done on CNB<br>Diagnosis of radial scar done on imaging and CNB<br>Every papillary lesion ascertained<br>Suspicion of malignancy on one or more investigations with indeterminate or inadequate CNB, usually in patient with screen-detected microcalcifications<br>Request by the patient | Preoperative triple diagnostic assessment should be achieved in most cases, but few conditions require an unquestionable definitive surgical diagnosis | A surgical biopsy has more physical and psychological consequences than other procedures<br>It is expensive and it will leave a scar<br>The more tissue removed, the more likely a change in the shape of the breast could be noticed<br>All biopsies can cause bleeding and swelling and carry a mild risk of infection |

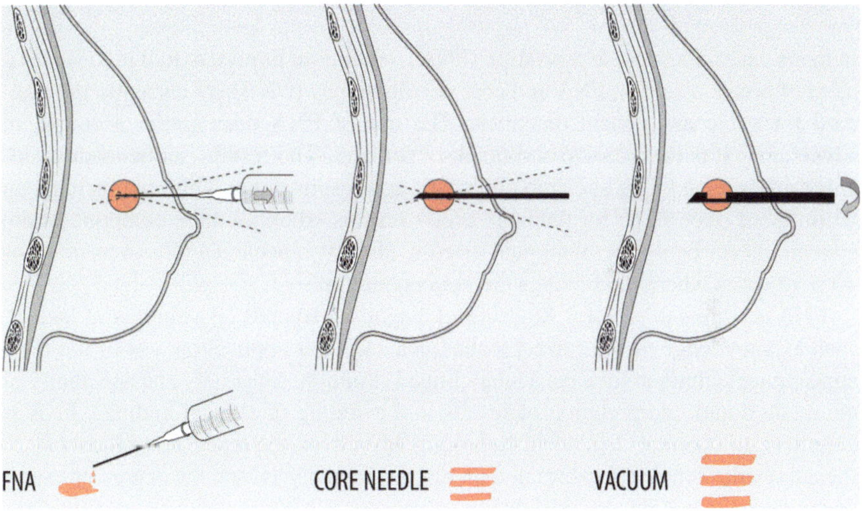


**Fig. 6.1** Different types of needle biopsy of the breast. FNA (fine needle aspiration): operator-dependent technique with multiple needle insertions and small samples. Core needle biopsy (CNB): few insertions, larger sample size and accurate histological diagnosis. Vacuum-assisted needle biopsy (VAB): several large samples with one needle insertion

Sampling techniques should be carried out with due regard to the imaging or to clinical finding, starting from the most suspicious features. Where there is a possibility of discordant clinical and imaging findings with regard to any lesion, it is worthwhile to carry out sampling under both imaging and clinical guidance.

Ultimately, each type of biopsy has its pros and cons (Fig. 6.1). The choice of which type to use depends on many factors: how suspicious the tumour looks, how big it is, where it is in the breast, how many tumours there are, personal preferences and other medical and ethical aspects related to the patient.

## 6.2 Cytological Samples

**Clinical Practice Points**

- FNA is an operator-dependent technique. Moreover, the reporting of breast cytological results is more demanding than histological analysis.
- Proper targeting of localisation by the operator and experience of the pathologist in handling and interpreting cytological samples make the difference in the results.
- FNA cannot reliably distinguish preinvasive from invasive cancer, nor does it provide sufficient tissue for testing cancer by immunohistochemistry.
- Besides FNA, cytological samples can be obtained by nipple discharge and by exfoliated cells of the surface of the nipple.

### 6.2.1 Fine Needle Aspiration (FNA)

In many cases, fine needle aspiration (FNA) remains an important tool in the assessment of breast diseases. FNA and core needle biopsy (CNB) are currently the standard for triple assessment diagnosis. The use of FNA does confer a couple of advantages: it is inexpensive and quick to perform. The results can be made available rapidly, enabling a one-stop diagnostic and results clinic. This approach has an accuracy of over 90 % for palpable breast lesions when all three components are concordant for benign or malignant disease. However, accuracy falls in as many as 40 % of cases where the findings are not concordant.

FNA is simple to perform, but truthful diagnosis depends on a number of factors, such as knowledge of the correct techniques and their application, use of the most appropriate technique for a particular clinical situation, sensitivity and specificity of the method and interpretation of results in the setting of clinical findings. FNA is definitely an operator-dependent technique. Moreover, the reporting of breast cytological results is more demanding than histologic analysis, and the degree of expertise required is not always available.

Findings from cellular samples are limited in that the reviewer may not be able to determine the grade or invasiveness of the tumour. It is also difficult to diagnose a lobular carcinoma on the basis of cytological results. Nevertheless, there is evidence to indicate that ultrasound and FNA biopsy are similarly useful for the axillary staging of patients with invasive carcinoma.

The technique of FNA is largely determined by the individual surgeon's preference, which may, in part, reflect hand size and individual technique. A 21-gauge (green) needle is used most commonly, although in expert hands, a 23-gauge (blue) needle can yield as much information, with less discomfort and bruising. Some clinicians opt for a hand-held 10-ml syringe, whereas others prefer a 20-ml syringe used with a syringe holder. Syringe holders allow a vacuum to be easily maintained but can make control of the needle tip less precise.

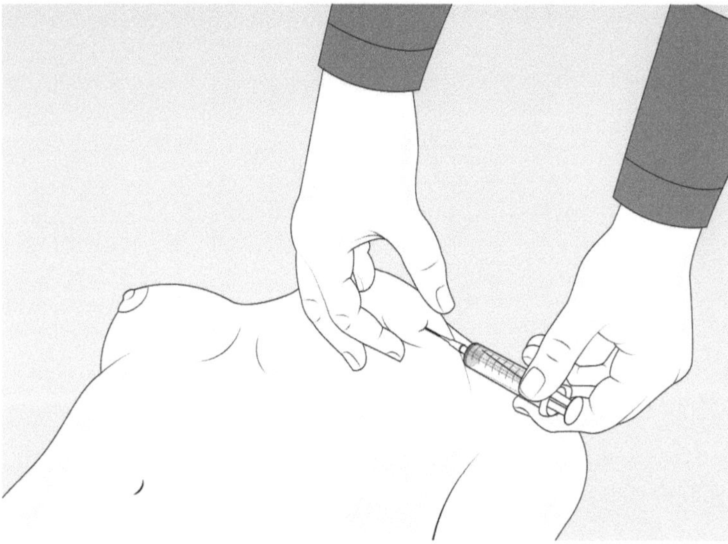

**Fig. 6.2** Fine needle aspiration of peripheral breast mass. In order to avoid a risk of pneumothorax, it is advisable to insert the needle diagonally

To perform FNA, the needle is passed through the lesion a number of times while maintaining suction and steadying the breast tissue with the other hand. Considering the potential risk of pneumothorax, it is important when performing needle biopsies of the breast, and wherever possible, to angle the needle tangentially to the chest wall (Fig. 6.2).

When the mass is near to the chest wall, it is better to move it laterally to a position over the rib (Fig. 6.3) or to use a needle alone (Fig. 6.4).

Sampling should be continued until aspirate is observed at the bottom of the plastic portion of the needle. Finally, the aspirate is transferred to slides and spread in a way thin enough to visualise individual cells. According to the preference of the local laboratory, the slides may be air-dried or fixed by immersing the slide(s) in alcohol for 30 s or by using the cytology spray fixative. In some cases, the presence of the cytologist is advisable at the time of sampling in order to immediately verify its adequacy.

*Free-hand insertion*. If the area to be biopsied can be felt, the needle is manually directed towards the suspicious area. The sample should be obtained with the needle inside the lesion by rapid and multiple inward and outward movements associated with rotations, to ensure a representative collection of cells. Before removing the needle, it is very important to take good care of interrupting the suction.

*Ultrasound (US) guidance* is generally preferred when the lesion is best visible with ultrasounds. In small lumps, the depth of the mass is misleading, and only US can guide the needle towards the centre of the lesion. An outpatient breast clinic should always have an US equipment. It is low cost and rapid and provides high-precision guidance in all kinds of sampling.

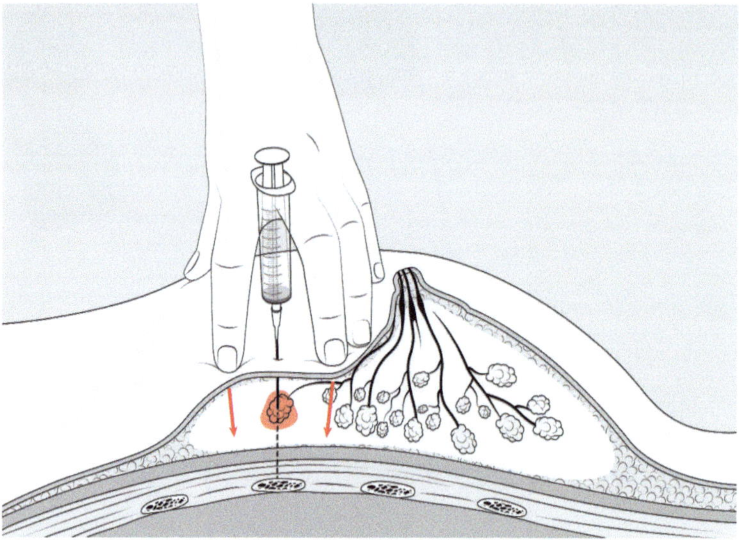

**Fig. 6.3** Fine needle aspiration of a breast mass. The mass is trapped between the pads of the index and the middle finger of the nondominant hand and the needle introduced vertically. In some cases, it is advisable to move the mass laterally to a position over the rib. For most lesions, it is cautious to use ultrasound guidance or outlining the lesion with a marker pen

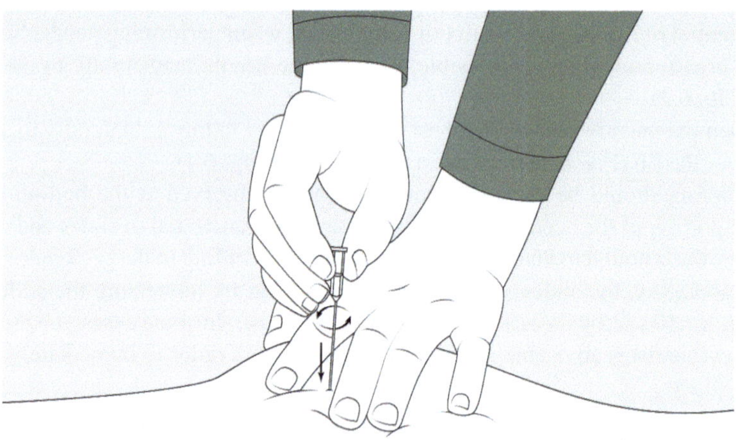

**Fig. 6.4** Fine needle aspiration of small superficial breast mass. A better control of the core insertion could be obtained using a needle alone. If the needle is slowly moved up and down with a little rotation, an appropriate sample could be obtained with no suction for negative pressure

*Stereotactic directional guidance.* In cases of non-palpable lesions visible only on mammograms, such as small opacities or small cluster of microcalcifications, stereotactic directional guidance should not be used, other than for a guided localisation (see Sect. 6.4).

### 6.2.2 Nipple Fluids

*Nipple discharge.* Nipple discharge occurs when fluid inside the ducts is elicited by expression of the nipple or when it spontaneously flows from the nipple. Nipple secretions can be expressed in up to 85 % of women and are generally the by-products of ductal epithelial cells undergoing cellular turnover.

Cytological investigation of nipple discharge is commonly done when spontaneous discharge comes from only one nipple orifice. The fluid is collected in one or more slides and immediately fixed by immersing the slide(s) in alcohol for 30 s or by using the cytology spray fixative. For cytology of nipple fluids, it is better to collect the final (not the first) fluid elicited by a gentle expression of the nipple and not to allow the material on the slide to dry prior to fixation.

*Nipple aspirate fluid (NAF) and ductal lavage (DL)* are considered new approaches to cancer prevention in high-risk patients with family history of BC. The majority of BCs originate in cells that line the inside of the milk ducts in the breast. The presence of atypical cells from nipple or fine needle aspiration has been linked to an increased risk of cancer within 3–5 years following testing, and it is generally assumed that atypical cells obtained using ductal lavage would indicate a similar risk. However, because fluid is not usually collected from all of the milk ducts during these procedures, it is unclear what conclusions can be drawn if no atypical cells are present in a sample.

Nipple aspirate fluid (NAF) is a minimally invasive procedure based on gentle suction to collect fluid from the nipple. This is done with a device similar to breast pumps used by nursing women. Fluid containing cells from the lining of the ducts can be obtained from about 75 % of women, but only a tiny amount of fluid and a few cells can be obtained.

Larger number of ductal cells can be collected by ductal lavage (DL) to detect abnormal intraductal breast cells. Moreover, DL is more sensitive than NAF in detecting cellular atypia. In this procedure, nipple aspiration is first used to draw a tiny amount of fluid to the surface of the nipple to locate the milk ducts. A slender catheter is then inserted into the duct through the natural opening. A small amount of anaesthetic is infused into the duct through the catheter, followed by a small amount of saline. This saline rinses through the duct, collecting cells, and is then withdrawn. As above-said, this minimally invasive procedure produces many more cells than the other methods, but practical usefulness of this procedure is still unclear.

**Table 6.5** Cytological categories

| | | |
|---|---|---|
| Cl | Insufficient cells for cytological analysis, i.e. fewer than five epithelial cell groups | The cause shall be indicated: poor cellularity with less than five epithelial cell clusters, artefacts making interpretation difficult (blood-stained or thick smears, vigorous spreading…) |
| C2 | Cells present all benign; non-suspicious features | Bare bipolar nuclei, stromal fragments, cohesive cluster of uniform epithelial cell. Sometimes specific diagnosis can be formulated (i.e. fibroadenoma) |
| C3 | Cells suspicious but probably benign | Increased cellularity, nuclear cytological atypia, loss of cohesion, and scanty bare bipolar nuclei |
| C4 | Cells suspicious but probably malignant | The cytological features are suggestive but not diagnostic of malignancy (i.e. lesions borderline or low-grade ductal carcinoma) |
| C5 | Definitely malignant | The cytological features are diagnostic of malignancy and, where possible, indicate the nuclear grade and report the presence or absence of microcalcifications |

### 6.2.3 Scrape Cytology

Scrape cytology is accomplished in eczematous skin changes of the nipple-areola complex that could be associated with an underlying in situ or invasive carcinoma, as in Paget's disease (see Sect. 14.1). The usefulness of cytology in the diagnosis of Paget's disease has been suggested only in a few studies despite the fact that in many cases, it offers definitive informative advantages over surgical excision biopsy.

Proper cytological smears are obtained by an apposition of the slide over the nipple with or without a gentle scrape. Easy practicability, rapidity, cost-effectiveness and non-invasiveness stand opposite to a limited sensitivity as a disadvantage.

### 6.2.4 Cytological Categories

All results of cytological sampling should be given by the cytologist as a numerical category. Cytological categories are shown in Table 6.5.

*Checking results*. Lesions which are challenging are mostly C3 results. They can be due to:

- Flourishing fibroadenoma
- Highly differentiated carcinoma
- Sampling made in the immediate premenstrual phase
- Hormonal replacement therapy in progress or suspended for no more than 15 days

Uncertain findings indicate the need for further investigations. If in the instrumental findings benignity predominates, it is indicated to perform a core needle biopsy rather than a surgical biopsy.

## 6.3 Histological Samples

**Clinical Practice Points**

- The most appropriate and definitive diagnosis is obtained with histological characterisation, allowed by a core needle biopsy (CNB) or an open surgery.
- A 14-gauge (or wider) CNB can provide a definitive diagnosis in more than 90 % of cases and should be the preferred method.
- While simple CNB removes one sample of breast tissue per needle insertion, CNB connected to a vacuum-powered instrument (vacuum-assisted biopsy, VAB) is accomplished to collect multiple tissue samples during only one needle insertion.
- Radiological microcalcifications or parenchymal distortions are best assessed with VAB because of the number and the width of samples.
- Since core biopsy has improved the accuracy of image-guided needle biopsy, the purpose to avoid histological underestimation and potential for sampling error has led to more invasive and larger-volume percutaneous biopsy devices.

Alongside open surgery, a definitive histological diagnosis can be obtained with core needle biopsy (CNB). In preoperative diagnosis of BC, a 14G core biopsy can provide both histological and biological characterisation of the lesion, outlining also grading and biomarkers (ER, PR, HER2, Ki67) useful for a suitable plan of treatment, as neoadjuvant therapy, where indicated.

### 6.3.1 Core Needle Biopsy (CNB)

A core needle biopsy (CNB) is much like an FNAB, but also something more. A larger hollow needle is used to withdraw small cylinders (or cores) of tissue from the abnormal area in the breast. CNB is most often done with local anaesthesia, and the needle is inserted two to six times to get the samples according to the nature and the size of the lesion. As said before, fewer passes are required for solid lesions compared with microcalcifications. CNB takes longer than an FNAB and can cause some bruising but usually does not leave scars inside or outside the breast.

The needle is usually placed under image guidance (ultrasound or x-rays) to be sure it's in the right place [2]. In cases of a large and easily felt area, free-hand insertion is feasible. The diagnostic ability of CNB depends on the type of lesion (mass or calcifications only), the width of the needle used (from 14G to 16G) and the amount of tissue taken.

CNB is particularly indicated in assessing findings highly suggestive or suspicious for malignancy (BIRADS 4/5), findings assessed as probably benign

(BIRADS 3, C1 and C3 cytological class), multicentric lesions in order to plan timing and way of treatment.

*Checking results.* It could be considered that with CNB, 10–30 % of intraductal carcinoma could not present foci of invasiveness as in the definitive surgery. Moreover, because of their characteristics of morphological complexity, some benign diseases such as atypical epithelial hyperplasia, sclerosing adenosis or radial scar require in any case excisional biopsy surgery.

## 6.3.2 Vacuum-Assisted Biopsy (VAB)

The need of multiple passes of the needle as in large areas of microcalcifications or in indefinite parenchymal distortion should give preference to VAB procedure. Only where resources allow, vacuum-assisted biopsy techniques offer significant advantages for biopsy in a large proportion of patients in achieving definitive preoperative diagnosis and reducing the need for surgical intervention. This technique can provide greater tissue volume for histological analysis with less risk of epithelial displacement or underestimation of disease such as DCIS or invasive tumours. In dedicated practices, VAB can also be used for the therapeutic excision of benign lesions measuring less than 15 mm.

With vacuum-assisted devices, an 8- or 11-gauge needle is positioned using ultrasound or mammographic guidance, and targeted breast tissue is drawn, cut and saved in a collecting chamber. There is potential risk of bruising with wide-bore needle biopsies, and anticoagulants should be stopped in some, but not all, cases. Minimal residual hematomas should be manually compressed for few minutes or handled with compressive bandages. Small incision does not require stitches for closure. In any case, CNB has a lower risk of hematomas and infection (less than 1 %) than open surgical biopsy where the rate of hematomas is 2–10 % and the rate of infections is 4–6 %.

The technique is safe, performed with the patient under local anaesthesia, with a low complication rate. As said before, the procedure is expensive, but with proper indications, it reduces intangible costs related to physical and psychological morbidity.

*Ultrasound localisation.* Modern, high-resolution ultrasound probe can detect even small mammographic densities. Approximately 50 % of all non-palpable lesions, usually detected by mammography, can be located by ultrasound. Only microcalcifications are hardly ever visualised (Fig. 6.5).

*Mammographic localisation.* Vacuum-assisted biopsies can be accomplished with dedicated equipment. Procedure is done in outpatient settings and performed under local anaesthesia. The patient usually lies face down on a moveable exam table, and the affected breast is positioned into an opening in the table. The breast will be compressed and held in position throughout the procedure. The table will then be raised and the procedure performed beneath it.

In all procedures, breast tissue is excised by a rotating cutter, and multiple harvests can be performed 360° around the lesion while the needle remains in the

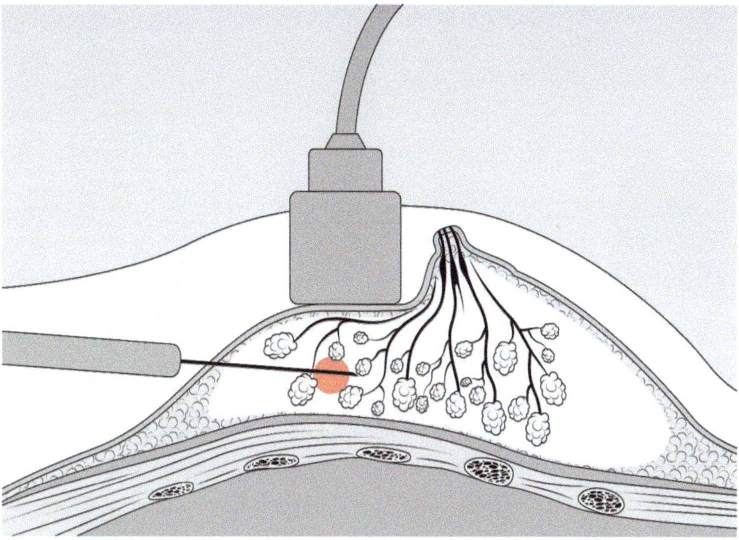

**Fig. 6.5** Core needle biopsy under US guidance. Under local anaesthesia, an ultrasound probe is placed over the site of the mass to guide the biopsy needle directly into the lesion

lesion during the whole procedure. Although 14-gauge needles were initially utilised, an 11-gauge probe (and in some cases a 9-gauge) is now widely used.

Finally, a VAB device can achieve the complete removal of the mammographic abnormality or of some small lesions up to 15 mm. Mammographic confirmation of complete removal or of removal of a major part of the lesion is important in the determination of the final diagnosis as representative. Lesions up to 10 mm in greatest dimension can be completely removed in almost all cases, while lesions from 11 to 20 mm can be completely removed in 50–70 % of patients, unless using other dedicated breast lesion excision systems.

### 6.3.3 Skin Punch Biopsy

In the case of lesions involving mainly the skin, especially with a suspicion of inflammatory BC or Paget's disease, a circular tool (skin punch) may be used to remove a small section of the skin and its deeper layers (Fig. 6.6). The wound is closed with one stitch.

### 6.3.4 Histological Categories

Histological categories are shown in Table 6.6.

*Checking results.* Undoubtedly, VAB is the best method to sample heterogeneous lesions that may have an associated component not otherwise demonstrated by CNB

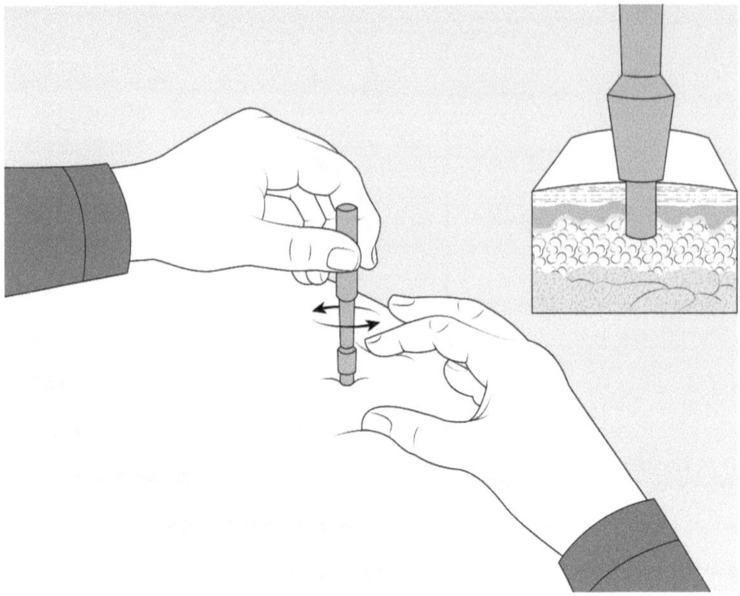

**Fig. 6.6** Skin punch biopsy. A circular tool is used to remove a small section of the skin and its deeper layers

**Table 6.6** Histological diagnostic categories

| | | |
|---|---|---|
| B1 | Normal tissue | Lipomas or hamartomas |
| | | Lesions not sufficiently predictable |
| B2 | Benign lesion | A wide variety of benign changes |
| | | Epithelial hyperplasia of usual type (HUT) |
| B3 | Lesion of uncertain malignant potential | Atypical ductal hyperplasia (ADH) with moderate degree of atypia |
| | | Atypical lobular hyperplasia (ALH) |
| | | Lobular carcinoma in situ (LCIS) |
| | | Papillary lesion |
| | | Phyllodes tumour |
| B4 | Suspicious of malignancy | Probable carcinoma cells but, where the sample is too small, crushed or poorly preserved for diagnostic certainty |
| B5 | Malignant | This should state whether invasive or in situ malignancy is demonstrated |
| | | Estimation of tumour grade and hormone receptor status can also be made |

as high-risk (ADH) and preinvasive (DCIS) lesions or preinvasive lesion (DCIS) and invasive cancer.

VAB is better than CNB in distinguishing ADH and DCIS in several reports. The volume increase in harvested tissue specimens resulted in a decreased sampling error in diagnosing ADH. Underestimation rates are lower for VAB than for CNB

(10–35 % vs. 45–55 %). However, use of the 11-gauge device cannot sufficiently exclude the discordance between ADH found after percutaneous biopsy and carcinoma found in subsequently excised tissue in order to reduce open surgery. About 25 % of patients are upgraded from ADH to DCIS, so that underestimation cannot be avoided completely. One explanation might be the subjective nature of the diagnosis of ADH using quantitative and qualitative criteria to distinguish ADH from DCIS. Moreover, ADH and DCIS can coexist in the same breast lesion; therefore, the recommendation that patients with ADH diagnosed by percutaneous biopsy should undergo surgical excision remains still valid.

Also in the diagnosis of DCIS vs. invasive BC, wide-bore needle biopsy has been demonstrated to be superior to CNB with about 10 % of vacuum-biopsy DCIS found to be invasive carcinoma at surgery compared with 20–30 % with 14-gauge core biopsy.

Finally, repeat biopsy rates for inadequate sampling of microcalcifications are also significantly lower when using VAB compared with CNB, although an equal proportion of malignancy is diagnosed following re-biopsy.

## 6.4 Localisation of Non-palpable Lesions

**Clinical Practice Points**

- Most non-palpable breast lesions can be successfully and accurately diagnosed using image-guided needle biopsy.
- Successful and effective excision of impalpable lesions is a combination of surgical and radiological skill. It is accepted that the only true reflection of excision adequacy is the subsequent rate of missing or recurrent lesions.
- Equipment and methods are the same required to accomplish a guided core needle biopsy, chosen starting from the simplest usable one, like US, to the more complex, like MRI. The modality of choice depends on the type of lesion and the operator's expertise.
- Inconclusive diagnosis, as well as BC and lesions frequently associated to cancer, should require appropriate surgery.

As BC screening with mammography increases, many non-palpable breast lesions are being detected. These lesions should first and foremost be definitively diagnosed by using image-guided needle biopsy. After needle biopsy, some of these lesions may require diagnostic or therapeutic surgical biopsy. If a malignant or indefinite diagnosis is obtained, surgical excision with uniform margins is indicated. This, in turn, requires accurate localisation of the lesion, which is required to ensure correct and adequate removal of the lesions and to minimise the degree of cosmetic disfigurement.

Preoperative localisation of the non-palpable breast abnormalities is accomplished by placing a marker or a hook wire in correspondence of the non-palpable lesion, using one or more positioning procedures.

### 6.4.1 Markers of Localisation

*Dye injection methods*, widely used in the past, nowadays are obsolete. Dye solutions, carried out at the time of cytological or micro-histological preoperative diagnosis, are easy to handle and produce a stained track that guides the surgeon to the targeted tissue. However, dyes tend to spread and diffuse, and localisation may become imprecise if too much time elapses between the dye injection and the surgery. Commonly, a sterile charcoal suspension is utilised that does not diffuse into the surrounding tissue and that stays in place for a long time. The trace goes from the lesion to the skin where a small spot is evident.

*Marker clip*. At the time of core needle biopsy or VAB, a tiny stainless-steel marker clip is put at the end of the procedure within the core biopsy site, just in case a subsequent surgery would be necessary. These small safe devices show up on mammograms or ultrasound and are often used to identify the area of surgical biopsy. Limits of markers are their displacement, especially if hematoma occurs, or migration in fatty breasts. In a dense breast, markers are more easy to detect and, moreover, to check in operative specimen.

*Preoperative hook-wire localisation* is another common preoperative approach to non-palpable lesions, feasible in at least 90 % of cases. An ultrasound- or mammography (rarely MRI)-guided hollow needle, containing the hooked wire, is inserted by the radiologist in the breast and placed within or near the lesion. After instrumental localisation, the hollow needle is removed, and the wire is left in place where it remains anchored by a small hook in its tip.

In cases of segmental microcalcifications, it may be advantageous for the radiologist to bracket the extent of the calcifications with two or more wires to allow complete surgical excision. The surgeon must be provided with a full and accurate description of the procedure performed and a precise report of the relative placement of the wire compared to the lesion. Relevant images correctly marked should also be provided.

The hook-wire method is particularly useful for deep lesions mainly in dense breasts where it can be anchored more securely. The choice of needles and wires used is dictated by the preference of the radiologist and the surgeons. A disadvantage of this procedure is the need for it to be carried out shortly before surgery and therefore to require accurate planning. Moreover, the hook wire may dislodge from its original position during patient transport or preoperative preparations, and this happens more frequently in fatty breasts.

Actually all localisation methods of hook wire are subject to potential inaccuracies, and it is important to confirm the correct placement of the guidewire. Ultrasonographic and mammographic wire localisations must be followed by mammography performed in two planes (latero-medial and cranio-caudal projections) to confirm that the correct lesion has been accurately targeted. Ideally, the guidewire should transfix the lesion on both projections, and the hook should ideally be placed no more than 1 cm from the target lesion.

Complications, including pneumothorax, have been described in the past. Wire fragments may also be retained following surgery. Published literature shows that the rate of needle localisation failure is in the range of 0–20 %. Factors associated with such failure include lesion size and type, increased distance of the needle from the lesion and decreased specimen volume, in addition to surgeon's expertise.

*Radio-guided occult lesion localisation (ROLL)* is a more recent method for localisation of non-palpable tumours. Before the operation, colloidal albumin labelled with technetium-99 m ($^{99m}Tc$) is injected directly into the lesion under stereotactic or ultrasonographic guidance. The accuracy of isotope placement is checked with scintigraphy.

Excision biopsy is then performed by using a gamma probe. After excision, the excised lesion and the cavity are checked for radioactivity, and the specimen is radiographed to ensure the radiographic adequacy of the excision. This technique is very accurate, more than the conventional wire localisation in large and fatty breast or other individual circumstances of possible dislocation of the wire. Although ROLL is considered superior to wire-guided localisation, the procedure is more complex and expensive in most common situation.

*Ink marker* drawing on the skin, finally, is the simplest method, but it does not indicate the depth of the lesion and should not be employed for small lesions.

### 6.4.2 Techniques of Localisation

*Ultrasound localisation.* If non-palpable lesions are visible under ultrasound, this is the preferred imaging for biopsy guidance. This technique provides the advantage of real-time imaging, allowing accurate placement of the needle. Being able to directly visualise the lesion and needle position results in a quicker procedure, reducing the risk of patient morbidity. As in all techniques, the lesion must be transfixed, and orthogonal mammography should be used to confirm the correct localisation. In individual cases, intraoperative ultrasound-guided excision of non-palpable BC could be performed, with results that are comparable to those reported with other methods.

*Stereotactic localisation.* The principles of stereotactic localisation involve mapping the distance between the geometric centre of the breast and the target lesion in two different planes and then projecting the coordinates onto the patient's breast. Earlier techniques in stereotaxis used mammographic projections to localise the target lesion within the breast [3]. Advances in digital mammography have since superseded manual computations. Dedicated stereotactic equipment that performs localisation with fixation of the breast is now in use. Stereotactic techniques have also been developed within other imaging modalities, including ultrasonography and magnetic resonance imaging (MRI). These techniques offer more options and greater flexibility in performing stereotactic biopsy but are less commonly available.

The main application of stereotactic localisation is for the small, indistinct lesions, particularly those occurring in association with surgical scarring, fibrosis or prosthetic implants. The procedure may be performed with the patient upright or prone, according with the practice of the breast unit, where adequate room is settled to lodge the device.

The prone position is more comfortable and it is also preferred for keeping the patient more stable. Although the vast majority of the published literature on stereotactic core biopsy involves the use of dedicated prone-biopsy units, with the advent of digital acquisition, the accuracy with upright stereotactic units could reasonably be expected to improve. In practice, if prone table is preferred for CNB, upright procedure is more advantageous for radiological localisation. For all cases, the best procedure is one that allows the patient lying in the supine chirurgical position.

*Prone table stereotactic procedure.* The needle is placed 1 cm beyond the lesion to ensure that it is adequately transfixed, but, because of the accordion effect (the thickness of the breast expands when compression is released), the hook-wire tip may migrate, causing the needle to be placed shortly off the lesion. As said before, the prone table position is better tolerated than the upright system, but boundary conditions and sometimes contraindications to stereotactic localisation are more or less the same for both techniques:

- Patients who cannot keep still for up to 30 min (anxiety, chronic cough, neurologic musculoskeletal problems)
- Weight greater than tolerated by the stereotactic machine
- Lesions too close to the chest wall or axilla to be accessed by the biopsy needle
- Indiscrete lesions or faint microcalcifications not seen clearly on stereotactic imaging
- Lesions uncomfortably close to blood vessels or breast implants
- Breast compresses to less than 2 cm from the chest wall

*Upright stereotactic procedure.* The woman is seated next to the stereotactic mammography unit, and the breast is compressed and held in position throughout the procedure. Dedicated stereotactic equipment estimates the site where the stiffer coaxial needle holding the hook wire is to be inserted at a depth calculated by a computerised system. Once the localisation is complete, the needle is removed leaving the wire in place, and mammograms are performed to confirm that the marker is in the proper position.

A normal mammographic unit technique requires a dedicated attachment. The breast lesion is located in a three-dimensional space (coordinates x, y and z) by means of a double radiological exposure obtained by tilting the arm of the mammography tube and measuring the coordinates of the lesion on two mammograms. Finally, a small mark is made on the skin and the needle inserted at the correct calculated depth.

*MRI localisation.* The use of MRI localisation reflects the increasing use of magnetic resonance mammography. Although a portion of MRI-depicted lesions can subsequently be localised with ultrasonography, some of them are occult in mammography and ultrasound, and they require MRI-guided needle biopsy or localisation.

All of the major manufacturers of MRI units have biopsy attachments available as an option; these require the patient to be kept in a semi-prone position. The MRI is then performed with the intravenous administration of a gadolinium-based contrast agent, and the lesion is localised by using MRI-compatible localisation needles.

Technical difficulties and challenges include the tendency of the MRI-visible lesion to fade over time. Moreover, because of the amount of time required to perform the procedure (more than half hour), the patient may begin to move, which could cause an error in needle placement. Nevertheless, MRI localisations have generally been as accurate as mammographic localisations, with miss rates of 2–9 %. Some investigators have suggested that postoperative MRI should be performed to verify complete excision of the lesion.

*Tomosynthesis* too allows radiologists to locate and accurately target regions of interest for biopsy and/or preoperative localisation. New tomosynthesis equipment offers a number of advantages over stereotactic procedures. They easily target lesions including those visible only in tomosynthesis images. Streamlined procedure steps and faster targeting are resulting in improved workflow and shorter patient procedure time. In some cases, fewer exposures are required, reducing dose exposure of the patient. Nonetheless, the technique is too recent for supported reports and, moreover, not widely available.

## 6.5 Open Surgical Biopsy

**Clinical Practice Points**

- The ratio of benign to malignant surgical excision biopsies performed for diagnostic purposes should not exceed 0.5:1, although a ratio of 1:1 is tolerated.
- The extent of benign biopsy should be minimised, and the most suitable discriminatory factor is the reduced weight of the specimen. Less than 30 g should be the standard in more than 90 % of cases.
- No frozen section should be performed if tumour diameter is less than 10 mm, with a minimum standard of about 95 % of cases.
- Proportion of impalpable lesions successfully excised without recourse to second operation requires a minimum standard superior to 90 % of cases.
- A true reflection of excision adequacy influences the subsequent rate of inadequate sampling or local recurrence.

### 6.5.1 Technique

A correct surgical standard provides for a mammogram to be carried out prior to almost any breast surgery as a matter of good practice to demonstrate the nature and extent of any disease that is identifiable.

The surgical procedure is carried out in the hospital's outpatient department under local anaesthesia, less commonly under general anaesthesia, and may be:

- An incisional biopsy, which removes only part of the suspicious area enough to make a diagnosis
- An excisional biopsy, which removes the entire mass or abnormal area, with or without trying to remove an edge of normal breast tissue, depending to the purpose of the biopsy

In order to limit the number of unnecessary biopsy procedures performed, it is recommended that the ratio of benign to malignant surgical excision biopsies performed for diagnostic purposes should not exceed 0.5:1. Benign lesions previously diagnosed and lesions removed due to patient choice are excluded. Nonetheless, considering the many factors that can influence the decision to perform the surgery, mainly due to the technical limits of previous procedures and to additional individual risks, a ratio of 1:1 is tolerated.

For cosmetic reasons, it is important to minimise the extent of benign biopsy for impalpable lesions, and at present, the most suitable discriminatory factor used is the weight of the specimen. Over 90 % of diagnostic biopsies for impalpable lesions, which subsequently prove benign, should weigh less than 30 g. All open surgical diagnostic biopsies which prove to be benign and weigh >40 g should be discussed at the postoperative MDT meeting and any mitigating reason recorded.

*Assessment of resection margins* is of outmost importance in high-risk (ADH) and preinvasive (DCIS) lesions. The surgeon should be discouraged from cutting specimens after removal before sending them to pathology. All specimens should be marked and oriented according to recognised local protocols. The surgeon should basically ensure completeness of excision, which may be achieved by the use of two-plane specimen radiography.

Macroscopic examination during surgery has only an orientation value. Only in those cases when it is considered to be useful enough, however unreliable in the absence of histological data, the pathologist could take care of cutting the specimens. After staining the outer surface of the specimen, the specimen is opened and inspected and the minimum distances measured and communicated to the operator.

At the time of surgery, the use of frozen sectioning is generally inappropriate, particularly in the assessment of clinically impalpable lesions. Microscopic extemporaneous examination of the margins is less reliable in general because of the possibility of dispersion of material useful for the diagnosis in case the tumour is located close to the margin. It may occasionally be justified in order to enable an ultimate diagnosis of invasive malignancy and to allow definitive surgery to be carried out in one operative procedure.

Touch prep, that is, cytology for apposition of the margins of resection, gives only approximate information. Microscopic examination after inclusion is the technique that provides the greatest number of diagnostic information from all the material in question.

*Checking the results.* After surgery, few false-positive results are reported. Some are only apparent, due to the complete removal of the lesion by means of core biopsy. Others are real, due to surgical failure to remove the lesion. On the other hand, surgery identifies some reported false-negative results for malignancy with core biopsy. These are in the range of 2–6 %, with a mean rate of 4.5 %, and more likely occur with microcalcifications. This variation may represent the wide range of experience and expertise in the technique found in different breast units.

### 6.5.2 Quality Outcomes

Quality outcomes of breast biopsy are highlighted in almost all guidelines. The most significant measures are reported below [4].

When the lesion is visible on x-ray, specimen radiographs must be available in or in very close proximity to the operating theatre so that confirmation of excision of the lesion can be confirmed without delay and prior to skin closure. Specimen radiographies should also be made available to the pathology department. In the case of open surgery, the lumpectomy specimen should be oriented in three planes so that the pathologist can use a multicolour staining system to identify close or positive margins.

Successful excision of impalpable lesions is therefore a combination of surgical and radiological skills, and the proportion of impalpable lesions successfully excised at the first operation and not requiring a second operation should be in excess of 90 %. It is accepted that the only true reflection of excision adequacy is the subsequent rate of missing and recurrent lesion.

Certain histologic results should be interpreted with caution. With core biopsy, a propensity to underestimate certain pathology exists. Over 50 % of all cases of atypical ductal hyperplasia (ADH) diagnosed with core biopsy prove malignant at surgery, and invasive carcinoma is found in up to 33 % of core biopsy-confirmed ductal carcinoma in situ (DCIS).

Radial scars diagnosed by means of core biopsy should also be regarded as high-risk lesions requiring excision. It is also more difficult to achieve a diagnosis using core biopsy in low-risk calcifications or where the underlying cause is subsequently proven to be benign.

Therefore, core biopsy results should always be carefully analysed to ensure that radiologic and pathologic concordance exists. Another concern is the potential malignant seeding of the needle track after core biopsy; however, the significance and true incidence of this phenomenon remain uncertain.

## References

1. Gutwein LG, Ang DN, Liu H, et al. Utilization of minimally invasive breast biopsy for the evaluation of suspicious breast lesions. Am J Surg. 2011;202:227–32.
2. Teh WL, Wilson AR, Evans AJ, Burrell H, Pinder SE, Ellis IO. Ultrasound guided core biopsy of suspicious mammographic calcifications using high frequency and power Doppler ultrasound. Clin Radiol. 2000;55(5):390–4.

3. Kettriz U, Rotter K, Schreer I, et al. Stereotactic vacuum-assisted breast biopsy in 2874 patients: a multicentric study. Cancer. 2004;100:245–51.
4. Perry NM. Multidisciplinary aspects of quality assurance in the diagnosis of breast disease EUSOMA. Eur J Cancer. 2001;37:159–72.

## Further Reading

Ciatto S. B3 core biopsies should be assumed as positive findings for accuracy purposes. Radiol Med. 2011;116:982–3.

Nakano S, Otsuka M, Mibu A, Oinuma T. Significance of fine needle aspiration cytology and vacuum-assisted core needle biopsy for small breast lesions. Clin Breast Cancer. 2015;15:e23–6.

Parkin CKE, Garewal S, Waugh P, Maxwell AJ. Outcomes of patients with lobular in situ neoplasia of the breast: the role of vacuum-assisted biopsy. Breast. 2014;23:651–5.

Querci della Rovere G, Patel A, Roche N, Grown G, Orzalesi L, Benson JR, et al. Preoperative localisation of impalpable breast abnormality. In: Querci della Rovere G, Warren R, Benson JR, editors. Early breast cancer – from screening to multidisciplinary management. London: Taylor and Francis; 2006.

Teh WL, Evans AJ, Wilson AR. Definitive non-surgical breast diagnosis: the role of the radiologist. Clin Radiol. 1998;53:81–4.

**Websites in Appendix**: *Surgery*, A-21.

# 7 Breast Pain

Giorgio Macellari and Giorgio Baratelli

## Contents



**Abstract**

• Breast pain alone or painful lumpiness is one of the most common breast issues and accounts for approximately 50–60 % of all referrals of new outpatients to clinics. • Although breast nodularity and lumpiness is sometimes associated with breast pain, it is a separate entity and should be assessed independently. • True breast pain is a rare symptom of BC. Sclerosing adenosis and postsurgery scar are uncommon but important causes. • Breast pain could be a problematic and

G. Macellari (✉)
Surgical Breast Clinic, Hospital "Guglielmo da Saliceto", Piacenza, Italy
e-mail: g.macellari@ausl.pc.it

G. Baratelli
Breast Unit, Hospital "Moriggia-Pelascini", Gravedona, Italy
e-mail: gmbaratelli@yahoo.it



A.M. Pluchinotta (ed.), *The Outpatient Breast Clinic: Aiming at Best Practice*,
DOI 10.1007/978-3-319-15907-2_7

baffling symptom. In the absence of suspicious elements, provide the woman with persuasive explanations. • The most challenging clinical issue is to determine the impact of breast pain on quality of life. • Most mild to moderate cases are seeking reassurance, and this is usually all that is required: this is successful in 80–85 % of patients. Few patients with breast pain need treatment with medications.

*Future directions*. Mastalgia is now accepted as a common cause of morbidity, occasionally severe enough to interfere with quality of life. Cases refractory to standard treatment need careful individual assessment, and some patient may benefit from psychological assessment and therapy.

## 7.1 Overview

**Clinical Practice Points**

- Mastalgia is now accepted as a common cause of morbidity, occasionally severe enough to interfere with quality of life and thus sufficient to justify careful investigation and treatment.
- Only a minority of breast pain is explained by breast pathologies. Most breast pain is of unknown cause.
- Careful examination can differentiate true breast pain, cyclic and noncyclic, from non-mammary pain arising from the underlying chest wall.
- A suspicion of cancer should be considered seriously in any patient complaining of a persistent and well-localised breast pain.
- In older women, pain associated to cancer is rare (2–3 % of all BC) and usually asymptomatic, in most cases suggesting an occasional finding.
- There is no evidence that mastalgia leads to an increased breast cancer risk.

In Western societies, mastalgia, or breast pain without underlying pathology, is a common complaint that may affect up to 70 % of women in their lifetime. Interestingly, it is less common in Asian cultures, affecting as few as 5 % of women.

*HISTORY AND PHYSICAL EXAM*. A patient history is directed toward identifying and characterising breast-related symptoms. The information gathered should include location and severity of pain, relationship to physical activities or the menstrual cycle, association with redness or warmth of overlying skin and impact on everyday activities, in particular sleep, daily routine and the use of medication. Hormonal influences, such as pregnancy, use of contraceptives and hormone therapy should also be reviewed.

Obtaining a history may also provide information useful for identifying non-breast sources of pain. The patient should also be asked about all medications she might be taking, and those that can be associated with breast pain should be noted.

Medications that may cause breast pain include: oxymetholone, chlorpromazine, diuretics, digitalis preparations, methyldopa and spironolactone.

A clinical examination of the breast should be performed with careful inspection and palpation of each breast, nipple-areolar complex and regional lymph nodes. Localised, generalised or bilateral breast tenderness should be noted. In addition to palpating the breasts while the patient is supine, examining the breasts while the patient is sitting or lying on her side may allow breast and chest wall tenderness to be distinguished (Fig. 7.1).

Laboratory studies are generally not useful. A pregnancy test, however, should be considered in women of reproductive age if the history or examination suggests pregnancy. Other hormone levels (e.g., oestrogen, progesterone and prolactin) are typically normal in patients with breast pain.

Imaging studies are frequently utilised in the evaluation of the breast. A mammogram should be considered especially in women with a family history of early BC. The risk of malignancy after normal findings on mammographic evaluation for breast pain is about 0.5–2 %, mostly in postmenopausal women. It is unclear whether the pain is related to the cancer or whether this symptom initiates a breast evaluation in which an asymptomatic cancer is identified. Breast pain secondary to malignancy is typically unilateral and persistent. In these cases, imaging with directed ultrasound may be a more valuable assessment tool.

A variety of conditions can result in pain perceived in the breast as a result of pregnancy, mastitis, trauma, thrombophlebitis, macrocysts, benign tumours or cancer; however, only a minority of breast pain is explained by these conditions. Most breast pain is of unknown cause, and the above conditions can be revealed as a result of a directed history and physical examination. As appropriate, an exam directed at the cervical and thoracic spine, chest wall, shoulders and upper extremities, sternum, heart, lungs and abdomen may be helpful in assessing other potential causes of the pain.

*CLASSIFICATION*. Breast pain is commonly categorised into three classifications: cyclic mastalgia, noncyclic mastalgia and non-mammary pain. Our personal classification scheme is shown in Table 7.1.

*Cyclic mastalgia* occurs in premenopausal women and is clearly related to the menstrual cycle. The pain is typically bilateral and diffuse, often located in the upper outer quadrants of the breasts with frequent radiation to the axilla and the ipsilateral arm. Occasionally, breast pain may be unilateral or more intense in one breast.

*Noncyclic mastalgia may* involve continuous or intermittent pain that does not concur with the menstrual cycle. The pain is more often unilateral and localised with the pain in the lower inner portions of the breast. Noncyclic breast pain generally occurs in older postmenopausal women.

*Non-mammary pain* may present with the symptom of breast pain. Following the history and physical exam, differentiating breast pain and pain radiating from the chest wall or another site is usually straightforward. Occasionally the origin of pain is not evident, or there are multiple origins of pain, making evaluation more challenging.

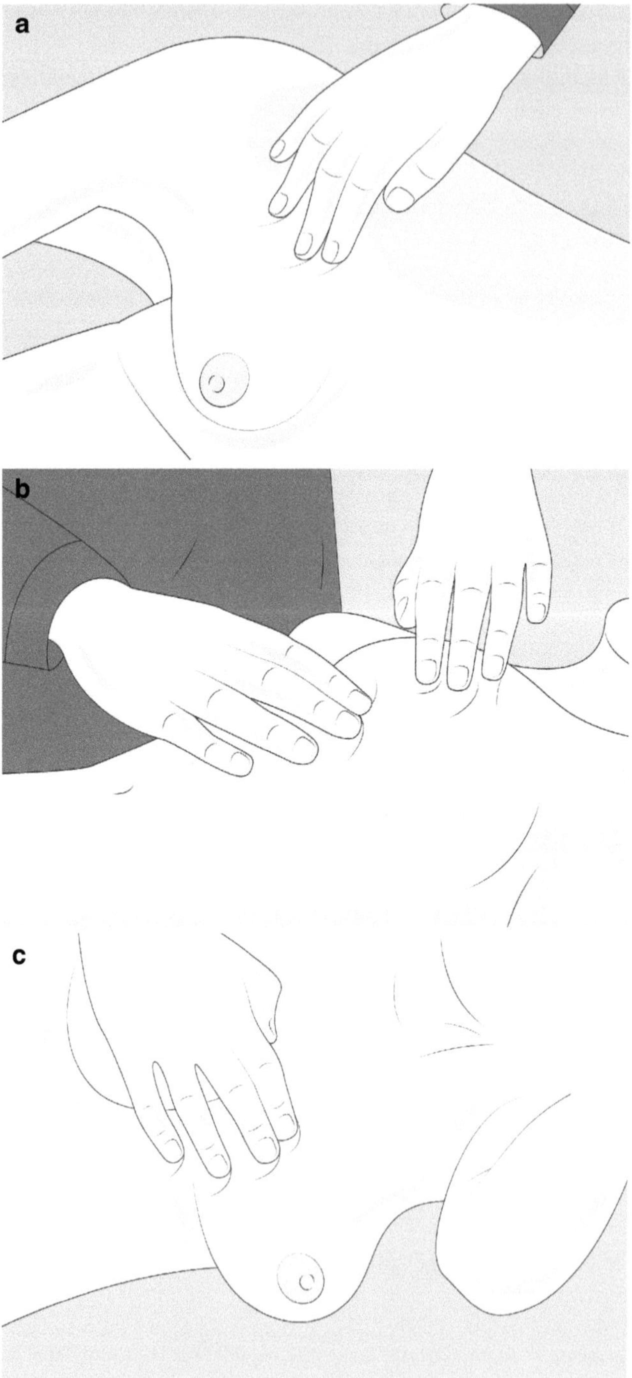


**Fig. 7.1** To identify any area of localised tenderness of the lateral chest wall, the patient is rolled on her side in order to let the breast fall away and to examine the site of the pain (*left*). Equally, to examine the medial chest wall tenderness, the patient is rolled on her side. The breast falls away and it is easier to palpate the costochondral junctions (*middle*). To examine the lower chest wall tenderness, the breast is lifted upward with one hand, while the other hand presses gently on underlying chest wall to identify the localised pain (*right*) [1]

**Table 7.1** Our personal classification of mastalgia

| Classification | Characteristics | Notes |
|---|---|---|
| Cyclic mastalgia (about 60–70 % of cases) | Pain varying with menstrual cycle, not to be confused with premenstrual syndrome | Pain charts are an important aid to assessment |
| | Women without periods, with ovarian function | |
| | Pain in the monthly patterns (women without periods or post hysterectomy) | |
| | Pain using cyclic hormone replacement therapy | |
| Noncyclic mastalgia (about 20–25 % of cases) | *Idiopathic mastalgia* | True mastalgia remains a mystery |
| | Usually a variable and unexplained symptom | |
| | *Painful breast pathology* | Many breast conditions could occasionally result in breast pain; however, only a minority of breast pain is explained by these conditions |
| | Stretching of Cooper's ligaments | |
| | Sclerosing adenosis | A highly significant association exists between the severity of mastalgia and the extent of ductal mammary ectasia |
| | Mondor disease | |
| | Pressure from brassiere | |
| | Fat necrosis from trauma | |
| | Hidradenitis suppurativa | |
| | Focal mastitis | |
| | Periductal mastitis | |
| | Stretch cyst(s) | |
| | BC (rare) | |
| Non-mammary pain (about 10–15 % of cases) | *Chest wall pain* | Underlying musculoskeletal pathology may be steadily symptomatic or occasionally exacerbated by lifestyle, increasing activities, and ill-fitting brassiere |
| | Tietze's syndrome (costochondritis) | |
| | Localised lateral chest wall pain | |
| | Diffuse lateral chest wall pain | |
| | Radicular pain from cervical arthritis | |
| | *Non-chest wall pain* | |
| | Gallbladder disease | |
| | Ischemic heart disease | |
| | Esophagitis and hiatal hernia, especially associated with abuse of alcohol | |

*PAIN CHART*. The main form of assessment to confirm the cyclical nature of the symptoms is a breast pain chart, a diary where to document and score pain on a daily basis as either severe, mild or no pain at all. The commencement of menstruation is also recorded, and after a couple of months, it becomes apparent if the symptoms are cyclical in nature.

A breast pain chart can be used to record the pattern and severity of the mastalgia, as well its relation to menstrual period. Many different models of breast pain record chart are available. Our personal chart takes account of three scores of

**Table 7.2** Our personal chart used to establish mastalgia [2]

| | Pain <30 % | Pain 30 up to 70 % | Pain more than 70 % |
|---|---|---|---|
| <7 days | Light | Light | Medium |
| 8–15 days | Light | Medium | Severe |
| >15 days | Medium | Severe | Severe |

mastalgia (light, medium and severe) according to intensity (assessed using the visual analogue scale) and to duration of the pain (Table 7.2).

## 7.2 Cyclic Mastalgia

**Clinical Practice Points**

- There are considerable overlaps between cyclical mastalgia and premenstrual syndrome, but there are also significant differences, requiring different approaches.
- A pronounced pain characterises cyclic mastalgia so that it should not be confused with premenstrual syndrome, even if cyclic mastalgia and premenstrual syndrome have substantial overlaps.
- Cyclic mastalgia includes pain varying with menstrual cycle as well breast pain in women without periods but with ovarian function (i.e. post hysterectomy) or even postmenopausal ones taking HRT.
- The basic cause of cyclical mastalgia is clearly endocrine in nature, but the precise mechanism(s) continues to elude investigators.
- In cyclic mastalgia, pain charts are an important aid to assessment.

Virtually all women will experience a degree of pain or discomfort in their breasts at some time of their lives. This is normal and most often occurs in the week prior to menstruation. Cyclical mastalgia is not to be confused with premenstrual syndrome (PMS), which, by definition, is associated with the menstrual cycle but differs in presentation, effective treatment and likely aetiology (see Chap. 3). In some women, however, the pain can become quite severe and in certain cases can result in problems with daily activities, quality of life and marital relationships. When this occurs, cyclic mastalgia should be treated.

Due to the relationship with the menstrual cycle or hormone replacement therapy, it is thought that the cause of cyclical mastalgia is hormonal. Actually the aetiology of mastalgia is not well understood. Hormonal assays of oestrogen, progesterone and prolactin have shown no consistent abnormalities despite the relationship to the menstrual cycle. Even so, pregnancy, lactation, menopause, oral contraceptives and hormone replacement therapy variously affect the course of breast pain. Some studies have shown hyperresponsiveness of prolactin to stimulation by thyrotropin-releasing hormone, while others have suggested elevated levels or abnormalities of lipid metabolism. It has been proposed that breast pain during the luteal phase of the menstrual cycle may be due to higher serum oestrogen-to-progesterone ratios. This may be related more to an insufficiency of progesterone rather than an excess of oestrogen.

One correlation between women with mastalgia and controls when determining total body water was not found. Therefore, as fluid retention is not a factor, there is no rationale for the use of diuretics or sodium restriction.

There are also other suggestions that consumption of too much caffeine or a deficient intake of essential fatty acids can also result in cyclical mastalgia. However, no explanation has been demonstrated with evidence, and in many cases cyclic mastalgia still remains a mystery.

*Symptoms.* Cyclic mastalgia affects up to 40 % of women before menopause, most often in the third decade of life. In the mildest form, the pain lasts only a few days prior to menstruation. The number of symptomatic days varies, however, and a few women can experience pain for virtually the whole month, with relief occurring only at the time of menstruation.

In approximately 10 % of these women, pain will be severe and interfere with their normal activities. A minority of women with the most severe pain will also experience it during menstruation. The pain can continue for many years but will usually disappear after menopause. In 20 % of women, it subsides without any intervention.

Cyclic mastalgia includes pain varying with menstrual cycle as well breast pain in women without periods but with ovarian function (i.e. post hysterectomy) or even postmenopausal ones taking hormone replacement therapy (HRT). Many women describe the pain as dull, burning, throbbing or aching, usually starting in the upper quadrant of the breast. Sometimes a shooting pain radiating to the arm and axilla may be present, probably secondary to glandular pressure on the intercostobrachial nerve (Fig. 7.2).

Even though both breasts can be involved, patient often claim one breast is worse than the other. On clinical examination, diffuse tenderness with lumpiness and nodularity in the breast is detected when the pain is present, and the upper outer quadrants of the breast are most commonly affected. There is no single discrete lump to feel and there are no abnormalities with the nipple. Mammography typically shows no abnormality, but the breast tissue can appear glandular and dense.

## 7.3 Noncyclic Mastalgia

**Clinical Practice Points**

- In noncyclic mastalgia, the pain in the breast is not related to the menstrual cycle and shows broad patterns and a poorer response to treatment.
- If any cause for chronic, severe and persistent breast pain is found, noncyclic mastalgia should be considered idiopathic.
- In some cases, differential diagnosis of overlapping symptoms of true noncyclic mastalgia and non-mammary pain turns out to be challenging.

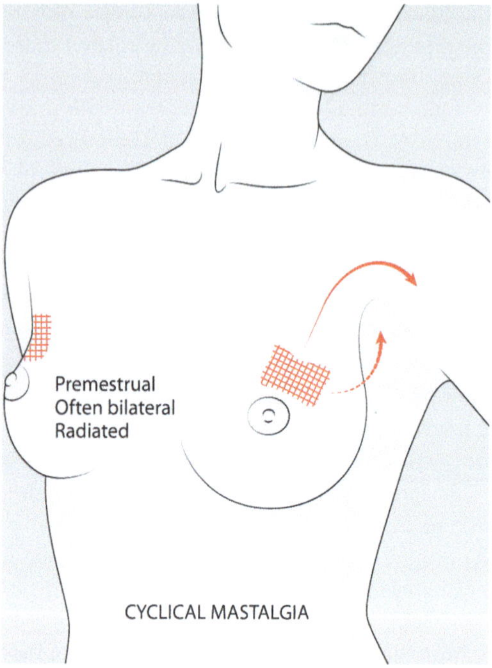


**Fig. 7.2** Symptoms and localisations of cyclical mastalgia. Symptoms may include a dull ache, heaviness, tightness, a burning sensation or breast tenderness. Pain is brought on by activity and may be reproduced by pressure on the upper outer quadrants, often associated with nodularity, radiated down the arm and toward the axilla, and relieved by menstruation [3, mod. with permission.]

Patterns of noncyclic mastalgia are: ill-localised pain not associated with menstrual periods. Symptoms usually are unilateral, involve upper quadrants and are described as heavy, aching, tender, concerning, burning, pulling, stabbing and pinching. True, or idiopathic, noncyclic mastalgia should be differentiated from breast pain due to specific pathologies as periductal mastitis or fat necrosis. Sometimes symptoms are so undistinguished that a challenging diagnosis with non-breast pain should also be done (Fig. 7.3).

### 7.3.1 Idiopathic Mastalgia

Idiopathic mastalgia is characterised by chronic severe breast pain that persist for years without any obvious cause. Pain can be bilateral or, more often, unilateral. Without any organic disease, aetiology is often misdiagnosed as psychological.

### 7.3.2 Breast Pain Due To Specific Pathology

A number of conditions can occasionally give rise to noncyclical mastalgia, each with certain additional symptoms or clinical signs that aid diagnosis. Inflammatory patterns are associated to focal mastitis, periductal mastitis, hidradenitis suppurativa and other chronic inflammatory diseases.

Stretching of Cooper's ligaments could be painful in large enlarging cyst as well in agglomerate of microcysts or also by pressure from brassiere. Trauma can be

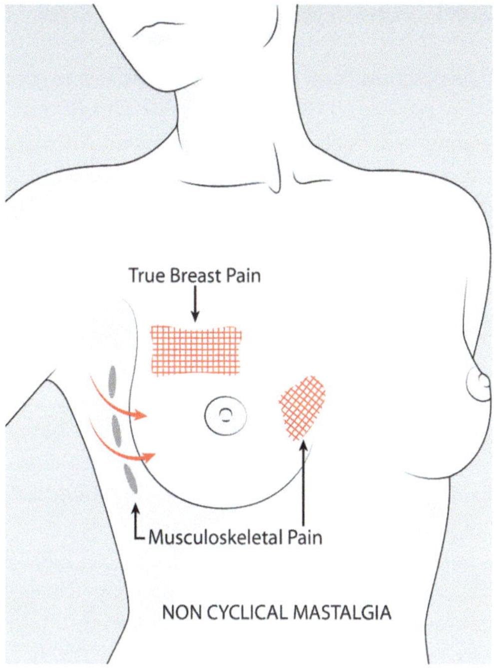


**Fig. 7.3** Localisation of noncyclical true mastalgia and of non-breast pain. Noncyclical true mastalgia arises from the breast tissue and usually involves the upper quadrants. Non-breast pain is usually a musculoskeletal pain, arising laterally from the ribs (radiated from the lateral edge of the breast toward the nipple) or medially from the chest wall as in Tietze's syndrome [3, mod. with permission]

followed by fat necrosis that can include nerve endings. In some way also, cancer is associated to fat necrosis and can result in breast pain.

Sclerosing adenosis is one of the most common (but infrequent) causes of true breast pain. It is characterised by over-proliferation of the terminal duct lobules and can cause impingement to adjacent nerve endings, thereby resulting in breast pain. It can present as a painful lump or be detected on routine screening mammography as a calcified opacity.

Radiological and ultrasound abnormalities found in the painful breast consist of small cysts (microcystic hyperplasia); however, it is doubtful whether pain can be attributed to a small, non-palpable cyst.

Finally, other causes of pain are Mondor disease (sclerosing periphlebitis of breast veins, see Chap. 8) or, rarely, breast cancer.

## 7.4 Non-mammary Pain

**Clinical Practice Points**

- Non-mammary pain, referred rather than originating in the breast, is the most common type of mastalgia in primary care.
- Non-mammary pain is worsened by activity and obliged working posture. It can be reproduced by pressure on a specific area of the chest wall.

### 7.4.1 Chest Wall Pain

Pain referred from the chest wall is the most common type of (untrue) breast pain in primary care. In outpatient breast clinics, its frequency is increasing, and even in women with a classic history of cyclical breast pain, the chest wall is more often the site of origin of the pain. Features suggesting that breast pain is referred rather than originating in the breast include pain that is unilateral and brought on by activity, very lateral or medial in the breast, and can be reproduced by pressure on a specific area of the chest wall.

Women who are postmenopausal and not taking hormonal supplements or who are known to have spondylosis or osteoarthritis are much more likely to have musculoskeletal pain rather than true breast pain. Women often report a recent increase in activities, such as gardening, decorating, lifting weights or increased visits to the gym, after which they become aware of pain. Lifestyle is important in relation to breast pain. It is more common in women who spend many hours sitting at a desk in front of a computer. Identifying any underlying behaviour and modifying lifestyle could be the keystone of treatment.

*Muscle-skeletal pain and radicular pain.* Non-mammary pain located in the lower outer quadrant of the breast may be secondary to vertebral, spinal or paraspinal problems. A radiculopathy can lead to both pain and hyperesthesia in this area and women often describe a burning pain. In localised or diffuse lateral chest wall pain musculoskeletal in origin, or also in radicular pain from cervical arthritis, the anterolateral and anteromedial branches of the intercostal nerves from T3 to T5 are involved. A branch of T4 penetrates the deep surface of the breast and runs up to the nipple. Irritation of this nerve can result in the shooting pain up to the nipple that many women describe. Pain can also be referred from the breast or chest wall through the intercostobrachial nerve to the inner side of the arm (Fig. 7.3).

Breast examination should include palpation of the underlying muscles and ribs with the woman lying on each side, allowing the breast to fall away from the chest wall (Fig. 7.1). The patient should indicate whether there is any localised tenderness on palpation of the chest wall and whether any discomfort evident during examination is similar to the pain normally experienced. If the patient has pain in the lower part of the breast, the underlying chest wall is examined by lifting the breast with one hand while palpating the underlying chest wall with the other hand. Allowing the woman herself to confirm that the site of maximal tenderness is in the underlying chest wall rather than the breast is an effective method of reassuring patients of the site of the pain.

*Tietze's syndrome.* Peristernal discomfort after direct pressure on the sternum suggests a Tietze's syndrome, a benign inflammation of one of the costal cartilages. Although Tietze's syndrome is also named costochondritis, it should be differentiated from costochondritis by swelling of the costal cartilages, which does not appear in Tietze's syndrome. The true causes of Tietze's syndrome are not well understood; it often results from a physical strain or minor injury, such as repeated coughing, sneezing and vomiting, or impacts to the chest. It has even been known to occur after hearty bouts of laughter. It can also occur by overexerting or by an injury in the chest and breast. Psychological stress can exacerbate Tietze's syndrome, but there is no evidence to suggest that it is a direct cause. Women who have had radiation therapy to the chest/breast will often experience this syndrome, which can occur shortly after therapy or years later.

*Surgical trauma.* Similar symptoms of chest wall pain are commonly reported in up to 50 % of women who underwent thoracic surgery. Pain following breast surgery is less common.

*Specific treatment of chest wall pain.* Besides the reassurance that there is no serious underlying cause for the pain and the use of nonsteroidal anti-inflammatory drugs (see over), if the pain is very localised to one specific spot, an appropriate local treatment should be considered.

Infiltrating the affected chest wall with prednisolone 40 mg in depot form combined with long-acting local anaesthetic can produce long-lasting pain relief. If the correct area has been targeted, the pain should disappear quickly. About half of women with a localised tender spot get enduring benefit from a single injection. Repeating the injection after 4–6 weeks increases both the number of women getting benefit and provides long-lasting pain control for two-thirds of women with much localised troublesome pain that interferes with regular daily activities.

In all forms of neuropathic pain such as intercostobrachial neuralgia or scar pain, recommended medicaments are gabapentin, pregabalin or amitriptyline. The use of external neuromodulation for postoperative neuropathic pain gives promising results. External neuromodulation consists of the application of electrical current through an external probe over the painful area, trigger zone or affected nerve. The pain reduction can be immediate, and the quality of life can be dramatically improved following regular applications. Further studies are required to establish the role of this treatment in chronic breast pain.

### 7.4.2 Non-chest Wall Pain

A respiratory infection may cause an intercostal neuralgia. If the pain is on the right side, gallbladder disease, esophagitis and hiatal hernia should be included in the differential diagnosis, and if it is on the left, a cardiac source should be considered.

## 7.5 Workup and Treatment of Breast Pain

**Clinical Practice Points**

- Mastalgia has a natural history of remission and relapse, and placebo response in most trials is significant, approaching 40 %.
- Only a small proportion (about 10 %) have problems of such severity and duration that specific treatment is necessary.
- Some interventions widely recommended in the past have not been found to have any useful effect and should be discouraged.
- Treatment should be considered when there is a history of mastalgia for at least sixth month or more than 7 days per menstrual cycle.

### 7.5.1 Workup for Breast Pain

The essentials of treatment of women with breast pain are making a diagnosis, excluding serious underlying pathologic processes, and communicating this to the patient to reassure the majority.

*Making a diagnosis*. Clinical examination of the breasts and assessment of the patient's individual risk for BC should be the main determinants of the need for imaging or other investigation. The information gathered should include the pain's relationship to menses, duration and location of pain, presence or absence of a mass, exacerbating factors (pregnancy, dietary fat and caffeine intake, history of fibrocystic breast disease, anxiety), impairment of daily activities and exogenous hormone use (hormone replacement therapy, oral contraceptive pills).

In severe cyclic mastalgia or scheduling of hormonal therapies, consider a gynaecological assessment and referral.

*Excluding an underlying pathological process*. Mammography and ultrasound should be obtained in any woman older than 35 years of age who has not had mammography within the past 12 months and is presenting with a new symptom. It is also advised in women younger than 35 if they have a family history or physical finding (see Sect. 2.3).

As appropriate, an exam directed at the cervical and thoracic spine, chest wall and upper extremities may be helpful in assessing other causes of pain. In case of chest wall severe pain, consider referral to appropriate specialists (physiotherapist, orthopaedist, neurosurgeon).

*Reassurance* is justified by the fact that mastalgia rarely is the only symptom of occult BC. Besides reassurance, lifestyle changes, a well-fitting bra and over-the-counter pain relievers should be considered for the treatment of breast pain before using prescription medication. The small group with severe, prolonged pain should be encouraged to keep a pain chart or daily calendar and return after 6–12 weeks. Consider that prospective daily calendar is more accurate for assessing breast pain severity than is patient recall.

*Treatment*. If breast pain interferes with daily activities and social relationships, prescription medications may be considered when reassurance and non-prescription modalities have failed.

*Follow-up*. Patients should be followed with serial breast examinations at 2–3 months and then every 4–6 months for 1 year to confirm that no further changes have appeared.

### 7.5.2 Treatment of Breast Pain

The first line of treatment for breast pain is to reassure the patient that she does not have BC. The risk of malignancy following a negative assessment (clinical and imaging) has been estimated to be only 0.5–2 %, so reassurance following a negative evaluation is appropriate.

Mastalgia has a natural history of remission and relapse. Often, cyclical mastalgia will settle over the course of a few months, returning to normal premenstrual breast discomfort without any specific treatment. If moderate or severe pain has been present for less than 6 months, a high probability exists of spontaneous remission after reassurance, and no specific treatment should be given.

Patients presenting with moderate to severe mastalgia fall into two broad groups: those accepting reassurance and those requesting treatment. The first group have scores for anxiety and depression similar to controls. The second group have cyclical variation in anxiety and depression scores, reaching pathological levels in the luteal period. It is not clear whether these luteal phase changes are the result of the pain or the cause.

Approximately 10 % of women choose a treatment to reduce the symptom of pain. During encounters for breast pain, the patient's description of the pain, quantitative assessment of the pain and decisions regarding reassurance, follow-up or therapeutic intervention should be documented.

Few women will require treatment with more than reassurance and well-tolerated medications such as evening primrose oil. For those with severe, refractory breast pain, the significant side effects of some of these medications must be balanced against the potential benefit in ameliorating breast discomfort and pain.

Non-pharmacologic interventions for breast pain are appropriate for women with breast pain. Although there has been little scientific investigation into the effectiveness of these non-pharmacologic approaches, they are frequently found to improve breast pain symptoms in clinical practice and are of low risk and expense to the patient. Guidelines for the treatment of mastalgia have been issued by SOGC [4].

#### 7.5.2.1 First-Line Treatment

*Reassurance and consideration of psychological factors*. Explanations and reassurance are enough for a large number of women with breast pain. In a randomised controlled study evaluating the intensity of the breast pain following a treatment based on explanations and reassurance, an overall success rate of 70 % was verified. Reassurance was found to be 85.7 % efficient in mild cases, 70.8 % in moderate cases and 52.3 % in severe cases. It was also found to be more effective for those whose symptoms were more intense in the premenstrual period. Relaxation therapy has been shown to have potential in the treatment of mastalgia, and this treatment might be more effective for cyclical rather than noncyclical mastalgia. *Recommendation*: education and reassurance are an integral part of the management of mastalgia and should be the first-line treatment (LoE II, 1 A).

Cases refractory to standard treatment need careful individual evaluation including psychological assessment, as women with severe mastalgia have psychological morbidity (in form of both anxiety and depression) that may be the result, rather than the cause, of their breast pain. Whether stress is a result of the pain or a contributing factor, psychological assessment and support is an integral part of the management of mastalgia. Levels of anxiety, depression and social dysfunction were also shown to be significantly higher in women with severe mastalgia compared with those who had non-severe mastalgia. Some of the women who had improvement after treatment continued to experience some residual anxiety that suggests psychosocial factors may also contribute to the complaint of mastalgia. Women with severe breast pain should be screened for psychological problems and provided with support.

*Mechanical support.* Although randomised controlled trials are lacking, there is evidence that a well-fitting bra may provide relief for mastalgia. A professionally fitted support bra, irrespective of age, cup size or underlying breast disease, has been shown to relieve breast pain even in patients who have not responded to hormonal treatments. Support bras are recommended for exercise. A soft supportive bra during sleep may also improve symptoms. In some prospective studies where women wore an individually fitted bra or a sports bra, a 75–85 % improvement in mastalgia was reported. *Recommendation* (LoE II, 3B): the use of a well-fitting bra that provides good support should be considered for the relief of cyclical and non-cyclical mastalgia.

What is a well-fitting bra? A badly fitting bra probably does not cause mastalgia, but pain can be increased by a badly placed underwire. A support bra is a simple, non-invasive treatment that is worth trying in women with persistent mastalgia. The strap around the chest should be firm but comfortable. When standing side-on at the mirror, the strap around the body should be horizontal and not ride up at the back. The underwear at the front should lie flat against the rib cage and not dig in and rub. The breast should be enclosed in the cups. There should be a smooth line where the fabric at the top of the cup ends and meets the breasts. There should not be any ridge or bulging over the top or sides of the cups.

*Reconsideration of contingent hormonal therapies.* When breast pain occurs in women taking oral contraceptives, it often resolves after a few cycles. In the case of severe pain that does not resolve, a lower dose or a different preparation could be tried. If this is not effective, consideration should be given to changing to alternative methods of birth control. Breast pain, described by 85 % of women as mild to moderate in severity, was cited by 18 % of those using transdermal therapy versus 5.8 % of those using oral therapy [5]. Moreover women receiving long-acting parenteral progesterone for contraception reported significantly less breast pain than the control group. *In conclusion*: until now it is unclear whether oral contraceptives relieve or cause cyclic mastalgia.

Mild and temporary to severe and persistent breast tenderness can result from taking hormone replacement therapies (HRTs). No methodical studies on modifying or eliminating hormone replacement therapy with regard to mastalgia have been reported. Suggested management includes discontinuing HRT if appropriate or trying a low dose and increasing slowly. *Recommendation* (LoE III, C): change in dose, formulation or scheduling should be considered for women on HRT. HRT may be discontinued if appropriate (LoE III, C).

#### 7.5.2.2 Second-Line Treatment

*Topical nonsteroidal anti-inflammatory drugs.* A prospective randomised blinded, placebo-controlled study demonstrated significant improvement with diclofenac diethylammonium (Voltaren Emulgel) in the treatment group for both cyclical and noncyclical mastalgia with minimal side effects. This is a reasonable alternative to a systemic analgesic for those who prefer topical therapy. In general, topical, non-steroidal anti-inflammatory gel, such as diclofenac 2 %, should be considered for pain control for localised treatment of mastalgia.

*Tamoxifen* is a selective oestrogen receptor modulator (SERM) utilised for the prevention and treatment of BC. Two randomised trials found tamoxifen superior to placebo in premenopausal women with cyclic or noncyclic mastalgia. Tamoxifen 20 mg daily alleviated pain (defined as 50 % reduction in linear analogue score) in 71 % of patients at 3 months, compared with 38 % who received a placebo. Tamoxifen 10 mg daily eliminated symptoms in 89 % of women at 6 months, compared with 38 % who experienced "partial improvement" in the placebo group [6]. The two doses were then compared directly and found to have equivalent response rates in a further trial, while side effects were significantly reduced at the lower dose. Response rates were superior in cyclic mastalgia: 94 % versus 56 % in the noncyclic group. Tamoxifen 10 mg daily is effective in the treatment of mastalgia. As it is significantly cheaper, it can be used as a first medication except in women with a history of thromboembolic disease.

Tamoxifen (*dose*: 10 mg daily for 3 months) should be considered when first-line treatments are ineffective. If this achieves pain relief, the dose can be further reduced to 10 mg on alternate days for a further 3 months. For the few who do not respond, a higher dosage of 20 mg/day should be given. The very few who do not respond to this treatment should be switched to danazol for 4 months. *Side effects* of tamoxifen commonly observed in short-term treatment for mastalgia include hot flashes (10 %), menstrual irregularity/amenorrhea (10 %), weight gain, nausea, vaginal dryness and bloating (5 % or less). Thromboembolic events, endometrial cancer and cataracts are rare but serious side effects of tamoxifen; their incidence in short-term, low-dose treatment regimens for mastalgia is not known. *Note*: barrier contraception must be utilised in order to avoid pregnancy.

*Danazol* is a derivative of the synthetic steroid ethisterone that suppresses the production of gonadotrophins and has some weak androgenic effects. Two randomised trials have compared danazol with placebo in premenopausal women with cyclic mastalgia, and one 3-arm trial compared tamoxifen with danazol with placebo. Treatment success was defined as >50 % reduction in mean pain score and was achieved in 65 % of those on danazol, 72 % of those on tamoxifen and 38 % of those on placebo [4]. Statistically, tamoxifen and danazol were equivalent, and both were significantly better than placebo. Danazol 200 mg daily is effective in the treatment of breast pain. To minimise side effects, it can be given in the luteal phase only.

Danazol (*dose*: 200 mg daily) should be considered when first-line treatments are ineffective. *Side effects* of danazol at the 200 mg daily dose included weight gain (30 %), menstrual irregularity/amenorrhea or menorrhagia (50 %), deepening of the voice (10 %) and hot flashes (10 %) (rarely, about 10 %, hirsutism, deepening voice, hot flashes). *Note*: barrier contraception must be utilised.

*Bromocriptine* is a dopaminergic agonist which inhibits the release of prolactin from the anterior pituitary. Bromocriptine, 5 mg daily, has been found effective in the treatment of cyclic mastalgia in 2 randomised, placebo-controlled trials. Both arms (bromocriptine and placebo) showed significant improvement in breast pain, but bromocriptine was more effective, with an absolute 45 % reduction in mean linear analogue score for pain. Overall, 11 % of patients in the bromocriptine group and 6 % in the placebo group discontinued treatment because of side effects [4].

Bromocriptine (*dose* 2.5 mg twice daily after gradual increase) should be considered in women with tamoxifen or danazol intolerance. *Side effects* of bromocriptine included nausea (32 %), dizziness (12 %) and vomiting (7 %) (rarely seizures, stroke or hypertension).

#### 7.5.2.3 Changes in Lifestyle and Diet

*Lifestyle changes*. Lifestyle changes such as smoking cessation, stress control, sedentary behaviours reduction, getting more exercise and improving coping skills may be possible low-risk interventions. Physical actions as hot packs, cold packs and massage may also relieve symptoms.

*Dietary changes*. The effectiveness of dietary measures is unclear. The most promising nutritional supplement is *flaxseed*. A Canadian study examined the effects of dietary flaxseed in women with severe cyclical mastalgia. One hundred sixteen women were enrolled in the double-blind placebo-controlled trial with the treatment group receiving 25 g of flaxseed daily, in a muffin, and followed for up to four menstrual cycles. However, there was no long-term follow-up. Breast pain was alleviated in both treatment groups but was reduced to a significantly greater degree in the flaxseed group. This one study shows promise and merits further research.

*Caffeine*. Interest in caffeine as a causative agent in fibrocystic breast disease arose from old observational studies in which resolution of signs and symptoms occurred in 85 % of subjects who abstained from methylxanthines for a period of 8 weeks or more. In additional randomised studies, no benefit was observed after 6 months of a caffeine-free diet, so that women with breast pain should not be advised to reduce caffeine intake.

*Vitamin E and Vitamin B6* are not proven to reduce breast pain and should not be considered for the treatment of mastalgia.

*Evening Primrose Oil (EPO)*. Three randomised, placebo-controlled, double-blind clinical trials have shown no or low efficacy for EPO in the treatment of cyclic mastalgia. Noncyclic mastalgia showed no response to EPO. Patients with cyclic mastalgia had significant improvement in pain after 3 months on EPO, but not on placebo. Pain levels returned to baseline by 6 months, despite continued therapy in the EPO group, and the placebo group showed no reduction in pain when they were treated at "crossover" with open-label EPO. In conclusion, there is presently insufficient evidence to recommend the use of EPO in the treatment of breast pain.

*Dietary Fat*. There is support for lipid metabolism playing a role in the pathophysiology of cyclical mastalgia. However, only one small randomised single-blinded controlled study assessed the effect of a low-fat diet (15 % energy from fat) on severe cyclical mastalgia. Reduced swelling, tenderness and nodularity were reported in six out of ten patients in the intervention group. More research is needed before any recommendation can be made.

*Isoflavones.* It has been demonstrated isoflavones reduced cyclical breast pain, but more studies are required before any recommendation can be made about the use of isoflavones to treat cyclical mastalgia.

*Topical Progesterone.* Topical progesterone locally applied to the breast in a small randomised controlled crossover trial has not proved superior to a placebo. However, a vaginal cream of micronised progesterone was found to be effective in reducing pain in 65 % of cases compared with 22 % of controls in a randomised double-blind placebo-controlled study.

*Topical nonsteroidal anti-inflammatory drugs.* A further development in the treatment of mastalgia has emerged from a trial of the efficacy of topical nonsteroidal anti-inflammatory drugs [6]. Diclofenac diethylammonium gel was applied every 8 h for a minimum duration of 6 months. Although a large placebo effect was demonstrated, both cyclical and noncyclical mastalgia groups demonstrated a change in pain values significantly higher than the control group. While the authors note that care should be taken in asthmatic patients, the ease of use with minimal side effects should ensure appeal of the regime to both patients and clinicians and warrants further study.

*Other medications* that have been found to be in some ways effective for the treatment of breast pain include goserelin, gestrinone, buserelin, leuprolide, quinagolide and cabergoline. In general, antibiotics, diuretics and vitamins have not been effective in the treatment of breast pain.

## References

1. Iddon J, Dixon JM. Mastalgia. In: Dixon JM, editor. ABC of breast diseases. 4th ed. Oxford: Wiley-Blackwell; 2012.
2. Baratelli GM. A simple and quick method to evaluate mastalgia. Breast J. 2006;12:95.
3. Mansel RE, Webster DJT, Sweetland HM. Hughes, Mansel & Webster benign disorders and diseases of the breast. London: Elsevier; 2009.
4. SOGC clinical practice guideline. Mastalgia. http://sogc.org/wp-content/uploads/2013/01/170E-CPG-January20061.pdf. Accessed 20 July 2014.
5. Barros AC, Mottola J, Ruiz CA, Borges MN, Pinotti JA. Reassurance in the treatment of mastalgia. Breast J. 1999;5:62–5.
6. Colak T, Ipek T, Kanik A, Ogetman Z, Aydin S. Efficacy of topical nonsteroidal antiinflammatory drugs in mastalgia treatment. J Am Coll Surg. 2003;196:525–30.

## Further Reading

ICSI health care guideline. Evaluation of breast pain. In: Diagnosis of breast disease. 14th edn. 2012. www.icsi.org. Accessed 30 Jan 2015.

Noroozian M, Stein LF, Gaetke-Udager K, Helvie MA. Long-term clinical outcomes in women with breast pain in the absence of additional clinical findings: mammography remains indicated. Breast Cancer Res Treat. 2015;149:417–24.

Scurr J, Hedger W, Morris P, Brown N. The prevalence, severity, and impact of breast pain in the general population. Breast J. 2014;20:508–13.

**Websites in Appendix**: *Breast Pain*, A-4.

# Inflammatory Diseases of the Breast

8

Alfonso M. Pluchinotta

## Contents



**Abstract**

• The grouping of inflammatory breast diseases is arbitrary but usually justified by the different aetiology. • Our personal classification of inflammatory breast diseases includes lactating, non-lactating and surface (mostly skin-related) mastitis. • Most chronic inflammatory conditions can mimic malignancy. • For non-lactating women over 35 years presenting breast changes with unexplained

A.M. Pluchinotta
Breast Surgery, Policlinic of Abano Terme, Padova, Italy
e-mail: pluchinotta.alfonso@gmail.com



A.M. Pluchinotta (ed.), *The Outpatient Breast Clinic: Aiming at Best Practice*,
DOI 10.1007/978-3-319-15907-2_8

inflammation, investigations are necessary to exclude ductal carcinoma in situ (usually peripheral) or inflammatory BC.

*Future directions*. Some inflammatory conditions of the breast are basically reactive so that the boundary between an abnormal and a true pathological condition may be difficult. Usually reversible and non-infectious, reactive conditions may be due to stimuli such as stasis of secretions (e.g. symptomatic mammary duct ectasia), trauma (e.g. fat necrosis) and metabolic (e.g. diabetic mastopathy) or autoimmune reactions (e.g. granulomatous lobular mastitis). Reactive changes can mimic malignancy so that it is important to identify the gross and microscopic versions in order to achieve appropriate treatment and avoid unnecessary surgery.

## 8.1 Overview

**Clinical Practice Points**

- Mastitis is an inflammation of the breast that can be accompanied or not by infection. For this reason, non-infectious and infectious mastitis should be considered separately.
- Infectious mastitis may be simple (anyway, antibiotics are necessary) or complicated, when an abscess formation occurs (antibiotics and aspiration are needed).
- Usually, true lactating mastitis is infectious and may resolve with antibiotics, while non-lactating mastitis is not always accompanied by microbial infections and may not resolve with antibiotics.
- For all mastitis factors of risk (as diabetes) and tendency to recur should be properly considered.

The definition of mastitis refers to the inflammation of the breast tissue that may be non-infectious or infectious. However, this distinction may be not that evident in the majority of cases. A wide array of breast infections could be observed, schematically represented in Fig. 8.1, but very few are common.

Inflammatory breast disorders are usually classified as lactating and non-lactating. A third group is constituted by surface, mostly skin-related, mastitis. This grouping is arbitrary but justified by the different aetiology.

*Lactating mastitis* (Fig. 8.2) is very common, mostly in the first 2–3 weeks of lactation but can occur at any stage of lactation. If infectious, lactating mastitis is usually due to *Staphylococcus aureus*.

*Non-lactating mastitis* (Fig. 8.3) is less common and rarely infectious and has a variable microbiology and may not resolve with antibiotic therapy.

Main characteristics of acute peripheral lactating abscess and acute subareolar non-lactating abscess are portrayed in Fig. 8.4.

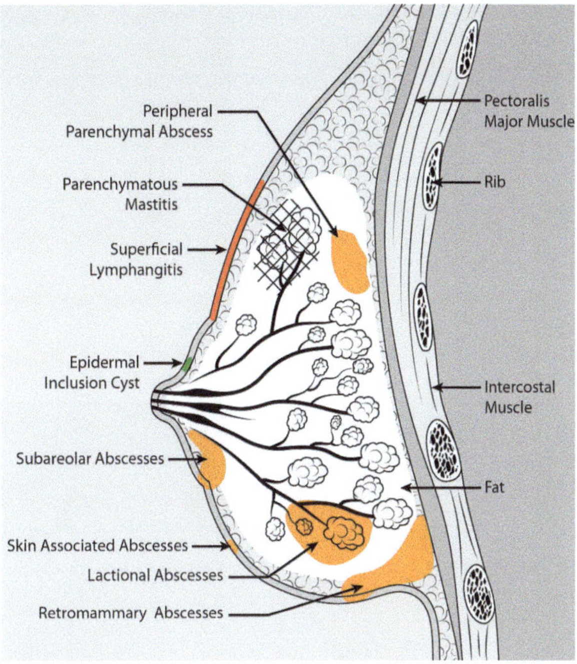


**Fig. 8.1** Schematic drawing depicting the most common types and locations of breast infections. In addition, other surface mastitis should be considered as breast cellulitis, breast lymphangitis, breast oedema and Mondor disease

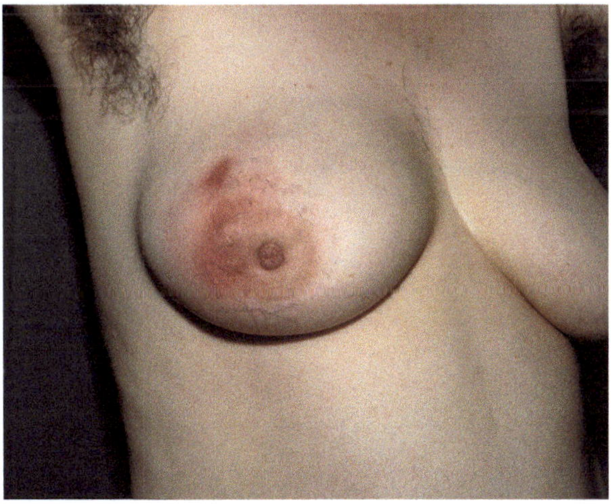

**Fig. 8.2** Plurifocal lactating mastitis

*Surface mastitis* mostly includes skin-related mastitis, a grouping of lesions common anywhere in the body and occasionally found in the breast. Actually, the simple term skin-related does not take into account breast inflammations that can originate from subcutaneous tissues as breast cellulitis, breast lymphangitis or breast oedema. With the term surface mastitis, we intend to encompass these superficial inflammatory lesions with skin-related lesions. In our opinion, Mondor disease too should be included in this group for its characteristic superficial presentation in the breast. Our classification for mastitis is shown in Table 8.1.

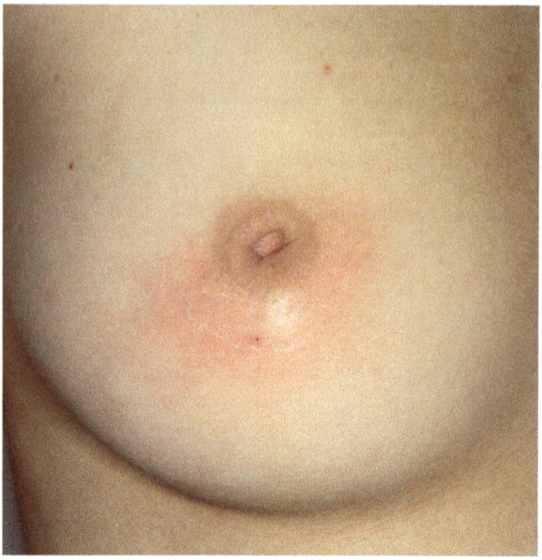

**Fig. 8.3** Non-lactating mastitis (subareolar mastitis) associated to nipple inversion

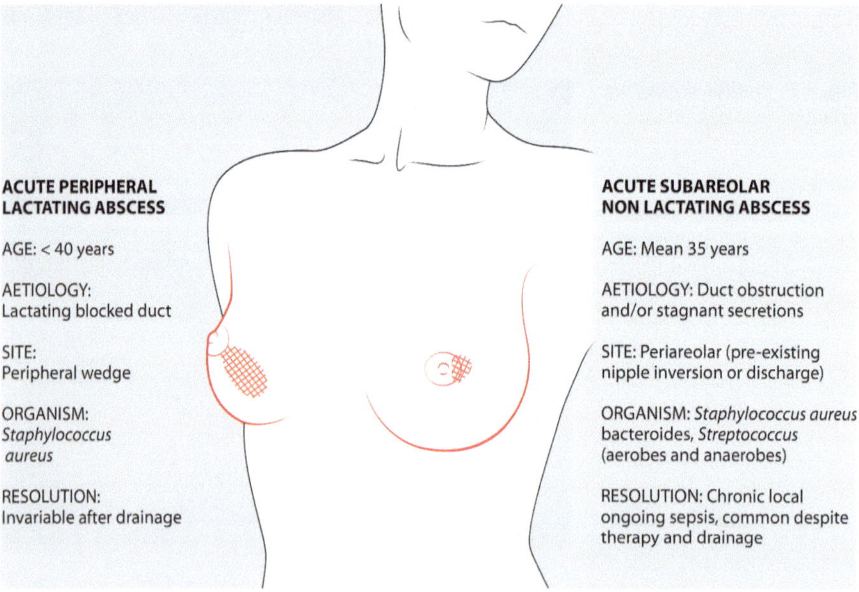


**Fig. 8.4** Main characteristics of acute peripheral lactating abscess and acute subareolar non-lactating abscess

*History*. In the presence of mastitis, the diagnosis is based primarily on the history and clinical symptoms. The general history should investigate generic factors of risk for infection as diabetes, chronic diseases, HIV infection, or an impaired

**Table 8.1** Personal classification of mastitis

| *Lactating mastitis* |
|---|
| Non-infectious (engorgement) |
| Infectious simple |
| Infectious complicated (abscess) |
| *Non-lactating mastitis* |
| Neonatal and pubertal |
| Subareolar mastitis |
| Peripheral mastitis |
| Postsurgical infections |
| Mastitis associated with malignancy |
| *Surface mastitis* |
| Skin-related infections |
| Breast cellulitis |
| Breast lymphangitis |
| Breast oedema |
| Mondor disease |

immune system. Since almost all kinds of mastitis tend to recur, an anamnestic record of prior episodes is equally important.

*Clinical presentation.* A breast infection is usually diagnosed based on physical examination. Features may be various. In general, a painful, swollen lump in the breast is found, sometimes with redness, heat and swelling of the overlying skin. Fever and malaise may or may not be present according to the nature of infections, but symptoms could subside in case the woman took antibiotics early.

*Assessment.* In general, an ultrasound may be useful to determine the liquid or solid nature of the lesion and guide a fine needle aspiration, if appropriate. Mammography in the acute phase is of little use.

*TREATMENT OF INFECTIOUS MASTITIS (principles)* – Classification between epidemic and sporadic (or endemic) mastitis is still used but has given way to recognition that these infections form a spectrum of illnesses, depending upon the virulence of the infecting organism and the degree of bacterial colonisation of the milk.

*Epidemic mastitis* is a hospital-acquired infection caused by virulent strains of *Staphylococcus aureus*. This infection is rare, and it usually occurs within 4 days of delivery. Even with prompt antibiotic therapy, progression to abscess formation may occur.

*Non-epidemic* (or sporadic) mastitis, in contrast, is a milder infection with less virulent organisms and generally responds well to treatment without hospitalisation. Hospitalisation may be required, however, if the infection fails to respond. Keeping the breast empty of milk promotes healing by helping to drain the culture medium that facilitates growth of organisms. Hence, the earlier recommendations that breastfeeding cease while mastitis is being treated have been superseded by the knowledge that breastfeeding is generally not harmful to the infant – when using appropriate antibiotics – and may speed resolution of the infectious process.

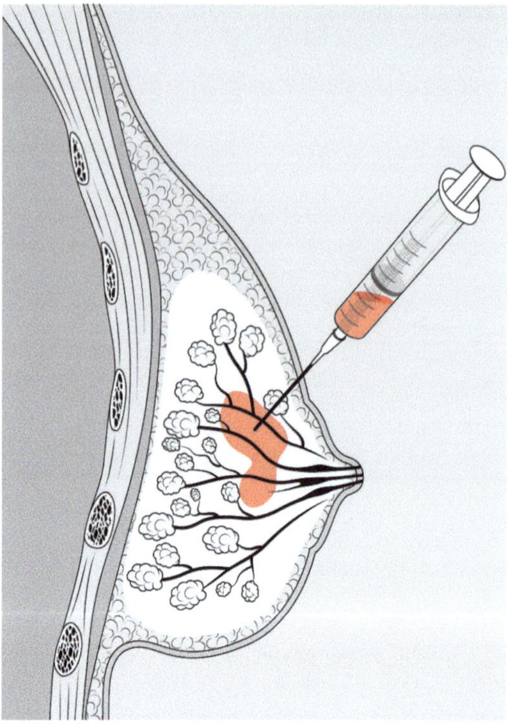

**Fig. 8.5** Needle aspiration of a deep breast abscess in order to evacuate pus and wash the cavity with local anaesthetic

Antibiotics are effective in lactating mastitis. In mastitis outside of breastfeeding, antibiotics may be disputable and, if indicated, should cover the spectrum of both aerobic and anaerobic bacteria, be administered for not less than 15 days and sometimes extended up to 2 months.

In the presence of an infection that does not respond to treatment, more investigations should exclude the presence of an underlying pathology as a BC.

*TREATMENT OF BREAST ABSCESS* (*principles*) – Any abscess should be managed by aspiration or incision and drainage preceded and followed by a course of antibiotics. In deep abscess, aspiration should be preferred, while in superficial abscess, incision is recommended. If the skin overlying the abscess is suffering, then the impaired skin should be excised [1].

*Aspiration* is best performed with ultrasound guidance with the abscess cavity being washed with local anaesthetic to dilute out and to help aspirate pus and reduce pain (Fig. 8.5). Repeated aspiration two to three times every 2–3 days is required to achieve resolution of most breast abscesses. Only for larger abscesses aspiration may need to be repeated five or more times.

*Incision and drainage*, if indicated, can almost always be performed under local anaesthesia or slight sedation. Only a small incision is required to drain a breast abscess adequately (Fig. 8.6) when feasible. An incision is made usually at the lower edge of the abscess to allow the pus out and ensure that it will continue to

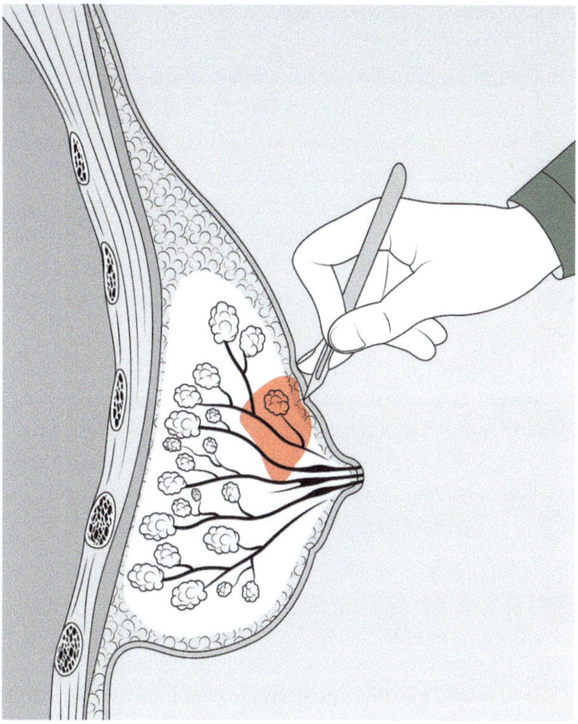

**Fig. 8.6** Drainage of a superficial breast abscess with a small incision

drain when the patient is sitting upright in the post-operative period. After incision, the abscess is irrigated with the same local anaesthetic solution to wash out residual pus and to limit the pain of the procedure. Placement of a drain or packing the abscess cavity after incision and drainage is usually unnecessary.

However, if a large abscess is present, surgical drainage may require general anaesthesia. In this case, the wound is packed initially with a wick soaked in antiseptic such as iodine solution and will not normally be closed with sutures. This helps to better clean the wound and prevent bleeding. It also ensures that the wound stays open to allow any remaining infection to drain out. If the skin is closed immediately or soon after surgery, there would be a high chance that the infection would persist and the abscess would recur. For this reason, it is wise to let the wound close in its own time.

*WORKUP* – In conclusion, *if an infectious mastitis is suspected*:

- Treat as soon as clinically suspected.
- Re-evaluate every 3 days until completely cleared.
- Change the antibiotic prescription if no response after 1 week.
- Consider minimal biopsy (skin punch) if not responding to second antibiotic therapy.
- Culture is usually not indicated.

*If an abscess is suspected*:

- Aspirate and drain with local anaesthesia under ultrasound guidance.
- A large (14–18 gauge) cannula needle is advisable.
- Following ultrasound could confirm the presence of small or residual abscess.
- Re-evaluate every 3 days until completely cleared.
- Treat with antibiotic if there are systemic symptoms (fever) or local cellulitis.
- Cultures are not necessary, unless there is no response to treatment.
- Minor surgical incision for drainage is reserved to very superficial abscess
- Major surgical drainage is rarely necessary.

A complete overview on mastitis, aimed to bring together available information on lactational mastitis and related conditions as well as their causes, is published by World Health Organization (see *Useful Websites* at the end of this chapter).

## 8.2 Lactating Mastitis

**Clinical Practice Points**

- Lactating mastitis is the most common form of infectious mastitis, even if a real infection during breastfeeding is less common than believed to be.
- Early prescription of appropriate antibiotics in case of true infection limits abscess formation.
- In lactating mastitis, drainage may be a minor procedure performed by needle aspiration or minimal surgical incision.
- Delay in referral to breast clinics of patients with lactating infection that does not settle rapidly with antibiotics continues to be a problem.

### 8.2.1 Non-infectious Lactating Mastitis

Non-infectious lactating mastitis is an engorgement of mammary ducts that can occur during breastfeeding as well as after weaning.

*Breastfeeding engorgement* is more common than infectious mastitis. Symptoms of simple engorgements are painful breast; tender, red, swollen and hard area of the breast, usually in a wedge-shaped distribution; slight or no fever; and no general malaise.

Milk removal and local packs may help to solve the symptoms, while investigations are not routinely required. For milk removal, breastfeeding is often more effective in pain control than using a breast pump and is more influential at encouraging milk flow. The pain of lactation mastitis is relieved by the application of gel packs or cold cabbage leaves to the breast, both are equally effective. Also, paracetamol may give some relief. Long-lasting milk removal and better maternal and infant hygiene may reduce the recurrence.

*Weaning engorgement.* Breast engorgement may occur also after weaning. The pregnancy-/lactation-related hormones usually return to normal levels shortly after weaning, but for some women, it can take several months to rebuild non-lactating state and there is an increased risk of rebound lactation and mastitis before hormone levels settling.

Most cases of postweaning mastitis or breast engorgement are solved with relatively little treatment. Recurrent postweaning mastitis on the other hand can be an indicator of a developing hyperprolactinemia or thyroid disorders and endocrinological examination must be considered.

Cold wraps or also warm, lactation-inhibiting herbs or medications can be used. Avoiding stress is equally important. *Salvia officinalis* and chasteberry extract can improve prolactin levels, which may reduce risk of recurrence, but no established data are available for its use in weaning engorgement. Bromocriptine may be effective in the prescribed dose but this rarely justifies the unpleasant side effects. Other prolactin-lowering medications (cabergoline, lisuride) are effective and appear safe but should be cautiously used for weaning.

### 8.2.2 Infectious Lactating Mastitis

Infectious lactating mastitis is rather common during breastfeeding, but less than believed to be. It is more frequent following a first child and most commonly seen within the first 6 weeks of breastfeeding, although some women develop it later or during weaning. Some blocked ducts could reduce drainage of milk from the affected area [2]. Moreover, there is usually a history of a cracked nipple or skin abrasion, although this is not always the site of entry of organisms. *Staphylococcus aureus* is the most common organism responsible, but *Staphylococcus epidermidis* and *Streptococci* are occasionally isolated.

*Clinical presentation.* The symptoms of lactating infection can develop more or less quickly. Most women first experience flu-like symptoms and just after a while, they may notice a sore red area on the breast, an abnormal discharge from the nipples or a prolonged, unexplained breast pain. Increasing pain is followed by other symptoms, as erythema, swelling and induration of the breast, associated with general symptoms of infection including nausea, fever 38 °C or higher, shivering and chills, fatigue and tachycardia. Some women do experience Raynaud's of the nipple during breastfeeding, which can cause more considerable pain.

*Treatment.* If symptoms do not improve, or are worsening after 12–24 h despite effective milk removal, and there is severe deep burning breast pain, a ductal infection should be highly suspected.

Promotion of milk drainage and early antibiotic therapy are the cornerstones of treatment. A 10-day course of a penicillinase-resistant antibiotic such as flucloxacillin (or erythromycin if penicillin allergic) is required. Tetracycline, ciprofloxacin and chloramphenicol should not be used to treat lactating breast infection as they may enter breast milk and can harm the baby.

Antibiotics give satisfactory resolution in many cases. If the infection does not settle after one course of antibiotics, if no pus is detected on ultrasonography and if clinical and imaging assessments indicate that the lesion is actually infective, antibiotics should be changed to cover other possible pathogens.

The role of associated mycosis and the value of fluconazole in breast pain and infection associated with breastfeeding are controversial. The evidence that fungal infections are important causes of mastitis is largely anecdotal. There are no data from properly controlled clinical studies showing the value of fluconazole and it should not be prescribed until further clinical trial evidence shows it to be beneficial.

Frequent emptying of both breasts by breastfeeding is essential. Also essential is adequate fluid supply for the mother and the baby. Use of pumps to empty the breast is somewhat controversial and anyway not as efficient as breastfeeding. In cases of minor mastitis, massage and application of heat prior to feeding can help as this may help unblock the ducts. However, in more severe cases of mastitis, heat or massage could make the symptoms worse and cold compresses are better suited to contain the inflammation.

At this point, investigations are not routinely required. Culture of the breast milk is proposed only when:

- Antibiotics have been prescribed and there has been no response after 48 h.
- Mastitis is severe enough also before any antibiotics are prescribed.
- Mastitis is recurrent.
- Infection is likely hospital acquired (endemic).
- The woman is unable to take standard antibiotics (such as flucloxacillin and erythromycin).

*Breast abscess* develops only rarely, in about 0.5 % of breastfeeding women. Known risk factors are age over 30, primiparous and late delivery. No correlation was found with smoking status; however, this may be in part because much fewer smoking women choose to breastfeed. If a breast abscess is suspected, or needs to be excluded, an initial ultrasound is useful in assessing the presence of collection of fluids.

An established abscess, usually in the middle or in the peripheral part of the breast tissue, should be treated either by repeated aspiration every 2–3 days until no more pus is aspirated or by incision and drainage. With ultrasound-controlled aspiration, minor fluid collection can also be evacuated. Surgery should be reserved for the minority of cases that do not resolve with antibiotics and repeated aspiration or those where the abscess is superficial with an involvement of the overlying skin (see Sect. 8.1 above).

Breast infections in lactating women can be distressing and debilitating and can interfere with early baby bonding. Women who want to continue breastfeeding should be encouraged to feed with the unaffected breast and, once letdown occurs in the affected breast, feed with the affected breast until it is completely empty. Warm compresses and paracetamol may give some relief.

For those women who present with multiple areas of breast infection, and are exhausted by breastfeeding, a consideration should be given to stopping breastfeeding and halting milk flow. Stopping milk production is achieved by prescribing cabergoline 2.5 mcg given twice a day for 2 days.

## 8.3 Non-lactating Mastitis

**Clinical Practice Points**

- As in lactating infection, non-lactating mastitis may be non-infectious or infectious without or with abscess formation.
- Non-lactating mastitis can be separated into those that occur centrally in the subareolar region and those that affect the peripheral breast tissue.
- Subareolar breast abscesses are slightly trickier. In subareolar periductal mastitis, cigarette smoking is a powerful facilitator of severe inflammatory complications.
- In mastitis outside of breastfeeding, the administration of antibiotics, which cover the spectrum of both aerobic and anaerobic, must not be less than 10–15 days, also being able to extend up to 2 months.
- In the presence of an infection that does not respond to treatment, it is good to do investigations to exclude the presence of a BC.

Besides neonatal and pubertal mastitis, non-lactating mastitis falls into two main groups:

- Subareolar mastitis, related to periductal inflammation, independent or related to duct ectasia
- Peripheral mastitis, sometimes related to systemic diseases, as diabetes and rheumatoid arthritis, or infections, as tuberculosis.

### 8.3.1 Neonatal and Pubertal Mastitis

Neonatal breast infection is not common but can occur in the first few weeks of life when the breast bud is enlarged (see Sect. 3.4). Although *Staphylococcus aureus* is the usual organism, occasionally, infection is due to *Escherichia coli*. If an abscess develops, a small incision placed as peripherally as possible to avoid damaging the breast bud leads to rapid resolution [3].

Prepubertal girls may also develop breast abscesses and this topic is treated in Chap. 3. Also as in neonatal infection, the decision for surgical drainage should be carefully made because future breast deformation may occur.

### 8.3.2 Subareolar Mastitis

Almost 90 % of nonpuerperal mastitis is represented by subareolar mastitis. This inflammation is sustained by a periductal mastitis, a rare occurrence associated to duct ectasia. Actually, periductal mastitis should be considered a separate entity from duct ectasia, which affects young women (as well as men), while only few older women with duct ectasia have experienced prior episodes of periductal mastitis.

The causes of periductal mastitis and its relations to duct ectasia are not well identified and widely discussed in *Mammary Duct Ectasia and Related Conditions* (Chap. 9). As is known, the majority of patients who get periductal mastitis are smokers. It is postulated that smoking leads to or is associated with damage of the subareolar ducts. It seems probable the breast concentrates substances in cigarette smoke (but, maybe, other substances originating from the diet or the environment) in subareolar ducts in higher concentrations than in plasma. These toxic substances may damage the ducts directly or there may be a localised hypoxic effect, with consequent subareolar duct damage and subsequent infection [4].

Periductal mastitis has been also associated with squamous metaplasia, which is likely a consequence of the enduring inflammation and infection. Squamous Metaplasia Of Lactiferous Ducts (SMOLD) breast disease typifies *Zuska's breast disease*, breast abscesses and fistulae as the result of obstruction and inflammation of lactiferous ducts by squamous metaplasia. Actually, it is recognised that squamous metaplasia leads to partial duct obstruction with subsequent duct dilatation and secondary inflammation and infection. However, duct dilatation, squamous metaplasia and duct obstruction blocked by keratin, nowadays, are not more considered precursors of periductal inflammation or relevant aetiologic factors. In conclusion, dilated ducts with collection of secretions and debris with stasis changes characterise the pathologic appearance of some but very few cases of duct ectasia.

Anyway, bacteria undoubtedly play a major role in established abscesses. The fact that the bacteria are the same as the flora of the mouth and vagina and that flare-up of abscesses can follow vaginal manipulation suggests that sexual stimulation may be responsible for the organisms reaching the ducts. Ectatic ducts provide the soil in which the bacteria can persist or from which they can invade. It is also possible that oral bacteria may be transferred to the nipple and provides a possible explanation for the frequency of involvement of the contralateral breast.

*Symptoms.* Subareolar infection is most commonly seen in young women between 30 and 40 years of age. Clinical manifestations include recurrent inflammation of the periareolar area, abscess and in late stages fistula. Pain is very common, while nipple discharge (usually non-bloody, only sporadically bloody) is rare. Congenital inverted nipples are considered a condition facilitating inflammation and sometimes bilateral involvement.

In the late stages, but uncommonly, subareolar ducts may become widely open and creamy or cheesy or purulent (Fig. 8.7) nipple discharge is observed. In most cases, damage to the subareolar ducts with ongoing chronic inflammation and resulting scarring of periductal tissues lead to fibrosis with nipple retraction.

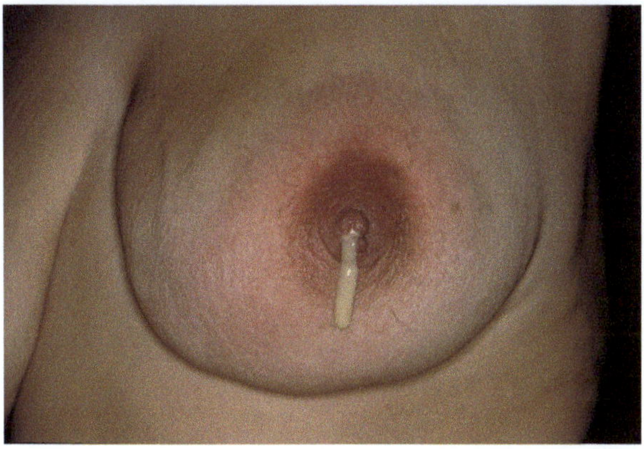

**Fig. 8.7** Spontaneous drainage of a subareolar abscess

When inflamed ducts become secondarily infected, duct damage and subsequent rupture lead to abscess formation. Such abscesses often drain spontaneously and, because of the tough muscle of the areola skin, the spontaneous drainage tends to burst through the skin at the edge of the areola. Recurrent abscesses and a draining fistula may occur so that the patient should be informed of this possibility.

Gram stain and culture of nipple aspirate should be obtained for cases of inflammation or infection. The percentage of cases with cultures positive for pathogenic or potentially pathogenic organisms has been reported as 60–80 % of cases. The most common organisms are *Staphylococcus* species, *Bacteroides*, *Streptococci* (*aerobes and anaerobes*) and *Proteus vulgaris*.

Leading features of acute subareolar abscess, compared to those of acute peripheral lactating abscess, are shown in Fig. 8.4.

*Antibiotic treatment*. Therapy should be tailored to results of culture test when available. In the absence of risk factors for methicillin-resistant *Staphylococcus aureus* (MRSA), outpatient therapy may be initiated with amoxicillin-clavulanate (875 mg orally every 12 h). Reasonable alternative regimens include dicloxacillin (500 mg oral every 6 h) or cephalexin (500 mg orally every 6 h), with metronidazole if anaerobes are suspected or in recurrent inflammation. In the setting of beta-lactam hypersensitivity, clindamycin (300 mg to 450 orally every 8 h) is a reasonable alternative while, if risk for MRSA is high, either trimethoprim-sulfamethoxazole (1 to 2 tabs orally twice daily) or doxycycline is appropriate.

In recurrent episodes, treatment should consist of a prolonged course (4–8 weeks) of antibiotics that target both aerobic and anaerobic bacteria and, if necessary, repeated aspirations, in order to avoid surgical intervention. Also in cases with negative or unavailable culture results, empiric therapy with amoxicillin-clavulanate (875 mg orally every 12 h) is advisable. The management should include, if the case, smoking cessation.

*Surgical treatment*. Antibiotic treatment alone or incision and drainage plus antibiotics lead to a recurrence of the subareolar abscess in up to half of the patients. For patients who develop repeated episodes of periareolar infection or a well-established mammary duct fistula, surgical removal of all affected ducts by a total duct excision is the preferred treatment. Patients who undergo a total duct excision for periductal mastitis should receive appropriate antibiotic treatment before surgery and the antibiotics should be continued post-operatively for at least 5 days or until all signs of infection have resolved.

Some discrepancies in clinical evolution are best explained by at least two separate pathologies underlying mammary duct fistula: a patchy mucosal ulceration of the lining of collecting major ducts giving an inflammatory (mostly chemical) response and a stagnation of duct contents due to duct ectasia with minimal periductal mastitis. The first is commonest in young women and is frequently accompanied by congenital nipple inversion. The second is seen in older patients, without nipple inversion. It is important to recognise this dual pathology because treatment of multiple duct disease by operation directed towards one duct will lead to recurrence, while failure to recognise the solitary congenital duct abnormality may lead to unnecessarily radical surgery.

*Drainage*. The methods of drainage of acute abscesses are described in *Overview* above.

*Total ductal excision* can often be performed with local anaesthesia and sedation as an outpatient procedure. The recommended surgical approach usually is via a circumareolar incision at the 6 o'clock position. Dissection is performed underneath the areola and a 2 cm portion of duct should be removed. In some cases, multiple ducts may be involved with multiple skin openings, so that all fistulae need resecting for a complete resolution of the issue.

When performing surgery for periductal mastitis, the back of the nipple must be cleared of all ducts right up to the nipple skin as infection may recur unless all residual diseased ducts are removed. Patients should be warned that this operation may result in reduced nipple sensitivity in almost 40 % of women.

*Fistulotomy/fistulectomy*. A fistula can develop after incision and drainage of a non-lactating abscess, following spontaneous discharge of a periareolar inflammatory mass or resulting from biopsy of a periductal inflammatory mass. Treatment is performed under antibiotic cover by opening the fistula (*fistulotomy*) or excising the fistula (*fistulectomy*) and diseased duct or all ducts. The best results are obtained from fistula excision rather than fistulotomy. Specialist breast surgeons achieve the lowest rates of recurrence and best cosmetic results.

Recurrence is not uncommon, often due to inappropriate or inadequate surgery. Up to one-half of patients with periareolar infection experience recurrent episodes of infection and recurrent abscesses with or without fistula. Repeated infections are much more common in women who continue to smoke but are also seen in diabetic and immune-compromised patients.

### 8.3.3 Peripheral Mastitis

Peripheral mastitis is less common than subareolar mastitis and usually has a chronic course. The majority has no obvious cause and can be associated with an underlying condition such as diabetes, rheumatoid arthritis, steroid treatment and trauma. Different types are considered.

*IDIOPATHIC GRANULOMATOUS MASTITIS* is defined as granulomatous mastitis without any other attributable cause such as systemic infections or foreign body reactions. It occurs on average 2 years and almost exclusively up to 6 years after pregnancy, and usual age range is 20–40 years.

Patients mostly present with a hard lump in one breast without any sign of a systemic disease. Other possible symptoms include nipple retraction, pain, inflammation of the overlying skin, nipple discharge, fistula, enlarged lymph nodes and in rare case peau d'orange-like changes. Presentation is mostly unilateral although a significant share of cases is bilateral. In few cases, contralateral or bilateral recurrences were documented.

Characteristics for idiopathic granulomatous mastitis are multinucleated giant cells and epithelioid histiocytes forming non-caseating granulomas around lobules. Often, minor ductal and periductal inflammations are present. The lesion is in some cases very difficult to distinguish from other causes such as multisystemic infections (tuberculosis), autoimmune diseases (sarcoidosis, Wegener's granulomatosis), foreign body reaction (silicone injection) and granulomatous reaction to carcinoma.

An established diagnosis should be obtained only with a core needle biopsy or an incisional biopsy. Treatment protocol is not well established. Some sources report that approximately half of the patients will fully recover after lengthy (range 2–24 months) expectant management. Treatment with steroids is lengthy and usually requires about 6 months. While some source reports very good success with steroids, most reports a considerable risk of recurrence after a treatment with steroids alone. For surgical treatment, recurrence rates of 10–50 % have been reported.

*DIABETIC MASTOPATHY* – Diabetic mastopathy (also known as *lymphocytic mastitis* or *lymphocytic mastopathy*) is seen almost exclusively in young women with insulin-dependent diabetes mellitus long standing for over 10 years. The exact mechanism remains unknown and is not related to poor control of the diabetes, and in fact, these changes are (rarely) seen in patients without diabetes. The pathogenesis is unknown, but it may represent an autoimmune reaction as the histologic features are similar to those seen in other autoimmune diseases.

Diabetic mastopathy often presents as one or more slightly irregular, dense masses. Sometimes, masses are bilateral and, over time, some formations tend to change in appearance or even to shrink. The diagnosis is supported primarily by history of prolonged treatment with insulin. Mammogram shows a suspicious breast mass with a dense mammographic pattern but often is normal with minimal changes. On the contrary, ultrasound features are worrisome for malignancy.

Core needle biopsy is recommended for diagnostic confirmation. Pathology shows dense keloid-like fibrosis and periductal, lobular or perivascular infiltration by predominately B lymphocytes. Surgical excision is not recommended if the diagnosis is confirmed on needle biopsy and there is no increased risk of subsequent BC. In addition, excision is associated with a high rate of recurrence.

*LYMPHOCYTIC LOBULITIS*, also known as *sclerosing lymphocytic lobulitis*, is similar to diabetic mastopathy and it is often associated with autoimmune disorders.

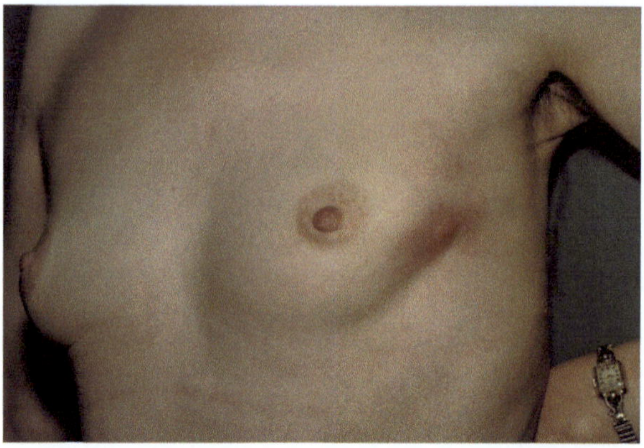

**Fig. 8.8** Pulmonary tuberculosis infection with fistula through the chest wall and abscess in retroglandular fatty space of the left breast

This condition presents clinically as a mass that can resemble malignancy. Histologically, it is characterised by intense fibrosis associated with lymphocytic infiltration around lobules and epithelioid fibroblasts in the stroma. Diagnosis is usually possible on core biopsy only. No specific treatment is required once a specific histological diagnosis is established.

*TUBERCULOSIS* of the breast is rare. It can be primary or, more commonly, secondary. Clinical presentation is a solitary, ill-defined, unilateral hard lump, but tuberculosis can also present with nipple discharge, skin thickening or discharging sinuses in the breast or axilla. A common presentation of tuberculosis nowadays is with an abscess resulting from infection of a tubercle cavity by an acute pyogenic organism such as *Staphylococcus aureus*. In rare cases, a retroglandular peripheral abscess may originate from a pulmonary cavitating infection with a chest wall fistula (Fig. 8.8).

Mammographic imaging may show a dense tract connecting an ill-defined breast mass to an area of skin thickening with a skin bulge. Ultrasound may demonstrate a complex, predominantly cystic mass. Solid caseating granulomata may be seen on biopsy. The diagnosis of TB is made by finding *Mycobacterium tuberculosis* bacteria in a clinical specimen taken from the patient. Treatment should follow standard recommendations for systemic tuberculosis and surgery is rarely required.

*OTHER INFECTIONS* – Primary actinomycosis, syphilis and mycotic, helminthic and viral infections have all been reported in the breast but are extremely rare.

## 8.3.4 Postsurgical Infections

*INFECTIONS FOLLOWING BREAST SURGERY* – Breast surgery often results in the formation of cavities within the breast where breast tissue has been removed. These fill up with inflammatory fluid and blood in the post-operative period, all as part of the normal healing process. Usually, this would settle with time, but if infection sets in, an abscess and wound infection can occur.

This has a number of consequences for the patient. Firstly, an infection in the breast after surgery will take longer to heal and the final scar may look less cosmetic than a non-infected wound scar. Secondly, since many operations are done for cancer, the presence of a wound infection can significantly delay the use of adjuvant therapy that may not be withheld until the infection has settled.

The reason for this is that the chemotherapy, as well as killing off residual tumour cells, will also suppress the patient's immune system to such an extent that their wound infection could worsen or indeed become life-threatening. In such cases, chemotherapy has to be postponed until it is safe to be administered.

*Infections of breast implants* – Infections of breast implants occur in approximately 2–3 % of cases. Postmastectomy implantation is associated with a higher risk of infection compared with breast augmentation alone. The use of particular surgical approaches or acellular dermal matrix may also increase the risk of infection [5].

Most acute and subacute breast implant infections are due to Gram-positive pathogens such as coagulase-negative staphylococci, *Propionibacterium* species, *Staphylococcus aureus* and Streptococci. Non-tuberculosis mycobacteria are also an important cause of subacute infections. Both Gram-positive and Gram-negative bacteria have been associated with late-onset infections, often secondary to bacteraemia.

Saline breast implant infections usually present in the acute post-operative period (6 days to 6 weeks after surgery); in contrast, silicone implant infections usually occur more than 6 months after surgery. Acute infections are usually associated with fever and breast pain, erythema and drainage. Subacute infections may present with chronic pain, persistent drainage, failed healing of the incision site or migration of the implant.

Diagnosis of implant infections is generally made by microbiological analysis of peri-implant fluid, which should be aspirated under ultrasound guidance and sent for Gram stain, aerobic and anaerobic bacterial cultures and fungal and acid-fast bacilli cultures.

There are no randomised trials or large cohort studies evaluating the management of breast implant infections. Some bacterial breast implant infections can be treated successfully with medical therapy alone. However, implant removal is often necessary for cure, particularly in case of mycobacterial and fungal infections.

For patients with breast implant infections who present acutely or have evidence of systemic toxicity, an empiric but strong parenteral antibiotic therapy should be given with a regimen effective against methicillin-resistant *Staphylococcus aureus* (MRSA), coagulase-negative staphylococci and Gram-negative bacteria.

An oral empiric regimen or deferment of antibiotics pending culture data is appropriate in subacute cases with localised infection. Patients who respond to initial parenteral therapy can switch to an oral regimen tailored to culture results. The duration of antimicrobial therapy depends on the infecting organism but should be continued for up 1–2 months.

The use of perioperative antibiotic prophylaxis with a single dose of cefazolin is widely used to prevent surgical site infections despite the lack of evidence regarding the efficacy of this practice.

### 8.3.5 Mastitis Associated with Malignancy

Inflammatory BC, comedo DCIS and locally advanced BC can be confused with an infection. In absence of specific symptoms, cancer should be suspected if an apparent breast infection does not respond to appropriate treatment.

*Inflammatory BC* (see Sect. 14.2) causes pain, redness and induration of the skin, usually affecting a large portion of the breast. Symptoms progress very rapidly, and within a month, the breast may have the *peau d'orange* appearance. An associated axillary lymphadenopathy is often present.

*Comedo DCIS* (see Sect. 12.1) can become infected and present with signs and symptoms of peripheral inflammation or of an abscess. After antibiotic treatment or aspiration of pus, the area can resolve completely and leave no residual mass. Nonetheless, all patients aged more than 35 years should have a mammogram after resolution of an episode of breast infection for which there is no obvious cause.

*Advanced BC* can present with skin ulceration and secondary infection of necrotic tissue can be malodorous. Successful treatment will require excision of all necrotic tissues along with appropriate local and systemic therapy coordinated with the medical oncologist. Metronidazole gel is valuable for eliminating odour generated by the anaerobic organisms that grow in the dead tissue.

## 8.4 Surface Mastitis

### 8.4.1 Breast Cellulitis

**Clinical Practice Points**

- Surface mastitis presents as a series of changes of cutaneous and subcutaneous tissue due to fluid stasis, extensive dermatological disease as eczema or inflammation of skin and cutaneous annexes.
- As other types of mastitis, surface inflammations could be non-infectious or infectious up to the formation of abscess.
- Although most surface inflammations are present everywhere in the body, some are common in the breast for its fatty texture or for the slender thickness of its skin.
- Slowing down of fluid circulation in the breast may facilitate superficial inflammatory changes as oedema and cellulitis.

*Primary cellulitis* is an uncommon infection in the breast, difficult to distinguish from other benign erythematous condition. It affects the skin of the lower half of the breast and is often recurrent in women who are overweight, have large breasts or have poor personal hygiene. In primary cellulitis, *Staphylococcus aureus*, including

**Fig. 8.9** Cellulitis following breast-conserving surgery

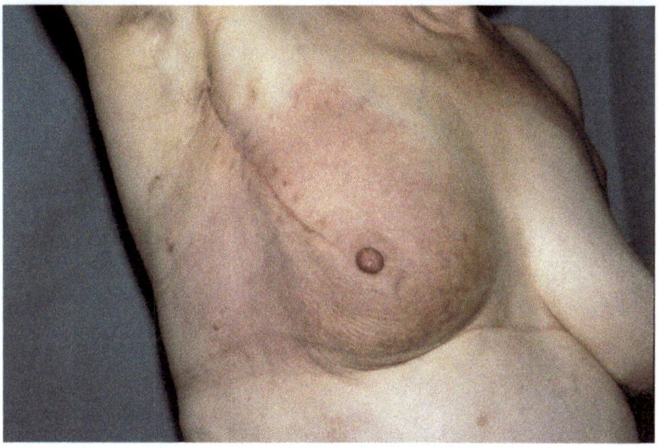

methicillin-resistant type, is the usual causative organism, while fungi such as *Candida albicans* are not important organisms, contrary to what commonly believed.

*Secondary cellulitis* is quite common. Independent risk factors for breast cellulitis include breast surgery both conservative (Fig. 8.9) and demolitive within previous 30 days, radiation treatment, prior breast cellulitis or infection, trauma (e.g. bites, nipple piercing, tattoos) and infected skin lesions (e.g. eczema, severe dryness, dermatitis). *Beta-haemolytic streptococcus* is the most common pathogen for post-operative cellulitis of the breast, although in many cases, no pathogen is isolated from skin aspirates or blood cultures. These germs have a proclivity to produce soft tissue infections in the setting of venous and/or lymphatic compromise [6].

Pain is a prominent feature of breast cellulitis and is associated with diffuse erythema, swelling, tenderness and warmth. Systemic symptoms (e.g. fever, chills) are uncommon, occurring in about 10 % of cases, and, when present, most often consist of low-grade fever. Axillary nodes can be enlarged and tender.

Diagnostic evaluation for breast cellulitis includes a history to assess for trauma, problematic breastfeeding, previous breast surgery, diagnosis and/or local radiation treatments. The clinical evaluation includes a breast examination to assess for extent of erythema, swelling and tenderness, and an axillary examination to assess for tender and/or enlarged lymph nodes.

Neither laboratory tests nor skin aspirates are required. Laboratory tests may identify a leucocytosis in patients with systemic symptoms (e.g. fever, chills). Blood cultures are typically negative in patients without systemic symptoms as a reflection of the low concentration of organisms present in the involved tissue. Beta-haemolytic streptococcus or *Staphylococcus aureus* may be identified in a small minority of patients, who usually have systemic symptoms of infection and sometimes sepsis.

Histopathologic evaluation of a full-thickness skin biopsy (punch or elliptical) can reveal a leucocyte infiltration, capillary dilatation, soft tissue inflammation and possible bacteria.

Radiographic imaging is useful if there is any clinical suspicion of an underlying fluid collection, abscess and malignancy or if there is no improvement in signs and symptoms from oral antibiotic therapy after 48–72 h of use. Mammogram and ultrasound may show no specific radiographic abnormality for cellulitis other than mild skin thickening and oedema.

Patients with uncomplicated breast cellulitis may be treated with empiric oral antibiotic therapy. Patients with signs of systemic toxicity or rapidly progressing erythema should be treated with parenteral antibiotics. Courses are the same of other non-lactating mastitis, that is, amoxicillin-clavulanate (875 mg orally every 12 h), dicloxacillin (500 mg oral every 6 h) or cephalexin (500 mg orally every 6 h).

The optimal duration of oral antibiotic therapy is uncertain; 10–14 days is generally appropriate for most patients, but the duration of antimicrobial therapy can be shorter or longer, depending on patient response. In general, antibiotics are continued until the clinical signs of infection have resolved, including pain, fever, erythema and oedema. In general, patients report improvement in pain before there is a noticeable decrease in erythema and swelling.

If the infection does not show evidence of a response (e.g. pain resolution, partial clearing of erythema and oedema) within 48–72 h of antibiotic therapy, further evaluation is necessary, including a mammogram and/or ultrasound to assess for a fluid collection (all abscess should be drained) or findings suspicious for cancer.

Treatment for patients with recurrent cellulitis should be guided by microbiologic data, if available. Otherwise, the approach to antibiotic selection is the same as for an initial episode of cellulitis. Chronic dermatologic conditions that predispose to cellulitis should be treated aggressively, and the skin of the lower breast should be kept as clean and dry as possible.

For some patients with multiple recurrent episodes, long-term suppressive antibiotic therapy may be appropriate. Management of these patients should be done in concert with infectious disease specialists or others with extensive expertise in the management of patients with long-lasting cellulitis.

### 8.4.2 Breast Lymphangitis

Lymphangitis is an inflammation of lymphatic channels due to infectious or non-infectious causes. It commonly develops after cutaneous inoculation of microorganisms into the lymphatic vessels through a skin wound or an abrasion or as a complication of a distal infection. Potential pathogens include bacteria, mycobacteria, viruses, fungi and parasites [7].

Lymphangitis can occur in the setting of normal lymphatic channels, but more frequently in presence of damaged lymphatic channels or anatomic abnormalities. Lymphatic damage and anatomic abnormalities can result in tissue protein and fluid accumulation, leading to non-pitting lymphoedema with induration and predisposing to invasion of microorganisms.

The clinical manifestations of lymphangitis are variable and may be *troncular*, characterised by erythematous streaks with pain and rapid spread, or *nodular* as swellings along the course of the lymphatic vessels (Fig. 8.10).

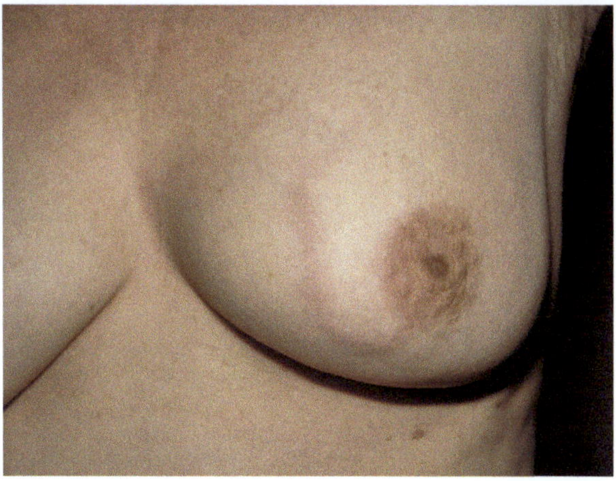

**Fig. 8.10** Troncular lymphangitis starting from the areola

*Troncular lymphangitis*. The causes of acute troncular lymphangitis include *Streptococcus pyogenes*, *Staphylococcus aureus* and Gram-negative organisms. Animal exposure can confer risk for lymphangitis due to *Pasteurella*, *Erysipelothrix* and anthrax.

Assessment for lymphangitis may include swab, aspirate and/or biopsy of the primary site for histology, microscopy (including Gram, fungal and acid-fast staining) and culture (including bacterial, fungal and mycobacterial cultures).

*Nodular lymphangitis*. The causes of nodular lymphangitis include *Sporothrix schenckii*, *Nocardia* (most often *N. brasiliensis*), *M. marinum*, leishmaniasis, tularaemia and systemic mycoses. Assessment is that above mentioned and treatment includes targeted medical therapy. Only few cases of nodular lymphangitis may require surgical debridement. In the setting of lymphoedema with significant lymphatic obstruction, surgical intervention may also be appropriate.

### 8.4.3 Breast Oedema

*Primary breast oedema* is very rare and usually is bilateral. It is observed in large, pendulous breasts and should be considered a sort of orthostatic oedema in absence of systemic pathological condition. It is detectable after a period of time in the sitting or standing posture and disappears slowly but spontaneously in recumbency. Orthostatic elevation of hydrostatic pressure within venous and/or lymphatic vessel is the probable mechanism in some cases. Episodes of cellulitis may foster its appearance. Pitting oedema is readily demonstrable in the lower quadrants. After ruling out the more trivial causes, including imbalance of fluid with sodium retention, no treatment is required.

*Secondary breast oedema* may be the comprehensive symptom of conditions due to heart failure (Fig. 8.11), nephrotic syndrome or inanition. The changes in the skin are thickening which may progress to ulceration, so that in unilateral pattern, even

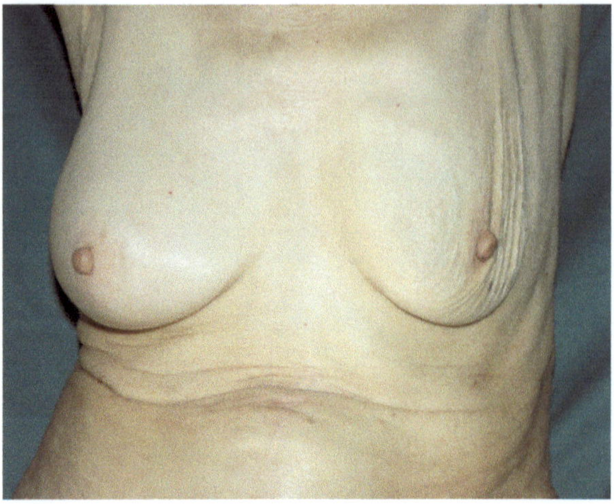

**Fig. 8.11** Marked oedema of the right breast due to heart failure

if no mass is palpable and nipple reaction is absent, a diagnosis of carcinoma should be excluded.

Breast oedema is also a more common situation after breast-conserving surgery, especially following axillary lymphadenectomy, radiation therapy or recurrent cancer in axillary lymph nodes. In fact, it is a lymphoedema caused by a disruption or blockage of lymphatic flow to the breast or axilla. There are several risk factors that increase the incidence of developing breast oedema, which include seroma, post-operative infection, large pendulous breast, cording development after surgery on the chest wall or axilla and marked reaction to radiotherapy. The position and orientation of the scar can be a risk factors; a vertical scar is more likely to develop lymphoedema than a horizontal scar.

Breast lymphoedema can present as swelling and hardening of the tissues with pain to the breast. Skin changes may include redness, discolouration and sometimes the appearance of *peau d'orange* due to fibrosis and trapped lymph fluid.

Nonsteroidal anti-inflammatory agents and analgesics are given for symptomatic relief. A correct bra fitting to offer support to the swollen breast should be advised. In very symptomatic cases, *treatment can include m*anual lymphatic drainage and measures as in the treatment of lymphoedema (see Sect. 21.3).

### 8.4.4 Mondor Disease of the Breast

Mondor disease of the breast is a rare benign breast condition characterised by a spontaneous thrombophlebitis of the superficial/subcutaneous veins of the chest wall. Mondor disease is rarely reported in the literature, and this is likely in part due to lack of awareness of the entity. It tends to prevail on individuals between 30 and 50 years of age, and males can also be affected in approximately 10–15 % of cases. Rarely, both synchronous and metachronous bilateral syndromes have been reported.

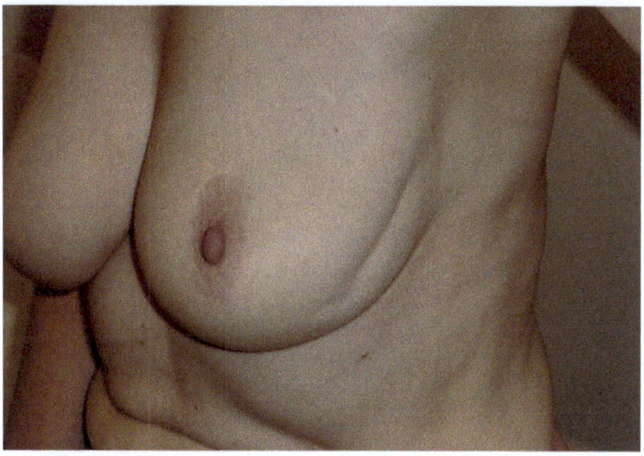

**Fig. 8.12** A case of spontaneous (idiopathic) Mondor disease of the left breast in a 35-year-old woman

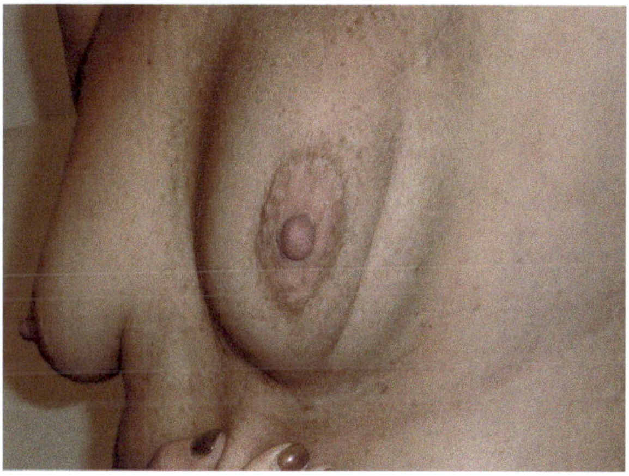

**Fig. 8.13** Episode of Mondor disease of the left breast in a 46-year-old woman, following and probably related to surgery and radiation therapy

An all-inclusive incidence rate of 0.5–1 % has been reported; however, it reflects only the symptomatic population [8].

Patients usually present an acute pain with a tender breast cord-like mass in the location of the affected vein, sometimes with an overlying skin erythema (Fig. 8.12). The evidence of cord may be accentuated when the ipsilateral arm is raised or the skin pulled downwards (Fig. 8.13).

The vessels most commonly involved are the lateral thoracic vein towards the upper outer quadrant and the thoraco-epigastric vein and the superior epigastric vein (Fig. 8.14). The upper inner quadrants of the breasts are almost never involved.

In most cases, the syndrome is idiopathic and its pathogenesis is not attributable to secure local or systemic factors, although it is conceivable an increased venous pressure due to a temporary condition of stasis. Associations with systemic diseases as rheumatoid arthritis are sporadically reported. In some cases, it is secondary to direct local injury, thoracic trauma (but also physical exertion and muscle strains) or breast surgical procedures (usually 3–4 weeks after surgery), ultrasound-guided or stereotactic core biopsies, previous central venous catheters, coagulative factors and

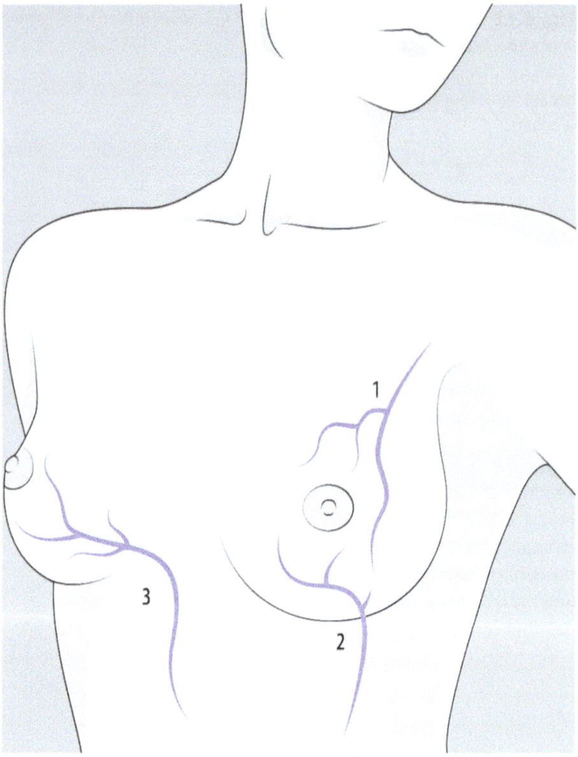


**Fig. 8.14** Main superficial veins of the anterior chest wall involved in Mondor disease: lateral thoracic vein (*1*), thoraco-epigastric vein (*2*) and superior epigastric vein (*3*)

dehydration. An association with BC has been reported but the veracity of this claim can be to confirm, although an infiltration of the vein or a secondary venous stasis could be a causative factor.

The pathogenesis includes formation of venous thrombosis with total or partial occlusion, vascular recanalisation causing fibromuscular hyperplasia of vessel wall and infiltration plus fibrosis of surrounding subcutaneous cellular tissue. The thrombotic vessel can adhere to the subjacent skin causing retraction and formation of characteristic cordiform grooves secondary to local fibroblastic proliferation.

Mammogram is justified only to exclude an associated pathology. Typically, Mondor disease appears as superficially located tubular-beaded density corresponding to a palpable ropelike mass. Mammography can be normal in a significant proportion of cases.

On breast ultrasound, Mondor disease appears as a tubular anechoic or iso-echoic structure with multiple areas of narrowing, giving a beaded appearance. Sometimes, low-level internal echoes may be present representing clots. The surrounding soft tissues may be hyper-echoic due to associated inflammatory response. No flow is present on colour or spectral Doppler studies, and in some situations, an abrupt cutoff within the normal vessel may be seen.

Mondor disease is a benign self-limiting condition and the natural history is for the thrombosed vein to recanalise and for clinical symptoms to resolve gradually in about 6 weeks. Nonsteroidal anti-inflammatory agents rubbed over the area of tenderness and analgesic medications are sometimes given for symptomatic relief. Otherwise, management with anticoagulants, antibiotics or surgical intervention is not indicated due to the thrombophlebitis subsiding spontaneously and without complications or persistent deformity. A close interval follow-up scan is usually recommended to ensure resolution and to exclude any other entity.

### 8.4.5 Skin-Related Infections

Skin disorders of the breast can be difficult to differentiate from true breast infections and should be taken into account when evaluating a patient with inflammation of the breast. A pragmatic grouping of localised superficial breast infections includes mainly epidermal cyst, intertrigo and hidradenitis suppurativa.

*EPIDERMAL CYST* – For epidermal cyst, several (almost) interchangeable synonyms exist including *epidermal inclusion cyst*, *epidermoid cyst*, *infundibular cyst* and *keratin cyst*. Epidermal cysts are also improperly referred to as *sebaceous cysts*, when in fact there is no sebaceous component.

Epidermal cyst is typically a discrete subcutaneous masses fixed to the dermis that can occur quite ordinarily within the skin of the breast as well as anywhere in the body. Examination usually reveals an overlying pore and keratinaceous material ('cottage cheese' with 'foot odour smell') can often be expressed.

On mammography, epidermal cyst shows up as a discrete density, although careful directed imaging with a lead marker over the palpable abnormality can help differentiate this from a suspicious lesion within the parenchyma.

Often, these inclusion cysts become infected, typically with *Staphylococcus aureus* forming local abscesses that require incision and drainage. Clinically, this condition presents as a tender, warm, erythematous mass. Patients may report a previous spontaneous drainage of the cyst with improvement in symptoms.

Management is aimed at resolution of the acute infection followed by surgical resection to prevent recurrence. If only inflammation is present, oral antibiotics and warm packs are appropriate. If an abscess is present, incision and drainage are indicated with evacuation of the pasty contents. Once the acute infection resolves, the patient is often left with a small indurated area with an overlying scar. Because epidermal cysts are susceptible to repeated cycles of inflammation and infection, they should be excised electively.

Finally, two specific types of epidermal cysts are observed, within the skin of the nipple and just below the nipple, which features are discussed in Sect. 11.1.

*HIDRADENITIS SUPPURATIVA* is a condition that affects the apocrine sweat glands and can result in infection and abscess formation of the skin of the lower half of the breast as well as of the axilla. This is often a smoking-related condition.

Infection should be controlled with appropriate antibiotics and drainage of any pus. Excision of the affected skin is effective at stopping further infection in about half of patients; the remainder goes on to have further episodes of infection despite surgery.

*INTERTRIGO* is inflamed skin in mammary folds, often due to moisture and maceration. This is often a recurrent problem in women with large ptotic breasts that make contact with the chest wall, usually affecting the skin of the lower half of the breast.

The primary management of intertrigo is to educate the patient about keeping the area as clean and dry as possible. The skin should be washed gently two times a day with simple soap, a mild cleansing solution or hypoallergenic skin wipes and then dabbed dry with a towel or dried with a hair dryer at a low setting. Preventive measures to keep skin clean and dry in susceptible areas include wearing a cotton bra or a cotton T-shirt or vest inside the bra. Steroids, skin creams and talcum powder should be avoided. Non-comedogenic oils may result emollient, hydrating and protective reinforcing the skin's barrier function. Antifungal agents should *not* be prescribed, as there is no evidence that they are effective or that fungi play an important role in this condition.

*OTHER SKIN-RELATED INFECTIONS* involving the nipple (as nipple ring infection due to piercing, runner's nipple and sinus pilonidalis) are discussed in Sect. 11.1.

## References


1. Dixon MJ. Breast abscess. http://www.uptodate.com. Accessed 30 Jan 2015.
2. Dixon MJ. Lactational mastitis. http://www.uptodate.com. Accessed 30 Jan 2015.
3. Banikarim C, De Silva NK, Fortunov R. Mastitis and breast abscess in infants, children, and adolescents. http://www.uptodate.com. Accessed 16 Jul 2014.
4. Dixon JM, Ravisekar O, Chetty U, Anderson TJ. Periductal mastitis and duct ectasia: different conditions with different aetiologies. Br J Surg. 1996;83:820–2.
5. Lalani T, Zenn MR, Sexton DJ. Breast implant infections. http://www.uptodate.com. Accessed 14 Nov 2014.
6. Dixon MJ, Baddour LM. Breast cellulitis: clinical manifestations, diagnosis, and management. http://www.uptodate.com. Accessed 30 Jan 2015.
7. Spelman D. Lymphangitis. http://www.uptodate.com. Accessed Apr 10 2014.
8. Schwartz RA. Mondor disease. http://emedicine.medscape.com/article/1087099-overview#showall. Accessed 20 Sept 2014.


## Further Reading


Kaviani A, Noveiry BB, Jamei K, Rabbani A. How to manage idiopathic granulomatous mastitis: suggestion of an algorithm. Breast J. 2014;20:110–2.

Naveen KN, Pai VV, Sori T, Kalabhavi S. Erysipelas after breast cancer treatment. Breast. 2012;21:218–9.

Pandey TS, Mackinnon JC, Bressler L, Millar A, Marcus EE, Ganschow PS. Idiopathic granulomatous mastitis—a prospective study of 49 women and treatment outcomes with steroid therapy. Breast J. 2014;20:258–66.

Salemis NS, Vasilara G, Lagoudianakis E. Mondor's disease of the breast as a complication of ultrasound-guided core needle biopsy: management and review of the literature. Breast Dis. 2015;35:73–6.

World Health Organisation. Mastitis causes and management. Geneva; 2000. http://whqlibdoc.who.int/hq/2000/WHO_FCH_CAH_00.13.pdf. Accessed 30 Jan 2015.

**Websites in Appendix**: *Mastitis*, A-4.3

# Benign Lesions of the Breast

# 9

Alfonso M. Pluchinotta, Giorgio Macellari, and Gigliola Lodovichetti

## Contents




A.M. Pluchinotta (✉)
Breast Surgery, Policlinic of Abano Terme, Padova, Italy
e-mail: pluchinotta.alfonso@gmail.com

G. Macellari
Surgical Breast Clinic, Hospital "Guglielmo da Saliceto", Piacenza, Italy
e-mail: g.macellari@ausl.pc.it

G. Lodovichetti
Multicentric Pathological Laboratory, Accredited to Health Local Service USL16, Padova, Italy







A.M. Pluchinotta (ed.), *The Outpatient Breast Clinic: Aiming at Best Practice*,
DOI 10.1007/978-3-319-15907-2_9

**Abstract**

• Benign breast diseases come to attention as imaging abnormality or as clinical symptom or as incidental pathological finding. Since most breast discoveries are benign, any new symptom can cause a natural anxiety that leads women to fear the worst. • For benign breast diseases, clinical classifications should be abandoned in favour of a simpler and comprehensive classification based on three histological categories: nonproliferative lesions, proliferative lesions without atypia and proliferative lesions with atypia. • Most benign breast disorders derive from minor aberrations of the normal processes of development, cyclical activity and involution. • Diagnostic assessment of benign lesions is planned to rule out cancer or associated high-risk lesions. Surgery of benign lesions is aimed at symptomatic relief. A good part of treatment is patient information and education.

*Future directions.* In the clinical practice, benign breast diseases represent a mostly negligible risk factor for BC. However, various studies demonstrate variability among the actual degree of risk, depending on whether lesions are proliferative and nonproliferative, with and without atypia, more or less associated with family history. The potential for research in benign breast diseases is endless. Studies on the link between benign breast disease and BC may help in discovering one of the many causes of BC.

## 9.1 Overview of Breast Benign Disorders and Diseases

**Clinical Practice Points**

- Since discordance may occur between clinical manifestations of benign lesions and their histologic modifications, pathological criteria should prevail on their classification.
- The simplest categorisation of benign epithelial breast lesions includes three histological categories: nonproliferative, proliferative without atypia and proliferative with atypia.
- Aberrations of normal development and involution (ANDI) classification embraces all aspects of benign disorders of the breast and may be helpful in both understanding the pathological process and guiding rational management.

### 9.1.1 Introduction

Benign conditions of the breast have improperly been neglected in comparison to cancer, despite the fact that only one out of ten patients presenting to a breast clinic suffers from cancer. Without the emotional implications as cancer, benign diseases have been improperly neglected, as it is evident in standard textbooks. Moreover, the sporadic nature of their investigations and the insularity of the resulting

**Table 9.1** A classification of benign conditions of breast according to clinical and pathological criteria

| Clinical criteria | Pathological criteria |
|---|---|
| Cyclical nodularity | *Nonproliferative lesions* |
| Mastalgia | Cysts |
| Nodule (localised, cyclic) | Mammary duct ectasia |
| Fibroadenoma | Other nonproliferative lesions |
| Galactocele | *Proliferative lesions without atypia* |
| Cyst | Adenosis and Fibrocystic changes |
| Secretion | Fibroepithelial (fibroadenoma) and related lesions[a] |
| Galactorrhea | Papilloma and benign papillary lesions |
| Abnormal secretion | Myoepithelial lesions |
| Infections | Sclerosing lesions (sclerosing adenosis, radial scar) |
| Milk stasis | *Proliferative lesions with atypia* |
| Lactating mastitis | Atypical ductal hyperplasia (ADH) also known as DIN 1b |
| Non-lactating mastitis: | Atypical lobular hyperplasia (ALH) also known as LIN 1 |
| Periductal mastitis | Flat epithelial atypia also known as DIN 1a |
| Complicated cysts | Lobular carcinoma in situ (LCIS)[b] also known as LIN 2 |
| Extramammary infections | |

[a]Except phyllodes tumour with borderline or malignant features
[b]Risk of pleomorphic LCIS (also known as LIN 3) is debatable

publications had led to much confusion, which in the past has had more serious consequences than neglect alone.

Until a few years ago, benign breast lesions were classified mainly according to clinical and macroscopic symptoms. This classification had the advantage of simplifying terminology in favour of more frequent symptoms and pathologies.

However, clinical manifestations are not always supported by histologic modifications. This leads to the observation of lesions which are mainly clinical and have little histologic confirmation (such as benign cyclical nodularity or cystic modifications) or that of lesions which, instead, are mainly histologic, but present few clinical symptoms or are asymptomatic (such as the rarely symptomatic atypical hyperplasia).

*CLASSIFICATION BASED ON PROLIFERATIVE CATEGORIES*. The simplest categorisation of benign epithelial breast lesions in general terms should be outlined as three histological categories: nonproliferative, proliferative without atypia and proliferative with atypia (Table 9.1). However, it is worthwhile to consider that all proliferative lesions usually without atypia (as fibroadenoma or papilloma) may occasionally present different degrees of atypia and of cellular proliferation, as well as incidental association with other pathologies. In general, benign lesions are classified on the degree of cellular proliferation and on the different response to hormonal stimulation in time [1].

As shown in Fig. 9.1, nearly all breast pathology originates in the terminal ductal lobular unit (TDLU), considered the *functional unit* of the breast and the most actively proliferating part. So that, for instance, cysts may be the consequence of the

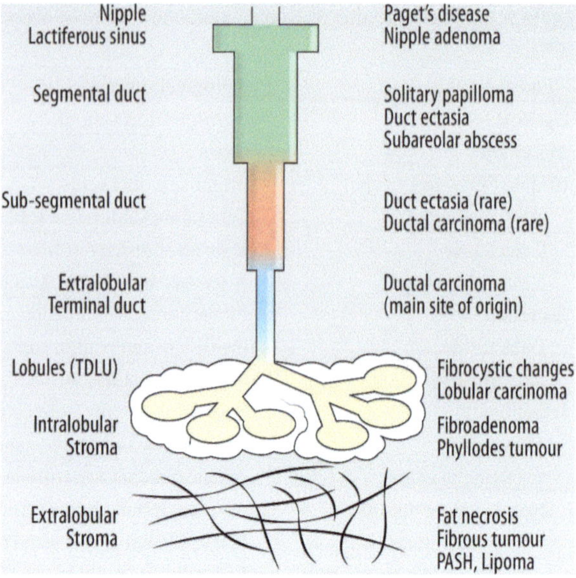


**Fig. 9.1** Schematic drawing illustrates the site of origin (on the *left*) for the most common breast diseases (on the *right*)

unfolding of the terminal ducts and lobular units, adenosis is a lobulocentric proliferation of ductules with epithelial and myoepithelial cells, fibroadenoma arises from the epithelium and intralobular stroma, myoepithelioma has a tubular structure surrounded by myoepithelial cells, and so on. Indeed, the only common lesion believed to be strictly of ductal origin may be the larger solitary intraductal papilloma.

*ANDI CLASSIFICATION.* Aberrations of normal development and involution (ANDI) classification is designed to embrace all aspects of benign disorders of the breast, starting from breast development and physiology to clinical symptoms and signs, up to histological patterns [2]. New sound concepts of pathogenesis clearly show that:

- Benign breast conditions are practically a universal phenomenon among women.
- Benign pathological states account for approximately 90 % of the clinical presentations related to the breast, and these diseases are more common in females 30–50 years old; thus, they are hormonal in nature.
- Previously there was a tendency to include almost all benign breast disorders and pathology under the designation of fibrocystic disease or mammary dysplasia, but today these terms are unsuitable.
- The term fibrocystic disease applied to a biopsy or a palpable breast mass is nonspecific and often includes normal physiologic and morphologic changes in the breast along with specific benign disease processes.
- Almost all benign breast disorders simply are relatively minor aberrations of the normal processes of development, cyclical hormonal response and involution.

On account of these principles, the ANDI classification, asserting that most benign disorders are related to normal processes of reproductive life, replaces the

**Table 9.2** Benign changes of the breast according to clinical and pathological criteria, in the ANDI (aberration) and non-ANDI (disease) classification [2]

| Stage | *Normal process* | *Aberration* | *Disease* |
|---|---|---|---|
| Early reproductive (15–25 years) | Lobular development | Fibroadenoma | Giant fibroadenoma |
| | Stromal development | Adolescent hypertrophy | Gigantomastia |
| | Nipple eversion | Nipple inversion | Subareolar abscess/ mammary duct fistula |
| Mature reproductive (25–40 years) | Cyclical changes of menstruation | Cyclical mastalgia | Severe mastalgia |
| | | Nodularity | |
| | Epithelial hyperplasia of pregnancy | Blood nipple discharge | |
| Involution (35–55 years) | Lobular involution | Macrocysts<br>Sclerosing lesions | |
| | Duct involution<br>Dilatation<br>Sclerosis | Duct ectasia<br>Nipple retraction | Periductal mastitis/ abscess |
| | Epithelial turnover | Simple epithelial hyperplasia | Epithelial hyperplasia with atypia |
| Non-ANDI | Condition of well-defined extramammary aetiology, such as fat necrosis or lactational abscess, together with extrinsic precipitating factors such as trauma, infection, smoking, etc. | | |

conventional view between 'normal' and 'disease'. Since there is a spectrum ranging from normal through slight abnormality (aberration) and occasionally to disease, the definition of normal and abnormal should be considered pragmatic (Table 9.2). Therefore, the purpose of the term ANDI is to prevent the use of the word disease for normal changes and to eliminate confusion.

The ANDI classification deserves to be reported, as it is most helpful in understanding pathological process and in guiding rational clinical management. Nonetheless, the currently used grouping based on proliferative/nonproliferative changes with/without atypia is preferable but not essential.

## 9.2 Nonproliferative Benign Breast Lesions

**Clinical Practice Points**

- Macrocysts represent the most common palpable benign breast mass in premenopausal women.
- The common subset of simple cyst is very easy to detect, but other subsets of cyst may be difficult to diagnose as benign.
- Fibrocystic changes are not a disease as such, but instead a general term that refers to a group of anomalies, symptoms and conditions that form part of the spectrum of benign breast pathology.
- Minor nonproliferative lesions do not cause palpable mass but are occasional findings on pathological samples or on mammogram.

### 9.2.1 Cyst of the Breast

Cysts are the result of a period of fluctuating involution of lobules extending over 20 years. The exact mechanism is not well understood, but it appears that the normal epithelial involution of the lobule is dependent – and not always integrated – on the continuing presence of the stroma around it. If the stroma disappears too early, the epithelial acini remain and may form microcysts, setting the pattern for macrocyst development by obstruction of the efferent ductules.

Some descriptions still do not provide adequate clarity and consistency. Also the fact that macrocysts appear to develop in two directions – apocrine and non-apocrine cysts – is something which is as yet poorly understood, but it is evident both develop from a common origin of microcystic involution.

*Macrocysts*. They constitute the most common discrete benign breast mass, estimated to occur in 7–10 % of all women. Simple cysts are fluid filled, round or ovoid masses derived (but not always) from apocrine metaplasia of the terminal duct lobular unit (TLDU). They are common in the premenopausal women between 35 and 50 years old and in women who take hormone replacement therapy at any age.

*Microcyst*. Asymptomatic microcysts are often found mainly in ultrasound scanning at any age, but mostly in the last decade of reproductive life.

Cysts are clinically significant for many reasons. As macrocysts cause considerable anxiety, mainly for the localised pain due to sudden onset in acute enlargement. Moreover they present as lumps in women of an age where BC is more likely to occur, so they are assumed to be cancers when first discovered.

Furthermore, there is some evidence that recurrent macrocysts may increase the risk of BC slightly, though opinions about, and evidence for, the details of the associated cancer risk are not uniform. Actually macrocysts fall into two comprehensive groups: those with a persisting apocrine cell lining and active secretion/concentration of many substances and those lined by flattened cells and metabolically much less active. In any case cysts may cause diagnostic confusion and psychological consequences, mainly when they are often recurrent and bilateral, requiring several visits to the outpatient clinic for assessment.

Finally, there are many kinds of cysts, and, because BCs only rarely present as a cystic appearance, some of them could be due to intracystic papillary tumours of benign histology or low-grade malignancy.

Cysts present as a lump in the breast that is normally smooth and fluctuant on clinical examination. If it is in tension or fast recurrent, simple macrocyst may be adequately treated by aspiration (Fig. 9.2). Upon aspiration the fluid within a breast cyst is normally either clear or turbid and can be any colour from pale to black, while no blood is seen.

The amount of fluid varies, generally between 2 and 10 ml, but can be considerably more. Usually the mass disappears after aspiration leaving a temporary defect. Afterwards the breast is re-examined, and if no further palpable abnormality is felt and if there is nothing on ultrasound to cause concern, the diagnosis is confirmed and no more steps need be done. Patients are reassured and warned that the cyst may recur or that they may develop further cysts in the same or other breast.

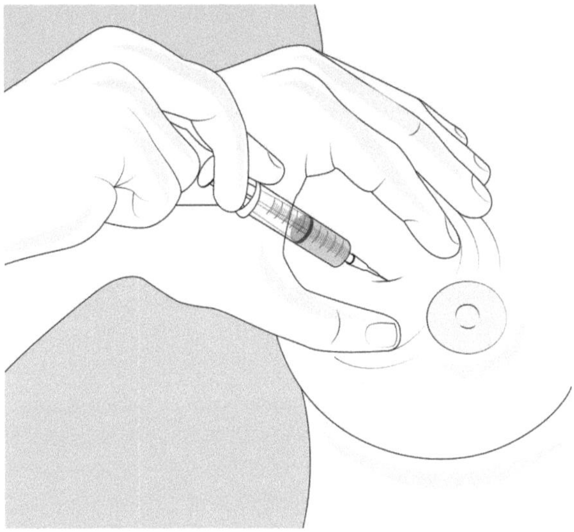

**Fig. 9.2** Fine needle aspiration of a cyst. The removal of cyst fluid by fine needle aspiration is somewhat therapeutic if there is no residual mass after aspiration and no recurrence in approximately 3 months

Since cystic lesions are furthermost common, true breast cysts should be classified as simple, complicated or complex based upon the characteristics identified by ultrasound evaluation. Moreover it is worth to remember some cysts may be secondary to a trauma or infection or associated with proliferative (as papilloma or carcinoma) or necrotic conditions, or may be false cyst (Table 9.3).

*Simple cyst.* It is well circumscribed with ultrasonic features that include posterior acoustic enhancement, without internal echoes (anechoic), solid components or Doppler signal. Subsets of simple cysts are:

- *Clustered microcysts* – a cluster of simple anechoic cysts, each smaller than 2–3 mm, without discrete solid components
- *Cysts with thin septa* that are less than 0.5 mm in thickness
- *'Juvenile' cyst* – a clinical term attributed to cyst in young girls up to the age of 20

*Complicated cyst.* It is defined by ultrasound criteria as a mass with homogeneous low-level internal echoes due to echogenic debris; without solid components, thick walls or thick septa; and without vascular flow. Some cysts will refill after 2–3 aspirations because of their thick walls, but a suspicion of intraluminal proliferation should be considered.

*Complex cyst.* It is defined by ultrasound criteria as a mass with thick walls and/or septa greater than 0.5 mm; presence of cystic and solid components, internal echoes, fluid debris level, irregular borders and septation; and absence of posterior wall enhancement. The ultrasound appearance of complex cysts can demonstrate anechoic and echogenic components. Needle aspiration can show atypical fluids (bloody or purulent). All complex lesions should be investigated.

**Table 9.3** Primary and secondary cysts of the breast

| | |
|---|---|
| True breast cysts | Simple cyst |
| | Typical ultrasonic features: well circumscribed, no internal echoes, posterior acoustic enhancement, no vascular flow |
| | Subsets are: |
| | Clustered microcysts |
| | Cyst with thin septa |
| | Juvenile cyst |
| | Complicated cyst |
| | Low-level internal echoes, thick wall or internal septa, no solid components, no vascular flow |
| | Complex cyst |
| | Thick wall and/or septa more than 0.5 mm, presence of cystic and solid components, no posterior acoustic enhancement |
| Secondary cysts | Galactocele |
| | Oil cyst of fat necrosis |
| | Abscess associated with periductal mastitis |
| | Liquefied haematoma |
| | Postsurgical fluid collection |
| Cysts associated with proliferative or necrotic conditions | Papillary tumour |
| | Papillary carcinoma |
| | Phyllodes tumour |
| | Necrotic carcinoma |
| False cysts | Epidermal cyst |
| | Parasitic cyst |

*Workup of cystic masses*. Ultrasound is beneficial for showing the cystic nature of these lesions and even more helpful with poorly defined or complex cysts. It is also valuable to ensure complete emptying of recurrent cysts in order to exclude the presence of intraluminal masses. It should be considered anyhow that leakage from a cyst gives causes surrounding inflammation with altered ultrasound appearances and may leave a residual mass after aspiration [3].

Mammogram usually detects cysts only if size is sufficient and breast density allows it. If indicated, mammogram should be performed before aspiration since image usually appears normal after aspiration, but only if the aspiration has been not traumatic.

Only a bloody aspirate needs to be investigated, whereas normal cystic fluid could be usually discarded. Cysts yielding blood-stained fluid should be submitted for cytological evaluation and in any case carefully followed even if triple assessment is negative. Surgical excision should be considered for any suspicious lesion, when multiple recurrences need repeated aspirations and when the patient refuses such repeated manoeuvres.

When blood is aspirated from a cyst (even if the cyst totally disappears) or when there is a residual palpable abnormality, a histological sampling is needed, though a period of observation for a short time may be justified in certain cases, depending on the results of mammography and cytopathology. Under these circumstances, a delayed diagnosis of a cancer mistaken for a cyst can be a serious cause of legal litigation.

### 9.2.2 Mammary Duct Ectasia and Partly Related Conditions

*OVERVIEW*. Mammary duct ectasia is basically a dilatation of the main ducts more or less associated with stasis of the secretions and ensuing reactive, inflammatory or infectious conditions. These various processes, individual but interrelated, explain the protean clinical presentations of the so-called mammary duct ectasia/periductal complex.

There are four main theories that try to explain duct dilatation:

- A progressive failure of the muscle wall of the duct, perhaps due to the relaxation effect of progesterone.
- A failure of absorption of the duct secretion due to inadequate lymphatic flow.
- An obstructive phenomenon due to blockage of the ducts at their termination by squamous cell debris, with leakage of highly irritant lipid material into the periductal tissue.
- A periductal inflammation as the primary process, perhaps a form of autoimmune disease, with muscle damage and duct dilatation as secondary phenomena. Obviously this theory contrasts sharply with the others.

Duct ectasia may indeed be involved in a number of processes that may exist alone or in combination with it. Some are subclinical minor variants of normality, as physiological involution, while others have a spectrum of clinical and pathological manifestations, which extends to disease with severe morbidity. A large spectrum of conditions is possible, where much confusion still arises due to failure to differentiate between histological findings and clinical disease entities.

In the attempt to include the clinical manifestations within a single all-embracing disease process, definitions as *duct ectasia/periductal mastitis* (DE/PM) complex and *mammary duct-associated inflammatory disease sequence* (MDAIDS) have been proposed. Actually all approaches are incompatible with the breadth of clinical manifestations or the observed pathology, and, furthermore, all conditions could also be regarded as one aspect of fibrocystic changes.

Mammary duct ectasia-related conditions present clinically in many ways, at times giving rise to all common breast symptoms (nipple discharge, pain, mass), as well as to other less common manifestations including inflammation, abscess, fistula, chronic persistent mastalgia and nipple inversion or sometimes retraction (for this distinction, see Sect. 11.1.1). As told before, all conditions may present by themselves or in combination with others. Afore dealing with the different phases of the pathogenesis connecting them to each other, it is useful set them out separately, as in Table 9.4.

**Table 9.4** The clinical spectrum of presentations of minor reactive duct ectasia to duct ectasia associated with inflammatory diseases

| Disorders/ process | Influential factors | Main clinical symptoms | Frequency |
|---|---|---|---|
| Duct ectasia *regressive* | *Constitutional* (fatty breasts, congenital nipple inversion, etc.) | *Asymptomatic* | By the age of 70, 40 % of women have substantial, bilateral and almost never symptomatic duct ectasia |
| | *Hormonal* (unclear action) | *Nipple discharge*: only elicited, coloured, thick, creamy, sometimes bloody | |
| Periductal fibrosis *reactive or mild inflammatory* | *Duct obstruction* with stagnant fluids | *Asymptomatic* or poorly symptomatic | Not common, sometimes unilateral |
| | *Nipple inversion* | *Nipple inversion*, more noticeable if pre-existing | |
| | | *Paraesthesias* | |
| Periductal mastitis *inflammatory* | *Environmental* (as smoking nicotine) | *Pain* (usually noncyclical mastalgia) | Rare, more common in young women (mean age 35 years) |
| | *Other reported elements* (as nutritional) not fully proven | *Subareolar inflammatory mass* (common) | Two–three times more common in smokers as compared to age-matched control subjects |
| | | *Nipple inversion* (rarely, retraction) | |
| Subareolar breast abscess *infectious* | (see Sect. 8.3) | *Abscess* that usually drains spontaneously | About 20–30 % of patients with severe periductal mastitis |
| | *Mixed flora* (aerobes and anaerobes) usually typical of (and probably coming from) those in the mouth and vagina | | |
| Periareolar fistula *complicated* | (see Sect. 8.3) | *Sinus opening* to fistula | About 20 % of patients with subareolar breast abscess |
| | *Inappropriate or inadequate surgery* of subareolar abscess | *Recurrence* with repeated discharge via fistula | |
| Secondary conditions *associated* | *Persistent nipple discharge* | *Crusting* of the nipple | Very rare, except crusting |
| | *Stasis of secretions* | *Dermatitis or eczema* of the areola | |
| | | *Inflammatory chronic diseases* (only in part) | |

*Duct ectasia* is a *regressive*, involutional process, a normal breast change. As women reach menopause and the breasts age, the major ducts get shorter and wider. By the age of 70, 40 % of women have substantial, bilateral and only slightly symptomatic duct ectasia.

*Periductal fibrosis* is a *reactive* or *mild inflammatory* condition, less common, usually without symptoms and occasionally found on biopsies done for another problem. Accumulation of detritus in the widened duct lumen can cause a fibrous thickening of the many elastic fibres of the wall.

*Periductal mastitis* is an *inflammatory* process, usually due to fibrous obliteration of the ducts, reported under many terms (*comedomastitis*, *mastitis obliterans*, etc.). Periductal mastitis can affect women of all ages, but most cases occur in premenopausal women (mean age about 35 years), two to three times more common in smokers as compared to age-matched control. These data suggest periductal mastitis and duct ectasia are separate conditions which affect different age groups, have different aetiologies and should be considered as separate entities. In few cases it can be accepted as part of the normal involution which may lead to the otherwise asymptomatic nipple retraction in the older woman.

Periductal mastitis is usually symptomatic. The breast becomes tender and hot to touch, and the skin may appear reddened. In almost all cases a subareolar inflammatory mass is palpable. Pain (usually noncyclical mastalgia) is common too, also in the absence of other symptoms. Nipple retraction, inversion or discharges are present in approximately 20 % of patients.

*Subareolar breast abscess* is an *infectious* nonreversible process, which occurs in about one out of five patients with periductal mastitis, but can also occur without previous symptoms. Purulent collection tends to drain spontaneously, and a recurrent *periareolar fistula* is a complication in about 20 % of cases (see Sect. 8.3).

*Other conditions*, secondary to persistent nipple discharge or stagnant secretions, may be occasionally observed as persistent crusting of the nipple, dermatitis or eczema of the areola (see Sect. 11.1).

Finally, there are a number of other chronic inflammatory conditions, such as lymphocytic mastopathy and granulomatous mastitis, which may be unrelated, but which also may overlap with periductal mastitis. If that were true, at least some cases are best managed by surgery directed to proximal ectatic ducts.

*PATHOGENESIS*. The pathogenesis of duct ectasia/periductal mastitis complex is doubtful, given that it can be considered from three different points of view.

*A primary dilatation of the ducts* due to hormone-induced muscle relaxation or to hypersecretion or failure of absorption of duct fluid. According to this classic theory, duct ectasia is the primary event, leading to stagnation of secretion, epithelial ulceration and leakage of duct secretions containing chemically irritant fatty acids into periductal tissue to give a chemical inflammatory process. This sequence starts when one or more of the larger ducts dilate, reaching a diameter of 5 mm in gross examples. This is commonly restricted to the portion of the duct deep to the areola. Typically, three or four ducts are dilated, the remaining ducts being normal. In a few cases, dilatation extends peripherally to involve segmental and even subsegmental ducts.

*An obstructive phenomenon* due to squamous metaplasia, either congenital or acquired with secondary duct dilatation and leakage of contents to give secondary inflammation. However, this view does not keep into account all aspects of the clinical pictures. Moreover the age distribution is contradictory if we consider the fact that inflammatory patterns classically occur in an earlier age group.

*A primary inflammatory condition*, autoimmune or due to bacterial invasion, with secondary duct wall destruction leading to dilatation. This alternative theory explains the primary process as periductal mastitis – perhaps on an autoimmune basis – leading to weakening of the muscle layer of the ducts and secondary dilatation.

The pathogenesis of combined duct ectasia and periductal mastitis is a more difficult problem, and it is likely that more processes may occur separately or in conjunction, thus explaining the wide spectrum of clinical presentations. The basic classic sequence – not valid in all cases – is set out below.

1. *Duct ectasia* with ducts filled with stagnant secretions. These may vary in colour and consistency and may be squeezed out leading to nipple discharge, usually of small amounts but sometimes sufficient to cause embarrassment.
2. *Ulceration* of the epithelial lining of the ducts and ulceration, due to stagnation of secretions, that may result in blood-stained nipple discharge and in leakage of stagnant secretions into the periductal tissue.
3. *Inflammatory response*, in the early stages chemical rather than bacterial, to secretions that contain fatty acids which are chemically irritant. Usually seen beneath the edge of the areola, dilatation may – but rarely does – extend into the subsegmental ducts, more peripherally in the breast, where stasis could contribute to the growing of some chronic inflammatory conditions.
4. *Abscess formation* – when this occurs, simple drainage is unlikely to be curative, and a persistent or recurrent *fistula* is likely to result. In some cases a massive fibrotic reaction stops abscess formation leading to a mass which may simulate a cancer.
5. *Fibrosis* – the periductal inflammation leads to fibrosis, and, as the fibrous tissue matures and contracts, it leads to nipple retraction.

However, a number of clinical aspects are incompatible with the classic view of the disease, and it is unlikely that this sequence is correct. It seems more likely for the duct ectasia/periductal mastitis complex to encompass several different processes which nevertheless may coexist and interact in some cases.

In particular, there are distinct processes affecting the young and the old women and perhaps a third process affecting all ages. Nipple discharge in the premenopausal woman and nipple retraction of the postmenopausal woman may be separate variants, while younger women tend to demonstrate the full picture with the exception of nipple discharge. Perhaps there is a greater obstructive element in young women, and this minimises nipple discharge while improving leakage of duct contents into the periductal tissues.

Moreover, in order to provide a pragmatic approach to the understanding and management of the disease, a number of facts must be taken into consideration.

- Simple duct dilatation with secretory stagnation can arise as an asymptomatic development, best regarded as an aberration of involution.
- Pregnancy and breastfeeding have frequently been considered as important in the aetiology of duct ectasia; however, this relation is hardly noticeable.

- Periductal fibrosis can occur in the absence of duct ectasia or of inflammation and probably represents part of the normal involutional process in the breast.
- The dilatation, too, may result from the same periductal inflammation that may cause duct fibrosis or obliteration, from the effect of some hormones or from simple muscle atrophy.
- The inflammatory complications are more common in young women, while nipple discharge and nipple retraction often occur in older women without overt inflammatory episodes.
- Acute inflammation occurs frequently in young women with a congenital inverted nipple, but in other subjects of this same age group, inflammation leads to retraction of a previously normal nipple.
- Some patients with recurrent subareolar abscess show a definite squamous metaplasia of the terminal duct, while a similar clinical picture can develop in women with grossly ectatic ducts without evidence of squamous epithelial replacement of the terminal ducts.
- The mammary duct fistula associated with squamous epithelial replacement is one entity, probably congenital in most cases and then usually associated with inverted nipple, while in other cases the squamous epithelium may occur as a secondary down-growth.
- There is increasing evidence for a bacterial role in severe forms of periductal mastitis, although at present this would appear to be secondary rather than primary.

*In conclusion*, firstly, clinical manifestations of minor degree can be regarded as a benign breast disorder, while they become a disease only when complicated by the development of severe inflammation. Then, whether it is primarily the inflammation leading to duct damage and dilatation or the duct dilatation giving rise to ulceration and leakage of contents still cannot be determined. There is evidence that both mechanisms are involved, by one or other in some cases, and together in others. Finally, it is also difficult to be certain at what stage a bacterial infection becomes more important than a chemical reaction to leaking duct contents. In each case, a symptomatic disease – inflammation, nipple discharge or retraction – must be regarded as the tip of the iceberg of a subclinical histological change.

*CLINICAL SPECTRUM*. In the mammary duct ectasia/periductal mastitis complex, all common breast symptoms are detectable either alone or interconnected (Fig. 9.3). *Pain*, usually noncyclical, is discussed in Chap. 7. *Nipple Discharge* in plain duct ectasia can be coloured, thick, creamy, or temporarily bloody (see Sect. 10.1). If inflammation is present, the most common complaint is a small amount of purulent discharge, which is confirmed by the patient expressing material from the nipple.

*Evanescent mass*. It is a common presentation of periductal mastitis. The patient notices a small, slightly tender mass in the subareolar region. By the time she is seen in a clinic 7–10 days later, the mass has often disappeared. Such rapid development and regression of a breast mass is uncommon in any other breast condition. These masses, tender and not fixed to surrounding tissues, are typically 1–2 cm in diameter and may progress to reddening of the overlying skin and still regress in a few days.

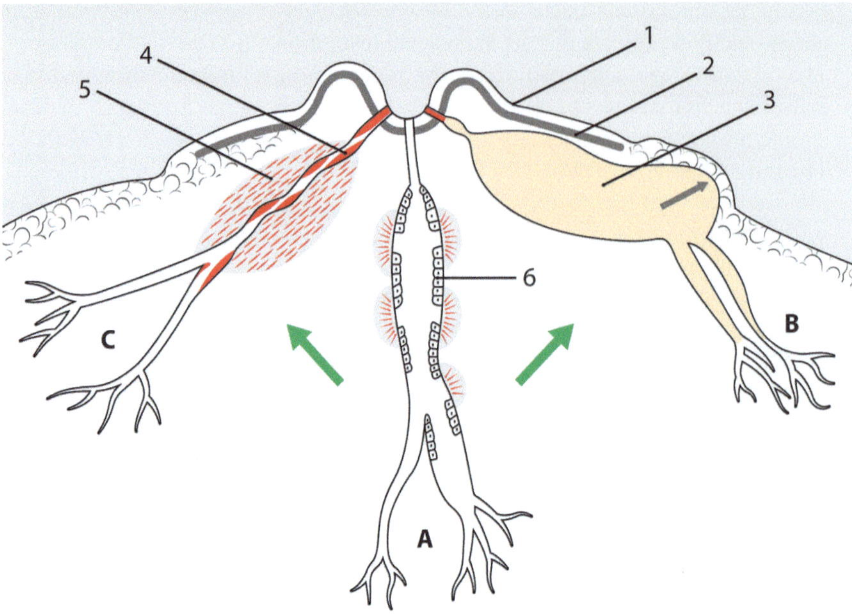


**Fig. 9.3** The classic, albeit questionable, view of the pathogenesis of the clinical spectrum of mammary duct ectasia/periductal mastitis complex. (**a**) The stagnant secretions lead to patchy mucosal ulceration, and the contents leak through giving a chemical inflammatory response into periductal tissue. (**b**) Blockage of duct, sometimes but not always produced by squamous debris, leads to dilatation of the subareolar portion; because of the tough muscle of the areola, an abscess tends to burst through the skin at the edge of the areola (*black arrow*). (**c**) Inflammation leads to fibrosis of the duct wall that contracts producing more nipple retraction and (rarely) a chronic mass. *1*, inverted nipple; *2*, muscle of the areola; *3*, subareolar abscess; *4*, duct thickened by fibrosis; *5*, fibrotic chronic mass (clinically rare); *6*, schematic representation of the epithelial lining of the duct, with patchy ulcerations

The patients have often been given antibiotics and naturally attribute their improvement to the treatment.

An evanescent mass may not recur or have a tendency to do so at the same site at intervals of a few months to 10 years or more. The *recurrent mass* has a tendency to become more severe with each recurrence. There is an appreciable incidence of bilateral involvement, and it is not uncommon for the opposite breast to become involved shortly or years after successful recovery of one breast.

*A persistent mass*. It endures for some weeks, and it is usually firm and fairly well defined. Cancer cannot be excluded, but cytological appearance (foamy macrophages and inflammatory cells without epithelial cells) is highly characteristic and justifies a short course of appropriate antibiotics. If the mass does not resolve rapidly, core needle or excisional biopsy is desirable in women of cancer age group. Provided there is no overt abscess formation, a periareolar biopsy wound will heal satisfactorily, and there is no need to perform a formal duct excision. In fact, macroscopically dilated ducts are not particularly common in the presence of a simple periductal mastitis mass.

*Subareolar abscess*. Any of the above subareolar masses may proceed to abscess formation (see Sect. 8.3). The underlying mass becomes attached to the skin, which first becomes reddened and then shows bluish discolouration. Nipple retraction will often develop if not already present, and nipple oedema may be marked. These abscesses are associated with discomfort which varies from mild to severe, but not usually as severe as with pyogenic abscess. Aspiration will yield creamy or dirty, watery pus, and bacteriological culture may be sterile on the first occasion. If not treated, it will burst spontaneously with considerable relief, but a persistent sinus will remain, or the abscess will recur sooner or later and usually at the same site.

*Mammary Duct Fistula* (see Sect. 8.3). It may result after simple drainage with persisting discharge or recurrent abscesses presenting at the same point.

*Fibrosis*. It is usually the ultimate result of inflammatory process. As fibrous tissue matures and contracts, it leads at minimum to *nipple inversion/retraction*. Therefore, even if a high incidence of congenital nipple inversion in young girls with recurrent subareolar abscess is common, a more progressive retraction of a previously normal (or already inverted) nipple during the evolution of severe periductal mastitis is commonly observed.

In few cases, fibrosis yields a hard oedematous *chronic mass*, fixed to the skin and with nipple retraction, sometimes with axillary node enlargement. The lesion simulates cancer closely, so that it may be impossible to distinguish the two on mammography, but core needle biopsy will yield the typical macrophages and inflammatory cells with no epithelial cells, so a presumptive diagnosis can be made and a trial of antibiotics given before biopsy. In these cases, the typical large ducts with their pultaceous contents are more likely to be present. A formal duct excision procedure under appropriate antibiotic cover, together with excision of the mass, is usually indicated.

### 9.2.3 Other Nonproliferative Lesions

Other nonproliferative lesions do not usually cause a palpable mass but can cause changes that are seen on cytology of discharge (as papillary apocrine changes) or on mammogram (as calcifications or minimal opacities corresponding to areas of mild hyperplasia).

*Papillary apocrine change* is a proliferation of ductal epithelial cells showing apocrine features, characterised by eosinophilic cytoplasm.

*Epithelial-related calcifications* are benign calcifications that are observed in the breast tissue and can be seen in normal ducts and lobules, stroma or blood vessel walls.

*Mild hyperplasia of the usual type* is an increase in the number of epithelial cells within a duct that is more than two, but not more than four, cells in depth. With five or more cells in depth, the hyperplasia of the usual type is defined as 'moderate'. Mild hyperplasia is associated with no risk of developing cancer, whereas the moderate form shows a slightly increased risk (1.5–2 times). The pattern of epithelial cells is very close to normal.

## 9.3 Proliferative Lesions Without Atypia

**Clinical Practice Points**

- The growth patterns of fibroadenoma and related subtypes may have static or regression phases.
- Biologic behaviour is very constant in hamartomas, while it may change from benign to malignant in phyllodes tumours.
- Papillary lesions of the breast incorporate a large spectrum of benign (solitary papilloma, multiple papillomas, papillomatosis, juvenile papillomatosis) as well as malignant lesions, relatively uncommon and still not well understood.
- In solitary papilloma atypical hyperplasia is less commonly seen, if compared to multiple papillomas.
- Sclerosing lesions can be seen as a component of other proliferative lesions (such as a sclerosing papilloma or a complex fibroadenoma), but also as a component of coexisting both in situ and invasive cancer.

### 9.3.1 Adenosis and Fibrocystic Changes

*ADENOSIS*. The term *adenosis* is used to describe a non-neoplastic lobulocentric proliferation of ductules with epithelial and myoepithelial cells, usually formed from the terminal duct lobular unit. The clinical presentation and microscopic variants are several, but mostly occurring in two forms: as a palpable mass or as a lesion seen only on microscopic examination. These two forms correspond to present terminology of *tumoral adenosis*, used when adenosis takes the form of a palpable or macroscopically recognisable mass, and *simple adenosis*, a microscopic lesion that is most often detected clinically because it contains calcifications seen on mammography.

*Clinical presentation*. Tumoral adenosis is more common in premenopausal women as part of fibrocystic changes. It may present as a mass of medium diameter (2–4 cm), more developed in width, without pathognomonic signs or appearances so that diagnosis is based on exclusion of other similar diseases.

*Imaging*. On mammogram the majority of masses appear as an irregular density, some with a lobulated appearance. Other masses are well circumscribed and some appear as stellate masses. Associated calcifications could be also identified. Ultrasound examination may reveal an oval mass, lobular or irregular. The masses are most likely to be hypoechoic and have posterior acoustic enhancement.

*FIBROCYSTIC CHANGES*. The description of fibrocystic breast changes is confused by the number of different terms (*fibrocystic disease*, *diffuse cystic mastopathy*, *mammary dysplasia* and so on) used to describe various conditions, many of which are similar and many of which are not.

The exact mechanism of this condition is not fully understood, though it is known to be tied to hormone levels, mainly oestrogens. Fibrocystic changes should be

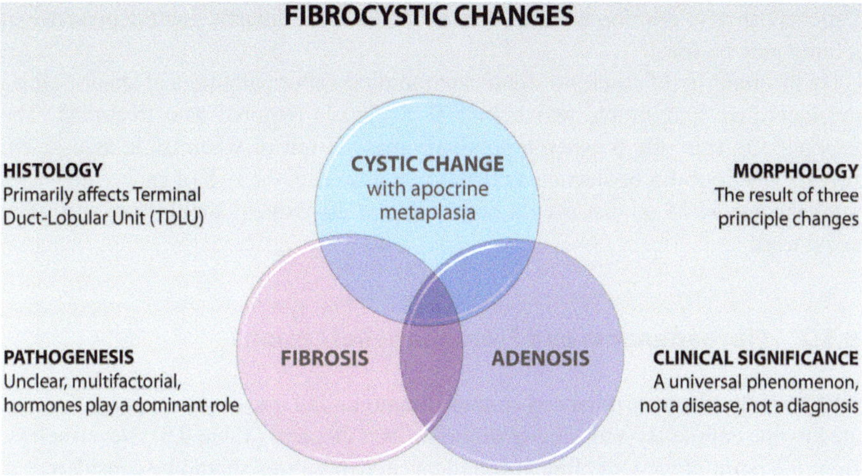


**Fig. 9.4** Main components and characteristics of fibrocystic breast changes

considered a cumulative process, starting from the terminal duct lobular unit (TDLU). Basically the symptoms are the result of the appearance of fibrous tissue, forming nodularity in the texture of the breast, associated with different grades of cystic changes with apocrine metaplasia and areas of adenosis (Fig. 9.4).

Fibrocystic changes are not a disease as such, but instead is a general term that refers to a group of anomalies, symptoms and conditions commonly observed in women of the 30–40-year age group. Main considerations about fibrocystic changes are the following [4]:

- Most women have hormone-related changes in their breasts, so that the term *fibrocystic changes*, rather than disease, should be considered an acceptable medical diagnosis.
- Fibrocystic changes are most common in the late woman's reproductive years but may be observed also in very young or older women.
- Nodularity is mainly localised, but minor features are observed in a scattered pattern.
- Most fibrocystic changes are focal normal variations also in histology.
- Only proliferative epithelial changes with atypia have an associated increased relative risk of cancer.

Broadly speaking, if young women get fibroadenomas as their main benign complaint and premenopausal women get breast cysts as theirs, then the gap in women between 30 and 40 is filled with fibrocystic changes.

Main symptoms of fibrocystic changes are cyclical mastalgia, lumpiness and nodularity. The symptoms may change as the woman moves through different stages of the menstrual cycle. As age progresses, cysts become more frequent.

Patients can also develop areas of such pronounced nodularity that the presence of a lump may be felt.

In the majority of cases, no significant radiological or pathological abnormalities are identified, and simple reassurance is all that is required as a treatment. The exception to this rule is when a dominant mass is felt or when triple assessment reveals any doubtful or suspicious feature. In any case, the risk of cancer increases after the age of 35 so that even a false-negative assessment should to be properly considered.

### 9.3.2 Fibroadenoma and Fibroepithelial Lesions

*OVERVIEW*. Mixed stromal and epithelial tumours fall into several types differentiated by the cellularity and activity of the stromal element (Table 9.5). Nevertheless, from the point of view of clinical significance, two groups should be considered:

- No-risk group: common simple fibroadenoma and less common fibroadenoma-like lesions as adenoma and hamartoma
- Potential risk group: phyllodes tumour, for its changing behaviour of the stroma, and fibroadenoma complex, for its association with other proliferative lesions, sometimes with atypia

*Assessment* of fibroadenomas as of other benign well-circumscribed breast masses in young females could be challenging due to normal glandular variance and density as well as the location (depth and size of the breast). The major diagnostic steps are a detailed history, physical examination and ultrasound. Triple assessment is usually by clinical examination, ultrasound and pathology, with fine needle aspiration (FNA) cytology or core needle biopsy (CNB). Mammogram is indicated in women older than 35 years of age.

*Treatment of fibroadenoma*. Routine excision is no longer appropriate, and most fibroadenomas can be treated conservatively in cases provided the diagnosis is confident and the patient compliant.

Surgery depends on a number of factors. These include the size and the position of the mass, whether or not there is any associated pain or discomfort, the anxiety of the patient and whether there are any unanswered questions from triple assessment.

If a safe diagnosis is established, size of the lump is the main influencing factor. Large fibroadenomas can often be confused with phyllodes tumours, which have a propensity for malignancy. Therefore, even though fibroadenomas are benign, if there is any doubt that the patient may have a phyllodes tumour, excision biopsy should be performed. Tumours over 4–5 cm in diameter can fall into this category, and usually tumours of this size are removed routinely. In the woman with small breasts and a large fibroadenoma, the tumour may be cosmetically unsightly, and therefore excision is required.

**Table 9.5** Classification and behaviour of fibroadenomas classified by their stromal components

| Simple fibroadenoma | Simple fibroadenoma |
|---|---|
| *Low stromal cellularity* | Symptomatically rubbery discrete mass<br>High mobility due to encapsulation and pliability of breast tissue<br>Incidental finding during the first breast imaging<br>In two out of three cases, it does not change in size<br>Juvenile fibroadenoma<br>Rare, characterised by rapid growth, usually seen in adolescent age<br>Giant fibroadenoma<br>So-called when fibroadenoma is larger than 10 cm<br>Pseudoangiomatous stromal hyperplasia (PASH)<br>Stromal proliferation that simulates a vascular lesion<br>Usually does not show progressive growth<br>In most cases core biopsy is accepted as final diagnosis |
| Tubular adenoma | Non-lactating adenoma |
| *Very low stromal cellularity* | Clinically similar to simple fibroadenoma<br>On mammography punctate microcalcification may be visible<br>Lactating adenoma (*mamma lactans*)<br>Occurs in the pregnant or lactating women<br>Often multiple<br>Tends to regress following cessation of breastfeeding |
| Hamartoma | Usually asymptomatic, may be palpable and similar to fibroadenoma |
| *Aggregate of mixed adipose, glandular and fibrous tissue* | On core biopsy is often reported as normal breast tissue |
| Complex fibroadenomas | About 10 % of fibroadenoma in the last decade of reproductive life<br>Contains other proliferative changes so that risk is unpredictable<br>Complete removal is advised |
| Phyllodes tumour | One out of 40 fibroadenomas |
| *High stromal cellularity and mitoses* | Age of onset 15–20 years later than fibroadenoma<br>Can grow fast, sometimes producing marked distortion<br>Classification identifies benign, borderline and malignant ones<br>Recurs in roughly 20 % of patients<br>Preoperative diagnosis avoids inadequate excision |

Fibroadenomas can sometimes be associated with breast pain. This is uncommon, and in most cases pain is not related to the presence of nodule so it may persist also after the removal of the fibroadenoma. The patient should be informed about that possibility.

Patient anxiety is another important factor in determining surgery. Despite reassurance from negative triple assessment, some women are unhappy with the prospect of a lump being left in their breast, and in order to relieve this understandable anxiety, excision can be performed.

*Absolute indications* for surgical removal of fibroadenomas are:

- Diagnosis not so unquestionable
- Progressive growth, since a much larger excision may be required at a later date
- Suspicion of a phyllodes tumour
- Strong desire expressed by the woman

*Relative indications* for surgical removal are:

- Volume as to create aesthetic or psychological problems
- Volume larger than 3–4 cm, but this parameter should be related to breast size and location of the nodule

If surgery is not performed, one of the three things may happen to the fibroadenoma. Firstly, it may simply resolve of its own accord over a period of months or years, but this is an uncommon event and happens in about 10–15 % of cases. Secondly, it may stay the same and remain in the breast for many years in most cases (about 80 % of cases). Finally, it may continue to increase in size in 5–10 % of cases, so that excision is recommended as outlined above.

*SIMPLE FIBROADENOMA* arises from the terminal duct lobular unit, probably as the result of increased sensitivity to oestrogen. The clinical onset may be sudden, but most fibroadenomas do not show further progressive development. The growth phase is followed by a static phase in about 80 %, regression in about 10–15 % and progression.

Simple fibroadenomas are typically smooth, but can be lobulated and feel like many small lumps bundled into one. Their size varies typically from 1 to 3 cm in diameter, but fibroadenomas up to 4 cm in diameter are not uncommon (Fig. 9.2). Solitary fibroadenomas are more common, but in one-third of cases, they are multiple. They are usually highly mobile on examination, so they have earned the description name of *breast mice*. Subsets of simple fibroadenoma are *juvenile fibroadenoma*, *giant fibroadenoma* and *pseudoangiomatous stromal hyperplasia* (*PASH*).

*Juvenile fibroadenomas* are distinguished from adult fibroadenoma by presenting a more glandular component and greater stromal cellularity. They occur in young women between the ages of 10 and 18 and vary in size from 3 to 10 cm or more in diameter (Fig. 9.5). Masses are usually painless, solitary, unilateral and may grow rapidly. Excision is recommended, but in some prepubertal girls there is a risk of damage to the breast bud, and this should be discussed with the patient and family.

*Giant fibroadenomas* refer to histologically typical fibroadenoma over 10 cm in size (5 cm in some nomenclatures). Excision is recommended. The primary challenge for the pathologist is to differentiate these from phyllodes tumours, which have a more cellular stromal component than fibroadenomas.

*Pseudoangiomatous stromal hyperplasia* (*PASH*) is a rare benign stromal proliferation that simulates a vascular lesion. PASH may present as a mass or thickening on physical examination.

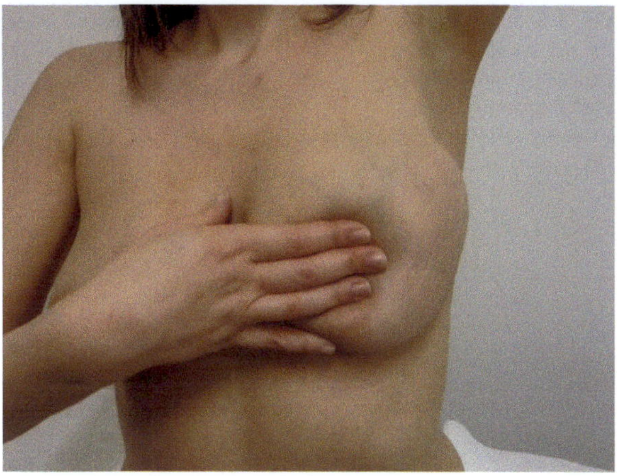

**Fig. 9.5** Very moveable mass in the left breast without skin involvement (histologically, juvenile fibroadenoma)

If there is any suspicious feature on imaging, the diagnosis of PASH on a core biopsy should not be accepted as a final diagnosis and excisional biopsy should be performed. However, in the absence of suspicious imaging characteristics, a diagnosis of PASH at core biopsy is considered sufficient, and surgical excision is not always necessary.

*TUBULAR ADENOMA* is a pure epithelial neoplasm of the breast. It is distinguished from fibroadenoma by its sparse stromal elements. Adenomas are divided into two main groups: non-lactating and lactating adenomas.

*Non-lactating adenoma* is usually solitary with clinical and instrumental features similar to a simple fibroadenoma. Mammogram may show punctate microcalcifications.

*Lactating adenoma* occurs commonly in pregnancy (see Sect. 3.4). Adenomas are often multiple, well circumscribed and lobulated. They tend to regress following cessation of breastfeeding, but sometimes may require excision because of their persistence and size.

*HAMARTOMA*, or *mastoma*, is characterised by an excessive growth of an abnormal mix of normal mammary tissues (see Sect. 3.2). It is encapsulated and can grow quite large, often presenting as a discrete, mobile mass. Hamartomas have varying amounts of glandular, adipose and fibrous tissue. In most cases, the fatty component prevails with embedded epithelial elements, for which it is also defined as *adenolipoma*, *fibroadenolipoma* or *lipofibroadenoma*.

Even if hamartomas can reach massive dimensions, their clinical manifestations are negligible. On mammograms, hamartomas have a distinctive appearance; they are smoothly circumscribed and separated from the surrounding breast by a lucent halo.

If the diagnosis is uncertain or if the patient is bothered by the mass, excision is recommended. If they are asymptomatic and a definitive diagnosis can be made based on mammography and biopsy, plain observation is a safe option.

*Complex fibroadenoma* represents about 10 % of all fibroadenomas and is more frequent in the last decade of reproductive life. It presents as a mass on physical

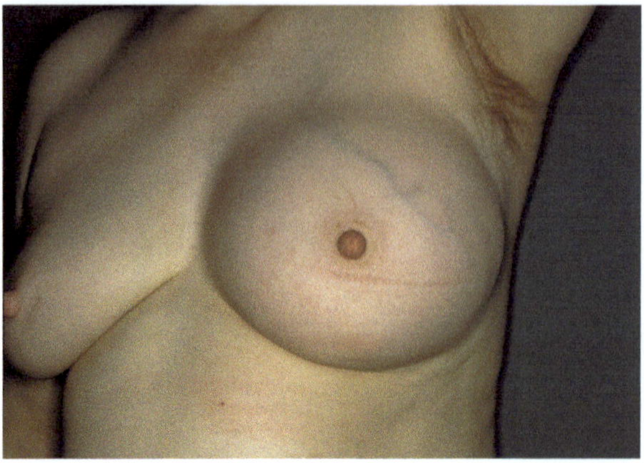

**Fig. 9.6** Enlarging mass in the left breast with skin distension and visible vascular involvement (histologically benign phyllodes tumour)

examination and a circumscribed nodule on mammogram or ultrasound. However, on pathology, complex fibroadenoma may contain other proliferative changes, such as sclerosing adenosis, duct epithelial hyperplasia, epithelial calcification or papillary apocrine changes. For this reason this lesion is associated with a slightly increased risk of cancer when multicentric proliferative changes are present in the surrounding glandular tissue.

Appropriate management of complex fibroadenoma is controversial. Some clinicians warrant its complete removal for histological examination. Others consider the risk of biological interest, but not that much to influence management; they suggest complex fibroadenoma can be managed conservatively, provided that diagnosis is established with a suitable core biopsy.

*PHYLLODES TUMOUR* is a fibroepithelial breast tumour characterised by a diverse range of biologic behaviour, from benign to malignant. In comparison with fibroadenoma, phyllodes tumours are 40 times less common (2.5 %), and the age of onset is 15–20 years later [5].

The typical appearance of phyllodes tumour is a smooth, multinodular, painless bulky breast lump. It is also possible to find phyllodes tumours that are of little/medium size and clinically not different from fibroadenomas. Less commonly, breast mass may grow rapidly causing pressure in the skin, leading also to dilated veins and shiny stretched skin. Anyway, suspicion for a phyllodes tumour should be increased with large tumour size and rapid growth (Fig. 9.6).

*Assessment.* Clinical examination and mammography do not detect phyllodes pathognomonic features. On ultrasound scanning these lesions are a solid, hypoechoic, well-defined bulky mass with some fluid areas inside. The presence of cystic areas within the mass may increase the level of suspicion for phyllodes tumours. FNA is always questionable, not able to make a specific diagnosis. The best procedure for a preoperative diagnosis of phyllodes tumour is yield with a core needle biopsy. If the results are indeterminate, excisional biopsy should be completed. Main clinical features and management of simple fibroadenoma and phyllodes tumour are listed in Table 9.6.

**Table 9.6** Main clinical features and management of simple fibroadenoma and phyllodes tumour

| | Features | Management |
|---|---|---|
| Simple fibroadenoma | Smooth, few lobulated homogeneous mass | An FNA is feasible in young women |
| | Changes cyclically | Local excision or enucleation is sufficient |
| Phyllodes tumour | Like fibroadenoma but usually (not always) larger size and rapid growth | A CB rather than an FNA should be performed |
| | Presence of cystic areas at ultrasound (not always but often) | Excision with a margin of at least 1 cm is highly recommended, mandatory in borderline and malignant subtypes |

*Histologically*, the mass is well circumscribed but lacks a true capsule. The skin is never involved. Leaf-like projections and stromal cellularity differentiate phyllodes from fibroadenoma. The mitotic rate of the stromal component determines whether the phyllodes is benign, borderline or malignant. Approximately 10–20 % of phyllodes tumours are malignant, although this figure varies significantly depending on the series.

Histologic distinction between benign and malignant phyllodes may be very difficult at times, and therefore there is thence the definition of *borderline* phyllodes tumour. The most commonly accepted criteria used for classification of benign versus malignant tumours are degree of stromal cellular atypia, mitotic activity, infiltrative as compared to circumscribed tumour margins and presence or absence of pure stroma devoid of epithelium. Ki 67 and p53 are predictors of malignant phyllodes.

*Treatment.* Incidental finding of phyllodes tumour after removal of a fibroadenoma can occur; if established as benign tumour, a wider excision of margins can be avoided and close follow-up planned.

A wide resection is mandatory for malignant and borderline phyllodes tumours with a margin of at least 1 cm of healthy tissue. Enucleation and/or local excision alone has inacceptable recurrence rates, reported in about 20 % of cases. Phyllodes tumours are not multicentric, since there is no biologic rationale for routine mastectomy, which can be reserved for cases where breast conservation cannot be achieved with an acceptable cosmetic result. Features and treatment of malignant phyllodes tumours are discussed in Sect. 14.4.

### 9.3.3 Papilloma and Benign Papillary Lesions

Papillary lesions of the breast include a variety of lesions that are characterised by a papillary configuration on gross or microscopic examination or both. Typically papillary lesions occur in women in their late reproductive or postmenopausal years (with an average age at presentation of 48 years). Papillary lesions are relatively uncommon and still not well understood. Even though benign papillomas are mostly safe, the likelihood of a future BC (papillary DCIS and invasive papillary carcinoma) is correlated with the presence and degree of atypia (see Sect. 10.2).

**Table 9.7** Classification and behaviour of intraductal papillomas classified by their proliferative epithelial components

| Solitary intraductal papilloma | Occurs in a large duct within 5 cm from the nipple |
|---|---|
| | Can be palpated in one-third of patients |
| *Hyperplasia of the major duct epithelium with a papillary configuration* | Bloody discharge is observed in half of cases and serous discharge in the other half |
| | Because of its thin stalk, it has the potential to tort completely leading to self-destruction (rarely) |
| | *Sclerosing papilloma* is a histological subtype with a dominant sclerosing architecture |
| | *Intracystic* (or *encysted*) *papilloma* is a clinical subtype where papilloma is encysted in a much enlarged duct or a giant cyst |
| | *Nipple adenoma* is a rather distinctive clinical (restricted to nipple) and histologic (also called *florid papillomatosis* or *erosive adenomatosis*) variant |
| Multiple intraductal papillomas | Many, at least five, intraductal papillomas in an area within a localised segment of the breast, usually in a peripheral location |
| *Hyperplasia of terminal ductulo-lobular units – atypias are more frequently seen* | Often palpable whereas nipple discharge is rare |
| | Occurs at a younger age than solitary papilloma |
| | Associated with an increased risk of malignancy if areas of atypical hyperplasia are found |
| | In some reports multiple papillomas are improperly named papillomatosis |
| Juvenile papillomatosis (Swiss cheese disease) | A very rare condition occurring in young women <30 years old (mean age 23) |
| *Atypical hyperplasia and multiple lesions are usually associated* | Usually a painless, mobile mass, similar to fibroadenoma |
| | High risk of cancer, found in about 4 % of patients |

Types of papilloma are *solitary papilloma*, *multiple intraductal papilloma* and *juvenile papillomatosis*. It is worth to remember that the histological classification of multiple papillomas should not include papillomatosis, small areas of cell growth not as focused as with papilloma (see above in nonproliferative lesions). In some pathological reports the description is still controversial also because similar or identical lesions have been classified using different terms, including epitheliosis or epithelial hyperplasia.

Classification and behaviour of intraductal papillomas classified by their proliferative epithelial components are listed in Table 9.7.

*SOLITARY PAPILLOMA* (or *central* papilloma) appears to be formed from hyperplasia of the duct epithelium supported by a fibrovascular core and that results in a pedunculated, single, friable tumour within the duct. Solitary papilloma is not thought to be a premalignant lesion and is considered by some to be an aberration rather than a true disease process.

Solitary papilloma is most frequently observed in women 30–50 years old. It grows to about 1 cm in size, dilating the duct, and the friable epithelium often bleeds, causing a spontaneous bloody nipple discharge. Sometimes a small palpable mass can be felt near the nipple, and gentle pressure on it causes a clear or bloody nipple discharge, easily to recognise especially when it comes from only one breast. Solitary papilloma is primarily located in one duct, usually one major duct beneath or next to the nipple (Fig. 9.4), but more single papillomas can be found more distant, even in both breasts. In rare cases solitary papilloma twists on its stalk causing severe ischaemia and necrosis, leading to the self-destruction with disappearance of the symptoms.

On galactography (or ductoscopy), most detectable solitary intraductal papillomas are often present in the subareolar region, within 1 cm from the nipple in 90 % of cases. They are few millimetres in size and appear as broad-based or pedunculated polypoid epithelial lesions that may obstruct and distend the involved duct. They may cause cysts by obstructing the duct.

With ultrasound, papillomas may be seen as a well-defined, smooth-walled, solid, hypoechoic mass or a lobulated, smooth-walled, cystic lesion with some solid components. A dilated duct can be frequently visible sonographically.

*Sclerosing papilloma* is a histological subtype of solitary intraductal papilloma. It is so termed when a papillary lesion forms a well-defined solid mass with dominant sclerosing architecture. It is usually a histological diagnosis and usually cannot be differentiated from a non-sclerosing papilloma on breast imaging.

*Intracystic papilloma* is a clinical subtype. Generally, the intracystic papilloma is the result of a very enlarged duct, so that this condition is better defined as *encysted* papilloma. Only in few cases papilloma is encysted in a large cyst (Fig. 9.4). Diagnosis is based on ultrasound, which shows a solid component within a cyst, or on observation that, in spite of many aspirations of the cyst fluid, its size does not change.

*Nipple adenoma* is an unusual variant of intraductal papilloma, a rather distinctive benign proliferative lesion restricted to the nipple (Fig. 9.7), largely discussed in Sect. 11.1.2.

*MULTIPLE PAPILLOMAS* are located in the periphery of the breast and are associated with the terminal duct lobular units (Fig. 9.7). They are usually multiple and present clinically as a palpable mass, but may also be clinically occult, detected as an abnormal density on breast imaging. These tumours are less likely to cause nipple discharge, on the contrary of solitary papilloma.

For the patient who presents with clinical symptoms, ultrasound can often demonstrate the lesion, as well as the dilated duct. In the presence of nipple discharge, galactography or ductoscopy may demonstrate, but only in an approximate way, the extension of the filling defect within the ductal system [6].

Compared to solitary papillomas, multiple papillomas are five- to eightfold less common. They tend to occur in younger patients and are less often associated with nipple discharge, more frequently peripheral and occasionally bilateral. Many clinical records report that peripheral papillomas, unlike solitary central papillomas, may be highly susceptible to malignant transformation.

*Diffuse papillomatosis* should be detached by multiple papillomas. Papillomatosis is a term used to describe microscopic foci of intraductal hyperplasia that have papillary architecture and therefore included among proliferative lesions without atypia.

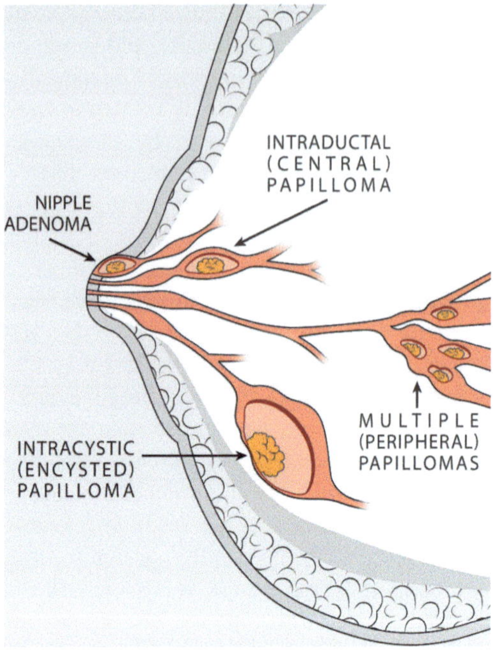


**Fig. 9.7** Main benign intraductal proliferative lesions of the breast: nipple adenoma, intraductal (central) papilloma, multiple (peripheral) papillomas and intracystic/encysted papilloma

Actually in this type of hyperplasia, there are very small areas of cell growth within the ducts, but not as focused as in papillomas. In addition, the histological classification of multiple papillomas /papillomatosis is somewhat controversial because similar or identical lesions have been classified using different terms such as *epitheliosis* and *epithelial hyperplasia*.

*JUVENILE PAPILLOMATOSIS* (or *Swiss cheese disease*) is a very rare condition, which, as the name implies, is mainly seen in young women (mean age between 19 and 23 years) and is unusual in women over 30 years old. Patients present with a firm, circumscribed, painless and mobile mass often in the periphery of the breast, most often thought to be a fibroadenoma. There is usually no nipple discharge.

Juvenile papillomatosis is a papillary proliferation of the ductal epithelium, which partly fills up smaller ducts and distends them to a degree. Gross pathology often shows a well-circumscribed mass containing multiple small cysts (<2 cm) within a dense fibrous stroma, therefore sometimes termed *Swiss cheese disease* by pathologists. Lesions can vary in size, usually ranging from 1 to 8 cm.

Juvenile papillomatosis is usually negative on mammography, albeit occasionally mammograms may show pleomorphic or amorphous microcalcifications, an asymmetric density or a prominent intraductal pattern. At ultrasound it can appear as an ill-defined, uneven hypoechoic mass with multiple small predominantly peripheral cysts. Galactography, when feasible, may show multiple irregular filling defects within the breasts.

Follow-up studies have suggested that juvenile papillomatosis should be considered a marker for familiar BC, being associated with an increased risk of BC in the patient's female relatives. The patient herself may be at increased risk (approximately 10 % in lifetime) for developing carcinoma, particularly if the lesion is bilateral and there is a family history of BC.

*TREATMENT* of papillary lesions is unquestionably surgical. When associated to nipple discharge, these lesions are usually small and mildly symptomatic, so that appropriate operations are planned, as microductectomy or retro-areolar major duct resection or duct-lobular segmentectomy (see Sect. 10.2). However, when a mass is detectable, main concerns are related to differential diagnosis with papillary carcinoma, especially in postmenopausal women [7].

*Differential diagnosis with malignant papillary lesions.* There is an overlap in the clinical and imaging patterns of benign papilloma and malignant papillary lesions, so that a thorough assessment is needed.

Papillary carcinoma of the breast is common in women with the mean age of approximately 65 years old; therefore, any circumscribed mass in a patient over 60 years old, especially if retro- or subareolar, should be considered suspicious.

Papillary carcinoma may manifest clinically as a palpable mass or nipple discharge, with the latter present in 20–35 % of patients. As benign papillomas, papillary carcinomas may be solitary or multiple, central (retro-areolar) or peripheral in almost the same ratio. As for benign papilloma, papillary carcinomas are usually well circumscribed and often contain haemorrhagic and cystic areas.

Imaging assessment may result as indistinct or controversial. The most common mammographic pattern (a round, oval or lobulated mass) is similar in benign papilloma and invasive papillary carcinoma. The mass margins are usually circumscribed but may be obscured or indistinct. Accompanying microcalcifications or a dilated ductal pattern may also be present. At mammography, like intraductal papillomas, papillary carcinomas may be evident as ductal obstructions, filling defects, or focal or diffuse ductal wall irregularities.

Also ultrasound shows minimal dissimilarities between papilloma and papillary carcinoma: a hypoechoic and solid mass, often with posterior acoustic enhancement, or otherwise complex cystic and solid masses may be evident. As they are relatively vascular, there are often colour flow components on Doppler investigation.

An intracystic papillary carcinoma, as well an intracystic papilloma, usually appears on MRI as a round or oval mass with well-defined margins. The internal composition is typically heterogeneous, with multiple nodular masses of intermediate signal intensity projecting from the periphery into the lumen.

In such circumstances, diagnosis in older women is rather uncertain until histological sections. Besides typical benign lesions, when the epithelium has diagnostic features of intraductal carcinoma, the lesion is classified as *papillary ductal carcinoma in situ*. If a cystic component is present, the lesion is described as an *intracystic papillary carcinoma*. In the absence of an appreciable cyst, a diagnosis of *solid papillary carcinoma* is appropriate. Invasive elements arising in a papillary carcinoma are almost always detected at the periphery of the lesion.

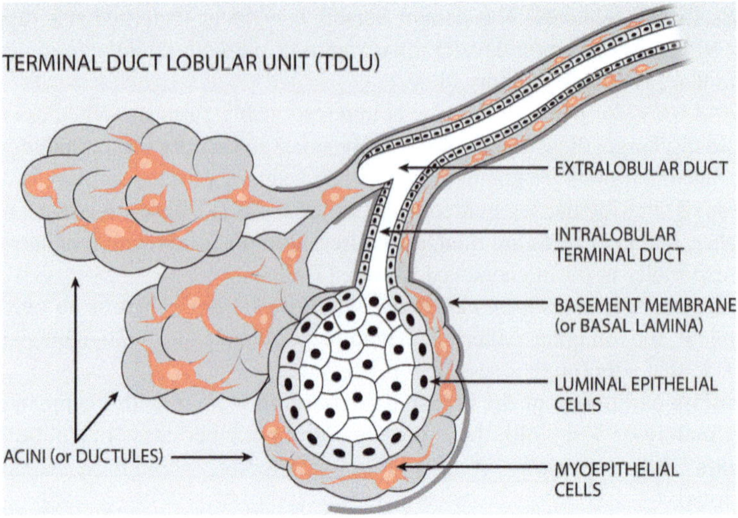


**Fig. 9.8** Tridimensional drawing of terminal ductal lobular units (TDLUs). Each TDLU is lined by two epithelial cell types, inner luminal secretory cells and outer contractile myoepithelial cells. Basement membrane is only partially represented

### 9.3.4 Myoepithelial Lesions of the Breast

Myoepithelial cells are known to be components of both benign and malignant tumours of mammary as well as sweat and salivary gland origin. Tumours containing glandular elements are called *adenomyoepitheliomas*, while pure myoepithelial cell tumours are called *myoepitheliomas*.

*ADENOMYOEPITHELIOMA* has a biphasic cytoarchitecture composed of tubular structures lined by duct luminal epithelial cells, surrounded by myoepithelial cells that have spindle or polygonal shapes (Fig. 9.8). Epithelial/myoepithelial proliferation begins as intraductal proliferation and develops along several lines: the myoepithelial cells may predominate, necrosis may be present and epithelial proliferation may include regions of papillary proliferation, including apocrine metaplasia. It can be said that adenomyoepithelioma and intraductal papilloma represent opposite ends of a spectrum of intraductal proliferations of the breast.

Histologic, ultrastructural and immunohistochemical features of benign adenomyoepithelioma overlap with those of metaplastic breast carcinoma, and sometimes the distinctions between these entities are poorly defined, arbitrary and not likely reproducible. Increased mitoses, marked atypia and spindle cell overgrowth are hallmarks of malignant transformation, while all lack in benign lesions. Malignant transformation may involve epithelial cell, myoepithelial cells or both.

*Clinical presentation.* Adenomyoepitheliomas present as a circumscribed breast mass (on average 2–3 cm) in the same age range as for patients with BC. Masses are firm to rubbery, generally circumscribed, but can grossly mimic carcinoma. The lesions may be palpable depending on size and location. Occasionally, they are seen as small opacities on mammographic imaging. The majority of adenomyoepitheliomas have been considered benign and appropriate therapy is local excision with a rim of uninvolved breast. After excision, however, they can recur locally.

*MYOFIBROBLASTOMA* of the breast, a tumour showing myofibroblastic differentiation without epithelial features, simulates spindle cell adenomyoepithelioma and other spindle tumours of the breast.

*Clinical Imaging*. Myofibroblastoma has a predilection for occurring in men, but it is a benign tumour in either sex. Like adenomyoepithelioma, it presents as a circumscribed mass, which may be palpable (especially in men) depending on size and location. Occasionally, it is seen as mass on mammographic imaging. Local excision with a rim of uninvolved breast is indicated.

*PLEOMORPHIC ADENOMA* of the breast is a benign tumour characterised by an admixture of epithelial and myoepithelial cells embedded in abundant myxomatous stroma. It occurs rarely and closely resembles its counterparts in the salivary glands and skin, where it is also known as *chondroid syringoma*. Other authors consider pleomorphic adenomas of the breast to be variants of intraductal papilloma with myxomatous osteocartilaginous stromal metaplasia. Recognition of pleomorphic adenoma in the breast is important because it can be overdiagnosed as malignant and result in inappropriate surgery.

*Clinical Presentation*. Pleomorphic adenomas of the breast occur in broad age range, with most tumours ranging from 1 to 5 cm (mean, 2 cm). Although pleomorphic adenomas can occur anywhere within the breast, they have a predilection to develop near the areola. Most are well circumscribed but can show multifocal growth or satellite lesions.

Appropriate therapy is local excision with a rim of the uninvolved breast. Pleomorphic adenomas of breast show little tendency to recur and even lesser tendency to metastasise.

### 9.3.5 Sclerosing Lesions

*SCLEROSING ADENOSIS* is a type of adenosis, a spectrum of benign alterations of breast tissue, which retains an exaggerated lobular architecture. In more detail, sclerosing adenosis is a distortion of epithelial, myoepithelial and stromal elements arising in a terminal duct lobular unit.

Prominent myoepithelial differentiation is most commonly encountered in sclerosing adenosis. It is also observed as a component of other proliferative lesions (such as intraductal and/or sclerosing papilloma, complex fibroadenoma) and can coexist with both in situ and invasive cancers.

*Clinical presentation*. In most cases, sclerosing adenosis is detected during routine mammograms or following breast surgery. On mammography, sclerosing adenosis may consist of architectural distortion, indeterminate microcalcifications (present in about the half of cases) or both. At times, a mass lesion or asymmetrical density may be present. It can be therefore very difficult to mammographically distinguish sclerosing adenosis from an infiltrating BC.

Sclerosing adenosis can appear as focal or diffuse. A clinically definite lump is palpable in 20 % of the cases, and it might cause skin retraction. In many cases women experience recurring pain that tends to be linked to the menstrual cycle. In few cases multiple small, firm, tender lumps as well as extensive fibrous tissue and sometimes small cysts (simple or complex) are found in the breast.

For sclerosing adenosis, if the mass is circumscribed or indistinctly marginated and the core biopsy clearly confirms the diagnosis, it may be reasonable to wait and see because the relative risk is low (RR = 1.5–2). However, if the spiculated mass is enlarging on short-term follow-up mammogram, or if there are fine linear or branching calcifications in a segmental or linear distribution, excision is mandatory.

*RADIAL SCAR* is a benign hyperplastic proliferative disease of the breast. Lesions smaller than 10 mm are referred to as *radial scar* and those larger than 10 mm, or with several fibro-elastotic areas in close contiguity, as *complex sclerosing lesions*.

Radial scar more commonly presents as a radiological finding, usually small and detected by mammography when reach at least 5 mm in size. Reported prevalence is in about 3–9 per 1,000 screening mammograms and 4–8 % in population-based pathology databases.

*Clinical presentation*. Radiologically a radial scar has a spiculated density similar to cancer, typically seen in one view only, but the centre tends to be a translucent, low-density area rather than a mass. The breast tissue behind the lesion is almost visible through the lesion. The relative low density of the centre is an important and visible difference between carcinoma and a radial scar. With the radial scar there is no dense centre, as in the cancer, and in fact, the lesion is usually as dense centrally as peripherally without an attempt at forming a mass. Microcalcifications are possible but rare. Ultrasound may show irregular, hypoechoic mass with acoustic shadowing.

Proposed possible causes include localised inflammatory reaction and/or chronic ischaemia with subsequent slow infarction. Pathology of radial scars displays hyperplastic tissue cells and a central fibrous core, with radial extension of tubular structures (the spiculated peripheral borders), mimicking infiltrating carcinoma. These tubular formations have two rows of cells, epithelial and myoepithelial.

In approximately 30 % of cases, a radial scar is associated with either ductal carcinoma in situ or tubular carcinoma. The occurrence is higher when there is associated atypia on histology. Other associations include atypical ductal or lobular hyperplasia.

Radial scar is very rare in women younger than 40 years old or older than 60. Clinical examination is often normal, although in about 25 % of cases radial scars can be palpable without any skin thickening or retraction.

*Treatment*. When radial scars are found on core biopsy, surgical excision is needed. In addition to the possibility of finding an unrecognised in situ or invasive cancer in about one-third of cases, radial scars without atypia have a slight relative risk (RR = 2–3), while with atypia the RR = 6, which increases to 8 if the lesions are greater than 5 mm. However, there is no clear evidence that these are premalignant lesions.

No additional treatment beyond excision is needed for radial scars. Although the presence of these lesions does increase the risk of BC, in the absence of atypia, the magnitude of this risk does not justify risk-reduction measures. Only in the presence of large lesions with atypia, the patient should be referred for counselling and consideration of chemoprevention. A comparison between sclerosing adenosis and radial scar is outlined in Table 9.8.

**Table 9.8** Comparisons between sclerosing adenosis and radial scar

| *Sclerosing adenosis* | *Radial scar* |
|---|---|
| Nodularity often painful | Only a mammographic finding |
| Definite lump in 20 % of cases | Clinically non-symptomatic |
| Compact density on mammography | Radiological findings are critically suspicious |
| Relative risk low (RR = 1.5–2) | Relative risk varies from 3 to 8 |
| Surgery indicated only if symptomatic and/or associated to atypical hyperplasia | Surgery always indicated for its frequent histological association to pre-invasive or invasive BC |
| *Common features* | |
| Are the same ANDI process characterised by overproliferation of the TDLUs? | |
| Core needle biopsy (not FNA) is always indicated | |
| Histologically may be difficult to distinguish from malignancy | |
| Even if more rarely in sclerosing adenosis, both lesions may be involved by atypical hyperplasia, LCIS or even | |
| DCIS or invasive cancer | |
| The likelihood of coexisting pathology (hyperplasia, non-invasive or invasive carcinoma) is related to the size of the lesion and the age of the patient | |

### 9.3.6 Other Lesions

*COLUMNAR CELL LESIONS (CCLs)* are a spectrum of lesions characterised by architectural and cytological alterations of the terminal duct of lobular units which become irregular or mildly dilated and lined by a layer of epithelium with apical snouts. The lesions are usually detected mammographically due to the presence of microcalcifications but are also frequently present in biopsies sampled for investigation for other breast lesions, benign or malignant.

CCLs have been reported in the literature under different names, but there is now an acceptable unifying terminology: columnar cell change, columnar cell change with hyperplasia, columnar cell change with atypia and columnar cell hyperplasia with atypia.

Columnar cell change and columnar cell change with hyperplasia are within the framework of proliferations without atypia and should be classified as B2 lesions in the same category as fibrocystic change.

Columnar cell change with atypia and columnar cell hyperplasia with atypia may have an advanced end of the spectrum till DCIS and are included within the framework of proliferations with atypia, collectively classified as flat epithelial atypia (FEA) by the WHO classification 2003 (see Sect. 9.4.2). When there is prominent architectural alteration, the designation of columnar change lesion – atypical ductal hyperplasia (CCL-ADH) should be applied.

The biological significance of columnar cell lesions is still evolving, and further information is required on long-term follow-up of these lesions. For the management, see Sect. 9.6 at the end of this chapter.

*MUCOCELE-LIKE LESIONS (MLL)* consist of duct-lobular units that are dilated and distended with mucin, which extravasates into the surrounding stroma. An MLL is frequently detected mammographically as indeterminate microcalcifications or a mass lesion which will lead to a needle core biopsy. Like the columnar cell lesion, the MLL is histologically heterogeneous. The histological features of an MLL in a needle core biopsy include mucin-filled ducts lined by benign epithelium, extravasated mucin containing benign epithelium or extravasated mucin without epithelium. Studies on screen-detected MLLs which were excised following CNB diagnosis report the association of MLL with ADH, DCIS and mucinous carcinoma, so that there is a general consensus to recommend excisional biopsy when a diagnosis of MLL is made on core biopsy.

*MICROGLANDULAR ADENOSIS* is a rare lesion of haphazardly infiltrating, small, uniform, rounded, open glands with eosinophilic secretions. It can be diagnosed only on excision biopsy. Furthermore, there is some evidence that microglandular adenosis may be a precursor for BC with atypical microglandular adenosis as an intermediate lesion. As a CNB only samples a fraction of the lesion, definitive diagnosis can be achieved only with an excisional biopsy.

## 9.4 Proliferative Lesions with Atypia

**Clinical Practice Points**

- Proliferative lesions with atypia are generally uncommon pathological findings considered both as a non-obligate precursor of invasive BC and a marker of increased risk. In fact, cancers that subsequently develop may occur anywhere in the breasts, not necessarily at the site of the atypia.
- Proliferative lesions with atypia identified by a core needle biopsy should have a wide excision as an attempt to identify a concomitant malignancy.
- For patients with a proliferative breast lesion with atypia identified by an excisional biopsy, no further resection of the lesion is indicated. A wider excision may be recommended when there is a radiologic-pathologic discordance and when the diagnosis indicates a less common histologic variant as pleomorphic LCIS.
- AHs are associated with a relative risk of BC four- to sixfold greater than the general population. A diagnosis of LCIS confers a long-term cumulative risk of a subsequent BC that averages 1–2 % per year and remains steady over time, resulting in relative risk of BC that is eight- to tenfold greater than the general population risk.
- Patients with AH and LCIS should be informed of their increased risk of BC and counselled regarding both medical and surgical risk-reducing options.

Proliferative lesions with atypia include atypical ductal hyperplasia (ADH), atypical lobular hyperplasia (ALH), flat epithelial atypia (FEA) and lobular carcinoma in situ (LCIS). These lesions are considered high risk because they are associated with an increase in the patient's future risk of developing BC. They are generally not considered premalignant lesions, as the cancers that subsequently develop may occur anywhere in the breasts, not necessarily at the site of the atypia [8]. Therefore, when these high-risk lesions are discovered, the focus should be on careful surveillance and consideration of risk-reduction strategies.

### 9.4.1 Atypical Hyperplasias

Atypical hyperplasias (AHs) are more a pathologic diagnosis than a clinical entity. They are usually discovered as an incidental finding on biopsy of mammographic abnormalities or breast masses. These lesions have some, but not all, of the features of ductal carcinoma in situ (DCIS) or lobular carcinoma in situ (LCIS).

*Atypical ductal hyperplasia* (*ADH*) is characterised by a proliferation of uniform epithelial cells with monomorphic round nuclei filling part but not the entire involved duct. ADH shares some of the cytological and architectural features of low-grade ductal carcinoma in situ (DCIS).

*Atypical lobular hyperplasia* (*ALH*) is characterised by monomorphic, evenly spaced, dyshesive cells filling part, but not all, of the involved lobule. ALH can also involve ducts. ALH shares some of the cytological and architectural features of lobular carcinoma in situ (LCIS).

Atypical hyperplasias (ADH and ALH), especially in multifocal lesions, confer a substantial increase in the risk (RR=4–6) of subsequent both ipsilateral and contralateral BC. AHs provide evidence of underlying breast abnormalities that predispose to BC this high-risk group. The cumulative incidence of BC along a period of 30 years approaches 35 %.

Some studies have shown that the risk of developing BC is higher with ALH than ADH; however, the data are disputed. There is a higher risk of subsequent BC when the ALH involves both lobules and ducts (RR ~ 6) as compared to lobules alone (RR ~ 4) or ducts alone (RR=2).

Data on the effect of family history of BC in women with atypical hyperplasia are conflicting. Some past studies showed that a family history of BC substantially increased the BC risk in women with AHs. However, subsequent studies have not confirmed this and did not show that a family history further increased the BC risk in women with AHs.

### 9.4.2 Flat Epithelial Atypia

Flat epithelial atypia (FEA), sometimes referred to as *columnar cell hyperplasia with atypia*, is a separate entity from ADH or ALH. Typically, flat epithelial atypia is diagnosed on breast biopsies done for calcifications found on screening mammograms. The relationship between flat epithelial atypia and cancer is still being defined, but the available data suggest that the risk of local recurrence or progression to invasive cancer is low.

### 9.4.3 Lobular Carcinoma In Situ

Lobular carcinoma in situ (LCIS) is a non-invasive lesion that arises from the lobules and terminal ducts of the breast (see Sect. 12.2). It almost always represents an incidental finding that is diagnosed on a breast biopsy that is performed for some other reason, such as an area of fibrocystic change or a fibroadenoma. In most instances, LCIS is not identified clinically, mammographically or by gross pathologic examination. Like AHs, LCIS is currently managed as an indicator lesion for the subsequent risk of developing invasive ductal or lobular carcinoma. The subsequent risk is conferred on both ipsilateral and contralateral breasts.

Some researchers, with the term *lobular neoplasia*, refer to a spectrum of proliferative changes within the breast lobule that includes both atypical lobular hyperplasia (ALH) and LCIS. Although both are associated with an increased risk of invasive BC, the magnitude of risk with LCIS is much greater than with ALH. Because of this difference and the implications for treatment, most experts continue to separate the two entities rather than using the all-encompassing term lobular neoplasia.

In the same way, pleomorphic lobular carcinoma in situ (LIN3, see Sect. 12.2) should be considered a distinctive entity. Because of its unpredictable and aggressive behaviour, it should be managed as a pre-invasive rather than a high-risk lesion.

### 9.4.4 Workup of Proliferative Lesions with Atypia

Classification, features and management of proliferative lesions with atypia are listed in Table 9.9.

**Table 9.9** Classification, features and management of proliferative lesions with atypia

| | Features | Management |
|---|---|---|
| Atypical hyperplasias (AHs):<br>Atypical ductal hyperplasia (ADH)<br>Atypical lobular hyperplasia (ALH) | AH shares some cytological and architectural feature of low-grade DCIS (LCIS)<br>Mostly diagnosed with CNB | If identified by CNB or incisional biopsy → wide excision<br>If identified by an excisional biopsy → no further resection recommended<br>Close surveillance or counselling may be indicated in women with family history of BC |
| Flat epithelial atypia (FEA) | FEA is less characterised in terms of future risk | |
| Lobular carcinoma in situ (LCIS) | Pleomorphic LCIS, for its uncertain behaviour, should be considered at distinctive risk (see Sect. 12.2) | |

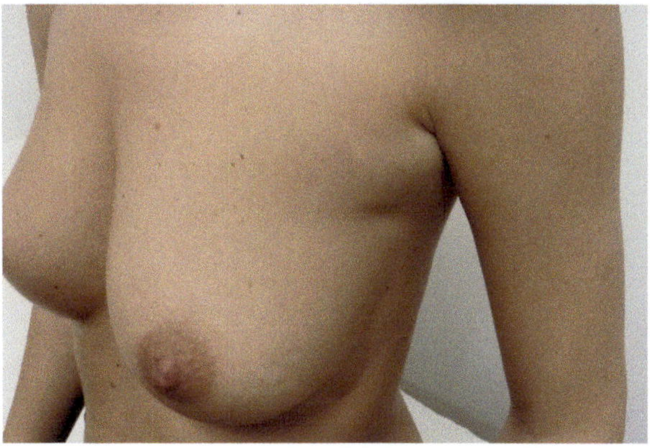

**Fig. 9.9** Mass in the left axilla (lipomatosis, even in the presence of a supernumerary gland, should be ruled out)

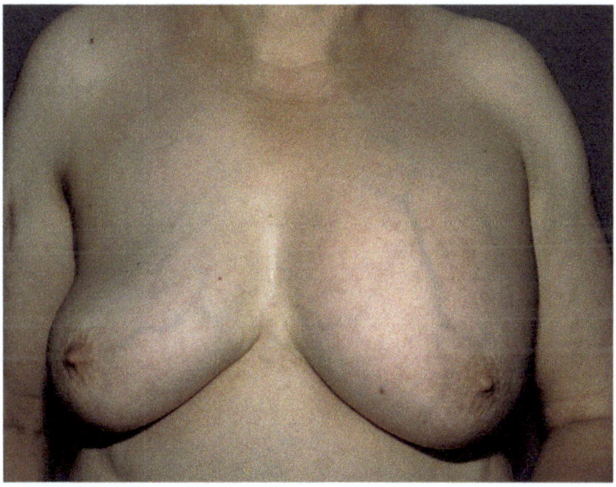

**Fig. 9.10** Enlarging mass in the left breast without skin involvement. Assessment showed a diffuse overgrowth of mature adipose tissue

If the core needle biopsy (CNB) identifies a proliferative lesion with atypia, papilloma, a surgical excision should be performed mainly to avoid underestimation of the diagnosis. Based upon retrospective reviews, analysis of a larger tissue sample removed by a surgical excision results in an upgrade in diagnosis from atypia to ductal carcinoma in situ (DCIS) or invasive BC in 10–30 % of patients.

For patients with a high-risk proliferative breast lesion identified by an excisional biopsy with negative margins, no further resection of the lesion is indicated. The excision should be wider for patients with pleomorphic LCIS (a pre-invasive lesion), for more local control (see Sect. 12.2), even if the increase of the risk is referred to subsequent both ipsilateral and contralateral BC.

In all cases, women with atypical hyperplasia should be closely monitored and counselled regarding risk-reduction strategies, especially in the presence of family history of BC.

## 9.5 Miscellaneous Benign Lesions

**Clinical Practice Points**

- Fat necrosis is becoming increasingly common with greater incidence of breast-conserving surgery and mammoplasty procedures, including lipofilling.
- Lipoma of the breast is easily documented on mammography by its very clear appearance. Core needle biopsy is less helpful since it shows normal fat cells, so it is unclear whether or not the examiner misses the mass.
- In some cases trauma with haematoma may alert a patient to the presence of a mass that was there before the event.

Note that some unusual lesions as galactocele (subset of cyst), hamartoma and pseudoangiomatous stromal hyperplasia (subsets of fibroadenoma) in most classifications are included among miscellaneous benign breast lesions. In regard of their aetiology, it is preferable to locate them in their proper sets.

*SARCOIDOSIS*. Breast symptomatology in sarcoidosis is rare and seen primarily in patients with systemic involvement. Sarcoidosis of the breast presents as firm hard masses, mimicking carcinoma. The mammographic appearance is also suspicious with irregular, ill-defined, spiculated masses that are solid on ultrasound. Core needle or excisional biopsy is needed for confirmation of diagnosis. There is no increased risk of subsequent BC associated with sarcoidosis of the breast.

*FIBROMATOSIS*. Fibromatosis is a manifestation of the dermoid tumour, which is an abnormal proliferation of mesenchymal tissue. It is relatively frequent in the breast following a trauma or an injury to the chest wall or shoulder. Clinically, the lesion in the breast tissue gives a greatly increased consistency and is presented with irregular margins. Histologically the same morphology of similar lesions of other districts is observed: a fibroblast proliferation of infiltrative nature, absence of capsule and high tendency to local recurrence.

*AMYLOIDOSIS*. It is very rare and occurs in association with amyloidosis of other organs and sometimes even systemic diseases such as rheumatoid arthritis. Amyloid deposition occurs around ducts, blood vessels and in the stroma, causing an inflammatory reaction including giant cells, lymphocytes and plasma cells.

*LIPOMA*. Breast lipoma is a benign, usually solitary tumour composed of mature fat which presents as a soft or semifirm, well-marginated indolent masses (Fig. 9.9) that may feel either smooth or lobulated. Patterns of lipoma may occur in a large variety of clinical settings from well-defined nodule to lipomatosis (Fig. 9.10). Because of their clinical softness, it is not difficult to distinguish lipomas from other conditions.

Lipomas may occur anywhere on the body, including the breast. The typical physical findings strongly support the diagnosis, especially if the mass has been present for a considerable time or other similar masses are present elsewhere in the breast or rest of the body.

They can be multiple and/or bilateral, usually well encapsulated and must be distinguished from subcutaneous fat of the breast region or also from subcutaneous panniculitis, usually ill shaped and bruising with overlying rosy and thicker skin.

Generally lipomas persist unchanged for a long time or have a very slow growth, sometimes as to deform the breast profile. In instrumental assessment, lipoma is typically recognisable as a very clear image on mammography. Ultrasound appears to be a solid ipoechogenic area with well-defined margins in the absence of a true capsule.

Evenly, core needle biopsy is not usually helpful because the mass provides little resistance to the needle, making it difficult to be sure the biopsy came from the mass. The cytology shows normal fat cells, so for the pathologist it is unclear whether this was a lipoma or the examiner missed the mass.

Histologically lipoma is composed of mature fat. A lipoma that contains ductal structures is defined as *adenolipoma*; since it is a normal epithelium trapped in the adipose tissue, this lesion may be due to an embryonic modification, as a hamartoma (see above). Other variants are the *angiolipoma*, in which there is a vascular component with capillary structures, and the *chondrolipoma*, which consists of adipose tissue and lobules of mature cartilage.

Excision is recommended only in cases in which the dimensions are such as to deform the profile of the breast or if the patient is bothered by its presence. Lipomas are usually well circumscribed and pliable so that they can be easily excised through a small incision. However, incomplete excision can be associated with recurrence.

*FAT NECROSIS*. Fat necrosis (or *steatonecrosis*) of the breast is a benign condition that most commonly occurs as a secondary symptom of various causes, the most recognisable of which are trauma or previous surgery. It above all occurs in voluminous and adipose breasts, especially in older women when sometimes, curiously enough, trauma may go unnoticed. Aside from accidental trauma (direct or indirect as those caused by seat belts) with formation of a little haematoma, even iatrogenic, surgical (plastic surgery and lipofilling) or instrumental causes (core needle biopsy, but also mammography) should be considered.

The cases in which an obvious cause could not be recognised are rare; as such fat necrosis is defined as, although with some doubts, *idiopathic*. In some cases it could represent an event secondary to rupture of dilated ducts or cysts, which may lead to necrosis of the surrounding fatty tissue with secondary inflammatory response. Beyond this hypothesis, fat necrosis should not be ruled out as a manifestation of a systemic disease such as a Weber-Christian (fever, arthralgia, liponecrotic multiple nodules) or Rothmann-Makai (multiple knots in the trunk and limbs) disease.

The traumatic action causes a necrosis of subcutaneous fat, leading to the formation of an irregular thickening content of blood and cellular debris. In time, the lipophagic granuloma could be reabsorbed at all or form a fibrotic mass, hard and irregular ill-defined margins, sometimes with skin retraction. Only rarely in some women, mostly young, the process leads to the formation of a cyst clear and oily in content that can be treated with simple suction.

Macroscopically fat necrosis yields a yellowish nodule, of different texture and without a defined nucleus of densification. Microscopically it is an observed lipid material surrounded by macrophages with foamy cytoplasm and a lymphocytic infiltrate with large presence of foreign body giant cells. In the context of fat necrosis, depositions of calcium salts in the form of calcifications of varying shape and size may be observed.

Fat necrosis can be confused with a malignancy on physical examination and may mimic malignancy on radiological studies. It is sometimes necessary to biopsy these lesions to confirm the diagnosis, although experienced radiologists can usually determine that a lesion represents fat necrosis based on mammographic findings such as low-density centre and ultrasound findings such as oil cysts.

If the clinical and instrumental assessment is suspicious, and even if the lesion persists unchanged over time, it is advisable to investigate the nature of the lesion without considering the cause of the symptoms. Factors affecting diagnostic uncertainty are inadequate cytological preparations which, although indicative of fat necrosis, have a decent amount of insignificant acellular material; long time to resolution of a posttraumatic thickening; and suspicion of recurrence in cases arising out of surgical scars.

Some methodological aspects still remain to be clarified, such as the duration of clinical observation and whether the regression of clinical symptoms only or even just their stabilisation should be considered prognostically favourable. The wait is anyway justified by the availability of reliable instrumental examinations that may exclude the presence of a proliferative process, first of all MRI.

Once the diagnosis is established, excision is not necessary, and there is no increased risk of subsequent BC.

Surgical treatment is required for diagnostic purposes only, although when deciding to proceed surgically, it is important to consider the possibility that, after surgery, a new necrotic mass might occur.

*HAEMATOMA*. Haematomas are typically the result of trauma or iatrogenic injury. Spontaneous haematomas are extremely rare, and only sporadic cases have been described during breastfeeding or therapy with anticoagulants.

Rarely, in the course of anticoagulant therapy with warfarin (usually after 5–6 weeks of treatment), aseptic ischaemic necrosis may be observed corresponding to a partial infarction of the gland, manifested by a sudden and painful oedema, followed by the appearance of bruising skin with erythematous halo. Management consists of replacement of dicumarolic medicaments with heparin and use of steroids and antibiotics. The possible excision of necrotic tissue may be postponed for a few days to allow adaptation to therapy.

In posttraumatic haematoma, the mass is typically painful and associated with ecchymosis. However, assuming that a mass present in the breast after a trauma is a haematoma and disregarding it could be a mistake. Often a minor trauma will simply alert a patient to the presence of a mass that was there before the event.

If the story matches the physical findings, the haematoma will resolve with time. Treatment includes a good supportive bra and analgesics. Some haematomas may need large-needle evacuation, while few expanding haematomas need surgical drainage and haemostasis. Likewise, conservative management of a haematoma after a reported trauma is reasonable.

Immediate imaging can be painful, and it is reasonable to avoid it. However, careful follow-up is mandatory to assure that the haematoma is resolving. If there is any suspicion of a residual mass or a failure to resolve, imaging and biopsy are recommended. Likewise, if the story and the findings raise any suspicion of malignancy, a thorough evaluation is warranted.

## 9.6 Workup of Benign Diseases of the Breast (Overview)

**Clinical Practice Points**

- Nowadays most challenging benign breast lesions are detected mammographically, or are incidental histological findings in specimens resected for cancer or any other radiological and clinical feature.
- Emphasis on screen-detected lesions, as indeterminate microcalcification and soft tissue densities, highlights the heterogeneous array of benign diseases, and, in fact, produces significant workloads in Breast Clinics.
- Due to the complicated nature of the studies required to determine the risk of subsequent malignancy, the majority of the risk assessment is relative rather than absolute, and however overall risk is very small in most benign diseases.
- At least one-third of indeterminate B3 lesions, diagnosed with a CNB, contain in the excisional biopsy one or more high-risk lesions.
- Results of CNB are considerably related to width of needles, minimum number of effective samples, and use of the vacuum-assisted device.

*OVERVIEW*. The assessment of the potential risk of progression to malignancy is increasingly playing an important part in the management of patients with benign breast disease. Nomenclature of benign breast lesions is still confusing with the use of a large variety of pathological terms. Our terminology used for benign breast diseases is based on the classification by the College of American Pathologists, which is used by the UK NHS Breast Screening Programme [9]. According to this institution, the B3 category lesions include ADH, lobular neoplasia, radial scar, columnar cell lesion (CCL), mucocele-like lesion (MLL), microglandular adenosis, and papillary and fibro-epithelial lesions.

With the exception of lesions such as atypical ductal hyperplasia, there is no consensus among investigators as to the level of risk associated with most benign lesions. Moreover, the clinician should not apply these risk factors to patients without taking into account other parameters such as family history, previous history of cancer, menopausal status or use of hormonal therapy.

B3 lesions represent the group which is more likely to be submitted to the assessment of the MDT. Starting to distinguish management between *necessary* because of a real risk and *advisable* for the chances to find out an associated high-risk lesion is essential. Indeed, at least 30 % of indeterminate B3 lesions diagnosed with a CNB contain a high-risk lesion in the excision biopsy.

The most challenging assessment is related to histological findings in CNB specimens and considerations to follow mainly surround this topic. There are three main issues.

- Which diagnosis can be considered secure enough to not require any other subsequent treatment? (Some of these aspects have been already considered earlier in other subchapters.)
- Which lesions have a long-term risk for cancer so as to suggest preventive measures? (See also Sect. 2.3.)
- Which lesions have a high likelihood of being associated with other lesions that require a surgical excision?

Moreover, other questions should be considered. Do we follow up the patient and re-biopsy if there is a change in the lesion? Do we repeat the biopsy immediately? Will the repeat biopsy give the answer we want? What if we miss the lesion on repeat biopsy and put the patient under unnecessary distress? As you would expect, each patient should be managed on an individual basis because there are no correct answers to these questions.*Workup*

*THE QUANTIFICATION OF THE RISK.* Figures shown here are based on leading and latest studies. Small variations observed in different studies may be due to the percentage of premenopausal patients in each study. Additional references in full may be found elsewhere [9, 10, 11].

- *Proliferative lesion* (overall): without atypia, RR = 1.9; with atypia, RR 5.3 [12].
- *Atypical ductal hyperplasia (ADH)*: no family history, RR = 4.3 (RR = 6.5 in presence of calcifications); with family history, RR = 9.7 [13].
- *Atypical lobular hyperplasia (ALH)*: no family history, RR = 4.2; with family history, 8.4 [13].
- *Columnar cell change*: without atypia RR = 1.5; with atypia/FEA, RR = 20.2 [14].
- *Fibroadenoma simple*, RR = 1.7–2.17; *Fibroadenoma complex* RR = 3.1–3.7 [12].
- *Hyperplasia (moderate or florid) without atypia*, RR = 1.5–2 [12] not linked to family history.
- *Papilloma* (solitary): without atypia, RR = 2.04–2.1; with atypia, RR = 5.1–13.1 [12, 15].
- *Papillomas* (multiple): without atypia, RR = 3.01–3.54; with atypia, RR = 4.4–7.0 [15].
- *Radial scar*: single NOS, RR = 2.5; single with ADH, RR = 3.5; multiple, NOS RR = 4.3; multiple with ADH, RR = 8.4 [16].
- *Sclerosing adenosis*: NOS, RR = 1.5–3.7; with ADH, RR = 6.5–6.7 [17].
- *Other lesions with unknown risk. Columnar cell lesion (CCL)* has a relatively recent background and their biological significance is still evolving, *mucocele-like*

*lesions (MLL)* are rare, can be associated with ADH, DCIS or mucinous carcinoma, but the risk of progressing to malignancy is unknown [10]. *Microglandular adenosis* is unusual and not clearly related to cancer even though there is molecular evidence that it may be linked to triple-negative BC.

- *Lesions with risk utterly irrelevant*: Ductal ectasia, most of fibrocystic changes, fat necrosis, focal fibrosis.

*CORE NEEDLE BIOPSY OUTCOMES*. The papers on CNB are relatively recent and a lack of concordance may be observed due to different diameter of needles, increasingly larger, and to great advantage of the vacuum assistance. For instance, in some misleading lesion as radial scars, an 11-gauge vacuum core biopsy may be adequate to sample the scars, while the use of a smaller 14-gauge CNB may miss a 5 % of cancers [11].

- *Lesions that never need excisional biopsy*, unless they are associated to other serious or indeterminate lesions.
  - Hyperplasia (moderate or florid) without atypia.
  - Columnar cell change and columnar cell hyperplasia without atypia, included in B2 classification.
  - Non-proliferative and secondary lesions, as fat necrosis, or mild proliferative lesion as focal fibrosis.
- *Lesions that need excisional biopsy.*
  - *Atypical hyperplasia*, either ADH or ALH. In biopsies following CNB, BC can be found in 14–31 % of specimens.
  - *Flat epithelial atypia (FEA)*, even when reported as columnar cell change with atypia and columnar cell hyperplasia with atypia.
  - *Lobular carcinoma in situ (LCIS)*, see also 'Lobular Carcinoma In Situ', Sect. 12.2.
  - *Mucocele-like lesion* to exclude not uncommon associated high-risk lesions [10]. Actually, the risk of associated malignancy is low in MLL without atypia, where an excision with a vacuum-assisted device could be a reasonable alternative to surgical excision. The risk is much higher if there is atypia, where excision is mandatory.
  - *All common benign lesions with atypiae*, including papilloma, radial scar, sclerosing adenosis, fibroadenoma complex.
  - *All B3 categories* if pathologically indeterminate.
- *Lesions that require a clinical judgment on whether to perform excisional biopsy*, other than the mentioned above.
  - Lack of concordant results with imaging.
  - When volume of lesions and the presence of calcifications do not provide a reliable result.
- *Lesions that require to be addressed to high-risk screening*. High-risk screening (see Sect. 2.3) should be associated to genetic testing (if appropriate as in patients with family history) and/or to one of predictive risk models (Gail, Claus, Boadicea, etc.). Only in relation to the pathological results and the imaging assessment the discussion of risk/benefits of chemoprevention or bilateral prophylactic mastectomy should be:

- Recommended, in atypical hyperplasias, multiple papillomas with atypiae, FEA, LCIS;
- Discretional, in other B3 lesions with a RR >2, and, in the opinion of some researchers, in marked hyperplasia without atypia (B2).

*OTHER CONSIDERATIONS*

- *Margins of excision.* In most benign diseases, margins of excision do not appear to be important as long as malignancy has been properly ruled out.
- *Mild atypiae* may be found in premenopausal women, due to hormonal influences, or in early menopausal women taking hormonal replacement therapy.
- *Atypical hyperplasia* (either ADL and ALH) and *lobular carcinoma in situ* (LCIS) imply increased risk for cancer in either breast.
- *Fibroadenoma.* Atypiae found within simple fibroadenoma do not seem to increase the risk for cancer.
- *Papilloma* should be considered on the basis of two factors: the number of lesions and the presence or absence of atypia.
- *Radial scar.* Small samples with CNB may underestimate the presence of cancer. A major risk is seen in lesions with coexistent proliferative disease. Radial scars may be also associated with tubular cancer, and in the past some tubular neoplasms have been identified with radial scars.
- *Sclerosing adenosis.* Diagnosis of sclerosing adenosis in a CNB is usually accurate if there is no radiological-pathological discordance.

## References


1. The Royal College of Surgeons. The breast clinic: benign breast diseases. https://www.rcsed.ac.uk/fellows/aaasalem/BenignbreastdiseaseDr.htm. Accessed 12 July 2014.
2. Mansel RE, Webster DJT, Sweetland HM. Aberrations of normal development and involution (ANDI): a concept of benign breast disorders based on pathogenesis. In: Hughes, Mansel & Webster's benign disorders and diseases of the breast. London: Elsevier; 2009.
3. Laronga C, Tollin S, Thurlow M. Breast cysts: clinical manifestations, diagnosis, and management. http://www.uptodate.com. Accessed 18 Oct 2014.
4. Hindle WH. Fibrocystic changes. In: Hindle WH, editor. Breast care: a clinical guidebook for women's primary health care providers. New York: Springer; 1999.
5. Grau AM, Chakravathy AB, Chug R. Phyllodes tumors of the breast. http://www.uptodate.com. Accessed 20 Feb 2014.
6. Al Sarakabi W, Worku D, Escobar PF, Mokbel K. Breast papillomas: current management with a focus on a new diagnostic and therapeutical modality. Int Semin Surg Oncol. 2006;3:1–8.
7. Warrick JI. Pathology of small, peripheral intraductal papillomas. http://emedicine.medscape.com/article/1873858-overview. Accessed 5 Jun 2013.
8. Sabel MS, Collins LC. Atypia and lobular carcinoma in situ: high risk lesions of the breast. http://www.uptodate.com. Accessed 20 Aug 2014.
9. NHSBSP Publication No 58: Oct 2005. NHSBSP Guidelines for Pathology Reporting in Breast Disease. http://www.cancerscreening.nhs.uk/breastscreen/publications/nhsbsp58.html. Accessed 30 Jan 2015.
10. Chinyama CN. Benign Breast Diseases. Berlin Heidelberg: Springer; 2014.
11. Kiluk JV, Geza A, Hoover SJ. High-Risk Benign Breast Lesions: Current Strategies in Management. Cancer Control. 2007;14:321–9.

12. Dupont WD, Page DL, Parl FF, et al. Long-term risk of breast cancer in women with fibroadenoma. N Engl J Med. 1994;331:10–5.
13. Page DL, Dupont WD, Rogers LW, Rados MS. Atypical hyperplastic lesions of the female breast. A long-term follow-up study. Cancer. 1985;55:2698–708.
14. Verschuur-Maes AH, Witkamp AJ, De Bruin PC, et al. Progression risk of columnar cell lesions of the breast diagnosed in needle core biopsies. Int J Cancer. 2011;129:2674–80.
15. Lewis TJ, Hartmann LC, Maloney SD, et al. An analysis of breast cancer risk in women with simple multiple and atypical papillomas. Am J Surg Pathol. 2006;30:665–72.
16. Jacobs TW, Bryne C, Colditz G, Connolly JL, Schnitt SJ. Radial scars in benign breast biopsy specimens and the risk of breast cancer. N Engl J Med. 1999; 340:430–6.
17. Jensen RA, Page DL, Dupont WD, Rogers LW. Invasive breast cancer in women with sclerosing adenosis. Cancer. 1989;64:1977–83.

## Further Reading

Castells X, Domingo L, Corominas JM, et al. Breast cancer risk after diagnosis by screening mammography of nonproliferative or proliferative benign breast disease: a study from a population-based screening program. Breast Cancer Res Treat. 2015;149:237–44.

Guray M, Sahin AA. Benign breast diseases: classification, diagnosis, and management. Oncologist. 2006;11:435–49.

Hartmann LC, Degnim AC, Santen RJ, Dupont WD, Ghosh K. Atypical hyperplasia of the breast–risk assessment and management options. N Engl J Med. 2015;372:78–89.

Moon HJ, Jung I, Kim MJ, Kim EK. Breast papilloma without atypia and risk of breast carcinoma. Breast J. 2014;20:525–33.

Morrow M, Schnitt SJ, Norton L. Current management of lesions associated with an increased risk of breast cancer. Nat Rev Clin Oncol. 2015. doi:10.1038/nrclinonc.2015.8.

Schwartz T, Cyr A, Margenthaler J. Screening breast magnetic resonance imaging in women with atypia or lobular carcinoma in situ. J Surg Res. 2015;193:519–22.

Wyss P, Varga Z, Rössle M, Rageth CJ. Papillary lesions of the breast: outcomes of 156 patients managed without excisional biopsy. Breast J. 2014;20:394–401.

**Websites in Appendix**: *Benign Conditions*, A-4.3.

# Nipple Discharge

# 10

Alfonso M. Pluchinotta and Barbara Gnocato

## Contents




**Abstract**

• Nipple discharge is the third most frequently reported breast complaint, after breast pain and breast mass. The vast majority of nipple discharges are physiological or otherwise benign. • In the presence of secretions, visual assessment is crucial while instrumental tests have often a negligible impact. • Physiologic discharges usually are bilateral, involve multiple ducts, are multicoloured or milky, are sometimes thick and are usually not spontaneous. • Pathologic discharges are spontaneous and usually blood-stained, serous or sometimes watery. They are unilateral, involve a single duct and are more worrisome in patients greater than 50 years old.

*Future directions.* Papillary lesions of the breast, a wide and heterogeneous group of epithelial lesions, encompass a spectrum of both benign and malignant lesions despite sharing a similar basic architecture. They represent one of the



A.M. Pluchinotta (✉) • B. Gnocato
Breast Surgery, Policlinic of Abano Terme, Padova, Italy
e-mail: pluchinotta.alfonso@gmail.com







A.M. Pluchinotta (ed.), *The Outpatient Breast Clinic: Aiming at Best Practice*,
DOI 10.1007/978-3-319-15907-2_10

more challenging diagnostic entities in breast pathology, where architectural features, cellular composition and distribution of myoepithelial cells as highlighted by immunochemistry are the major but not exclusive diagnostic criterion. Whether these lesions should be excised if diagnosed on incisional or core biopsy is still controversial.

## 10.1 Clinical Features of Nipple Discharge

**Clinical Practice Points**

- The clinical significance of nipple discharge is correlated to its visual assessment and persistence in time. A secretion should be considered physiologic or pathologic based on the appearance of the fluid and on the following characteristics: unilateral or bilateral, spontaneous or not spontaneous and mono- or pluri-orificial.
- The fluid is divided into three groups based on appearance; milky (galactorrhoea), coloured opalescent and blood-related (blood-stained, serous and watery) discharge.
- Almost all persistent unilateral secretions are related to different types of papillary lesions. A negative cytology is not sufficient to exclude the presence of proliferative lesions, and in any case the treatment cannot be based solely on cytological data.
- Tough rarely, some medicaments but also stresses such as trauma, surgical procedures and anaesthesia may also inhibit dopamine release, thereby causing hyperprolactinaemia and inducing galactorrhoea.
- Some non-physiological secretion, in women who are pregnant or are breastfeeding without other findings, should be placed in observation without taking action.

### 10.1.1 Visual Assessment and Grouping

Basic assessment of patient presenting with complaint of spontaneous nipple discharge should be started with a history aimed to detect and characterise symptoms, including whether discharge has been spontaneous, persistent, unilateral vs. bilateral, single or multiple ducts, and its relation to menses, pregnancy, exercise, trauma, medications and/or thyroid disorders [1].

The visual assessment of the discharge is of major importance because it correlates with clinical significance. The examination should attempt to obtain fluid from the nipple by using a gentle centripetal pressure at the base of the areola. The squeezing should be performed gently starting from the periphery of the areola in a radial manner (Fig. 10.1). Especially in the case of mono-orificial secretion, every

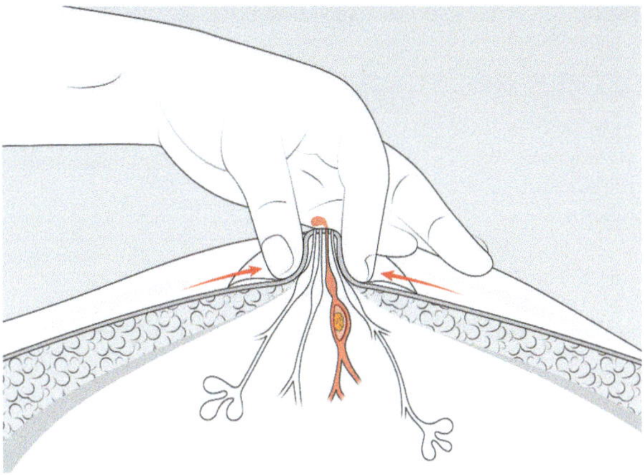

**Fig. 10.1** Secretions should be obtained from the nipple by a centripetal, gentle pressure at the base of the areola

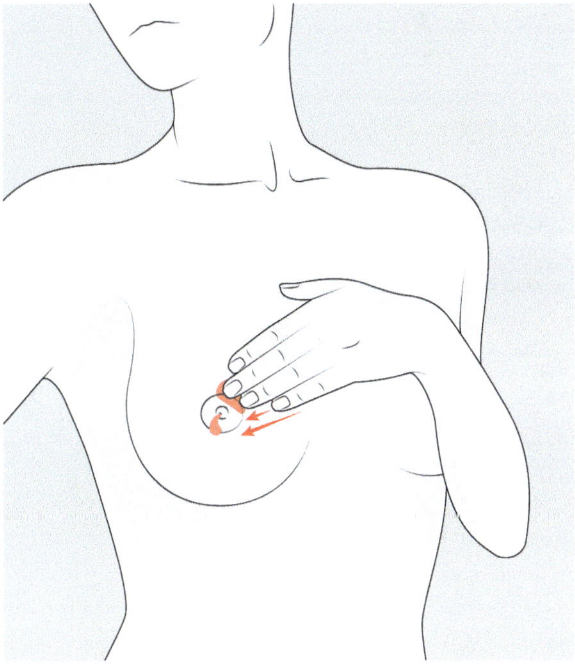

**Fig. 10.2** The woman may help in locating area the pressure of which can cause the secretion

quadrant should be palpated in order to identify the site where the lesion is presumably localised. In some cases the woman is cooperative and effective in locating the area where the pressure of which can cause secretion (Fig. 10.2).

Nipple discharge is considered spontaneous when it occurs easily, without a persistent stimulation. It should be considered spontaneous even when the woman reports a history of bloody discharge and supports it with the finding of stains of blood on her bra or underclothing.

**Table 10.1** Characteristics and clinical significance of the groups of nipple discharge

| | Groups | Characteristics | Significance |
|---|---|---|---|
| *Physiologic* in most cases of little significance; require no treatment | *Milky or milky white* (galactorrhoea) | Slight galactorrhoea | Slight galactorrhoea is idiopathic in most cases |
| | | True galactorrhoea | Only true galactorrhoea may be suggestive of prolactinoma |
| | *Coloured opalescent* (non-galactorrhoea and non-blood) | Fibrocystic changes | All appearances are the more or less extreme result of hormonal and/or involutional changes |
| | | Duct ectasia phenomena, from flawing to dense secretions | |
| *Pathologic* in most cases due to papillary lesions | *Blood or blood-related* (serous, watery) | Bloody or blood-stained | All appearances have the same significance with a high risk of papillary lesions (benign and malignant) |
| | | Serous | |
| | | Watery | |

*Grouping*. Different appearances of mammary secretions should be gathered in three groups:

- *Milky* or milky white (galactorrhoea), functional or idiopathic, of little significance
- *Coloured* opalescent (non-galactorrhoea and non-bloody), usually more or less brown-stained but also lipidic or comedones (cheesy appearance) as an expression of ductal ectasia, also of little significance
- *Bloody* or blood-related (serous, watery), the only really significant, especially if real, spontaneous, persistent and not related to breastfeeding

Milky and coloured opalescent secretions are physiologic in most of cases, while bloody or blood-related secretions are mostly pathologic. The main characteristics and clinical significance of the groups of nipple discharge are shown in Table 10.1.

*MILKY (GALACTORRHOEA)*. It is crucial to distinguish *slight* galactorrhoea from *true* galactorrhoea.

*Slight galactorrhoea*. The discharge is milky or more often serous-milky whitish or colourless, poorly consistent, depending on the content of proteins (serum albumin, globulins and lactalbumin), but especially of lipids. Discharge is bilateral, at low profusion, easy but non-spontaneous, while prolactinaemia is normal or slightly increased.

The symptom may be secondary to a reduced antagonism of progesterone lactogenic action of prolactin in the presence of anovulatory cycles or luteal insufficiency. It occurs bilaterally after a pregnancy, but also in the course of hormonal therapy with neuroleptics, especially in the presence of a marked breast involution (fatty breasts). In approximately 20–25 % of women, slight galactorrhoea has not any evident reason and is probably due to a greater glandular receptivity to low levels of prolactin, so that it should be considered idiopathic.

**Table 10.2** Medications that cause hyperprolactinaemia (effect may be dose-dependent)

| Medications |
|---|
| *Antipsychotics, first generation*: chlorpromazine, loxapine, perphenazine, pimozide, thiothixene, trifluoperazine, ziprasidone (moderate); fluphenazine, haloperidol (high) |
| *Antipsychotics, second generation*: aripiprazole, clozapine, iloperidone, lurasidone, olanzapine, quetiapine (none or low); asenapine (moderate); paliperidone, risperidone (high) |
| *Antidepressants, tricyclic*: nortriptyline (none); amitriptyline, desipramine (low); clomipramine (high) |
| *Antidepressants, SSRI* (selective serotonin reuptake inhibitor): citalopram, fluoxetine, fluvoxamine, paroxetine, sertraline (none or low) |
| *Antidepressants (others)*: bupropion, venlafaxine, mirtazapine, nefazodone, trazodone (none) |
| *Antiemetic and gastrointestinal*: prochlorperazine (low); metoclopramide, domperidone (high) |
| *Antihypertensives*: verapamil, methyldopa (none or low) |
| *Opioid analgesics*: methadone, morphine, others (transient increase for several hours following dose) |

Frequency of increase to abnormal prolactin levels with chronic use: high >50 %; moderate: 25–50 %; low: <25 %; none or low: case reports [2]

**Table 10.3** Potential causes of slight, normoprolactinaemic galactorrhoea

| Cause | Examples |
|---|---|
| Endocrine changes | Oral contraceptives |
| | Hypothyroidism |
| | End-organ hypersensitivity to normal or low levels of prolactin |
| Medicaments' effect | (See Table 10.2) antipsychotics, antidepressants, antiemetic and gastrointestinal, antihypertensives, opioid analgesic |
| Herbal supplements | Fennel, anise or fenugreek seed, cocaine or opioid |
| Mechanical causes | Excessive breast stimulation associated with sexual activity |
| | Frequent breast self-exams with nipple manipulation |
| | Skin rash on the chest or prolonged clothing friction |
| Neurogenic stimulation | Stresses |
| | Chest wall surgery, trauma or burns |
| | Spinal cord damage due to injury, surgery or tumours |

Galactorrhoea, idiopathic or otherwise normoprolactinaemic, usually not bothersome, requires no action. Treatment of galactorrhoea secondary to thyroid or ovarian dysfunction should be, as far as possible, etiological. If neuroleptics or other drugs are responsible (Table 10.2) [2], in some (few) cases it could be necessary to correct or restrict their use.

Nevertheless, the causes of slight galactorrhoea could be several and sometimes unpredictable. A synopsis of them, including also mechanical and neurogenic triggers, is listed in Table 10.3.

*True galactorrhoea* is always extramammary in origin and must be considered a manifestation of functional activity due to increased prolactin as a result of various causes that affect the pituitary gland. With high levels of prolactin, galactorrhoea is

**Fig. 10.3** Toothpaste-like secretions of the breast due to dense inspissation of the secretion (comedones)

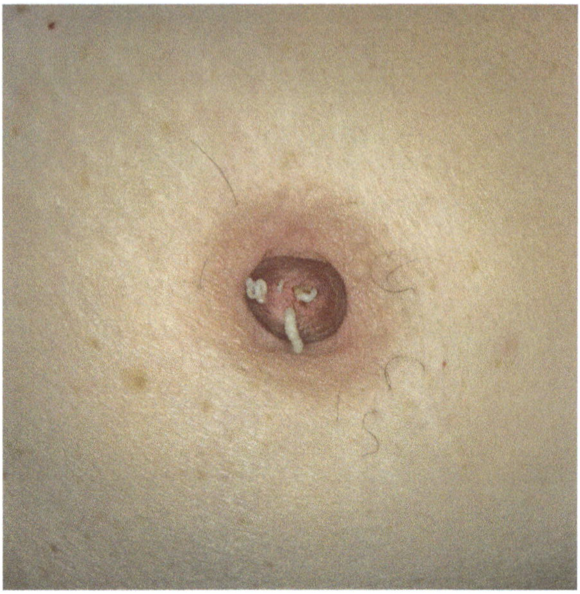

very clear and spontaneous, sometimes associated with amenorrhoea. Patients should undergo in-depth investigations including hormonal assay of prolactin after stimulation with TRH and, in case of abnormal levels, MRI of the sella turcica. An endocrinologist referral could be needed.

*COLOURED OPALESCENT DISCHARGE.* Coloured opalescent discharge may have many causes.

*Fibrocystic changes secretions.* In the group of coloured opalescent discharge, yellow, brown, green and grey fluids can be observed from multiple ducts. The appearance of the fluid is associated with fibrocystic changes in many patients, due to regressive, and at the same time secretive, phenomena. The initially clear and opalescent tone with time becomes more colourful with tinges that turn to beige, tan, grey or grey-green. Discharge occurs for an ectasia of the major ducts, which can be more or less marked and affect a variable number of them, initially limited and subsequently increased. Secretion is found in the same fluid component of the cyst and galactography can sometimes show a communication between cyst and dilated ducts.

*Mammary duct ectasia.* When duct ectasia phenomena are more marked, as observed with some fatty breasts, dystrophic secretions are mostly fluid or viscous, slightly opalescent with changeable patterns of consistency, which can range from flowing to very dense. In particular, when the dilation of main retroareolar ducts is strong and diffuse (ectatic dystrophy of retroareolar ducts), the secretion appears thicker and creamy, yellowish and ointment-like, due to an abnormal accumulation of cellular debris and lipids (Fig. 10.3).

Colostrum-like or foam cells, amorphous cellular debris, lipoid debris and crystalline bodies are the ultimate expression of involution and degeneration phenomena of the epithelium of the ducts (Fig. 10.3). In this complex symptomatology of

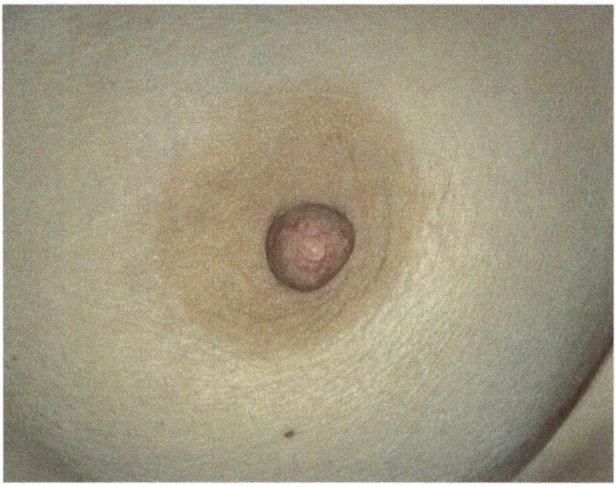

**Fig. 10.4** Serous discharge from the nipple. Serous (or watery) secretion is considered as an effective hematic-related secretion for all purposes

duct ectasia/periductal mastitis (see Sect. 9.2.2), episodes of galactophoritis can be observed with sporadic and momentary secretion of blood concomitant with the normal secretions.

As part of the same framework, the galactophoritis may evolve into an acute noninfective colliquation that can find a natural way out to the outside through a duct. A gentle pressure, in order to elicit the purulent discharge, sometimes allows complete drainage of the abscess-like collection (Fig. 8.6).

*BLOODY AND BLOOD-RELATED DISCHARGE.* Bloody or blood-stained discharge is more often due to one or more papillomas (see over), whereas it is rarely (10 %) indicative of a malignant papillary lesion. The risk of malignancy is increased in the presence of a palpable mass, or in relation to age, being greater in older women. Also a nipple adenoma (see Sect. 11.1.2) could cause a blood-stained secretion, mostly just in the initial stage or when the appearance of its efflorescence is predominant.

*Serous secretion.* The true serous secretion is clear but not very fluid, because of a more or less high content of proteins, so that in setting up the slide for cytology it looks tacky and sometimes slightly sticky.

*Watery secretion.* This rare form of secretion should be distinguished from serous secretions for its distinctive look: very light or watery as rock water (Fig. 10.4). As a serous secretion, it is slightly viscous. The serous secretions as well as watery secretions, when mono-orificial spontaneous and persistent, have the same clinical significance of blood-stained secretions and so are mostly associated with a benign or malignant papillary lesion.

In the presence of bloody or blood-related discharge, patients should be thoroughly examined for a palpable mass. In patients with no palpable finding, the site of potential intraductal papilloma (but, less commonly, of multiple papillomas) should be reported by locating the orifice of the affected duct on the surface of the nipple. A thorough manual pressure of the circumference of the areola could be determinant. The bloody or blood-stained secretion does not distinguish benign from malignant papilloma, even in the case of negative or benign cytology.

*INCIDENTAL NON-PERSISTENT NIPPLE DISCHARGE. Bloody discharge of pregnancy* occurs mainly during the third trimester of pregnancy, due to proliferative changes within the ducts of the breasts (Sect. 3.4).

*Blood-stained discharge*, due to an inflammation of one or more mammary ducts, is a transient result of the nuisance action of some hormonal changes, as in some (few) patients taking oral contraceptive pills. However, the majority of episodes are without recognisable causes. Usually the bloody component disappears in 7–15 days and it may be appropriate to make a brief wait-and-see to rule out other causes.

*Bloody chocolate-like discharge*. A bloody discharge, usually dark and brown as chocolate, can be an isolated occurrence secondary to an abnormal stimulating hormone action on main ducts with intraluminal micro-haemorrhages. Discharge comes out spontaneously or provoked by a slight squeezing. Sometimes a short but profuse pouring out causes an immediate alleviation of pain due to the engorgement and distension of retroareolar ducts.

Isolated episodes can be observed during puberty due to a sudden and important oestrogen stimulation of the ducts, or after the oestrogen overload of the *morning after pill*, or in the premenopausal hyper-oestrogenic phase especially during a significant delay of menses.

*Blood post-traumatic discharge* can be observed as outcome of a trauma, but also a mammography, a fine-needle aspiration and even a too energetic palpation. It is associated to a superficial bruising. Despite the apparent correlation between cause and effect, it is not always easy to exclude the presence of a concomitant breast lesion.

*Discharge due to mechanical stimulations*. Bleeding from a fissure of the nipple is a condition that can be observed in joggers (jogger's nipple). The persistent friction of a loose-fitting T-shirt can result in soreness, dryness or irritation to one or both nipples during or following running or other physical activity or exercise, especially in hot days (see Sect. 11.2).

### 10.1.2 Laboratory Testing

*Hemoccult test*. The presence of few red blood cells in the discharge, since indicative of bloody secretion, in some cases could be provoked by squeezing, which should never be forceful.

In darker secretions, especially if mono- or pauci-orificial, the presence of blood can be questionable so a strip for occult blood, as Hemoccult or similar test, should be employed. Bloody or guaiac-positive discharge raises the possibility of an intraductal proliferative lesion, although the character of the fluid is generally unreliable for a differential diagnosis among the various possible causes.

If the secretion is discrete, it can be put on a white gauze. In the presence of blood, staining appears slightly faded towards the periphery, while in case of coloration due to ductal ectasia staining appears to be completely uniform.

*Cytologic examination.* Cytology smears, obtained by squeezing the nipple and examined by means of Papanicolaou and/or May-Giemsa staining, provide information about normality, atypia, malignancy and also papillary pattern of the exfoliated cells.

However, in lesions with associated atypia, the cytomorphologic features may overlap with those of hormone-stimulated ducts (as in premenopausal women or who are taking HRT) or with those of low-grade DCIS. Therefore, in almost all cases a tissue biopsy is required for a definitive diagnosis.

Although useful in most case, as within imaging procedures, a negative result is not conclusive and should not stop further evaluation. Sensitivity of cytology in the presence of a malignant lesion is positive in 60–80 % of cases, but false negatives are observed in 15–35 % of cases and false positives in 3–4 % of cases. In conclusion a negative cytology is not sufficient to exclude the presence of malignancy, and in any case the treatment cannot be based solely on cytological data.

Sometimes secretion is poorly significant. Nevertheless, since the majority of non-obstructing malignant and premalignant breast diseases are associated with fluid production, cytological analysis of fluid produced in high-risk women is considered useful to identify subgroups at high short-term risk of development. In selected cases, procedures as nipple aspirate fluid (NAF) and ductal lavage (DL) could be indicated but only for early detection of BC (see Sect. 6.2).

*Hormonal assessment.* Monitoring of hormones to determine an endocrinologic basis of the nipple discharge is rarely indicated. Only for true galactorrhoea assay should be performed for prolactin and TSH as both of these pituitary hormones may induce galactorrhoea, may have a reversible cause and may likewise reflect further underlying pathology (e.g. pituitary adenoma, hypothyroidism, etc.).

### 10.1.3 Imaging

*Mammography.* Simple mammography should be performed in all patients aged 35 years and over complaining of bloody or blood-related discharge. Intraductal papilloma cannot be detected by conventional mammography, but mammogram can detect pathognomonic microcalcifications, so that further investigations are required, especially if calcifications are polymorphic, clustered or linearly distributed.

*Galactography* (*or ductography*) (see also Sect. 5.1) is a rather simple, safe but sometimes uncomfortable technique for the visualisation of the affected duct system in patients with discharge suspicious for an intraductal proliferation.

Solitary papilloma could be found in the major ducts as a filling defect within a dilated duct. Multiple papillomas could be observed in the branching ducts, located in a segmental or subsegmental distribution with sometimes a cystic dilatation of the ductal system. Distortion, narrowing or obstruction of the ducts may indicate the presence of malignancy.

Galactography, however, has considerable limitations in detecting lesions that do not completely obstruct the ductal lumen, as well in detecting multiple lesions in the same duct. Therefore, galactography does not exclude the presence of proliferative papillary lesions in patients with pathologic discharge and does not replace surgery for the diagnosis.

Although still controversial, galactography is gaining popularity, in spite of the few data on effectiveness, cost and therapeutic purpose with routine use. Galactography may be also combined with adjunctive techniques, such as hook-wire insertion and ultrasound-guided fine-needle aspiration (FNA) or percutaneous dye injection. High-resolution ultrasound, fibre-optic ductoscopy and MRI galactography appear to be promising developments.

*High-resolution ultrasound.* When the physical examination reveals a palpable abnormality in a localised area of the breast, ultrasound imaging may be useful in determining its characteristics, whether it is a cyst, an intracystic growth or a solid mass. Modem high-resolution ultrasound techniques with 3D views are helpful in visualising intraductal disorders and are becoming a good complementary approach if not an alternative to traditional radiology techniques. Furthermore, there is increasing evidence that ultrasound-guided percutaneous stereotactic vacuum core biopsy is a reliable minimally invasive diagnostic and therapeutic modality in some clinical scenarios.

*Ductoscopy.* New submillimetre fibre-optic micro-endoscopes, which measure between 0.55 and 1.2 mm in external diameter, may be inserted through the ductal opening on the nipple surface. The procedure is performed under local anaesthesia in the outpatient's clinic with minimal discomfort and no reported complications.

In skilled hands, ductoscopy allows direct visualisation of the mammary ductal epithelium, biopsy of intraductal lesions and guidance during duct excision surgery. It also provides working channels for insufflation, irrigation, ductal lavage and possible therapeutic intervention. The sharp clear magnified images viewed on a video monitor combined with the use of intraductal biopsy devices including microbrushes and other biopsy tools allow the retrieval of tissue specimens under direct visualisation for cytopathological analysis. If the procedure is adjunct to galactography, accurate localization of intraductal abnormalities has been reported as high as more than 95 % of cases.

Nevertheless, mammary ductoscopy has some limitations due to the fact that it examines only few ducts and furthermore is incapable of reaching the peripheral small branches of the ducts. Thus, it is unable to visualise the terminal duct-lobular unit (TDLU) where malignant lesions often originate. Moreover, the technique is still not widely used in clinical practice due to the high cost and limited expertise, so, for now, the technique is considered investigational [3].

*MRI* in the management of proliferative lesions is currently limited. Papillary lesions present with a variable appearance on MRI ranging from occult to small luminal mass or to irregular rapidly enhancing lesion that cannot be reliably distinguished from invasive malignancy. Conversely, starting with the assumption of high

**Table 10.4** Workup for nipple discharge related to its features

| Features | Measures |
|---|---|
| Non-spontaneous, non-bloody and bilateral (physiologic) | Consider endocrine changes or potential effect of medications and supplements |
| | Specific test not indicated |
| | Imaging if indicated in relation to age |
| Non-spontaneous, bloody and bilateral | Could be physiologic in pregnancy and with some endocrine storm. Follow-up is needed |
| Spontaneous, bloody (or serous or watery) and unilateral (pathologic) | Cytology helpful but not always discriminant |
| | If persistent for more than 2 weeks, imaging is indicated |
| | In persistent discharge surgery, also in absence of imaging and cytological abnormalities, is indicated |
| Spontaneous, non-bloody unilateral | Hemoccult test is required. If negative, a short follow-up is recommended to test the persistence for over 2 months |

sensitivity of MRI, the absence of enhancement typical of malignancy in women with papillary lesions can be reassuring and supportive of conservative management. However, in clinical practice, the high cost, limited expertise and suboptimal specificity of MRI remain obstacles to its widespread use. More recently, MR galactography has been shown to be of diagnostic value, but only in skilled hands.

*Core-needle biopsy*. If the proliferative lesion causing the discharge is detectable on mammography and/or ultrasonography, then imaging-guided vacuum-assisted biopsy can be both diagnostic and curative. In fact, imaging-guided vacuum-assisted core biopsy is a minimally invasive method of obtaining an accurate tissue analysis. Moreover, in selected cases, the technique has a high probability of completely removing the lesion and of eliminating the symptomatic (and worrisome for the patient) nipple discharge.

Clinically occult papillary lesions diagnosed by core-needle biopsy are rare, representing less than 1 % of core-needle biopsies. When the lesion is subsequently excised, cancer is found in about one-third of cases of previously diagnosed papillomas containing atypia. For this reason, despite some cases of definitive recovery reported in the literature with large-bore CNB, it is generally recommended that any papillary lesion diagnosed by core-needle biopsy be excised to rule out malignancy.

### 10.1.4 Workup

In conclusion, in the workup of mammary secretions the basis of assessment is the visual judgment of the discharge as well whether its appearance is unilateral or bilateral, by one or more ducts, spontaneous or provoked, sporadic or recurrent or persistent. The main measures of workup for nipple discharge are shown in Table 10.4.

## 10.2 Treatment of Nipple Discharge

**Clinical Practice Points**

- Surgical evaluation with major duct excision is required for mono-orificial discharge, unless thick or cheese, as a new symptom in a woman older than 35 years, even if imaging and cytological results are negative.
- Pathological discharge associated with a mass requires a preoperative ultrasound-guided core-needle biopsy or at least a fine-needle aspiration.
- In women older than 40 years, major duct excision appears to detect a higher percentage of occult malignant lesions when compared with minimally invasive microductectomy.
- In imaging suspicious of multiple papillomas, a duct-lobular segmentectomy should be considered as a more effective surgery.

### 10.2.1 Surgical Treatment of Nipple Discharge

When pathological nipple discharge occurs, in almost all cases it is caused by a papillary lesion. These proliferative lesions are widely discussed on Sect. 9.3; however, when associated to discharge, they are referred to as asymptomatic or mild symptomatic mass. That is why, for practical purposes, they should be considered separately.

Intraductal papilloma is the commonest pathological finding accounting for 50–80 % of cases followed by multiple intraductal papillomas (10 %). The incidence of malignancy (invasive or in situ) varies between 5 and 20 % depending upon the series study.

Every patient with pathologic nipple discharge should be referred for diagnostic imaging evaluation. While imaging may detect an underlying abnormality, negative results should not deter further evaluation. In women with this symptom, imaging studies are indeed not sufficiently reliable for identifying all papillary lesions, with or without atypia [4].

*CLINICAL PATTERNS are the most influential factors on assessment. Pathological discharge from a single duct.* Mono-orificial discharge as a new symptom in a woman older than 40 years, unless thick or cheese-like, should be strictly investigated and/or undergo surgery. After the accomplishment of the usual tests, also if their results are inconclusive, there is a surgical indication for spontaneous pathological discharge confirmed on clinical examination with one of the following characteristics: mono-orificial, bloody or blood-related (serous, watery) and persistent (occurs for at least 2 weeks). A higher incidence of malignancy was found in patient with blood-stained nipple discharge compared to those with non-bloody discharge or when compared to those with serous discharge alone [4].

*Pathological discharge associated with a mass*, especially in para-central or subareolar location and easily elicited by the manual pressure, should be highly considered. At age over 50 years, the presence of blood in the discharge and the presence of a clinical mass increase significantly the risk of associated malignancy, and it is recommended that these patients be fully investigated by conventional imaging and sampling techniques. Nevertheless surgery is mandatory, whichever are radiological and histological results [5].

*Non-bloody/blood-related discharge from multiple ducts.* Conservative management of non-bloody nipple discharge can be considered in patients with no other clinical or radiological sign of malignancy. Discharge requires surgery only when it causes distressing symptoms such as persistent staining of clothes.

*SURGICAL OPTIONS.* Three options are considered: *microductectomy*, *major duct excision* and *duct-lobular segmentectomy*. If the discharge can be localised to a single duct, microductectomy gives satisfactory results in younger patients with a minimal interference with breastfeeding. In older patients where breastfeeding is not required, major duct excision may be preferable irrespective of whether the discharge is localised to one duct, both to avoid inconvenience of further discharge from a different duct and to provide a more comprehensive histology.

*Microductectomy* is indicated:

- In young women, not to preclude the possibility of breastfeeding
- When the discharge is not otherwise suspicious
- With no cytological atypia

Prior to operation, methylene blue is injected in the affected duct. Ultrasonography can be used to localise the ectatic duct in cases where there is no secretion on the day of the scheduled operation. The blue colour enables the surgeon to excise the affected duct accurately. The excision of the duct system should be about 25 mm or as far as dilated ducts contain blood/serum discharge. Such a microductectomy preserves breast tissue and gives a better cosmetic result than with complete major duct excision.

*Major duct excision* appears to detect a higher percentage of occult carcinoma when compared with minimally invasive microductectomy. Results are related to the larger sample size of the resection specimen, but this motivation is widely disputable. At present, major duct excision is indicated:

- In women older than 40 years, although age should not be used in identifying women at risk of malignancy
- In otherwise morphologically abnormal discharge
- In recurrences after previous surgery
- In the presence of cytological atypia
- Under a cloud of suspicion of multiple papillomas
- In a large collection of discharges that suggest stasis in involved peripheral ducts

*Duct-lobular segmentectomy* is an alternative to the standard major duct excision, purposely indicated:

- In para-central mass associated to easy discharge elicited by the manual pressure
- In imaging suspicious of multiple papillomas, as in multilobulated mass detected with ultrasound

Recently, two more conservative approaches have been investigated:

- *Imaging-guided vacuum-assisted core biopsy*, which can be diagnostic and therapeutic for small papillomas seen on mammography and/or ultrasound
- *Ductoscopy-assisted microductectomy*, which could be considered the procedure of choice for a papilloma-related single-duct discharge. There is an increasing evidence that ductoscopy performed by (few) super-specialised operator has the potential to reduce the number of duct excision procedures and to minimise the extent of surgical resection.

## 10.3 Follow-Up

*Papillary hyperplasia* is a form of usual ductal hyperplasia not requiring any follow-up.

*Papilloma*. Patients who prove to have solitary duct papilloma have insufficient increase in the risk of subsequent malignancy to justify routine follow-up.

*Atypical papilloma*, synonymous with *intraductal papilloma with atypia*, refers to an intraductal papilloma involved by variable amounts of atypical ductal hyperplasia. The greater likelihood of recurrence or malignancy has been consistently reported to be higher when a papilloma with atypia versus without atypia is present on biopsy, underscoring the importance of noting atypia within a papilloma. Some studies suggest patients with single atypical papilloma necessitate additional surgery, whereas other studies conclude additional excision was not necessary.

Although the risk, small but real, could affect both breasts, long-term follow-up seems to be more appropriate than risk-reducing (prophylactic) measures. Only for patients with family history of BC, the benefits of chemoprevention may be comparable to those with proven atypical hyperplasia, although there is not enough data available to confirm this statement.

*Multiple papillomas*. Patients with multiple papillomas do have an increased risk of developing cancer and should be kept under annual review with regular digital mammography if conservatively treated. MRI may improve surveillance in view of its high sensitivity (but suboptimal specificity); however, its use is controversial unless in young high-risk women.

*Papillary ductal carcinoma in situ*, found by chance after major duct excision, usually requires a re-excision with more large free margins, since most often it is associated with a low-grade invasive carcinoma.

## References

1. Goodson WH, King EB. Discharge and secretion of the nipple. In: Bland KI, Copeland EM, editors. The breast: comprehensive management of benign and malignant disorders. 3rd ed. St. Louis: Saunders; 2004.
2. Golshan M, Iglehart D. In: Chapgar AB, editor. Nipple discharge. http://www.uptodate.com/contents/nipple-discharge. Accessed 20 Sept 2014.

3. Tang S, Gui G. Nipple discharge and the role of ductoscopy in breast diseases. In: Dixon JM, editor. Breast surgery. London: Elsevier; 2014.
4. Chen L, Zhou WB, Zhao Y, et al. Bloody nipple discharge is a predictor of breast cancer risk: a meta-analysis. Breast Cancer Res Treat. 2012;132:9–14.
5. Rampaul RS, Rakha EA, Robertson JFR, Ellis IO. Pathology and biology of breast cancer. In: Dixon JM, editor. Breast surgery. London: Elsevier; 2014.

## Further Reading

Huang W, Molitch ME. Evaluation and management of galactorrhea. Am Fam Physician. 2012;85:107e–80 ICSI. Health Care Guideline: Diagnosis of Breast Disease (14th edition, 2012) In: https://www.icsi.org/_asset/v9l91q/DxBrDis.pdf. Accessed 20 Jul 2014.

Mansel RE, Webster DJT, Sweetland HM. Nipple discharge. In: Hughes, Mansel & Webster's benign disorders and diseases of the breast. London: Elsevier; 2009.

Nelson RS, Hoehn JL. Twenty-years outcome following central duct resection for bloody nipple discharge. Ann Surg. 2006;243:522–4.

**Websites in Appendix**: *Benign Conditions*, A-4.3.

# Miscellaneous Minor Disorders of the Breast

# 11

Alfonso M. Pluchinotta and Rafaele Grigoletto

## Contents



**Abstract**

• Rudimentary mammary glands isolated or associated with sebaceous gland (as in Montgomery's glands) may be (rarely) found just below the areola. This condition should be taken into consideration, just like mammary glands (more rarely) found deeper, beyond the pectoral fascia. • The skin of the areola and the nipple, for its contents of subcutaneous glands, is more prone to different kinds of dermatological diseases. True dermatitis is generally bilateral and part of other localisations anywhere in the body. • Paget's disease should be taken in consideration in all cases of unilateral eczema of the areola. • Aside from the well-known and indolent dermatitis, radiation therapy may promote some dermatological diseases as herpes zoster and morphea. • For unexplained clinical observations, factitial diseases should be considered for patient with emotional and psychotic problems, who have a history of seeking frequent medical attention.

A.M. Pluchinotta (✉)
Breast Surgery, Policlinic of Abano Terme, Padova, Italy
e-mail: pluchinotta.alfonso@gmail.com

R. Grigoletto
Breast Unit, Istituto Oncologico Veneto (IOV), Padova, Italy



A.M. Pluchinotta (ed.), *The Outpatient Breast Clinic: Aiming at Best Practice*,
DOI 10.1007/978-3-319-15907-2_11

## 11.1 Disorders of the Nipple and Areola

**Clinical Practice Points**

- Normal congenital nipple inversion is common, but self-correcting changes often occur during pregnancy and lactation, allowing breastfeeding.
- The terms inversion and retraction of the nipple are sometimes used interchangeably, which may cause confusion.
- Montgomery's glands have a complex structure that includes sebaceous glands and rudimentary mammary glands, the latter joining in the same duct so that they may (rarely) sustain the same pathology of the breast.
- Nipple pain associated with breastfeeding may be associated with candidal or staphylococcal infection. Rare causes of nipple pain are Raynaud's phenomenon and postsurgical complex regional pain syndrome.
- Nipple adenoma, for its expanded and sometimes ulcerated appearance, is not easily differentiated from intraductal papilloma and Paget's disease.
- Raynaud's phenomenon and complex regional pain syndrome (CRPS) are rare causes of nipple pain, sometimes occurring after surgery.

### 11.1.1 Nipple Inversion and Retraction

*CLASSIFICATION OF NIPPLE TYPES* – The classification of nipple types should be based upon appearance, whether the nipple can be pulled out manually, and how well projection can be maintained [1]. Three main types should be considered: *everted* (normal), *inverted* (congenital or acquired), and *retracted* (Fig. 11.1).

*Everted nipple* is the common (normal) type, where nipple is held *erect* by a cylindrical column of small smooth muscles. Even if its projection is low or *flat*, when stimulated by touch or cold, it becomes erect.

*Inverted nipple* appears to be indented in the areola, and in congenital cases, this aspect is due a failure of the underlying mesenchymal tissue to proliferate and

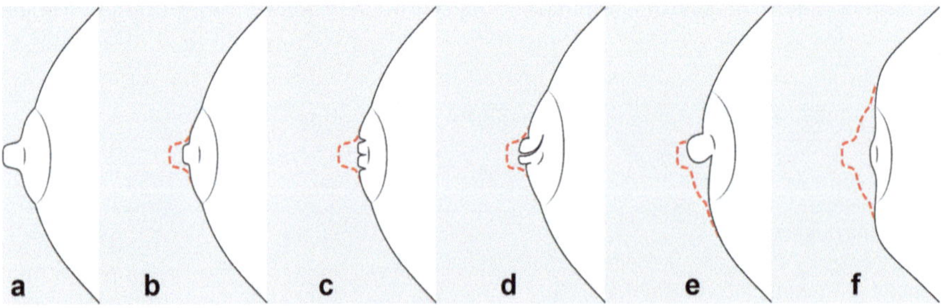


**Fig. 11.1** Diagram of types of nipple: (**a**) everted erect (normal); (**b**) everted flat (normal); (**c**) inverted umbilicated (normal congenital); (**d**) true inverted (pathologic usually benign); (**e**) partially retracted or deviated (pathologic, both benign and malignant); (**f**) fully retracted (pathologic, usually malignant)

project the nipple papilla outward. The nipple may be pulled out with gentle squeezing of the areolar skin, and the projection could be maintained for some minutes then the nipple reverts to an inverted state. Inverted nipples may be:

- *Congenital* (about 3–10 % of normal types, prevalence may change with age, pregnancies, and lactation) that may be *umbilicated* (more than 90 % of congenital forms, easy to pull out) or *invaginated* (3–10 % of congenital forms, more difficult to pull out)
- *Acquired* when a forceful manipulation is required to pull the nipple out, and inversion recurs quickly. This type of nipple inversion may occur because the nipples are stuck into scar tissue of the periductal mastitis (commonly presents as a slitlike inversion, Fig. 11.2) or into fibrosis due to aging or as late duct ectasia phenomenon (commonly presents as a circular inversion).

*Retracted nipples, unlike inverted nipples,* will not come back out when stimulated. The nipple is strongly deviated or buried below the level of the skin. Despite maximal manipulation, the nipple cannot be pulled out. Nipple retraction may be partial (deviated nipple), when a single duct is involved in a pathological process as periductal mastitis or invasive/ non-invasive ductal carcinoma (Fig. 11.3), or full, as result of severe fibrosis or pathological causes as chronic inflammatory diseases and carcinoma.

A synopsis of nipple types is showed in Table 11.1 that includes also a grading system for nipple inversion based upon how difficult it is to pull the nipple out manually and how well projection is subsequently maintained. The majority of patient with nipple inversion have grade II inversion.

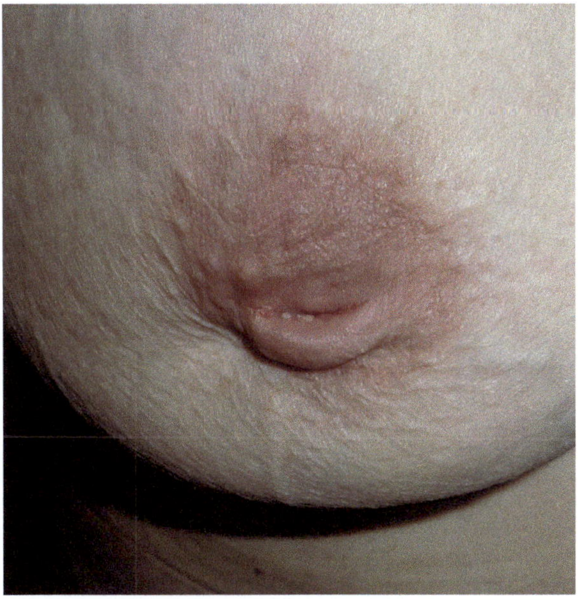

**Fig. 11.2** Slitlike nipple inversion, symmetrical and central, involving the nipple but not the areola

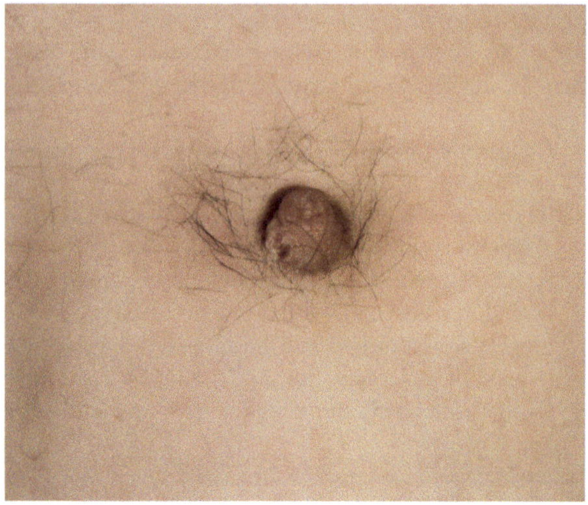

**Fig. 11.3** Nipple retraction, due to underlying BC in a man

**Table 11.1** Classification of nipple types

| Definition | Types | Causes and notes | Grade |
|---|---|---|---|
| Everted | *Erect* | Normal common | *Grade 0* |
| | *Flat* | Flat type became protractile when compressed or stimulated | |
| Inverted | *Umbilicated*<br>>90 % of congenital easy to pull out | Normal congenital<br>Due to a failure of the underlying mesenchymal tissue to proliferate and project the nipple papilla outward | *Grade I* – the nipple is pulled out with gentle squeezing of the areolar skin. Nipple projection is well maintained for several minutes, but then the nipple reverts to an inverted state |
| | *Invaginated*<br>5–10 % of congenital difficult to pull out | 3–10 % of normal types, prevalence may change with age, pregnancies, and lactation | |
| | *True inverted* | Acquired | *Grade II* – forceful manipulation is required to pull the nipple out, and inversion recurs quickly |
| | | *Slitlike inversion* (due to periductal mastitis) | |
| | | *Circular inversion* (fibrosis due to aging or as late duct ectasia phenomenon) | |
| Retracted | *Partially retracted (deviated)* | Acquired | *Grade III* – the nipple is strongly deviated or buried below the level of the skin. Despite maximal manipulation, the nipple cannot be pulled out |
| | *Fully retracted* | *Deviated* (scarring of a single duct due to periductal mastitis, prior surgery or breast cancer) | |
| | | *Fully retracted* (severe fibrosis due to aging, or duct ectasia phenomenon, pathological processes as chronic inflammatory diseases and BC) | |

*SURGICAL CORRECTION OF BENIGN NIPPLE INVERSION* – For many women, inverted or non-protractile nipples can be a source of aesthetic and functional concern, leading to self-consciousness and psychological distress.

The goal of surgical correction is to restore projection while maintaining the ductal anatomy as much as possible. For this purpose, the simplest nonsurgical technique is a plain device that can be used by women of any age to pull out inverted or non-protractile nipples. Using suction to gently stretch the ducts over time, it can achieve a permanent correction between 1 and 3 months of continuous use, for 8 h/ day.

The simplest surgical technique is a *purse-string suture*, which is placed around the neck of the nipple through a periareolar incision. This technique tightens the neck of the nipple and works well for those with less severe cases of nipple inversion.

*Selective division of ducts* is another technique that makes a blunt dissection through vertical spreading of fibrous tissue parallel to the lactiferous ducts through an inferior periareolar incision. Placing the nipple on traction for 2–5 days with a stent completes the repair. More severe cases of nipple inversion are treated with *triangular skin flaps*, which can be mobilised to add bulk to the base of the nipple and, when closed, tighten the neck of the nipple [2].

If ducts may be carved, percutaneous release of nipple inversion can be accomplished with a simple minimally invasive technique using a needle tip for lysis of retracted ducts. For this technique, an 18-gauge needle tip is inserted at the 6 o'clock position and used to lyse fibrous tissue and tethered glands until satisfactory nipple projection has been achieved. Following this, a monofilament purse-string suture is placed, starting at the entry site, with entry and exit through the same stitch point every 3–5 mm around the nipple base. The suture is then tied under moderate tension. In a series of 58 inverted nipples in 31 patients, there were 13 recurrences, of which 11 were successfully treated with a second purse-string suture and two required a third procedure [3].

### 11.1.2 Nipple Adenoma

*Nipple adenoma* is an uncommon and distinctive variant of intraductal papilloma, a benign proliferative lesion restricted to the nipple [4]. Alternative terms for this entity include mainly *florid papillomatosis* but also *erosive adenomatosis*, *syringomatous adenoma*, *superficial papillary adenomatosis,* and *papillary adenoma.* The spectrum of clinicopathologic features related to its unique location and heterogenous histopathology makes nipple adenoma a unique entity.

Nipple adenoma may occur at any age even though is most commonly seen in the middle aged to elderly. Asymptomatic nipple adenoma is found in 1–16 % of breast specimens obtained for carcinoma. It usually presents as a papilliferous lesion of the nipple, often with ulceration, which may be concealed under a crust. The condition is sometimes painful, the commonest descriptions being burning or itching.

On examination, the whole nipple may be indurated, has an expanded appearance, and may be ulcerated. The main differential diagnoses are prolapsing intraductal papilloma, Paget's disease of the nipple, factitial disease, and eczema.

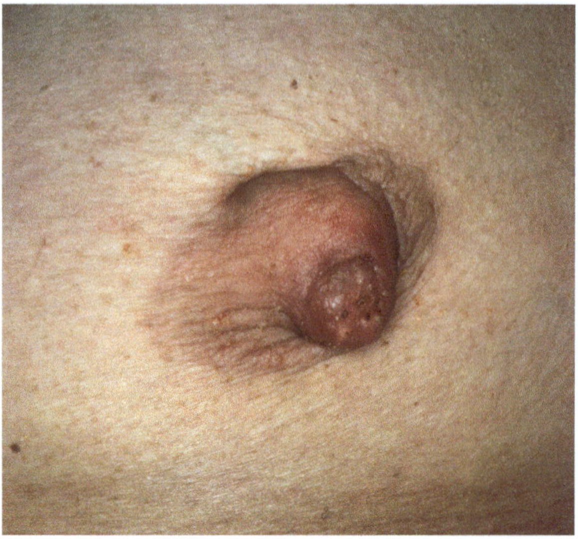

**Fig. 11.4** Nipple adenoma, involving only the nipple area

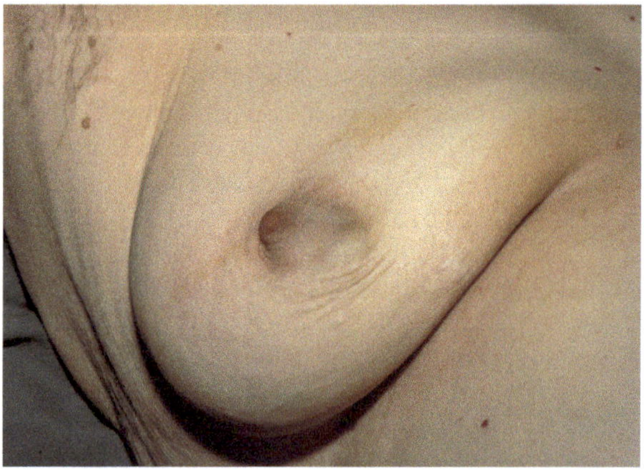

**Fig. 11.5** Large central papilloma deforming the areola with minimal involvement of the nipple

The differential diagnosis from Paget's disease can only be made with certainty by biopsy, although the characteristic clinical features are different. Nipple adenoma does not extend on to the areola like established Paget's disease, and it has the appearance of a deeper lesion eroding through the nipple. Early Paget's disease is more superficial in appearance.

Nipple adenoma erodes through the nipple duct (Fig. 11.4), while an intraductal papilloma, if (rarely) superficial and prolapsing through the duct, tends to expand the nipple rather than erode it (Fig. 11.5). If a papilloma prolapses through the opening of a duct, the nipple remains normal and never becomes ulcerated.

A comparison among clinical features of nipple adenoma, Paget's disease, and prolapsing intraductal papilloma is showed in Table 11.2.

Nipple adenoma is not itself regarded as premalignant, although, in about 5 % of cases, it has been found associated with BC. This incidence of associated BC needs

**Table 11.2** Compared clinical features of prolapsing intraductal papilloma, nipple adenoma, and Paget's disease

| *Prolapsing intraductal papilloma* | *Nipple adenoma* | *Paget's disease* |
|---|---|---|
| Does not extend on the areola | Does not extend on the areola | Areola is involved in most cases |
| Tends to expand the nipple rather than erode it | Erodes through the nipple as a deeper lesion | Is superficial in appearance |
| Never ulcerated | Sometimes ulcerated | Crusting but never ulcerated |
| Painless or slightly burning | Painful, sometimes burning or itching | Slightly itching |
| Benign at low risk (if no atypia) | Benign at low risk | Preinvasive cancer |

for careful assessment of both breasts. Another association of nipple adenoma is with intraductal papilloma that has also been reported to occur more commonly than would be expected by chance. Nipple adenoma is adequately treated by local excision of the affected part of the nipple, and in most cases there is no need to remove the whole nipple. This assertion is anyway still controversial.

### 11.1.3 Observations About Montgomery's Glands

Three types of glands are found in the areolar skin:

- *Apocrine sweat glands*, which are a normal finding, with no clinical implication
- *Modified sebaceous glands* (Montgomery's glands) which are similar to sebaceous glands elsewhere, except that they are associated with a lactiferous duct extending from a more deeply placed rudimentary mammary gland (Fig. 11.6)
- *Rudimentary mammary glands,* with a lactiferous duct blind or open in areola, that are very rare

The number of Montgomery's glands can vary greatly, usually averaging from 12 to 20 per nipple. The main function of these modified sebaceous glands consists of producing some lipoid fluids to keep the areola lubricated and smooth. Volatile compounds in these secretions may also operate as an olfactory stimulus for newborn appetite. Montgomery's glands and rudimentary mammary glands both undergo changes during pregnancy. The portion of the gland visible on the surface of the areola, looking as a round bump, is named *Montgomery's tubercle*. The tubercles become more pronounced during pregnancy and sometimes when the nipple is stimulated.

When the detailed anatomy of the glandular components of Montgomery's tubercles is considered, the occasional clinical problems of retention cysts (Fig. 11.7), milklike or also bloody discharge (Fig. 11.8), are not so surprising. If anything, it is more surprising that discharge from the tubercles is as rare as it seems to be in the literature. Occasionally, BC arising from areola are described [4], mostly tubular or well-differentiated subtypes (Fig. 11.9).

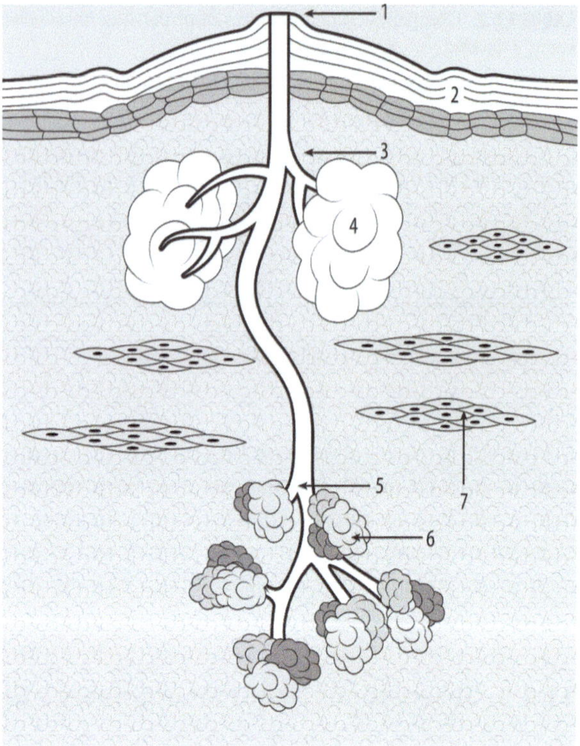


**Fig. 11.6** Schematic diagram of the Montgomery's tubercle and underlying modified sebaceous glands (Montgomery's glands) of the areolar skin. *1* tubercle of Montgomery, *2* areolar epidermis, *3* terminal duct, *4* sebaceous gland, *5* lactiferous duct, *6* mammary lobules, *7* areolar smooth muscle. Rudimentary mammary glands are underneath the areolar smooth muscle; their lactiferous ducts join sebaceous ducts within the areola and terminate at the Montgomery's tubercles (Adapted from Smith et al. [5])

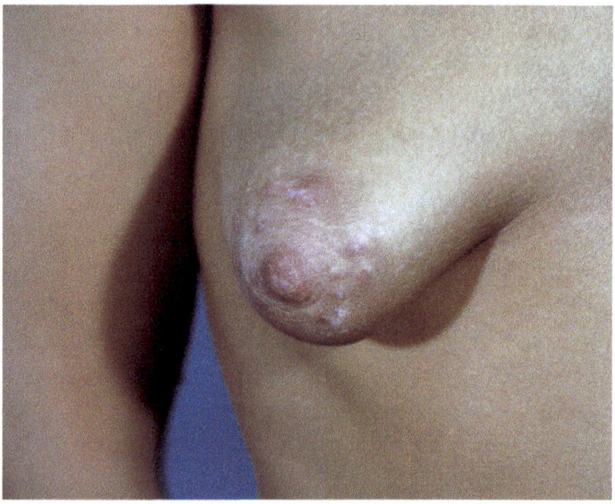

**Fig. 11.7** Several retention cysts of the Montgomery's glands, mostly observed in young women

Bleeding from Montgomery's glands is occasionally seen in young girls and may be confused with bleeding from the nipple. No obvious cause is usually found on biopsy and the bleeding may be due to trauma. For this reason, before surgery a wait-and-see attitude is recommended.

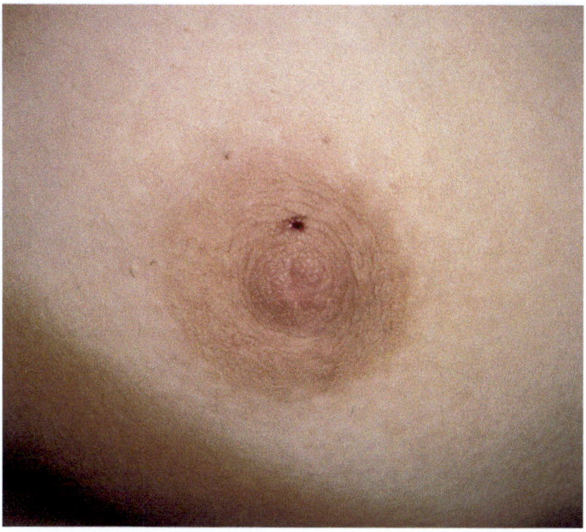

**Fig. 11.8** Bloody discharge from a duct open in the areola

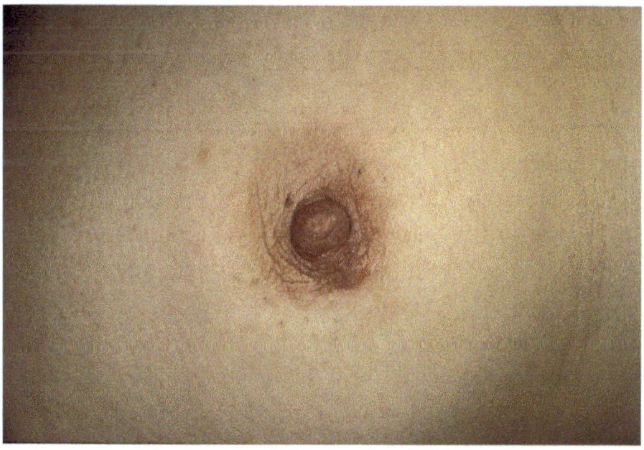

**Fig. 11.9** Very superficial BC, not involving the underlying gland, probably due to cancerisation of rudimentary mammary gland included in Montgomery's glands

Infection of the tubercles may mimic subareolar abscess associated with periductal mastitis and the persisting lesion suggests a mammary duct fistula, although it will present on the areola rather than at the periphery of the areola as occurs with mammary duct fistula.

Histologically, mammary elements of Montgomery's glands are found subject to many of the conditions affecting the breast, including hyperplasia, cyst formation, periductal fibrosis, apocrine metaplasia, as well papillary proliferations and cancer [6].

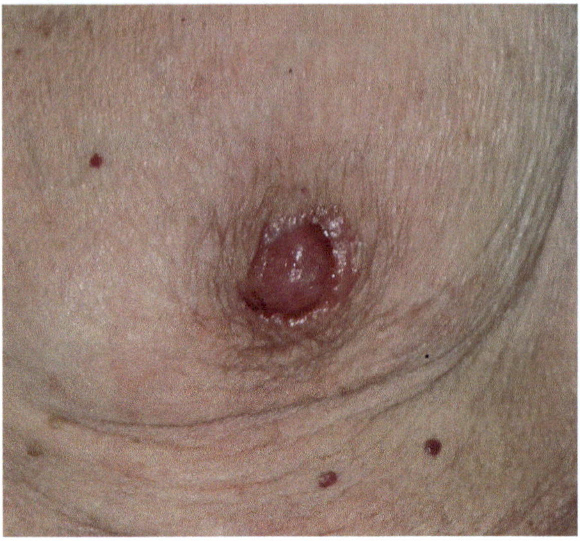

**Fig. 11.10** Nipple dermatitis underlying a nipple crusting

### 11.1.4 Minor Disorders of the Nipple and Areola

*NIPPLE CRUSTING* – Dried-up secretions may accumulate on the nipple's surface, particularly in association with inverted or retracted nipples. Thick secretions can cause the formation of crusts which is easily removable, sometimes accompanied by a modest fibrotic thickening of the dermis or by a real dermatitis (Fig. 11.10). Sometimes crusts hide an underlying nipple lesion such as eczema, Paget's diseases, or nipple adenoma. Having excluded these conditions, no action is required other than reassurance and advice about cleaning the nipple.

*VERRUCOUS NIPPLE* – The nipple and areola may be affected by verrucous change leading to verrucous nipple (or *naevoid hyperkeratosis*), a benign condition of nipple and areola that presents hyperkeratotic thickening with dark pigmentation. This rare condition takes a naevoid form, appearing in young women after puberty and is thought to be related to oestrogens. A similar condition may arise in males having oestrogen treatment for prostatic cancer. A verrucous nipple may cause itching, malodour, and interference with breastfeeding. A number of dermatological measures have been used, but treatment is difficult to assess because of the lack of reports in literature.

*FIBROEPITHELIAL POLYP* – Fibroepithelial polyp is an acrochordon, a usually small, soft, benign, pedunculated neoplasm of the skin. Other synonyms as *soft fibroma* or *pedunculated fibroma* have been used in the literature. Fibroepithelial polyps could be located in many sites of the body, but this rather common condition is found on the nipple and, less frequently, in the areola. They are pedunculated dry

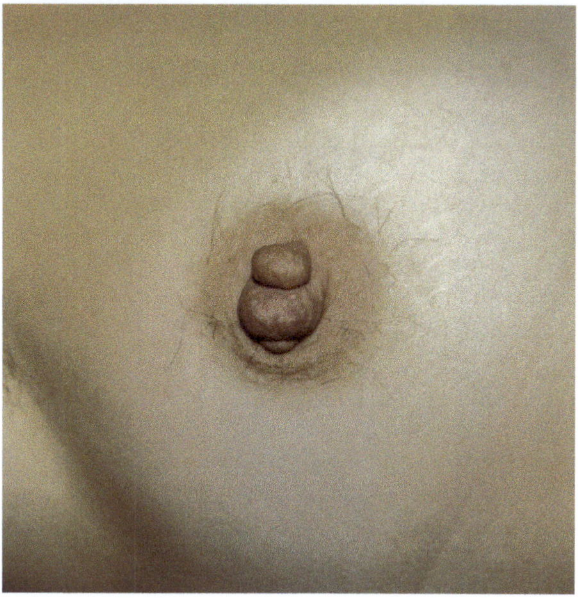

**Fig. 11.11** Pedunculated fibroepithelial polyp of the skin of the nipple, simulating a double nipple

lesions resembling skin tags sometimes so large to look like a double nipple (Fig. 11.11). *Angiofibromas* and *neurofibromas* occurring at this site have the same connotation and are more or less pedunculated. They are readily treated by local excision and do not recur.

*EPIDERMAL CYST.* Two specific types of epidermal cysts are observed within the skin of the nipple or just at the base of the nipple:

- *Superficial epidermal cyst*, clearly visible as a whitish bead of the skin of the nipple that can be only temporarily drained or surgically removed
- *Deep epidermal cyst*, just below the nipple, which corresponds to an inclusion cyst derived from modified sebaceous glands of Montgomery that occasionally flow into the collecting ducts. The second type is very rare and requires a wider excision than the first.

*LEIOMYOMA* – Leiomyoma of the nipple is surprisingly uncommon in view of the large quantities of smooth muscle present. Leiomyomas can be observed also in the areola where smooth muscular fibres are unpredictably well represented (see Fig. 11.6). Leiomyomas can occur at any age and appears as a smooth round lump within the skin of the areola or nipple, usually about 5–7 mm in size, most probably present for years before its detection. A distinction should be made between *superficial leiomyoma*, arising in the smooth muscle of the nipple and areola, and *deep leiomyoma* that arises from smooth muscle associated with blood vessels. If evolving in size, both are adequately treated by limited local excision without consequences.

*PERIMENOPAUSAL NIPPLE PAIN/PARESTHESIA* – Few years before and after the menopausal time, some women describe various sensations of irritation, pricking, and burning in the nipple region. No clear aetiological basis has been enunciated; the most likely explanation relates to the slight periductal inflammatory changes as part of the normal involutional process. Another possible explanation is hormonal imbalance associated with declining ovarian function, since similar nipple sensations may be experienced with hormone administration. Paget's disease must be considered and excluded, since itch, pricking, and irritation are commonly experienced in the early phase of this condition.

*RAYNAUD'S SYNDROME* – Raynaud's syndrome of the nipples causes vasospasm of the nipple, which leads to severe, uncomfortable, burning pain. This condition is characterised by blanching of the nipples, followed by cyanosis and/or erythema after exposure to cold temperatures. Strangely, the affection of the nipples does not seem to be associated with the typical changes of Raynaud's syndrome in the extremities, questioning whether or not it is the same condition.

The pain and throbbing of the nipples associated with Raynaud's phenomenon often mimics fungal infections as candidiasis, so that breastfeeding mothers with Raynaud's of the nipples are often treated inappropriately with topical or systemic antifungal agents.

Reynaud's phenomenon of the nipple is currently recognised as one of the causes of nipple pain during lactation, but it is raising the likelihood that such events may be associated with a previous breast surgery. Some reports refer that, in severe cases, a symptomatic relief could be obtained with calcium channel blockers, as nifedipine.

*COMPLEX REGIONAL PAIN SYNDROME (POSTSURGICAL PAIN)* – It is now recognised that complex regional pain syndrome may affect parts of the body other than the limbs, where it has long been recognised as a reflex sympathetic dystrophy of the causalgia type. Similar changes have been reported in the breast, especially in the nipple area after surgery.

Pain syndrome may appear after major duct excision, but some sporadic cases are reported after nipple-sparing mastectomy or minor surgery. The syndrome is uncommon, and before surgery, patients should be informed for the potential loss of sensitivity of the nipple as a potential complication and of pain syndrome as an exceptional event.

Pain syndrome may be also related to cold. Even though the patient was warmly clothed, the nipples were subjectively intensely cold and objectively so to examination. The attacks gradually abated over a period of 4–5 years. In severe pain, intravenous no selective alpha-adrenergic antagonist, as phentolamine, gave temporary relief, while long-term relief is provided by stellate ganglion blockade.

*NIPPLE RING INFECTIONS* – Nipple rings can cause subareolar breast abscess and recurrent nipple infections, particularly in smokers. In case of simple inflammation without a recognised infection, time of full healing (nipple piercing will take 2–4 months to repair) and metal allergies should be taken in consideration. *Mycobacterium fortuitum* infection should be suspected after nipple piercing if the infection fails to resolve with removal of the piercing and antibiotics directed against

*Staphylococcus aureus*. In recurrent infections, to foster antibiotic selection, a tissue sample rather than a simple swab should be submitted for culture. Rarely, excision of the nipple areolar complex is required to control enduring infection.

*RUNNERS/JOGGERS' NIPPLE* – The nipple is occasionally the site of friction trauma and the condition of runners' (or joggers') nipple is well recognised. This lesion is presumably the result of constant rubbing of an unprotected warm and moist nipple on ill-fitting clothing. It is sometimes severe enough to produce bleeding. Long-distance runners are especially predisposed, because they are exposed to the irritation on the nipple for the greatest period of time especially in hot days. Related conditions are cyclist's nipple due to the combined effects of perspiration and wind-chill producing a cold painful sensation lasting for several days. However, nipple friction is not only suffered by athletes; the inside of a badge, a logo on normal items of clothing, or breastfeeding can also cause the friction which results in this condition.

The condition is easily preventable and treatable with methods including: avoiding the use of loose-fitting T-shirt during exercise, wearing appropriate cotton shirts, applying a waterproof adhesive bandage or a surgical tape to act as a barrier between skin and cloth, and applying an anti-chafing balm or petroleum jelly prior to exercise.

*PILONIDAL SINUS* – Pilonidal sinus abscesses affecting the nipple have been reported in hairdressers and sheep shearers. These infections are a result of small pieces of cut hair that accumulate in the hairdresser's or shearer's clothes. The hairs penetrate the skin and cause inflammation and infection. Wearing closely woven clothing that prevents the passage of hair through clothing can prevent this contact with cut hair.

## 11.2 Other Dermatological Observations

**Clinical Practice Points**

- Dermatological observations of the mammary region are usually part of common systemic dermatitis and may range from simplest to complex or allergic. Depending on the evolving phases, it may be erythematous, oedematous, vesicular, groaning serous fluid, scaling, or – more often – polymorphic.
- Dermatitis is usually bilateral affecting especially the areola and the skin around it, while the nipple is involved to a lesser extent.
- Since most lesions are not painful and not associated with swelling or warmth, a diagnosis may be difficult and, if indicated, a biopsy is needed to support the diagnosis.
- Dermatitis artefacta of the breast is an uncommon expression of an underlying psychological problem.

*CANDIDIASIS* – Nipple pain in a breastfeeding woman may be a presentation of nipple thrush; however, confirmation of the diagnosis is very difficult. Clinical features suggestive of nipple thrush include:

- Pain that gets worse after a breastfeed and increases for up to 2 h
- Thrush, more likely after antibiotic usage, with a history of cracked nipples or a history of this condition
- No pyrexia and no redness so that areola may show no colour loss

Sore nipples are the most common breastfeeding problem in the first few days after birth, and only persistent pain without improvement needs to be evaluated for candidiasis or other possible causes including:

- Eczema of the areola and nipple
- Raynaud's syndrome of the nipple, which presents with typical changes of colour
- Bacterial infection of the nipple, which presents with red, inflamed, cracked nipples with or without exudates or fever

In a prospective cohort study [7] regarding signs and symptoms associated with mammary candidiasis between 2 and 9 weeks postpartum, positive predictive value (PPV) for candida colonisation was highest when there were 3 or more signs or symptoms simultaneously or when flaky or shiny skin of the nipple/areola was reported together or in combination with breast pain:

- Sore + burning + pain + stabbing + skin changes combination had 100 % positive predictive value (PPV).
- Burning + pain + stabbing + skin changes combination had 100 % PPV.
- Pain + stabbing + skin changes combination had 100 % PPV.

Treatment consists in applying miconazole cream after every feed, and remove any residual cream before the next feed. Treatment plan often includes a topical antibiotic ointment because candida of nipples can concurrently present with nipple fissure where *Staphylococcus aureus* could be often present. Also the baby should be treated concurrently, e.g. with nystatin suspension. If there is no improvement after 5 days, the diagnosis may be incorrect and should be re-examined.

*ECZEMA* – Eczema may occur in a form localised mainly or completely to the nipple and areola (Fig. 11.12) and requires to be distinguished from the eczema conditions of Paget's disease (Fig. 11.13) and nipple adenoma (Fig. 11.14) which also have a dried squamous appearance in its pre-ulcerative phase.

Paget's disease and eczema can usually be differentiated on clinical grounds (Table 11.3). In spite of this, Paget's disease is still often neglected because of an erroneous diagnosis of eczema. It is important to think of Paget's disease in every inflammatory condition of the nipple and areola and to be aware of the range of appearances of Paget's disease.

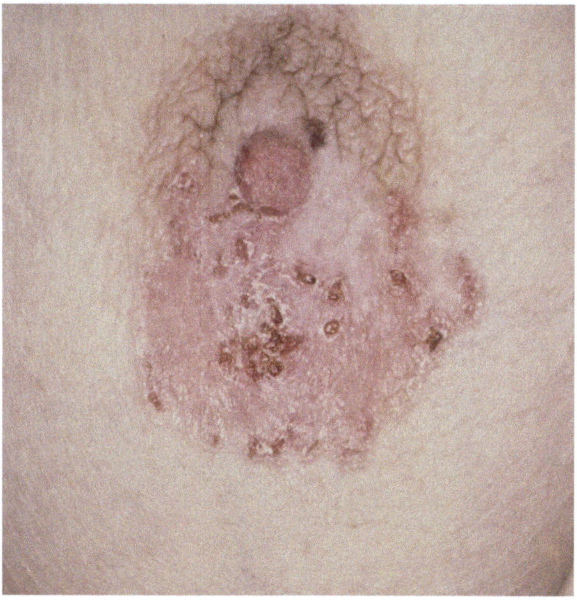

**Fig. 11.12** Eczema of the areola sparing the nipple

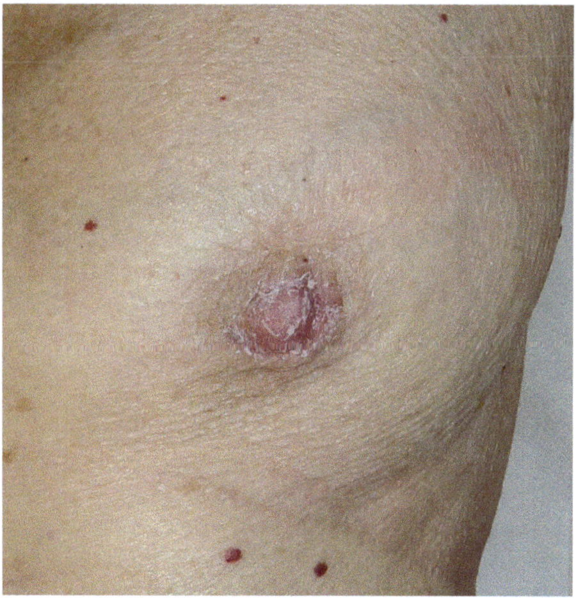

**Fig. 11.13** Paget's disease involving mainly the nipple with early extension to the areola

Usually, in patients with eczema of the nipple and areola, the condition is bilateral, and in many patients there is evidence of eczema elsewhere. When this is not the case, eczema is usually symmetrical and does not extend beyond the areola. The possibility of a factitial syndrome should be considered. Treatment in cases of eczema follows the same guidelines as eczema elsewhere in the body.

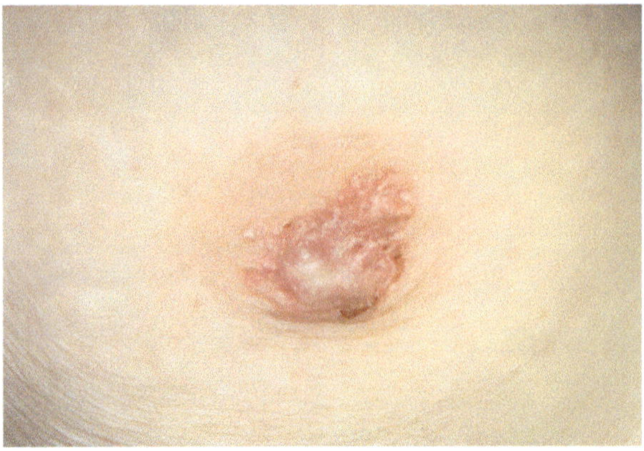

**Fig. 11.14** Nipple adenoma in late stages, with a squamous appearance

**Table 11.3** Clinical features of eczema of the nipple and Paget's disease [1, mod.]

| *Eczema of the nipple* | *Paget's disease* |
|---|---|
| Usually bilateral | Unilateral |
| Intermittent history with rapid evolution | Continuous history with slow steady progression |
| Moist, often with vesicles | Moist or dry, no vesicles |
| Indefinite edge | Irregular but definite edge |
| Nipple may be spared | Nipple always involved, disappears in advanced cases |
| Itching common | Itching common |
| Often history of atopy | Only occasionally a history of atopy |

*HERPES ZOSTER (POSTIRRADIATION)* – Herpes zoster is a viral disease characterised by a painful and blistering eruption in the skin (Fig. 11.15). It represents reactivation of latent varicella zoster virus infection. In high-risk groups such as elderly or immunocompromised patients, the incidence of zoster can be high.

Some reports suggest that radiation therapy is a risk factor for zoster; in fact the skin eruptions are often in or near the radiation treatment field. The diagnosis is typically made through clinical history and exam, but several tests are available to confirm the diagnosis and differentiate it from other infections or dermatitis.

Effective management consists of prompt antiviral medication, acute pain control, appropriate precautions to limit transmission, and referral to specialists in certain cases. Despite appropriate therapy, one out of five patients can develop persistent post-herpetic neuralgia, defined as pain more than 4 months after resolution of the rash. Several classes of pain medication are available to treat acute or long-term pain. Vaccination against zoster should be recommended for patients aged 60 years or older, in order to reduce the incidence and severity of zoster.

*MORPHEA (postirradiation)* – Breast-associated morphea, or localised scleroderma, is an idiopathic, often self-limiting, inflammatory cutaneous disorder that causes fibrotic changes in the skin through an early inflammatory stage followed by sclerosis and subsequent atrophy. The depth of involvement may be superficial

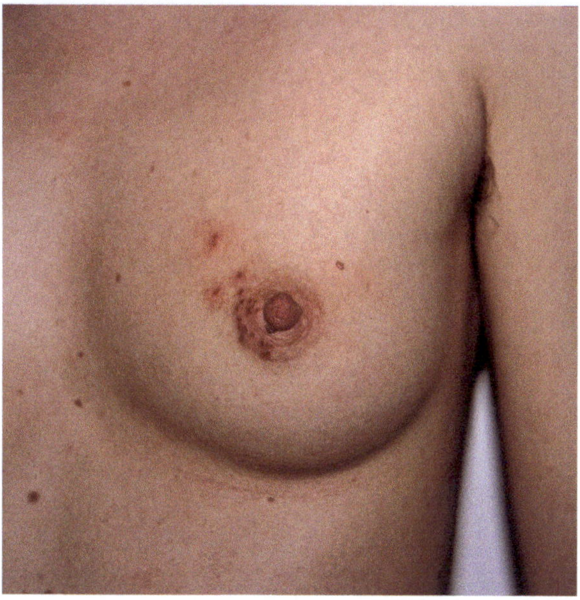

**Fig. 11.15** Herpes zoster of the left mammary region in a young woman, characterised by a painful skin rash with blisters in a limited area, often in a stripe figure

(primarily dermal) or deep (involving the deep dermis plus the subcutaneous tissue and fascia).

Breast-related aetiology includes radiation therapy, trauma, breast implants, and autoimmune disorders following chemotherapy. The interval between completion of radiation treatments and onset of the skin disorder is variable, ranging from 1 month to up 30 years. Post-radiation morphea is still a rare phenomenon and should be kept distinct from radiation-induced dermatitis or radiation-induced fibrosis.

The initial sign of morphea is an unexplained pain or itching at the site of disease followed by an abrupt development of an inflammatory, erythematous patch or oedematous plaque (Fig. 11.16). Sclerosis usually begins in the centre of inflammatory lesions, initially leaving an erythematous or violaceous border. Later, the skin becomes pale and glassy in appearance. The clinical manifestations of postirradiation morphea include moderate-to-severe mixed dermal inflammatory infiltrate, with hyperpigmentation, retraction, skin thickening, and dermal fibrosis extending into the subcutaneous adipose tissue.

*VIRAL INFECTIONS – Molluscum contagiosum* occasionally occurs in the skin of the nipple. Touching the affected skin spreads the virus that causes molluscum from person to person, as well as touching a surface with the virus on it, such as a towel, clothing, or toys. *Molluscum* can be spread from one person to another by sexual contact, just as herpes virus and genital warts of the nipple (*condyloma acuminatum*) that could be occasionally seen.

*STEATOCYSTOMA MULTIPLEX OF THE BREAST* is a rare familial hamartomatous malformation that is characterised by the presence of multiple intradermal cysts. The disease usually appears during adolescence and progresses with age and

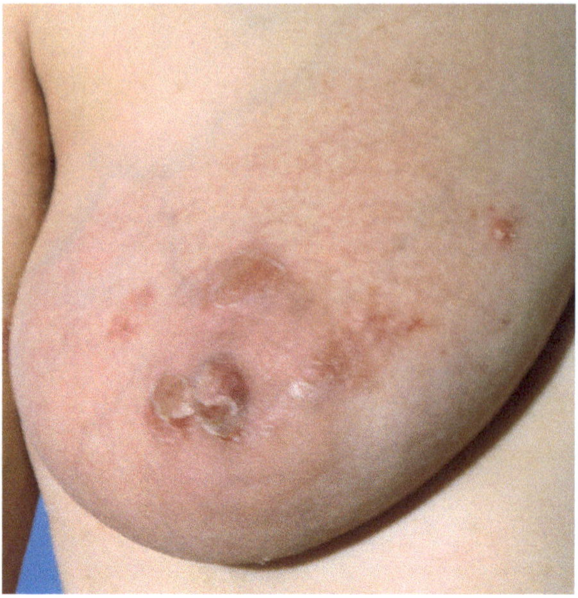

**Fig. 11.16** Bullous morphea of the right mammary region following radiation therapy. Clinical presentations of morphea are various. In this 44-year-old woman, disease is characterised by oedema with surrounding erythema and plaques, some of them with bullous appearance

presents as numerous palpable (usually mobile) intradermal oil cysts ranging from 2 to 20 mm in diameter. The cysts are usually asymptomatic although they can occasionally crack to the skin surface and may become infected.

Mammography shows characteristic subcutaneous oil cysts as multiple, small, round lesions with a circumscribed margin, central fat density, and a peripheral high-density rim. Ultrasound shows multiple nodules that are oval, relatively well circumscribed, and hypo-echoic with posterior enhancement.

*DERMATITIS ARTEFACTA* and *artefactual skin diseases* are intentionally created by the patient, sometimes very clever in producing and perpetuating skin lesions, which are not easy to classify. The diagnosis is difficult to establish but should be considered when the clinical situation does not conform to common appearances of pathological processes, especially in patients who had a history of seeking frequent medical attention.

The patterns include many superficial injures, mostly on the areolar and the nipple area, self-inflicted by the patient, by means of complicated or repetitive actions, for primary or secondary gains. First presentation may occur in adolescence and may continue undetected for many years with a history of multiple visits to both general practitioner and outpatient hospital [8]. Various symptoms are released, as infected lesions or unusual bumps, which may undergo many investigations and occasionally surgical procedures before the nature of the disease is recognised.

The need for a psychodermatology multidisciplinary team to treat some difficult conditions has been jokingly advocated. Psychiatric referral may help in establishing the emotional or psychotic problem that leads to this wilful or subconscious self-neglect. It may occur as a cry for help when emotional stresses become too great to endure. Precipitating events range from simple anxiety to interpersonal conflicts and severe personality disorders, including compulsive behaviour, depression, and psychotic disturbances. Often no obvious psychotic problem is found and there is no recognised effective therapy.

## References

1. Mansel RE, Webster DJT, Sweetland HM. Disorders of the nipple and areola. In: Hughes, Mansel & Webster benign disorders and diseases of the breast. London: Elsevier; 2009.
2. Killelea B, Sowden M. Nipple inversion. http://www.uptodate.com. Accessed 30 Nov 2014.
3. Szczerba SM, Paulius KL, Nadimi S, Maguina P. Wire subcision as a treatment for nipple inversion. Plast Reconstr Surg. 2009;123:206e–7.
4. Dabbs DJ, editor. Breast pathology. Philadelphia: Elsevier; 2012.
5. Smith DM, Peters DG, Donegan WL. Montgomery's areolar tubercle. A light microscopic study. Arch Pathol Lab Med. 1982;106:60–3.
6. Glazebrook KN, Morton MJ, Reynolds C. Carcinoma of the breast mimicking an areolar dermal lesions. J Ultrasound Med. 2007;26:1083–7.
7. Francis-Morril J, Heinig MJ, Pappajanis D, Dewey KG. Diagnostic value of signs and symptoms of mammary candidosis among lactating women. J Hum Lact. 2004;20:288–95.
8. Dixon JM. Breast infection. In: Dixon JM, editor. ABC of breast diseases. 4th ed. Oxford: Wiley-Blackwell; 2012.

## Further Reading

Bengualid V, Singh V, Singh H, Berger J. Mycobacterium fortuitum and anaerobic breast abscess following nipple piercing: case presentation and review of the literature. J Adolesc Health. 2008;42:530–2.

Rodríguez-Pichardo A, Hoffner MV, García-Bravo B, Camacho FM. Dermatitis artefacta of the breast: a retrospective analysis of 27 patients (1976-2006). J Eur Acad Dermatol Venereol. 2010;24:270–4.

Spyropoulou GA, Pavlidis L, Trakatelli M, et al. Rare benign tumours of the nipple. J Eur Acad Dermatol Venereol. 2015;29:7–13.

Val-Bernal JF, Diego C, Rodriguez-Villar D, Garijo MF. The nipple-areola complex epidermis: a prospective systematic study in adult autopsies. Am J Dermatopathol. 2010;32:787–9.

# Staging and Workup of the Noninvasive Breast Cancer

# 12

Virgilio S. Sacchini and David N. Anderson

## Contents



**Abstract**

• Mammography detects approximately one case of ductal carcinoma in situ (DCIS) per 1,300 examinations. Currently DCIS represents about 20–30 % of all breast malignancies. • In ductal carcinoma in situ (DCIS), the risk of systemic disease is virtual, but the real risk is of local recurrence (both in situ and invasive), more frequently in the same breast. • In lobular carcinoma in situ (LCIS), the risk of systemic disease is virtual, but the real risk is the development of multiple invasive lobular BCs with the same occurrence in both breasts.

*Future directions.* DCIS is not a single disease but rather many distinct diseases with different histopathologic and molecular characteristics, a propensity to progress to invasive disease, and differential response to treatment. Advances

V.S. Sacchini (✉) • D.N. Anderson
Breast Service, Department of Surgery, Memorial Sloan-Kettering Cancer Center (MSKCC), New York, NY, USA
e-mail: sacchinv@mskcc.org



A.M. Pluchinotta (ed.), *The Outpatient Breast Clinic: Aiming at Best Practice*,
DOI 10.1007/978-3-319-15907-2_12

in genomics and proteomics may provide improved understanding of the underlying biologic pathways of tumour progression and information to select the most targeted treatment approaches for the management of these lesions.

## 12.1 Ductal Carcinoma In Situ

**Clinical Practice Points**

- Ductal carcinoma in situ (DCIS) is a complex pathological entity, which presents challenges in terms of treatment and also in terms of support to the increasing number of women diagnosed with the condition.
- Localised DCIS can be treated by breast-conserving surgery (BCS) and usually with radiation therapy (RT). For patients with larger areas of DCIS, mastectomy with or without breast reconstruction is effective.
- DCIS treated with BCT should provide clear resection margins. Considering the potential propensity toward longitudinal rather than radial growth, glandular resection should be, if possible, full-depth.
- Factors that influence local recurrence in DCIS after BCS include completeness of excision, radiation therapy, patient age, and histological grade.
- Follow-up of women treated for DCIS is aimed at the early detection of local recurrence or a new contralateral cancer, but not the detection of systemic disease.
- Since most recurrences have a similar pattern to their initial appearance, tumours initially presenting with calcifications usually recur with radiologically detectable calcifications.

### 12.1.1 Overview

*Definition.* Ductal carcinoma in situ (DCIS) is defined as a malignant transformation and proliferation of the cells lining the duct with an intact basal membrane. As there are no blood or lymphatic vessels in the epithelial layer, DCIS, as well as LCIS, theoretically does not cause metastatic spread (Fig. 12.1). DCIS arises from the ductal epithelium in the region of the terminal ductal lobular unit (TDLU) and represents an intermediate step between atypical ductal hyperplasia (ADH) and invasive BC.

Because of the difficulties in separating low-grade DCIS from atypical intraductal hyperplasia, a different classification has been proposed where these proliferations are classified as *ductal intraepithelial neoplasia* (DIN), or also as *mammary intraepithelial neoplasia, ductal type.* The latest WHO Classification of Tumours of the Breast [1] includes this terminology (Table 12.1), however it still needs to be fully clarified. This could be the result of the failure to introduce new diagnostic criteria useful to reduce the inter-observer variability and the diagnostic difficulties between ADH and some cases of low-grade DCIS. Even now, for purposes of clinical management, when the DIN terminology is used, the traditional terminology should be mentioned as well.

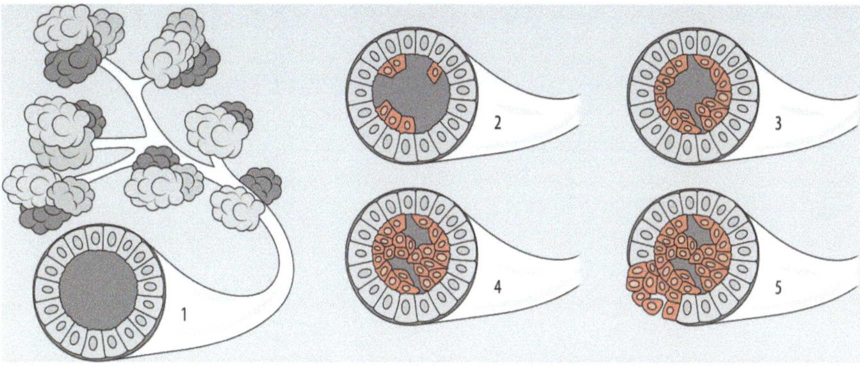


**Fig. 12.1** Breast duct with normal duct cells (*1*), with ductal hyperplasia (*2*), with atypical ductal hyperplasia (*3*), with carcinoma in situ (*4*), and with microinvasive ductal carcinoma (*5*)

**Table 12.1** Classification of DIN in comparison with traditional classification

| Traditional terminology | Ductal intraepithelial neoplasia (DIN) terminology |
|---|---|
| Flat epithelial atypia | *DIN 1a* – ductal intraepithelial neoplasia grade 1a |
| Atypical ductal hyperplasia (ADH) | *DIN 1b* – ductal intraepithelial neoplasia grade 1b |
| Low-grade DCIS (DCIS G1) cribriform or micropapillary | *DIN 1c* – ductal intraepithelial neoplasia grade 1c |
| Intermediate-grade DCIS (DCIS G2) cribriform or micropapillary with necrosis or atypia or other types | *DIN 2* – Ductal intraepithelial neoplasia grade 2 |
| High-grade DCIS (DCIS G3) with or without necrosis (comedo-type DCIS) | *DIN 3* – ductal intraepithelial neoplasia, grade 3 |

This approach obviates the current separation of ADH and low-grade DCIS into two very drastically different categories of noncancer and cancer without interfering with appropriate management of the various lesions. A more extensive use of this separation of terms would have many advantages in communication with the patient. The forms of noncancer would elicit less anxiety by the patient, while the forms of cancer would be considered the way they are perceived, i.e. as invasive.

The above classification (Table 12.1) comprises the traditional DCIS subtypes based primarily on architectural pattern: micropapillary, papillary, solid, cribriform, and comedo. Well-differentiated categories of DCIS are of the non-comedo subtype and poorly differentiated of the comedo subtype (Table 12.2).

*Non-comedo subtypes of DCIS* are low nuclear grade and have a positive ER status (ER+). Mitoses are relatively infrequent and the prognosis is good. In the non-comedo category, cribriform carcinoma has a better prognosis; micropapillary carcinoma has a favourable prognosis, while solid carcinoma is less favourable due to its intermediate grade. The developmental pathways for low- and intermediate-grade DCIS appear different from that for high-grade DCIS.

**Table 12.2** Subtypes of DCIS: histological characteristics, calcifications features, and prognosis

| Subtypes | Grade | Necrosis | Calcification | Prognosis |
|---|---|---|---|---|
| *Comedo* | High | Extensive | Branched | Worse |
| *Intermediate* | Intermediate | Limited | Limited | Favourable |
| *Non-comedo:* | Low | Absent | Inconsistent | Solid: favourable |
| Solid | | | | |
| Micropapillary | | | | Micropapillary: good<br>Cribriform: very good |
| Cribriform | | | | |

*Comedo-type DCIS* has high nuclear grade, shows pleomorphism, and has abundant central luminal necrosis. 80 % of comedo lesions are aneuploid, are ER negative, have a high rate of HER2 overexpression, and express p53 mutations. Moreover, they are associated with greater tumour size, increased incidence of multicentricity and microinvasion, and a higher rate of local recurrence. In conclusion, comedo-type DCIS has a worse prognosis.

DCIS proliferation in the ductal system has a propensity toward longitudinal rather than radial growth. Due to the complexity of its presentations, many terms have been coined to outline the unpredictable localisation, architectural characteristics, invasive potential, and prognostic significance of DCIS.

*Multifocal DCIS.* Multifocality is another important characteristic of a majority of DCIS. Actually, upon closer evaluation by three-dimensional reconstructions of the cross-sectional segments, almost all foci seemingly disconnected are in essence unifocal, harbouring disease arising from convolutions of the same duct system.

Confinement of DCIS to multiple TDLUs (multifocality) without extension into the major duct system would imply an earlier stage in the development and progression of DCIS, but current sampling and processing methods in no way could distinguish multiple TDLU involvement from duct progression. Furthermore, DCIS lesions that have extended some distance toward the nipple are more likely to develop subsequent recurrences or invasive carcinoma compared with those confined to the TDLU. Obviously, it is very important to assess how far along this route (along the major duct and toward the nipple) the DCIS has already extended at the time of initial resection.

*Multicentric DCIS,* on the other hand, refers to foci of disease present in different sectors of the breast arising simultaneously in separate ductal systems. On average, 30 % of cases are believed to be multicentric.

*Microinvasive DCIS* has been defined by the American Joint Committee on Cancer (AJCC) as the extension of cancer cells beyond the basement membrane into adjacent tissues with no focus more than 1 mm in greatest dimension. Lesions fulfilling this criterion are staged as pT1mic, a subset of pT1 BC. It is helpful to consider that in the presence of multiple foci of microinvasion, only the focus with the largest dimension is used to classify the lesion and the sizes of individual foci are not added together. However, this aspect is still controversial.

The importance of the structure and activity of the basement membrane is increasingly recognised – a complex lattice-like structure lying between stroma and epithelium, with a complex paracrine pathway between stromal, myoepithelial, and epithelial cells.

*Extensive intraductal component (EIC)* is referred to invasive BC with an additional extra-tumoural focus of DCIS. EIC is properly defined as intraductal carcinoma occupying more than 25 % of the area encompassed by an invasive tumour and extending beyond the infiltrating edge of the tumour into the surrounding breast tissue.

*Paget disease* (see "Paget Disease", Sect. 14.1) is a less common presentation of BC clinically characterised by eczematous, scaly skin at the nipple-areolar complex. It is associated with underlying (invasive and/or in situ) disease in 97 % of cases; therefore, it is important to consider Paget disease in any patient presenting with a persistent nipple-areolar complex abnormality.

Other considerations about multiple (multifocal and multicentric) BC are discussed in Sect. 15.1.

### 12.1.2 Diagnosis

*Mammography*. DCIS is often detected mammographically as microcalcifications. Currently, about 20–25 % of screening-detected malignancies are DCIS. Calcium deposition usually occurs in the areas of rapid growth and necrosis, leading to its typical mammographic appearance.

In mammograms with high-grade, comedo-type DCIS, calcium depositions resulting from increased necrosis are radiologically intense and often linear and branching. Low- and intermediate-grade DCIS are more likely to be discontinuous with gap areas typically small at <5 mm in 80 % of cases.

*Core or surgical biopsies* are the only reliable means in diagnosing DCIS, while fine-needle aspiration (FNA) should not be performed and moreover cannot distinguish DCIS from invasive carcinoma.

*Frozen section* has no role in the intra-operative diagnosis of non-palpable foci of microcalcifications or in the evaluation of margin status during glandular resection. This approach limits the ability of pathologists to evaluate the lesion overall.

*Histology*. DCIS may appear in different histological variants with specific cytonuclear, architectural, and molecular pathological features that can be recognised only by an expert histologist. The main differences between DCIS and infiltrating carcinoma are the disruption of the basal membrane and the way DCIS preserves the ductal/lobular anatomy.

DCIS accounts for about 80–85 % of non-invasive carcinomas. Lobular carcinoma in situ is not only less common (about 15–20 %) but also has different characteristics as compared to DCIS (Table 12.3).

### 12.1.3 Treatment

The great pathologist David Page, in one of his most popular paper (1996), defined DCIS as *understanding the misunderstood stepchild (that) has lagged behind our understanding of other elements of breast cancer.* Although non-invasive, it is clearly a malignant disease and recurs in about 33 % of cases within 10–13 years if treated with excisional biopsy alone. The recurrence, if it occurs, is invasive carcinoma in 50 % of

**Table 12.3** Features of ductal and lobular carcinoma in situ

| | DCIS | LCIS |
|---|---|---|
| Average age | Late 50s | Late 40s |
| Menopausal status | 70 % postmenopausal | 70 % premenopausal |
| Clinical signs | Breast mass or not, Paget disease, nipple discharge | None |
| Mammographic signs | Microcalcifications | None |
| Biomarkers | Comedo-type: ER negative, HER2 positive, high Ki67 | ER-positive, HER2 negative, low Ki67 |
| Risk of subsequent carcinoma | 30–50 % at 10–20 years | 25–30 % at 15–20 years |
| Site of subsequent invasive carcinoma | Same breast 99 % | Same breast 50–60 % |
| | Contralateral breast 1 % | Contralateral breast 40–50 % |

Adapted from Bundred et al. [2], with permission

cases. When axillary node dissection has been performed, metastases have been found in <3 % of DCIS cases. When mastectomy has been performed, the disease is often found to be multicentric (additional CIS lesions >2 cm away from the main lesion).

*SURGERY*. Surgical treatment of DCIS is aimed to achieve tumour-free margins. To reach this goal, all requirements related to the treatment of invasive cancer are applicable to DCIS, in particular:

- Optimal imaging, including magnification views in cases of microcalcifications
- Preoperative diagnosis of microcalcifications or density by histological core needle biopsy stereotaxis or ultrasound guided
- If necessary, discussion of the patient with the multidisciplinary team
- Guide localisation preceding any surgery of a clinically occult lesion
- Surgical resection targeted to at least 1 mm tumour-free margin
- Specimen radiography after diagnostic and/or therapeutic excisional surgery
- Marking of the specimen after excision to guide the pathologist
- Diagnostic workup by the pathologist according to established guidelines

Complete excision of DCIS is the ultimate goal in management of DCIS. Surgery must also consider that the distribution of DCIS is usually segmental and grows toward the nipple and that biopsies should be done by the surgeon in the shape of a cone and toward the nipple [3]. Moreover, the potential propensity toward longitudinal rather than radial growth should be considered; therefore, glandular resection should be full-depth.

Although it is accepted that the duct system forms segments represented by the branching of a major lactiferous duct, there is no proof that each segment is encased in a fibrous or fascial capsule. For this reason, surgeons cannot identify a mammary segment during operation, and they are obliged to focus their attention on removal of the areas of mammographically detected density or microcalcification. Nonetheless, attempts can and should be made to remove the lesion in a more or less conical shape along the segmental route of possible extension toward the nipple (Fig. 12.2). The resected specimen should have sutures identifying the direction of

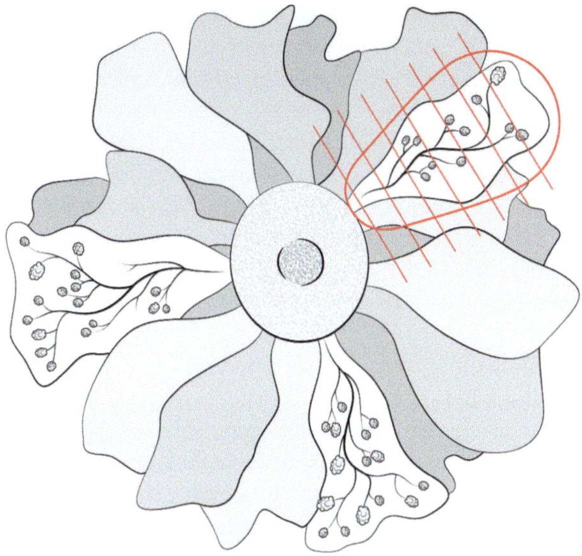

**Fig. 12.2** Graphic representation of the segmental distribution of mammary duct system, optimal conical excision of a segment involved by DCIS with the tip of the cone pointing toward the nipple, and optimal orientation and serial sectioning of the excised sample from the periphery toward the nipple (Adapted from Tavassoli [3]). This drawing also depicts as ductal-lobular segmental units radiate from the nipple in an unevenly and sometimes unpredictable arrangement

the nipple and the superior, anterior, and lateral margins. Regardless of their precise shape, these samples should be serially sectioned toward the direction of the nipple to evaluate the extent of the lesion's spread from the TDLU(s) of origin.

For all patients treated with BCS for DCIS, a minimum of 1 mm radial margin of excision, based on pathological examination (no malignant cells at the inked border), is recommended. Only if the excisional margin is less than 1 mm at the fibro-glandular border of the breast (i.e. skin or chest wall) the re-excision is not indicated.

If resection margins are involved, a re-excision guided by post-operative mammography (and if necessary again a guide-wire localisation) should be attempted. When a re-excision will result in poor cosmesis, a mastectomy (with or without reconstruction) should be considered and offered. If, on basis of mammographic findings, DCIS is considered to be too large for breast conservation (usually exceed ing a 3 cm area of microcalcifications), immediate mastectomy with or without reconstruction should be discussed.

Since BCS should be followed by a RT in almost all cases, mastectomy may be the preferred treatment if:

- DCIS presents multicentric or widely multifocal.
- Failure to achieve adequate margins on attempted surgical biopsy.
- The breast has previously received RT.
- The patient has scleroderma or another connective tissue disease, which can contraindicate RT.
- The patient lives in an area where RT is inaccessible or inconvenient.

High cellular grade is more common in DCIS than in invasive BC, but this factor does not contraindicate BCS. Moreover, in women under 40 years, this higher risk of local recurrence is not a contraindication to BCS.

*Surgery of the axilla*. In planning BCS, SLN biopsy should not be performed routinely in patients with a preoperative diagnosis of DCIS without suspicion of invasion. Nevertheless, patients with a mass on clinical examination or mammogram suggesting an increased risk of invasive or microinvasive disease should have SLN biopsy at the time of definitive operative procedure. In addition, SLN biopsy should be performed in all patients undergoing mastectomy, since mastectomy precludes SLN biopsy in the event invasive disease is subsequently discovered.

*Surgical*. A summary of quality objectives and outcome measures to follow in patients with DCIS have been drawn up by the British Association of Surgical Oncology (BASO) [4].

- *Informed options*. When appropriate, patients should be given an informed choice between BCS and mastectomy. This includes the difference in local recurrence rates between the two approaches. All patients undergoing mastectomy (by choice or on advice) should have the opportunity to discuss breast reconstruction options and have immediate breast reconstruction if appropriate. If breast conservation or breast reconstruction is not offered, the reasons should be documented in the medical record.
- *Specimen radiography*. To ensure adequate assessment of surgical excision of DCIS treated by BCS, intra-operative specimen radiography should be carried out for all cases. All specimens must be marked by the surgeon according to local protocols to allow orientation by the reporting pathologist.
- *Ink-free margin*. To ensure adequate surgical excision of DCIS treated by BCS, all patients should have their tumours removed with no evidence of disease at the microscopic radial margins. If the margin of excision is deemed to be inadequate, further surgery to obtain clear margins should be recommended.
- *Number of operations*. To minimise the number of therapeutic operations in women undergoing BCS for DCIS, as standard at least 95 % of patients should have three or fewer operations, while an optimum target should be all patients have less than three operations.
- *Recurrence*. To minimise local recurrence after BCS for DCIS, patients with extensive (>30–40 mm diameter in relation to glandular volume) or multicentric disease should usually undergo treatment by mastectomy.
- *Axillary surgery*. To minimise morbidity from axillary surgery, axillary staging surgery is not routinely recommended for patients being treated for DCIS alone. It may be considered in patients considered high risk of occult invasive disease. Axillary node dissection (AND) is contraindicated in patients with DCIS alone.

*RADIATION THERAPY* (RT) after wide excision reduces the risk of local invasive and non-invasive recurrences. Four randomised trials show that adjuvant RT significantly reduces the risk of in-breast tumour recurrence by 50 % or greater compared to excision alone. However, treating all women who undergo wide excision for DCIS with adjuvant RT may be overtreatment for some. The majority of cases of DCIS do not recur when treated with excision alone, and there may be subgroups of patients with DCIS in whom the risk of local recurrence is so low that RT may be of no benefit. The difficulty, however, is in reliably predicting those patients who would not recur in the absence of RT. Therefore, radiotherapy should always be discussed with the patient who desires to conserve her breast after complete excision of DCIS.

The NSABP B-17 trial randomised 818 women with DCIS treated by lumpectomy to no further therapy or breast RT [5]. The trial demonstrated a reduction in ipsilateral recurrence (invasive plus non-invasive) from 27 to 12 % with the use of RT at 8 years of follow-up. Half of the ipsilateral breast tumour recurrences were invasive for those who did not receive radiation. RT reduced the incidence of all non-invasive tumours from 13 to 8 % and of all invasive tumours from 13 to 3 %.

Equally, the European Cooperative Group Study randomised 1,010 women to receive either RT or observation following surgery. The relapse rate was 16 % without RT and 9 % with RT [6]. The benefit of RT for DCIS was also shown in other meta-analysis of RT compared to no further treatment following excision. In addition, the reduction in the risk of a local recurrence of RT appears to be long lasting, though this is not associated with a survival advantage. This was shown in a report of the long-term follow-up of the National Surgical Breast and Bowel Project Trial B-17 [6]. At 15 years, compared to excision alone, RT resulted in:

- A significantly lower rate of ipsilateral invasive recurrence (8.9 versus 19.4 %)
- Similar overall survival (83 versus 84 %) and cumulative all-cause mortality rate through 15 years

However, as mentioned before, although the decrease in the risk of local recurrence by RT is evident in all subtypes of DCIS, in some patients with low-risk DCIS (tumour size <10 mm, low/intermediate nuclear grade, adequate surgical margins), the risk of local recurrence following excision only is so low that omitting radiation may be an option (LoE IV, C). In this case, the annual recurrence rate amounts to >1 %. Randomised data on additional dose to the tumour bed (boost) are lacking, but a boost can be considered, for patients at higher risk for local failure (LoE III, B), APBI should only be carried out within a clinical trial [6].

*ENDOCRINE THERAPY.* For ER-positive patients treated with BCS, hormonal therapy for 5 years reduces the rate of subsequent in-breast tumour recurrence (IBTR) and the rate of contralateral BC. Adjuvant tamoxifen, if not contraindicated, is the first choice. Improved results are achieved with extended hormonal treatment with an AI following completion of 5 years of tamoxifen. The benefit of extended endocrine therapy is reduction in the incidence of IBTR and also reduction of the rate of contralateral BC. For patients with positive receptor status who undergo mastectomy, hormonal therapy is not mandatory, unless to reduce the risk of contralateral BC in high-risk patients [7].

Data from the NSABP B-24 trial involved 1,804 women who had lumpectomy and RT and were randomised to receive either tamoxifen (20 mg/day for 5 years) or placebo [8]. The cumulative incidence of breast cancer events was 8 and 13 %, respectively. These data, re-elaborated in 2012, show:

- ER was positive in 76 % of patients.
- Patients with ER-positive DCIS treated with tamoxifen (versus placebo) showed significant decreases in subsequent BC at 10 years and overall follow-up, which remained significant in multivariable analysis.

- Results were similar, but less significant, when subsequent ipsilateral and contralateral, invasive and non-invasive, BCs were considered separately.
- No significant benefit was observed in ER-negative DCIS.
- PR and either receptor were positive in 66 and 79 % of patients, respectively, and in general, neither was more predictive than ER alone.

The data support the use of adjuvant tamoxifen for treatment of ER-positive DCIS. The use of adjuvant tamoxifen for ER-positive DCIS, however, must be carefully weighed against the known toxicities of the drug because there was no survival benefit.

### 12.1.4 Recurrence

Although radiotherapy reduces tumour recurrences following BCS, there is still an overall recurrence rate of between 3 and 13 % at 5 years, and 50 % of which are invasive disease. Risk factors for IBTR are discussed in, Sect. 15.1. In general, poor clinical prognostic factors include younger age at diagnosis (<40 years) and presentation with a palpable mass. Histological poor prognostic factors include high-grade, noticeably present comedo necrosis, HER2 overexpression, and negative receptor status. Tumour size is considered a not significant factor [9].

A new tool to provide individualized estimates of the risk of local recurrence in women treated by breast conservation alone is represented by Oncotype DX DCIS. This is a 12-panel gene test with a scoring system that categorizes DCIS as low, intermediate, or high risk for local recurrence over 10 years following treatment with breast-conserving surgery alone. The DCIS Score can be used for discussions between patients and physicians to decide upon a course of further treatment, as radiation therapy. Hopefully this will improve individualized management of DCIS and reduce over-treatment of women at low risk of recurrence and reduce under-treatment of women at higher risk of recurrence.

A review of DCIS recurrences and their primary lesions from the EORTC 10,853 trial [6] found concordant histology (similar grade) in 62 % of cases and identical marker expression (ER, PR, HER2, and P53) in 63 % of both invasive and non-invasive recurrences. This high percentage of tumours with identical receptor profiles indicates that it is likely that residual disease after initial treatment recurs as detectable DCIS or progresses to invasive cancer.

After BCT for DCIS, patients should be followed carefully with at least annual mammography. It should be kept in mind that DCIS is a potentially curable disease by mastectomy, while BCT should carry a very limited risk for the development of invasive cancer. The outcome measures should be [10]:

- The breast relapse rate (invasive cancer) after BCT for DCIS should be less than 10 % at 10 years.
- The chest wall relapse rate after mastectomy for DCIS should be less than 5 % at 10 years.

## 12.2 Lobular Carcinoma In Situ

**Clinical Practice Points**

- Lobular carcinoma in situ (LCIS) continues to give significant difficulties in screening, diagnosis, assessment, and treatment.
- LCIS is generally considered a risk indicator, conferring an increased rate of developing invasive carcinoma of about 1–2 % per year with a lifetime risk of 20–30 %.
- Since most LCIS presents without specific abnormalities and calcifications on mammography, its discovery is often an incidental microscopic finding.
- Close radiological follow-up of women diagnosed with LCIS is indicated due to the increased risk of ipsilateral and contralateral invasive BC.
- In planning patient follow-up, the extended time span may have significant implications in communication. Moreover, chemoprevention with tamoxifen or raloxifene in postmenopausal women should be considered in select patients.

**Table 12.4** Proposed terminology of Lobular intraepithelial neoplasia (LIN) in comparison with conventional classification [10]

| Conventional terminology | LIN terminology |
|---|---|
| Atypical lobular hyperplasia (ALH) | *LIN 1* – lobular intraepithelial neoplasia grade 1 |
| *Classic*-type LCIS | *LIN 2* – lobular intraepithelial neoplasia grade 2 |
| High-grade or *pleomorphic*-type LCIS | *LIN 3* – lobular intraepithelial neoplasia grade 3 |

Note that the more common terminology of Lobular neoplasia (LN) include atypical lobular neoplasia and lobular carcinoma in situ. Pleomorphic lobular carcinoma in situ is considered a subtype of LN that has high-grade nuclei.

### 12.2.1 Overview

While we have known of LCIS for several decades, it continues to pose significant difficulties in screening, diagnosis, management, and treatment. This is partly due to its multifocal and bilateral presentation, incomplete understanding of its biology and natural history, and potential perpetuation of misconceptions gathered over the last decades.

*Definition.* Similar to DCIS, the difficulties in separating atypical hyperplasia from intermediate and high-grade categories in LCIS have led to these proliferations being classified as *lobular intraepithelial neoplasia* (LIN). The classification below (Table 12.4) distinguishes atypical lobular hyperplasia (LIN1), intermediate grade as "classic" type (LIN2), and high grade as "pleomorphic" type (LIN3). However, before reaching a final agreement, further pathological aspects need to be clarified. Even now as with DIN, when LIN terminology is used, the traditional terminology should be mentioned as well.

LCIS is five times less common than DCIS; however, recent literature suggests the incidence in postmenopausal women is increasing. In the literature, the diagnosis of LCIS is most frequent in women aged 40–50 years, a decade earlier than DCIS.

Calculating the true incidence of LCIS has always proved difficult, as there are no specific clinical abnormalities. In particular, there is no palpable mass, and most (but not all) LCIS is not associated with microcalcifications; thus, it is often undetectable by mammography. The diagnosis of LCIS is therefore often made as an incidental, microscopic finding in breast biopsy performed for other indications. For these reasons, the true incidence of LCIS in the general population is unknown, and many asymptomatic women presumably go undiagnosed.

A finding of LCIS should mandate more sections in order to exclude invasive lobular carcinoma, which is present in 5–15 % of all cases. LCIS is usually multifocal and shows a solid proliferation of uniform small cells within multiple breast lobules and occasionally in ducts; cells have small, uniform nuclei leading to dilatation of the involved acini of the lobules and loss of cohesion. Typically LCIS is ER positive, does not overexpress HER2, and has a very low proliferative rate expressed as Ki67.

In addition to being multifocal, LCIS is bilateral in a large percentage of cases. Over 50 % of patients diagnosed with LCIS show multiple distant foci in the ipsilateral breast, and roughly 30 % of patients have further LCIS in the contralateral breast. Such multifocality in a clinically non-detectable lesion is one of the reasons why planning subsequent management has proven problematic and contentious.

*LCIS as a risk indicator and a potential precursor.* LCIS has generally been considered a risk indicator, a marker of increased risk, conferring an increased rate of subsequent development of invasive carcinoma of about 1–2 % per year, with a lifetime risk of 20–30 %. This means one-third of women with LCIS would probably develop carcinoma with long-term follow-up, and the risks remain high for at least 20 years [11].

Women <40 years have the highest relative risk of developing invasive cancer. The risk decreases with increasing age at diagnosis, unless another incidental second biopsy is positive for LCIS during follow-up.

The literature suggests the risk for invasive carcinoma is greater for pleomorphic LCIS than classic LCIS. It has been documented that the relative risk for development of subsequent cancer is different in women diagnosed with ALH compared with LCIS. Patients diagnosed with ALH have a four to five times higher risk than the general population (i.e. women of comparable age who had a breast biopsy performed with no atypical proliferative disease). This relative risk appears to double to eight to ten times for LCIS. Although LIN is a helpful term for collectively describing this group of lesions, specific classification into ALH and LCIS may still be justified or preferable in terms of risk stratification and management decisions.

The development of contralateral BC is three times more likely in patients diagnosed with LCIS than in those without LCIS. The risk for development of BC is bilateral, and it was a common belief that this risk was equal for both breasts. However, more recent studies demonstrate carcinoma is three times more likely to develop in the ipsilateral compared with the contralateral breast, supporting the view that ALH and LCIS act both as precursor lesions and as risk indicators.

Both invasive ductal and lobular carcinoma occur with LCIS, a fact that some have used to suggest that LCIS is not a true precursor lesion. However, the incidence of invasive lobular carcinoma occurring with LCIS is significantly greater than without. The coexistence of DCIS and LCIS may explain the ductal component observed, whereby DCIS and not LCIS is the likely precursor lesion.

In one 775-patient study, Bratthauer and Tavassoli [10] report clinical implications of LCIS by utilising the DIN/LIN terminology. The frequency of associated invasive carcinomas (ductal and lobular) increased from 14 % in LIN 1 to 23 % in LIN 3. Remarkably, while the frequency of invasive lobular carcinoma increased dramatically from 11 % in LIN 1 to 86 % in LIN 3, the frequency of invasive ductal carcinoma markedly decreased with advancing grade of LIN from 89 % in LIN 1 to 14 % in LIN 3. This is the reason why an excisional biopsy should be performed when LIN 3 is observed in a core biopsy. Moreover, based on the higher frequency of invasive lobular carcinoma associated with LIN 3, biopsies with LIN 3 should be evaluated diligently for the presence of an associated invasive lobular carcinoma. According to the authors, the high frequency of DIN associated with LIN might suggest that the subsequent invasive ductal carcinomas originate from the associated DIN and that some of this may represent a different phenotype of the same cells that form the LIN lesion. It is also possible that the neoplastic cells may reflect or retain stem cell characteristics with plasticity and the capacity to attain or progress into either a ductal or lobular invasive phenotype.

Finally, the association of LCIS and lobular invasive cancer in those with a positive family history of BC has been clinically documented. However, up to date, any predisposition gene has been identified, and the current literature does not support a significant role for germ line mutations in BRCA1/2 or E-cadherin in its pathogenesis [12].

### 12.2.2 Diagnosis

The majority of women with a primary diagnosis of LCIS are premenopausal, 35–55 years old, and different patterns of fibrocystic changes have been found associated with LCIS in this population. Since most LCIS does not present as a mass nor contain microcalcifications, mammography and ultrasound do not appear to have a role in prospective detection of LCIS. Only in some cases will pleomorphic LCIS show microcalcifications that could be more easily picked up because of their similarities in presentation with DCIS [12]. Rarely LCIS is associated with contrast enhancement on MRI and may be visible, but this is usually masked by enhancement secondary to concomitant fibrocystic change. In conclusion, a reliable diagnosis may not be possible even with MRI.

Radiology, however, may have a role in subsequent surveillance of patients following a diagnosis of LCIS, to identify either other pre-invasive lesions such as DCIS or the invasive carcinoma for which the patient would be at risk. In particular, this may be important in high-risk women with a positive family history of BC. Although there are no data available on systematic randomised clinical trials regarding the efficacy of radiologic follow-up in women diagnosed with LCIS and it is not known whether it will improve the outcome of women who develop subsequent invasive BC, it seems reasonable to suggest at least the same degree of surveillance as is recommended in women at average risk.

Accordingly, women who are diagnosed with LCIS should undergo annual bilateral mammography; in women with dense breasts and a genetically increased risk, additional screening breast ultrasound should be considered. Whether high risk or not, women diagnosed with LCIS should undergo MRI for intensified surveillance if possible within one of the current European clinical trials (e.g. MARIBS).

### 12.2.3 Treatment

*Observation* is the preferred treatment for LCIS casually found in an excisional biopsy. Patients with pure LCIS following wide excisional biopsy shouldn't undergo further surgery. LCIS at margins should be reported, but surgical negative margins are not required, since it is presumed to be a multicentric lesion.

*Surgery* depends on the associated pathology, and pathological reporting and management based on excisional specimens is controversial.

- If the diagnosis of pleomorphic LCIS is in core biopsy and other high-grade lesions are associated with it, further surgery is recommended.
- If LCIS seen in an excisional biopsy is associated with lesions and/or a mass lesion on radiology and/or radiological-pathological discordance, patients should undergo further surgery.
- If LCIS associated with an invasive carcinoma is at the margins, no further excision is required if the invasive cancer is completely excised. It is important the multidisciplinary team and clinicians involved in the case understand the implications of such findings and do not over interpret this information in terms of requirement for further excision, which is not indicated in the majority of cases.

*Radiation therapy*. The literature on the use of RT for LCIS is limited, and currently there is little data to recommend its application in the management of LCIS. Therefore, in women diagnosed with LCIS, there is no role for radiation therapy or chemotherapy.

*Endocrine therapy.* Data from the National Surgical Adjuvant Breast Project (NSABP) show up to 50 % reduction in invasive cancer from in situ carcinoma after endocrine therapy [13]. Currently, the duration of treatment and long-term outcome data are pending.

- If a woman with invasive and coexistent LCIS chooses breast conservation as her surgical treatment option, some investigators consider tamoxifen indicated for the prevention of a second primary, regardless of the hormonal receptor status of the invasive cancer.

- If observation is the treatment option chosen, strong consideration should be given to chemoprevention with tamoxifen. Raloxifene may also be considered for postmenopausal women.

*Prophylactic simple or bilateral mastectomy,* usually with immediate reconstruction, is not justified, although it could be considered in high-risk patients (e.g. with family positive history) or if the patient has decided to have surgery (see 'High-Risk Woman', Sect. 2.3).

## References

1. Lakhani, SR, Ellis. IO, Schnitt, SJ, Tan, PH, van de Vijver M.J. WHO Classification of Tumours of the Breast (4th edition). Lyon: IARC Press, 2012.
2. Bundred N, Dixon JM. Carcinoma in situ. In: Dixon JM, editor. ABC of breast diseases. 4th ed. Oxford: Wiley-Blackwell; 2012.
3. Tavassoli FA. Ductal carcinoma in situ: introduction of the concept of ductal intraepithelial neoplasia. Mod Pathol. 1998;11:140–54.
4. Association of Breast Surgery at BASO. Surgical guidelines for the management of breast cancer. Eur J Surg Oncol. 2009;35(Suppl1):1–22.
5. Fisher ER, Dignam J, Tan-Chiu E, et al. Pathological finding from the National Surgical Adjuvant Breast Project (NSABP) eight-year update of Protocol B-17: intraductal carcinoma. Cancer. 1999;86:429–38.
6. Julien JP, Bijker N, Fentiman IS, et al. Radiotherapy in breast-conserving treatment for ductal carcinoma in situ: first results of the EORTC randomised phase III trial 10853. Lancet. 2000;355:528–33.
7. Wapnir IL, Dignam JJ, Fisher B, et al. Long-term outcomes of invasive ipsilateral breast tumor recurrences after lumpectomy in NSABP B-17 and B-24 randomized clinical trials for DCIS. J Natl Cancer Inst. 2011;103:478.
8. Allred DC, Anderson SJ, Paik S, et al. Adjuvant tamoxifen reduces subsequent breast cancer in women with estrogen receptor-positive ductal carcinoma in situ: a study based on NSABP protocol B-24. J Clin Oncol. 2012;30:1268–73.
9. Barbes NLP, Bundred NJ. Treatment of ductal carcinoma in situ. In: Dixon JM, editor. Breast surgery. London: Elsevier; 2014.
10. Bratthauer GL, Tavassoli FA. Lobular intraepithelial neoplasia: previously unexplored aspects assessed in 775 cases and their clinical implications. Virchows Arch. 2002;440:134–8.
11. Rutgers EJTH, on behalf of EUSOMA Group. Quality control in the locoregional treatment of breast cancer. Eur J Cancer. 2001;37:447–53.
12. Lakhani SR, Audretsch W, Cleton-Jensen AM, et al. The management of lobular carcinoma in situ (LCIS). Is LCIS the same as ductal carcinoma in situ (DCIS)? Eur J Cancer. 2006;42:2205–11.
13. Fisher ER, Costantino J, Fisher B, et al. Pathologic findings from the National Surgical Adjuvant Breast Project (NSABP) Protocol B-17. Five-year observations concerning lobular carcinoma in situ. Cancer. 1996;78:1403–16.

## Further Reading

Anderson BO, Calhoun KE, Rosen EL. Evolving concepts in the management of lobular neoplasia. J Natl Compr Canc Netw. 2006;4:511–22.

Bleicher RJ. Ductal carcinoma in situ. Surg Clin North Am. 2013;93:393–410.

Collins LC, Achacoso N, Haque R, et al. Risk factors for non-invasive and invasive local recurrence in patients with ductal carcinoma in situ. Breast Cancer Res Treat. 2013;139:453–60.

Georgian-Smith D, Lawton TJ. Calcifications of lobular carcinoma in situ of the breast: radiologic-pathologic correlation. AJR Am J Roentgenol. 2001;176:1255–9.

Lagios MD, Silvestein MJ. Ductal carcinoma in situ: recent history and areas of controversy. of ductal carcinoma in situ by oncotype Dx technology: some concerns. Breast J. 2015;21:21–6.

NCCN Guidelines Version 3.2013 Ductal carcinoma in situ. www.nccn.org/professionals/physician_gls/pdf/breast.pdf. Accessed 30 Jan 2015.

Nicholson S, Hanby A, Clements K, et al. on behalf of Sloane Project Steering Group. Variations in the management of the axilla in screen-detected Ductal Carcinoma In Situ: Evidence from the UK NHS Breast Screening Programme audit of screen detected DCIS. Eur J Surg Oncol. 2015;41:86–93

Petrelli F, Barni S. Tamoxifen added to radiotherapy and surgery for the treatment of ductal carcinoma in situ of the breast: a meta-analysis of 2 randomized trials. Radiother Oncol. 2011;100:195–9.

Siziopikou KP. Ductal carcinoma in situ of the breast: current concepts and future directions. Arch Pathol Lab Med. 2013;137:462–6.

Vargas AC, Lakhani SR, Simpson PT. Pleomorphic lobular carcinoma of the breast: molecular pathology and clinical impact. Future Oncol. 2009;5:233–43.

**Websites in Appendix**: search *DCIS* and/or LCIS in *Main Health Professional Websites*, A-1.

# Staging and Workup of Invasive Breast Cancer

# 13

Virgilio S. Sacchini and Alfonso M. Pluchinotta

## Contents



**Abstract**

• Breast cancer (BC) *is a* heterogeneous disease, comprising multiple entities associated with distinctive *histological* and *biological* features. • The heterogeneity may be decreased after stratifications by grade (especially for grade I and III tumours) or by ER/PR status; however, one *residual* unpredictable heterogeneity is still observed. • Among predictive factors, also race and cancer subtype could play a modifying role.

V.S. Sacchini (✉)
Breast Service, Department of Surgery, Memorial Sloan-Kettering Cancer Center (MSKCC), New York, NY, USA
e-mail: sacchinv@mskcc.org

A.M. Pluchinotta
Breast Surgery, Policlinic of Abano Terme, Padova, Italy
e-mail: pluchinotta.alfonso@gmail.com





A.M. Pluchinotta (ed.), *The Outpatient Breast Clinic: Aiming at Best Practice*,
DOI 10.1007/978-3-319-15907-2_13

*Future directions.* In theory, understanding which genes are amplified, which are deleted, and which are mutated in the BC cells provides the base for a rational, tailored medical treatment. Further studies on sources of still unknown heterogeneity of genetic/epigenetic characteristics could lead to a more stratification rather than unification of breast cancer assessment and treatment.

## 13.1 Pathology of Invasive Breast Cancer

**Clinical Practice Points**

- Approximately two of every three patients with invasive BC have a no special type (NST) carcinoma. Special types of BC are less common with a better (e.g. cribriform type) or worse (e.g. metaplastic type) prognosis.
- In some cases, a single BC can be a combination of these types (e.g. ductal and lobular BC) or be a mixture of invasive and in situ cancer (e.g. BC with extensive intraductal component).
- TNM system criteria have varied over time, so that reports in investigational studies may be discordant and should be related to the staging edition in place when the study began.

### 13.1.1 Overview

There are several types of BC, some of which are quite rare [1]. In some cases, a single breast tumour may be a combination of these types or a mixture of invasive and in situ cancer. One generic classification takes into account two main categories: non special type and special type BC.

*No Special Type (NST) BC.* The invasive NST BC, also known as ductal carcinoma NST, is the most common type, comprising between 50 and 75 % of cases in the various published series.

*Special type BC.* All the other types of BC that are not NST fall in this category. The most frequent histological types are lobular carcinoma, tubular carcinoma, mucinous carcinoma, cribriform carcinoma, medullary carcinoma, invasive micropapillary carcinoma, metaplastic carcinoma, and apocrine carcinoma. Rare special types include invasive papillary carcinoma, secretory carcinoma, carcinoma with neuroendocrine features, lipid- and glycogen-rich carcinomas, oncocytic carcinoma, salivary gland-like tumours, and skin adnexal-type tumours. Incidence and characteristics of the main histological types are showed in Table 13.1.

*Classification* of an invasive BC as special type is based on the finding of the typical morphological features of that special type in more than 90 % of the neoplasia. When a BC shows two different morphological aspects and none of these histological aspect is represented by more than 90 %, the tumour is classified as *mixed.* The most frequent mixed types of invasive BCs are represented by a combination of

**Table 13.1** Incidence, mean age, and prognosis of main BC types

| Types | Incidence (%) | Mean age range | Prognosis |
|---|---|---|---|
| Non special type | 50–75 | | Intermediate |
| Lobular | 5–15 | 63 | Better than NST |
| Tubular | 1–2.5 | 58–64 years | Good |
| Mucinous | 1–5 | 59–71 years | Very good |
| Cribriform | 0.5–3 | 53–58 years | Excellent |
| Medullary | 1 | 52 years | Variable |
| Micropapillary | 1.2–2.3 | 53–59 years | Similar to NST |
| Metaplastic | 1 | 50–60 years | Worse |
| Apocrine | 0.5–3 | | Similar to NST |

NST carcinoma and lobular carcinoma, NST carcinoma and tubular/cribriform carcinoma, or NST carcinoma and mucinous carcinoma.

*Microinvasive BC* is a rare occurrence representing 0.5 % of invasive BC. Microinvasive BC is an invasive carcinoma with an extension of cancer cells beyond the basement membrane with no focus greater than 2 mm or with no more than 3 foci of invasion each <1 mm in its greatest dimension. The size of the individual foci should not be added together, but the size of the largest focus only is used to classify the microinvasion.

Microinvasive BC is the first stage in the development of invasion and can be seen in association with DCIS and LCIS. Conversely, most of these lesions upon review turn out to be T1a lesions with an extensive intraductal component. Comedo was reported to be the most common histological subtype of DCIS associated with microinvasion and often has a poor prognosis. Usually microinvasion is not associated with axillary LN invasion.

*Coexisting lesions.* Most BC develops in the TDLU, and often, associated pathologies (proliferating atypia or borderline lesions) can coexist with the main pathology. These coexisting pathologies are more often statistically determined than properly diagnosed. Moreover may be difficult to distinguish the multifocal forms of breast cancer from the multicentric ones and, just as most of the synchronous forms from the metachronous ones (see Sect. 15.1).

### 13.1.2 Main Types of BC

*NST Carcinoma (Ductal Carcinoma NST).* It frequency rises with increased patient age and is very uncommon before the age of 30 in patients without a family history of BC. On gross examination, NST carcinoma is a firm, well-defined to poorly defined, sometimes stellate nodule. Microscopically, malignant epithelial cells with different grades of atypia are arranged in tubules, trabeculae, or sheets. The nuclear atypia, the extension of tubular pattern, and the frequency of mitoses vary with the degree of differentiation.

*Lobular Carcinoma (LIC).* The mean patient age at presentation is 63 years. In recent years, its incidence seems to be increasing over that of other types of BC. Macroscopically, the appearance is variable, from a grey or white, firm, well-circumscribed mass to a not well-defined area of thickening. Histologically, lobular carcinoma may be subdivided in the following variants: classical, alveolar, solid, tubule-lobular, pleomorphic, and mixed.

The neoplastic cells are typically uniform and non-cohesive, with regular, round or oval, eccentrically placed nuclei with small nucleoli. The majority (75 %) of lobular carcinomas are classified as grade 2, 5 % as grade 1, and only 10 % as grade 3. LIC is immunohistochemically negative to E-cadherin in more than 85 % of cases.

The histological variant of invasive lobular carcinoma seems to be important for prognosis; the tubule-lobular variant has a very low risk of local and distant recurrence, whereas the solid variant has a high risk of regionally and distant-site recurrence (82 and 54 %, respectively). Metastatic pattern of LIC differs from that of invasive ductal carcinoma NST. LIC frequently metastasizes to bone, serosal cavities, gastrointestinal tract, uterus, ovary, and meninges, while invasive ductal carcinoma NST shows preferential tumour extension to the lung. Prognosis is a slightly improved than invasive ductal carcinoma NST.

*Tubular Carcinoma.* On gross examination, tubular carcinoma is a hard nodule with a stellate appearance usually ranging from 10 to 20 mm. Microscopically, it is entirely composed of angulated tubules with a single layer of epithelial cells often showing apical snouts. More than 90 % of the tumour must be composed of these tubules to classify as tubular carcinoma.

By definition, tubular carcinoma is of histological grade 1 as it scores 1 for tubule formation, 1 or rarely 2 for nuclear atypia, and 1 for number of mitoses. Even if nodal metastases can be detected in 12–19 % of the T1 cases, the prognosis is good.

*Mucinous Carcinoma.* On macroscopic examination it appears as a soft, well-circumscribed mass with a gelatinous aspect on a cut surface. The characteristic histological features are nests, trabeculae, acini, or sheets of neoplastic cells dispersed in a pool of extracellular mucin. Intracellular mucin may also be present with the presence of some signet-ring cells.

Mucinous carcinoma may have nodal metastases in 14 % of cases, and this principally depends on the size; for example, tumours less than 1 cm in size have less than 4 % risk of lymph node metastases. The prognosis is very good with an overall 5-year survival of 80–86 %.

*Cribriform Carcinoma.* At presentation, cribriform carcinoma has a mean size greater than 2.0 cm and on gross examination is a moderately well-defined mass with a stellate/grey cut surface. Microscopically, the neoplastic cells are organized in a cribriform pattern and have a low or, rarely, an intermediate cytonuclear grade. As with tubular carcinoma, these invasive tumours are often of histological grade 1. Lymph node metastases may be present in a percentage of cases similar to that reported for tubular carcinoma with only one or two metastatic nodes. The prognosis is excellent with a 5-year survival rate of almost 100 %.

*Medullary Carcinoma.* The average age of affected patients is 52 years, but half are less than 50 years old. Macroscopically, medullary carcinoma is a well-defined and well-circumscribed mass with a grey/tan cut surface; its average size is greater than 2.0 cm. This tumour is characteristically composed by pleomorphic nuclear grade 3 cells, arranged in a syncytial growth pattern for more than 75 % of the nodule, without glandular structures and with a diffuse, moderate to marked lymphoplasmacytic infiltrate which is present into and all around the tumour. To classify an invasive BC as a *true* medullary carcinoma, *all* the histological features cited above must be present. Prognosis is dependent on pathological findings due to the problematic reproducibility of its diagnosis. Nevertheless, it has been recorded that women with medullary node-negative carcinoma have a better prognosis than node-negative patients NST grade 3 (10-year survival rate of 84 % versus 63 %).

*Micropapillary Invasive Carcinoma.* Macroscopically it is a grey/white, stellate nodule with a mean size greater than 2.0 cm. Histologically, invasive micropapillary carcinoma is composed of nests of eosinophilic cuboidal/columnar cells surrounded by an artifactual clear space. This lesion is typically of histological grade 3 (58–82 %) or grade 2 (18–33 %) and shows lymphovascular invasion in the majority of cases (from 63 to 76 % in different series). Lymph node metastases have been recorded in 69–95 % of cases. Despite some discordant data, the prognosis of patients affected by invasive micropapillary carcinoma seems to be similar to that of patients affected by NST cancer when matched for other prognostic features.

*Metaplastic Carcinoma.* This neoplasia usually arises in the sixth and seventh decades of life as a palpable breast mass or, sometimes, as inflammatory carcinoma. On gross examination, metaplastic carcinoma is a solid mass greater than 3.0 cm, which typically has a tan/white cut surface; cystic areas may be present. Microscopically, metaplastic carcinoma is composed of spindle cells in about 70 % of cases; the cells show moderate/severe nuclear atypia with a conspicuous number of mitoses and are arranged in fascicles, possibly with a storiform pattern. Many times a squamous differentiation and/or an association with intraductal carcinoma or NST invasive carcinoma is present. Metaplastic carcinomas are generally of histological grade 3, but the prognostic value of grading in metaplastic carcinoma is uncertain. This type of tumour is typically negative for ER, PR, and HER2. Lymph node metastases are less frequent in metaplastic cancers than in invasive carcinoma NST of similar size and grade. However, as in other triple-negative BCs, distant metastases, preferentially brain and/or lung metastases, can be found at the time of diagnosis. Metaplastic BCs have lower response rates to conventional adjuvant chemotherapy and a worse clinical outcome than those of other types of triple-negative BCs.

*Apocrine Carcinoma.* This tumour has clinical characteristics similar to those of NST invasive carcinoma. Also on gross examination, apocrine carcinoma lacks specific features. Microscopically, the neoplastic cells show typical apocrine differentiation with abundant eosinophilic granular cytoplasm and large nuclei with prominent nucleoli. Many studies have shown no difference in outcome, including survival, between apocrine carcinomas and NST invasive cancers when matched for standard prognostic parameters.

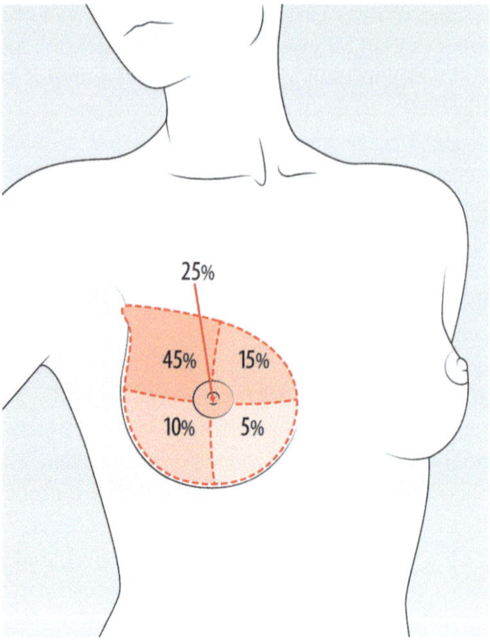


**Fig. 13.1** Clinical quadrants of the breast with the approximate percentage of all BC found in each

### 13.1.3 Location of Breast Cancer

Clinically, the breast is divided into five quadrants (upper outer, lower outer, upper inner, lower inner, and central). This arbitrary distinction may be impractical for big tumours, which occupied more than one quadrant, or small tumours located on the interface between two quadrants, e.g. at 12, 3, 6, and 9 o'clock, should be classified in a separate category. The approximate percentage of all BC found in each quadrant is represented in Fig. 13.1.

From a practical point of view, this spatial definition was based on the assumption that unicentric cancers arising in one quadrant of the breast were more likely to grow from the same ductal structures, while multicentric BC were more likely to occur in separate areas of the breast. The application of molecular biology techniques to this problem has provided some clarification of these issues. Molecular studies suggest that most, but not all, multicentric carcinomas arise from the same cells so that the terms multicentric and unicentric-multifocal do not indicate two biologically distinct processes. In general, the term multifocality indicates lesions in closer proximity than those designated as multicentric, but the therapeutic considerations for both groups are similar (see Sect. 15.1).

However, definitions of multicentric and unicentric-multifocal are problematic since the 'quadrants' of the breast are arbitrary external designations, whereas no internal boundaries exist. In addition, these definitions may result in similar lesions being classified differently, based on their location in the breast, irrespective of its size. For example, two lesions at 11 and 1 o'clock could be classified as multicentric because they occur in the upper outer and upper inner quadrants, whereas two lesions could be classified as multifocal if they are at 1 and 3 o'clock.

Finally, some considers the location of the tumour within the breast an important predictor. Tumours that develop toward the outside of the breast tend to be less difficult to treat than those that occur more toward the middle of the breast.

### 13.1.4 Staging of Breast Cancer

*TNM system.* TNM is the most widely used system for BC staging [2]. It works in a two-step procedure which first classifies cancer by several factors (T for tumour, N for nodes, M for metastasis) and then groups these TNM factors into overall stages. It is crucial to be aware that the TNM system criteria have varied over time, sometimes fairly substantially, so that reports often use the staging edition that was in place when the study began rather than the date of acceptance or publication. The AJCC Seventh Edition TNM Classification for Breast Cancer is presented in Table 13.2.

**Table 13.2** AJCC TNM Classification for Breast Cancer, 7th edition [3]

| *Primary tumour (T)* | |
|---|---|
| TX | Primary tumour cannot be assessed |
| T0 | No evidence of primary tumour |
| Tis | Carcinoma in situ |
| Tis (DCIS) | Ductal carcinoma in situ |
| Tis (LCIS) | Lobular carcinoma in situ |
| Tis (Paget) | Paget disease of the nipple not associated with invasive carcinoma and/or carcinoma in situ (DCIS and/or LCIS) in the underlying breast parenchyma. Carcinomas in the breast parenchyma associated with Paget disease are categorized based on the size and characteristics of the parenchymal disease, although the presence of Paget disease should still be noted |
| T1 | Tumour ≤20 mm in greatest dimension |
| T1mi | Tumour ≤1 mm in greatest dimension |
| T1a | Tumour >1 mm but ≤5 mm in greatest dimension |
| T1b | Tumour >5 mm but ≤10 mm in greatest dimension |
| T1c | Tumour >10 mm but ≤20 mm in greatest dimension |
| T2 | Tumour >20 mm but ≤50 mm in greatest dimension |
| T3 | Tumour >50 mm in greatest dimension |
| T4 | Tumour of any size with direct extension to the chest wall and/or to the skin (ulceration or skin nodules) |
| T4a | Extension to chest wall, not including only pectoralis muscle adherence/invasion |
| T4b | Ulceration and/or ipsilateral satellite nodules and/or oedema (including peau d'orange) of the skin, which do not meet the criteria for inflammatory carcinoma |
| T4c | Both T4a and T4b |
| T4d | Inflammatory carcinoma |

(continued)

**Table 13.2** (continued)

| *Regional lymph nodes (N)* | |
|---|---|
| *Clinical* | |
| NX | Regional lymph nodes cannot be assessed (e.g. previously removed) |
| N0 | No regional lymph node metastasis |
| N1 | Metastasis to mobile ipsilateral level I, II axillary lymph node(s) |
| N2 | Metastases in ipsilateral level I, II axillary lymph nodes that are clinically fixed or matted or in clinically detected[a] ipsilateral internal mammary nodes in the *absence* of clinically evident axillary lymph node metastasis |
| N2a | Metastases in ipsilateral level I, II axillary lymph nodes fixed to one another (matted) or to other structures |
| N2b | Metastases only in clinically detected[a] ipsilateral internal mammary nodes and in the *absence* of clinically evident level I, II axillary lymph node metastases |
| N3 | Metastases in ipsilateral infraclavicular (level III axillary) lymph node(s), with or without level I, II axillary node involvement, or in clinically detected[a] ipsilateral internal mammary lymph node(s) and in the *presence* of clinically evident level I, II axillary lymph node metastasis; or metastasis in ipsilateral supraclavicular lymph node(s), with or without axillary or internal mammary lymph node involvement |
| N3a | Metastasis in ipsilateral infraclavicular lymph node(s) |
| N3b | Metastasis in ipsilateral internal mammary lymph node(s) and axillary lymph node(s) |
| N3c | Metastasis in ipsilateral supraclavicular lymph node(s) |
| *Pathologic (pN)*[b] | |
| pNX | Regional lymph nodes cannot be assessed (e.g. previously removed or not removed for pathologic study) |
| pN0 | No regional lymph node metastasis identified histologically. *Note:* isolated tumour cell clusters (ITCs) are defined as small clusters of cells ≤0.2 mm, or single tumour cells, or a cluster of <200 cells in a single histological cross section; ITCs may be detected by routine histology or by immunohistochemical (IHC) methods; nodes containing only ITCs are excluded from the total positive node count for purposes of N classification but should be included in the total number of nodes evaluated |
| pN0(i−) | No regional lymph node metastases histologically, negative IHC |
| pN0(i+) | Malignant cells in regional lymph node(s) ≤0.2 mm (detected by hematoxylin-eosin [H&E] stain or IHC, including ITC) |
| pN0(mol−) | No regional lymph node metastases histologically, negative molecular findings (reverse transcriptase polymerase chain reaction [RT-PCR]) |
| pN0(mol+) | Positive molecular findings (RT-PCR) but no regional lymph node metastases detected by histology or IHC |
| pN1 | Micrometastases or metastases in 1–3 axillary lymph nodes and/or in internal mammary nodes, with metastases detected by sentinel lymph node biopsy but not clinically detected[c] |
| pN1mi | Micrometastases (>0.2 mm and/or >200 cells, but none >2.0 mm) |
| pN1a | Metastases in 1–3 axillary lymph nodes (at least 1 metastasis >2.0 mm) |

**Table 13.2** (continued)

| | |
|---|---|
| pN1b | Metastases in internal mammary nodes, with micrometastases or macrometastases detected by sentinel lymph node biopsy but not clinically detected[c] |
| pN1c | Metastases in 1–3 axillary lymph nodes and in internal mammary lymph nodes, with micrometastases or macrometastases detected by sentinel lymph node biopsy but not clinically detected† |
| pN2 | Metastases in 4–9 axillary lymph nodes or in clinically detected[d] internal mammary lymph nodes in the absence of axillary lymph node metastases |
| pN2a | Metastases in 4–9 axillary lymph nodes (at least 1 tumour deposit >2.0 mm) |
| pN2b | Metastases in clinically detected[c] internal mammary lymph nodes in the absence of axillary lymph node metastases |
| pN3 | Metastases in ≥10 axillary lymph nodes; or in infraclavicular (level III axillary) lymph nodes; or in clinically detected[d] ipsilateral internal mammary lymph nodes in the presence of ≥1 positive level I, II axillary lymph nodes; or in >3 axillary lymph nodes and in internal mammary lymph nodes, with micrometastases or macrometastases detected by sentinel lymph node biopsy but not clinically detected†; or in ipsilateral supraclavicular lymph nodes |
| pN3a | Metastases in ≥10 axillary lymph nodes (at least 1 tumour deposit >2.0 mm); or metastases to the infraclavicular (level III axillary lymph) nodes |
| pN3b | Metastases in clinically detected[d] ipsilateral internal mammary lymph nodes in the presence of ≥1 positive axillary lymph nodes; or in >3 axillary lymph nodes and in internal mammary lymph nodes, with micrometastases or macrometastases detected by sentinel lymph node biopsy but not clinically detected[c] |
| pN3c | Metastases in ipsilateral supraclavicular lymph nodes |
| *Distant metastasis (M)* | |
| M0 | No clinical or radiographic evidence of distant metastasis |
| cM0(i+) | No clinical or radiographic evidence of distant metastases, but deposits of molecularly or microscopically detected tumour cells in circulating blood, bone marrow, or other nonregional nodal tissue that are no larger than 0.2 mm in a patient without symptoms or signs of metastases |
| M1 | Distant detectable metastases as determined by classic clinical and radiographic means and/or histologically proven >0.2 mm |

The original and primary source for this information is the American Joint Committee on Cancer (AJCC) Cancer Staging Manual, Seventh Edition (2010) published by Springer Science+Business Media (with permission)

[a]*Clinically detected* is defined as detected by imaging studies (excluding lymphoscintigraphy) or by clinical examination and having characteristics highly suspicious for malignancy or a presumed pathologic macrometastasis on the basis of fine-needle aspiration (FNA) biopsy with cytologic examination

[b]Classification is based on axillary lymph node dissection, with or without sentinel lymph node biopsy. Classification based solely on sentinel lymph node biopsy without subsequent axillary lymph node dissection is designated (sn) for sentinel node – for example, pN0(sn)

[c]Not clinically detected is defined as not detected by imaging studies (excluding lymphoscintigraphy) or not detected by clinical examination

[d]*Clinically detected* is defined as detected by imaging studies (excluding lymphoscintigraphy) or by clinical examination and having characteristics highly suspicious for malignancy or a presumed pathologic macrometastasis on the basis of FNA biopsy with cytologic examination

A different effect on staging arises from evolving technologies that are used to assign patients to particular categories, such that increasingly sensitive methods tend to cause individual cancers to be reassigned to higher stages, making it difficult to compare a specific cancer's prognosis to the historical expectations for that stage. Finally, of course, a further important consideration is the effect of the improvement in treatments over time as well.

*T – Tumour.* The tumour values (TX, T0, Tis, T1, T2, T3, or T4) depend on the cancer at the primary site of origin in the breast. TX refers to an inability to assess that site; Tis refers to DCIS, LCIS, or Paget disease; T4d refers to inflammatory BC, a clinical circumstance where typical skin changes involve at least a third of the breast.

*L – Lymph Node.* The lymph node values (NX, N0, N1, N2 ,or N3) depend on the number, size, and location of BC cell deposits in various regional lymph nodes, such as the axilla (axillary lymph nodes), the collar area (supraclavicular lymph nodes), and inside the chest (internal mammary lymph nodes).

The axilla is divided into three levels: level I is the low axilla and is below or outside the lower edge of the pectoralis minor muscle; level II is the mid-axilla which is defined by the borders of the pectoralis minor muscle; and level III, or high (apical) axilla, which is above the pectoralis minor muscle.

There are some nuances to the official definitions for N0 disease, which includes N0(i+) which refers to isolated tumour cells (ITC), which are small clusters of cells no greater than 0.2 mm, or single tumour cells, or a cluster of fewer than 200 cells in a single histological cross section, whether detected by routine histology or immunohistochemistry (IHC); N0 also includes N0(mol–), in which regional lymph nodes have no metastases histologically but have positive molecular findings (RT-PCR).

*M – Metastases.* Previous editions featured three metastatic values (MX, M0, and M1) which referred, respectively, to the absence of adequate information, the confirmed absence, or the presence of BC cells in locations other than the breast and regional lymph nodes, such as to bone, brain, and lung.

The present TNM edition no longer uses the MX option and allocates tumours to one of three clinical categories: M0 refers to no clinical or radiographic evidence of distant metastases; cM0(i+) refers to molecularly or microscopically detected tumour cells in circulating blood, bone marrow, or nonregional nodal tissue, no larger than 0.2 mm, and without clinical or radiographic evidence or symptoms or signs of metastases, and which, perhaps counter-intuitively, does not change the stage grouping, as staging for M0(i+) is done according to the T and N values; and M1, which refers to distant detectable metastases as determined by classic clinical and radiographic means, and/or metastasis that is histologically larger than 0.2 mm.

## 13.2 Prognostic and Predictive Factors

**Clinical Practice Points**

- The single most important factor predicting a patients' prognosis is the presence or absence of axillary node metastases.
- Other powerful histological prognostic factors are tumour size, histological grade, and lymphovascular invasion.
- Biomarkers (ER, PR, HER2, and Ki67) are targets and/or indicators of highly effective therapies, and their assessment is essential and mandatory.
- Molecular subtypes (e.g. basal-like subtype) have a strong impact on prognosis, even in the presence of small tumours without nodal involvement.

### 13.2.1 Histological Factors

*Grading.* All invasive carcinomas (NST and special types) are morphologically subdivided according to their degree of differentiation which reflects how closely they resemble normal breast epithelium. Three tumour features are evaluated to assess the histological grade: tubule formation, as expression of glandular differentiation; nuclear pleomorphism; and mitotic counts. A numerical scoring system of 1–3 is used to separately evaluate each feature. To obtain an optimal evaluation of histological grade, high-quality tissue preservation and histological sectioning is required.

Histological grade is a powerful prognostic factor. In unselected BC series, the overall survival is significantly better in patients with grade 1 tumours (about 75 % of patients alive after more than 20 years from the diagnosis) than in those with grade 2 or grade 3 tumours (about 55 and 45 % of patients alive after more than 20 years from the diagnosis, respectively).

*Tumour Size.* The evaluation of tumour size is performed on the gross and microscopic examination. T classification depends on the maximum size of invasive carcinoma; concomitant DCIS should not be considered. If multiple areas of invasion are present, T classification is based on the largest focus. A small cancer and some special types of BCs are often best evaluated by measuring size on glass slides.

Increasing tumour size is independently associated with a worse survival, with a 15-year cumulative survival of 90 % in tumour less than 1 cm in maximum diameter, against a 15-year cumulative survival of less than 50 % in tumour more than 3 cm in maximum diameter (Table 13.3).

**Table 13.3** Fifteen-year Kaplan-Meier BC death rates and mean tumour sizes, sorted by tumour sizes and lymph node (LN) status [4]

| Tumour size (mm) | % LN+ | Average number of LN+ | 15-year death rate (%) |
|---|---|---|---|
| 1–9 | 11 | 0.35 | 10 |
| 10–19 | 30 | 0.97 | 20 |
| 20–29 | 40 | 1.23 | 30 |
| 30–39 | 50 | 2.87 | 50 |
| 40–49 | 52 | 3.15 | 64 |

**Table 13.4** Terms to define lymph node metastases with the corresponding TNM pathological stage

| Term | Definition | Pathological *N* stage |
|---|---|---|
| Isolated tumour cells | Tumour cell deposit ≤0.2 mm | pN0i+ |
| Micrometastasis | Tumour cell deposit >0.2 and ≤2 mm | pN1mic |
| Macrometastasis | Tumour cell deposit >2 mm | pN1 |
| Number of positive axillary lymph nodes | If there is one tumour cell deposit >2 mm, then all lymph nodes with micrometastases or macrometastases are counted as positive lymph nodes. Cancerous nodules in the axillary fat without histological evidence of residual lymph node tissue are counted as positive lymph nodes | pN1a (1–3 positive axillary lymph nodes) |
| | | pN2a (4–9 positive axillary lymph nodes) |
| | | pN3a (≥10 positive axillary lymph nodes) |

*Lymph Node Status.* Lymph node status is the most important single prognostic factor for all except a small group of BCs with haematogenous metastasis without the involvement of nodes. For example, basal-like carcinomas, a molecular subtype with a poor prognosis, are rarely associated with extensive nodal involvement, so that in this instance other prognostic markers are more important than nodal staging.

Nodal metastases are strongly correlated with tumour size and the number of invasive carcinomas. Studies show that overall survival is decreased as the number of nodes that are involved increases [5]. No significant correlation was found between nodal positivity and biomarkers (ER, PR, HER2, and Ki67). Remarkably, the association with in situ carcinoma is correlated with lower nodal positivity in tumours presenting equally sized infiltrating components. Age is an independent variable and significantly modifies the risk of nodal positivity in tumours <1 cm. In fact, in patients under 50 years old, the proportion of nodal positivity in pT1a tumours is significantly higher than in patients over 51 years old.

Definition of terms used to describe axillary lymph node metastases in most common situation is showed in Table. 13.4. While the presence of macrometastatic lymph nodes and the number of positive nodes are strongly related to prognosis, the presence of micrometastases or ITCs seems to have a limited impact on prognosis, estimable at less than 3 % at 5 and 10 years when compared with node-negative women. Moreover, positive nodes are a marker of distant dissemination, and surgical removal of lymph nodes does not appear to have a major effect on survival but only on local recurrence. Finally, even if negative nodes are a favourable prognostic factor, 10–30 % of node-negative patients will eventually develop distant metastases.

*Lymphovascular Invasion.* Lymphovascular invasion (LVI) can be present in up to 50 % of invasive BCs, but percentages vary in the medical literature, possibly because the findings are concentrated on the periphery of the tumour and not within it. LVI is microscopically seen as small groups of neoplastic cells within clear spaces lined by endothelium.

LVI is generally correlated with loco-regional lymph node involvement and is also an important independent prognostic factor, very useful in node-negative patients. Moreover, LVI can also predict local recurrence following BCS, as well as chest wall recurrence after mastectomy. Finally, LVI in the dermis is a particularly poor prognostic factor, being strongly associated with local recurrence and distant metastases. Recently, the presence/absence of LVI has been included as a component of the minimum data set for histological reporting of early invasive BC.

The prognostic value of LVI with node-negative BC and long-term follow-up demonstrated a strong association between poor histological grade and younger age with LV1-positive cancer. LVI is prognostically significant and was independent of grade, size, and type for overall survival [6].

Circulating tumour cells (CTCs) are cancer cells that are present in the blood of patients with solid cancers and are shed from existing tumour lesions into the blood stream. The enumeration of CTCs with sensitive lab tests has long been considered to hold great promise in guiding treatment decision-making in BC patients. However, guidelines on how to use CTC enumeration in clinical decision-making in primary breast cancer and metastatic BC are lacking. They may potentially be useful for women with advanced breast cancer to help tell if treatments are working.

## 13.2.2 Biological Factors (Biomarkers)

*ER and PR expression.* ER and PR tests are performed by immunohistochemistry (IHC) which is a sensitive and specific method that can be performed on formalin fixed paraffin-embedded tissue sections. The nuclear IHC staining of ER and PR is evaluated and expressed as a proportion of positive invasive neoplastic cells with respect to all the invasive neoplastic cells, the result ranging from <1 to 100 % positive cells.

Many clinical studies and randomized trials have shown that ER, in combination with PR, is a strong predictive factor of response to hormonal therapies such as tamoxifen and aromatase inhibitors. The former binds ER and blocks oestrogen-stimulated growth, while the latter suppresses the production of oestrogen.

There is a direct correlation between the likelihood of response to hormonal therapies and the level of ER and PR expressions. Positive ER and PR tumours are associated with the best rate of response (about 60 %). Those tumours with very low levels of ER and PR tumours may also respond well to hormonal therapies, while ER- and PR-negative tumours are essentially unresponsive. The remaining two discordant phenotypes of tumour are associated with intermediate response rates, although there is debate whether tumours with a negative ER associated with positive PR could actually exist.

*HER2 expression.* HER2 is very important in the growth and differentiation of normal epithelial cells. Many studies demonstrate that the HER2 gene is amplified in about 15 % of tumours in patients with primary BC and that amplification is strictly correlated with a very high expression of the receptor. In clinical practice, HER2 is determined by IHC and/or in situ hybridization (ISH) techniques, such as fluorescence (FISH), chromogenic (CISH), and silver (SISH) in situ hybridization. All methods provide equivalent results in terms of clinical efficacy.

Patients affected by HER2-positive (i.e. positive 3+ by immunostaining or positive 2+ by immunostaining with gene amplification by ISH) BC have a worse prognosis with respect to patients with HER2-negative BC. This is true also for patients with small-size BCs. Nevertheless, HER2-positive invasive BC responds favourably to biologic therapies (e.g. trastuzumab, lapatinib, pertuzumab) that specifically target the HER2 receptor.

*Ki67 expression.* Ki67 is a nuclear antigen expressed in all phases of the cell cycle other than the Go phase. IHC can reliably assess this antigen, and MIB1 is the most widely used antibody. The nuclear IHC staining of Ki67 is evaluated and expressed as the percentage of positively staining neoplastic cells among the total number of invasive neoplastic cells, the result ranging from <1 to 100 % positive cells. The evaluation of Ki67 should be performed on the invasive edge of the tumour, i.e. the neoplastic area in which there is highest positivity.

Many retrospective studies have demonstrated the prognostic value of Ki67, but the cut-off values to designate "low" and "high" Ki67 neoplastic populations differ widely. At the 2011 St. Gallen Consensus Conference, Ki67 value was considered important, together with ER, PR, and HER2, to subdivide luminal A tumour phenotype from luminal B, and <15 % was established as the suitable cut-off value [7].

Some data suggest that Ki67 predicts neoadjuvant and adjuvant chemotherapy response in negative ER tumours; in these cases, a straightforward hypothesis is that the higher rate of response to chemotherapy observed in patients with negative-ER tumours could be due to the consistently higher values of Ki67 in these tumours. If so, Ki67 levels may be very helpful to select those patients most likely to benefit from chemotherapy. Even if Ki67 expression should be associated with the more common histopathological parameters, it seems to be an additional independent prognostic parameter for disease-free survival (DFS) and overall survival (OS) in BC patients.

### 13.2.3 Molecular Subtypes

Hormone receptor status and HER2 and Ki67 expression can be used to roughly define the four major molecular subtypes (Table 13.5). Each subtype may contain subsets within it, such as the presence or absence of p53 or other gene mutations. In addition to the four major subtypes, another minor subtype (normal-like) may or may not be considered [8].

*Luminal A molecular subtype.* Most BCs are luminal A tumours, i.e. most cells start in the inner (luminal) cells lining the mammary ducts. Luminal A tumours tend to be ER and/or PR positive and HER2 negative and have low Ki67 expression or tumour grading (1 or 2). Fewer than 15 % of luminal A tumours have p53 mutations, a factor

**Table 13.5** Principal molecular subtypes of BC [7]

| Molecular subtype | Main features (with other subsets within it) | Prevalence (approximate) | Prognosis |
|---|---|---|---|
| Luminal A | ER+ and/or PR+, HER2–, low Ki67 | 40 % | Good |
| Luminal B | ER+ and/or PR+, HER2+ (or HER2– with high Ki67) | 20 % | Poor |
| Triple negative/ basal-like | ER–, PR–, HER2– | 15–20 % | Worst |
| HER2 type | ER–, PR–, HER2+ | 10–15 % | Fairly poor |
| Normal-like | Small size, indeterminate features | 6–10 % | Good |

linked with a poorer prognosis. Of the four subtypes, luminal A tumours tend to have the best prognosis with fairly high survival rates and fairly low recurrence rates.

*Luminal B molecular subtype*. Luminal B tumours tend to be ER+ and/or PR+ highly positive Ki67 and/or HER2 overexpressed. Women with luminal B tumours are often diagnosed at a younger age than those with luminal A tumours. Compared to luminal A, luminal B tumours tend to have factors that lead to a poorer prognosis including: poorer tumour grade, larger tumour size, positive lymph nodes, and p53 gene mutations in about 30 % of cases. In fact, women with luminal B tumours have fairly high survival rates, although not as high as those with luminal A tumours.

*Triple-negative/basal-like molecular subtypes* are ER, PR, and HER2 negative. There are several subsets of triple-negative BC. One subset is referred to as *basal-like* because the tumours have cells with features similar to those of the outer (basal) cells surrounding the mammary ducts. Most basal-like tumours contain p53 mutations. Most triple-negative tumours are basal-like and most basal-like tumours are triple negative. However, not all triple-negative tumours are basal-like and not all basal-like tumours are triple negative.

About 15–20 % of BCs are triple negative and/or basal-like. These tumours tend to occur more often in younger women. Most BRCA1 BCs are both triple negative and basal-like. Triple-negative/basal like tumours are often aggressive and have a poorer prognosis, at least within the first five years after diagnosis.

*HER2 molecular subtype*. The molecular subtype HER2 type is not the same as HER2+ and is not used to guide treatment. Although most HER2-type tumours are HER2+ (and named for this reason), about 30 % are HER2–. HER2-type tumours tend to be ER and PR negative and have positive lymph nodes and higher tumour grade.

About 10–15 % of BCs have this molecular profile. About 75 % of HER2-type tumours contain p53 mutations. HER2-type tumours have a fairly poor prognosis and appear to be diagnosed at a younger age than luminal A and luminal B tumours.

*Normal-like molecular subtype*. About 6–10 % of all BCs are classified as normal-like. Although called arbitrarily *normal-like*, these tumours are not more common than others. These tumours are usually small and tend to have a good prognosis. At this time, it is unclear whether normal-like tumours are a distinct molecular subtype. Some tumours are simply unable to be classified into another subtype because the tissue sample tested did not contain enough cancer cells.

## 13.3 Multimodal Therapeutic Plan

**Clinical Practice Points**

- Since approximately one third of patients with operable BC develop distant metastatic cancer in their lifetime, postoperative adjuvant treatments should be considered in almost all cases.
- In selected cases, neoadjuvant therapy could be proposed not only to downstage the tumour but also to allow a more rapid evaluation of therapies.
- Patient with metastatic BC from the beginning (de novo) may take advantage of primary surgery in some selected cases.
- For early breast cancer but with poor prognostic markers, treatment recommendations must be made with a blend of science and art all at the same time.

### 13.3.1 Preoperative Assessment

A first but incomplete preoperative assessment could be settled with data obtained from core needle biopsy, including: histological type, grade of tumour, and biomarkers (ER, PR, Ki67, and HER2). While lacking some factors, this data set, together with clinical features, allows for a first therapeutic strategy. In most cases, the preferred course of action is surgery, while in selected cases neoadjuvant systemic treatment is proposed.

*Surgery* is usually the primary standard treatment of BC (see Chap. 16). Surgery for BC must be carried out or directly supervised by a fully trained surgeon, dedicated to breast surgery. The aim of surgery in invasive BC is to achieve tumour-free margins with the least possible mutilation, in accordance with the needs of the informed patient. To reach this goal, the surgeon must have seen the patient before any surgery and have been completely informed about the clinical situation of the patient. Surgical procedures and technical skills in surgery of the breast and of the axilla are highlighted in Chap. 16.

In patients with unifocal operable tumours too large for BCS, downsizing it with neoadjuvant systemic therapy should be considered (LoE IA). Although there has been a suggestion of higher local relapse rates after neoadjuvant chemotherapy and breast conservation, especially in young women, there appears to be no long-term significant survival harm from neoadjuvant chemotherapy and subsequent conservative surgery in young women. A more articulated debate should be carried out for tumours >5 cm (T3), as discussed in Sect. 18.5.

*Neoadjuvant (or primary) systemic therapy*, defined as the first systemic treatment a patient receives when non-metastatic BC is diagnosed, needs to be reconsidered (see Sect. 18.4).

In the last two decades, preoperative chemotherapy has been performed in women with large operable BC in order to downstage the tumour and thus enabling

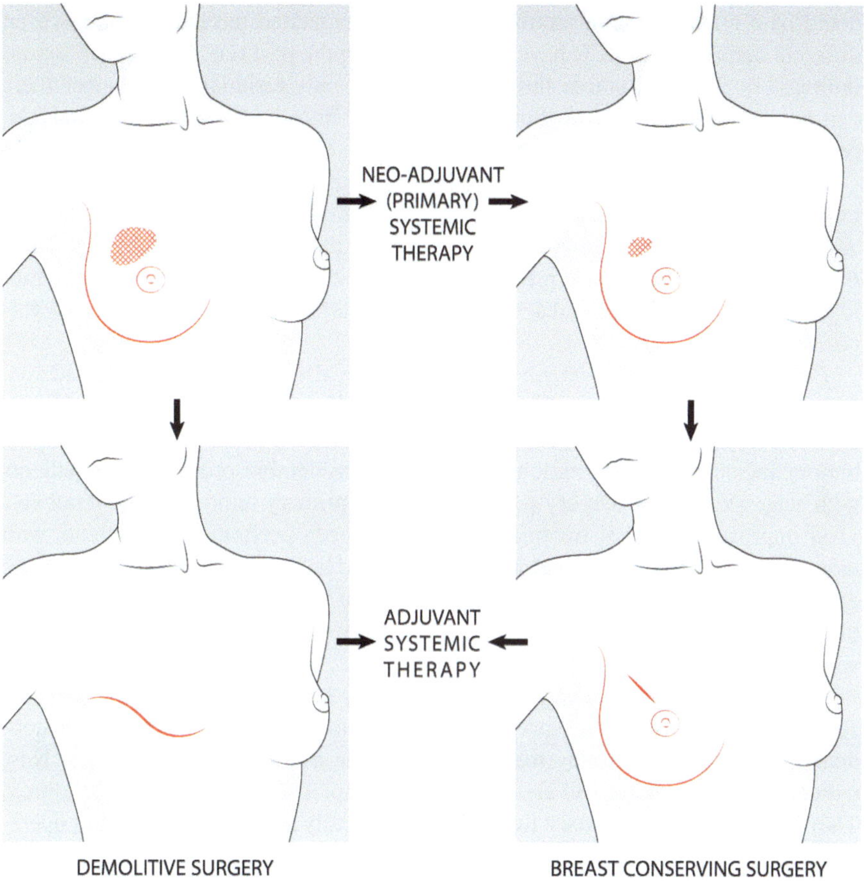


**Fig. 13.2** Neoadjuvant (primary) systemic therapy. A woman, whose large tumour is inoperable in its current state or can be removed only by a demolitive surgery (mastectomy), in most cases, may instead receive neoadjuvant therapy to shrink the tumour enough to allow breast-conserving surgery

breast-conservative surgery (Fig. 13.2). Aside from these results, several randomized trials have shown that in patients with operable BC, neoadjuvant chemotherapy achieves similar survival rates to adjuvant treatment.

More recently, the preoperative approach has also been tested in patients with early BC, irrespective of tumour size and suitability for conservative surgery, when adjuvant chemotherapy is indicated in order to allow a more rapid evaluation of new therapies without the need for long-term follow-up to demonstrate a survival advantage. In fact, the neoadjuvant setting gives the unique opportunity to get insights in BC biology in order to evaluate therapeutic comebacks and to find predictive factors for better individualization of treatment.

Pathologic complete response (pCR) of residual tumour after neoadjuvant treatment is associated with a very favourable long-term outcome, suggesting that pCR could be a marker for long-term effects on disseminated tumour cells. However, different definitions of pCR have been reported in the past (i.e. no residual tumour in breast, no residual tumour in breast and axilla, only residual DCIS), since there was not a general agreement about the prognostic impact of potential residual cancer cells.

Data from several retrospective analyses showed that the application of multimodal treatment consisting of neoadjuvant chemotherapy, surgery, radiotherapy, and hormonal therapy improved survival for patients with locally advanced BC. Moreover, the combined preoperative administration of chemotherapy and biological therapies with targeted agents can substantially improve prognosis in HER2-positive patients.

*Primary surgery of metastatic breast cancer* also needs to be reconsidered. Approximately 6–10 % of new BC cases are initially stage IV or metastatic. This is also called de novo (from the beginning) metastatic BC. In some retrospective tumour registries and institutional studies, a considerable proportion of patients with stage IV BC had surgery performed on the primary tumour with overall survival improved. Surgical treatment has mainly been performed on patients with more favourable prognostic factors and who would be expected to have a longer life expectancy. In addition, it has not been shown that surgery improves survival, as in published reports there are significant differences in the characteristics of patients who undergo surgery and patients who do not [9].

The first argument against performing primary surgery in metastatic BC is that surgery may not provide any survival advantage and may be associated with postoperative complications. Today that it is not true in a large number of cases. Now patients with metastatic BC are frequently asymptomatic and in good condition. They often have small primary BCs rather than locally advanced cancers. An operation may therefore not represent any increased surgical or anaesthetic risk compared to patients without metastases. Moreover, in some cases, the presence of distant disease is due to the improvements in imaging technology that enable the detection of minute foci of metastases that previously would have remained undetected.

Nonetheless, a few patients with metastatic BC may represent an anaesthetic challenge because of debilitation, as well as a surgical challenge because of locally advanced cancer with bulky lymph node involvement in most cases; the likelihood of adverse outcomes may be increased.

Another challenging argument against surgery in metastatic BC is that primary BC is easily accessible and provides measurable disease that can be used to scale the response to systemic treatment; removing the mass makes the clinical assessment of response to therapy more difficult. This argument is difficult to dispute, but it is a methodological aspect that does not preclude a minimal surgery in a multimodal approach to the disease.

An additional argument is that in a rodent cancer model, the primary tumour has been shown to inhibit its remote metastases. Following excision of the tumour, neovascularization and growth of metastases occurred; it suggests that this could also happen in patients after primary surgery in metastatic BC. The dispute remains challenging, even if the progression of metastatic disease noted in the rodent cancer model has not been observed in humans.

Several retrospective nonrandomized studies have shown an association between primary BC surgery and improved overall survival in metastatic BC. Moreover some expert panels suggest that removal of the primary tumour may be considered in selected patients. In an attempt to definitively answer the question, some prospective randomized trials are ongoing to compare the results of primary surgery to no surgery for patients with metastatic BC.

### 13.3.2 Postoperative Assessment and Planning

*Pathological assessment.* Postoperative assessment is mainly pathological on surgical specimens and should be carried out according to the pTNM system to include: number, location and maximum diameter of removed tumour(s), histological type and grade of the tumour(s), vascular and lymphovascular invasion, biomarker analysis, evaluation of the resection margins, total number of removed and number of positive lymph nodes, as well as the extent of metastases in the lymph nodes (Fig. 13.3).

*Staging of distant disease.* No evidence exist that any routine subset of tests is sufficiently accurate to exclude distant disease in primary operable BC. Therefore, any test will be performed on indication of symptoms and extent of local disease. For patients with tumours suitable for primary surgery, with no clinical evidence of dissemination, a preoperative screening test should be chest X-ray, full blood count, and liver function tests. For patients with clinically involved axillary nodes or being considered for neoadjuvant therapy by the size and extent of the primary tumour, further screening tests should be arranged. These include liver imaging (computed tomography (CT) scan or ultrasound) and skeletal survey (bone scan); tumour markers are optional [10].

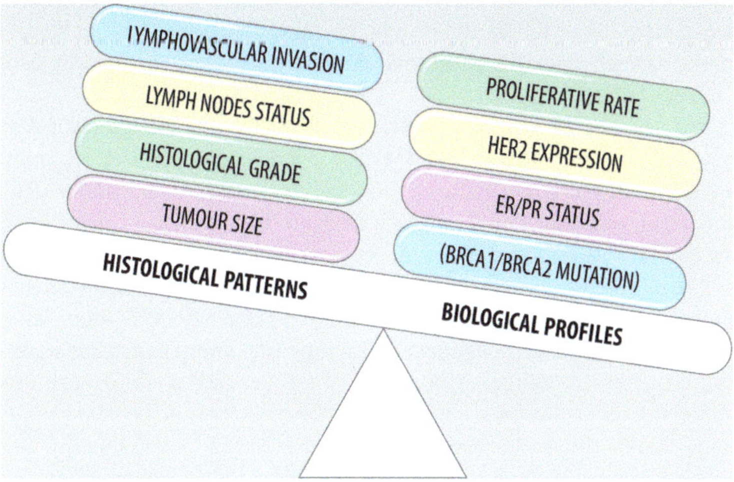


**Fig. 13.3** Main histological patterns and genetic profiles in the postoperative assessment of BC

*Treatment strategy* is based on the tumour extent/location (size and location of primary tumour, number of lesions, number and extent of lymph node involvement) and biology (pathology including biomarkers, gene expression) as well as on the age and general health status of the patient and personal preferences. Age should be taken into consideration in conjunction with other factors and should not be the determinant reason for withholding or recommending a treatment; age is a continuous variable and its cut-offs in clinical trials are always arbitrarily chosen. Overall, guideline recommends that 'younger' patients are not overtreated (see Sect. 15.3) and that 'older' patients are not undertreated because of age alone (see Sect. 15.4). Patients should be actively involved in all management decisions. The possibility of hereditary cancer should be explored and, if needed, prophylactic procedures discussed following appropriate genetic counselling and testing of the patient (see Sect. 2.3). In younger premenopausal patients, possible fertility issues should be discussed and guidance about fertility-preservation techniques provided before initiation of treatment [11].

*Systemic therapy.* Since approximately one third of patients with operable BC develop distant metastatic cancer in their lifetime, postoperative adjuvant treatments should be considered in almost all cases. Women at sufficiently high risk to warrant adjuvant chemotherapy include nearly all women with positive axillary lymph nodes and many with high-risk, node-negative disease as well. Historically, node-negative patients with sufficiently high risk to be considered as candidates for adjuvant chemotherapy tend to be those with tumours that: (1) are hormone receptor negative, high grade, or poorly differentiated; (2) overexpress HER2−; (3) have markers of increased proliferation (e.g. mitotic index, high Ki67, or elevated S-phase fraction); and (4) have evidence of angiolymphatic invasion. The relative benefit of chemotherapy depends on many factors, including the s age at diagnosis, presence of comorbidities, and hormone receptor status. A synthesis of the main systemic treatments is outlined in Chap. 18.

*Radiation therapy* (RT) following BCS or indicated in special situations should be started within 8 weeks of completion of surgery. However, if chemotherapy is indicated, the timing of RT should be adjusted in order to avoid the additive myelosuppressive side effects of both treatments. Indication and procedures of RT are briefly illustrated in Chap. 17.

*ONLINE ALGORITHM.* Computerized decision-making tools such as *Adjuvant! Online* (www.adjuvantonline.com) have influenced patient selection for appropriate systemic adjuvant therapy. Breast cancer outcome estimates are for patients who have unilateral, unicentric, invasive BC, undergone definitive primary breast surgery and axillary node staging, and no evidence of metastatic or known residual disease. In this algorithm, professionals enter age, comorbidities, ER status, tumour grade, tumour size, and the number of positive lymph nodes. Then that person selects for the type of adjuvant endocrine therapy (i.e. tamoxifen, aromatase inhibition) and adjuvant chemotherapy regimen (first, second, or third generation). A report is then generated estimating 10-year recurrence risk or 10-year mortality (a) with no systemic adjuvant therapy, (b) with adjuvant endocrine therapy alone, (c) with adjuvant chemotherapy alone, or (d) both endocrine and chemotherapy.

Graphic printouts of the results are available for counselling patients on both the risks and the benefits of adjuvant chemotherapy. Potential shortcomings of Adjuvant! Online include the relative lack of clinical data for patients who have very small lymph node-negative tumours or who are elderly and the absence of important known risk factors such as HER2 (although a new version will include data on HER2 and adjuvant trastuzumab).

*MULTIGENE PREDICTION ASSAYS.* There are a number of multigene assays (Onco*type* DX, MammaPrint, and Breast Cancer Index) that have been shown to reliably determine prognosis in patients with early-stage breast cancer. However, only Onco*type* DX has been studied for use in predicting chemotherapy benefit among patients randomized in phase III studies of chemotherapy plus tamoxifen versus tamoxifen alone [12]. Thus, this test is commonly used to help determine which patients with early-stage, oestrogen receptor-positive breast cancer should receive adjuvant cytotoxic chemotherapy to reduce the likelihood of recurrence and improve survival over and above the benefit from endocrine therapy alone.

Onco*type* DX and Breast Cancer Index are performed on formalin-fixed paraffin-embedded tissues, whereas MammaPrint requires fresh tissue in special RNA preservative. Roughly speaking, while Onco*type* DX and Breast Cancer Index are used in ER+, lymph node-negative breast cancer patients for determining prognosis and making chemotherapeutic decisions, MammaPrint is used to determine prognosis in early-stage breast cancers regardless of hormone receptor status.

## References

1. Santinelli A, Biscotti T. The pathology of breast cancer. In: Mariotti C, editor. Oncologic breast surgery. Milan: Springer; 2014.
2. Wasif N, Maggard MA, Ko CY, Giuliano AE. Invasive lobular vs. ductal breast cancer: a stage matched comparison of outcomes. Ann Surg Oncol. 2010;17:1862–9.
3. Edge SB, Byrd DR, Compton CC, et al. AJCC cancer staging manual. 7th ed. New York: Springer; 2010.
4. Michaelson JS, Silverstein M, Sgroi D, et al. The effect of tumor size and lymph node status on breast cancer lethality. Cancer. 2003;98:2133–43.
5. Rappel RS, Rakha EA, Robertson JFR, Ellis IO. Pathology and biology of breast cancer. In: Dixon JM, editor. Breast surgery. London: Elsevier; 2014.
6. Lee AH, Pinder SE, Macmillan RD, et al. Prognostic value of lymphovascular invasion in women with lymph node negative invasive breast carcinoma. Eur J Cancer. 2006;42(3):357–62.
7. Gnant M, Harbeck N, Thomssen C. St. Gallen 2011: summary of the consensus discussion. Breast Care. 2011;6:136–41.
8. Voduc KD, Cheang MC, Tyldesley S, Gelmon K, Nielsen TO, Kennecke H. Breast cancer subtypes and the risk of local and regional relapse. J Clin Oncol. 2010;28:1684–91.
9. Murphy JO, Sacchini VS. Primary surgery in metastatic breast cancer. In: Mariotti C, editor. Oncologic breast surgery. Milan: Springer; 2014.
10. Rutgers EJTH. Quality control in the locoregional treatment of breast cancer. (Eusoma group). Eur J Cancer. 2001;37:447–53.
11. Senkus E, Kyriakides S, Penault-Llorca F, et al. Primary BC: ESMO Clinical Practice Guidelines for diagnosis, treatment and follow-up. Ann Oncol. 2013;24(Supplement 6): vi7–vi23.

12. Marrone M, Stewart A, Dotson WD. Clinical utility of gene-expression profiling in women with early breast cancer: an overview of systematic reviews. Genet Med. 2014. doi:10.1038/gim.2014.140.

## Further Reading

Castle J, Shaker H, Morris K, Tugwood JD, Kirwan CC. The significance of circulating tumour cells in breast cancer: a review. Breast. 2014;23:552–60.

Fitzgibbons PL, Page DL, Weaver D, et al. Prognostic factors in breast cancer. College of American Pathologists Consensus Statement 1999. Arch Pathol Lab Med. 2000;124:966–78.

Kennecke H, Yerushalmi R, Woods R, et al. Metastatic behavior of breast cancer subtypes. Clin Oncol. 2010;28:3271–7.

Khazai L, Middleton LP, Goktepe N, Liu BT, Sahin AA. Breast pathology second review identifies clinically significant discrepancies in over 10 % of patients. J Surg Oncol. 2015;111(2):192–7.

Rampaul RS, Rakha EA, Robertson JFR, Ellis IO. Pathology and biology of breast cancer. In: Dixon JM, editor. Breast surgery. London: Elsevier; 2014.

Soerjomataramam I, Louwman MW, Ribot JG, et al. An overview of prognostic factors for long-term survivors of breast cancer. Breast Cancer Res Treat. 2008;107:309–30.

Vaz-Luis I, Ottesen RA, Hughes ME, et al. Outcomes by tumor subtype and treatment pattern in women with small, node negative breast cancer: a multi-institutional study. J Clin Oncol. 2014;32:2142–50.

Yerushalmi R, Hayes MM, Gelmon KA. Breast carcinoma-rare types: review of the literature. Ann Oncol. 2009;20:1763–70.

**Websites in Appendix**: *Predictive Markers,* A-4.17; *Second Opinion*, A-4.20.

# Breast Cancer Special Issues 14

Oreste D. Gentilini, Marta Cavalli, and Chiara Boccardo

## Contents




**Abstract**

• The key to diagnosis of Paget disease (PD) is a high index of suspicion. Paget disease should be strongly considered when any areolar or nipple lesion fails to heal with topical steroid therapy. • Inflammatory breast cancer (IBC) is a clinical diagnosis. Identification of warning signs and clinical symptoms is crucial to prompt diagnosis and appropriate referral. • Occult primary breast carcinoma (OPBC) should be differentiated from lymphoma or non-breast metastatic disease. • The most frequent non-epithelial breast malignancies, even if they are rare, are grade III phyllodes tumour, angiosarcoma and primary breast lymphoma.

*Future Directions*. Within breast oncology, Paget disease, inflammatory breast cancer and occult primary breast cancer should be considered *orphan diseases* for the heterogeneity of their immunohistochemical profiles and controversial treatments. These diseases affect very few patients, information is as well scarce, and therefore treatment can be difficult to plan. Nowadays, research is moving first meaningful footsteps toward these so far neglected diseases.



O.D. Gentilini (✉) • M. Cavalli • C. Boccardo
Division of Breast Surgery, European Institute of Oncology (IEO), Milano, Italy
e-mail: oreste.gentilini@ieo.it





A.M. Pluchinotta (ed.), *The Outpatient Breast Clinic: Aiming at Best Practice*, DOI 10.1007/978-3-319-15907-2_14

## 14.1 Paget Disease of the Breast

**Clinical Practice Points**

- Paget disease (PD) of the breast is a rare type of cancer involving the skin of the nipple and, usually, also the areola.
- Progression of PD is slow and extremely variable so that disease is often associated with delay in diagnosis. Typically, 10–12 months can pass before disease is correctly diagnosed.
- PD is associated to an underlying carcinoma of the breast, either preinvasive or invasive; in 82–100 % and in nearly 60 %, the carcinoma is a unifocal disease.
- Biopsy and assessment of extensive intraductal component may help in planning treatment if breast conservation therapy (BCT) is taken into consideration.
- If the nipple-areolar complex (NAC) and any associated lesion can be resected with negative margins, a lumpectomy is an option, with subsequent radiation and possible NAC reconstruction in the future. If not, a simple mastectomy is indicated.

*Incidence.* PD is rare and accounts for approximately 1–3 % of all patients with BC. It typically occurs in postmenopausal women, with a peak incidence among those who are 55–65 years of age. Disease has been found also in adolescents and in people in their late 80s. Men can also develop PD of the breast, but it is very rare and late, and average age at diagnosis is around 70 years of age.

*Clinical presentation.* Progression of PD is slow and extremely variable. It typically starts as a scaly erythematous patch on the nipple, then spreads to the areola. It is well demarcated from the surrounding normal skin. Early symptoms can include itchiness and burning sensations. Later skin conditions, such as dermatitis or eczema, appear with tingling or redness in the nipple (Fig. 14.1). Areola may be crusty with a thickened skin on or around the nipple that may appear flattened (Fig. 14.2). Discharge from the nipple, that may be, is uncommon. Clinical presentations of Paget disease and differential diagnosis with prolapsing intraductal papilloma, nipple adenoma and eczema are discussed in Sect. 11.1.2.

The eczematous status can temporarily be resolved with corticosteroid treatment. In addition, tiny vesicles can also appear and disappear on the nipple area. This adds to a delay in diagnosis. Typically, 10–12 months can pass before PD is correctly diagnosed. In the latter stages, PD can ulcerate and destroy the nipple or areolar complex. Bloody discharge, yellowish or bloody, is more common but only at this stage.

*Assessment.* Physical exam, mammographic X-ray and breast ultrasound are the first-line diagnostic steps in order to find any possible breast lesion or mass, which together with the clinical suspicion of PD can corroborate such a diagnosis. Physical

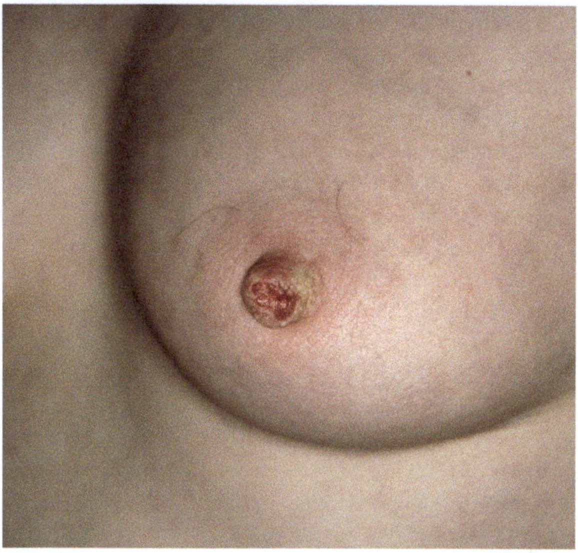

**Fig. 14.1** Paget disease: in its early stage, PD appears as an erythematous, scaly, crusted lesion of the nipple

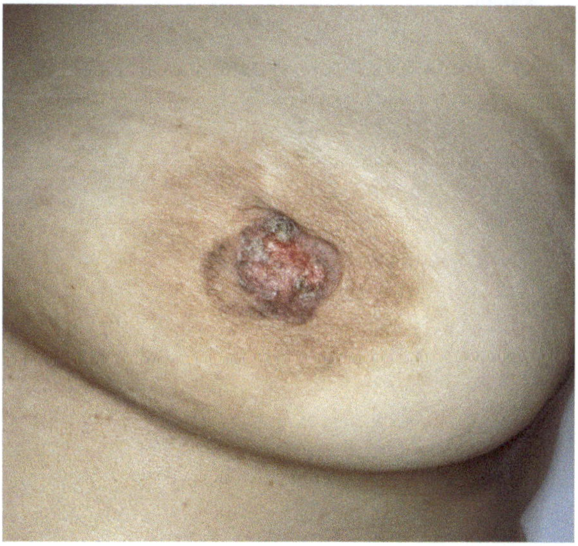

**Fig. 14.2** Paget disease: in more advanced PD, the lesion has spread to the areola, and the nipple appears flattened

examination can reveal a mass, which might then be seen as a nodule by mammogram or ultrasound. Even if neither masses nor nodules are palpable or visible, microcalcifications could be a possible finding seen at mammogram. It is important to consider that a concomitant tumour might be located several centimetres away from the nipple and areola complex. About 50–70 % of patients with biopsy-proven mammary PD show positive findings on mammography [1].

Ultrasound has no characteristic findings in PD, yet findings may include dilated irregular subareolar ducts, calcifications and a subareolar mass or flattening and/or thickening of the nipple.

MRI could be indicated in a dense breast or when an underlying DCIS or invasive cancer has not been identified by first-line investigations. MRI can also help in detecting multifocal/multicentric lesions and in better defining lesion topography with respect to the nipple-areola complex [1]. Any dubious breast lesion will be biopsied independently of PD suspicion.

Simultaneously, diagnosis of PD is established by cytology or wedge biopsy of nipple. For nipple sampling, there are several procedures including:

- Surface cytology: a glass slide is leaned against the surface of the nipple many times.
- Scraping cytology: the cutting edge of the glass slide is used to remove the top layer of skin.
- Punch biopsy: a circular cutting tool (punch) is used to remove a disc-shaped piece of tissue (see Sect. 6.3.3).
- Wedge biopsy: a lancet is used to remove a small wedge of tissue.

A mammogram should always be performed. However, it is usually negative in the case of a preinvasive cancer. It is important to consider that, in case tumour was present, that tumour could be located several centimetres away from the nipple and areola. In dense breasts, MRI could be indicated.

In the case of a negative cytology test for the nipple-areola eczematous lesion, if the PD suspicion remains high, a punch or wedge biopsy must be performed.

Typically, there are four possible clinical patterns of the disease:

- Changes in the nipple or areolar complex only (*true* PD)
- Changes in the nipple or areolar complex with an underlying breast mass
- Clinical presentation of a breast mass with histologic confirmation of PD
- Coexistence of typical PD with detached distant tumour (rare)

*True* PD is a variety of ductal carcinoma in situ (DCIS), associated to clinical eczema of the nipple and characterized by large, round "Paget cells" found in the epidermis of the nipple and the areola. The pathogenesis of PD still remains debatable: there are two theories about the origin of the Paget cells. In the first, it is thought that the cancer cells start growing inside the ducts within the breast and then make their way out to the nipple surface (*epidermotropic ductal theory*). This would appear to explain why so many people with the Paget disease of the nipple have an associated underlying breast carcinoma.

Another theory suggests that PD originates from the epidermis cells of the nipple itself (in situ *malignant transformation theory*). This theory would explain the small number of people who only have the Paget disease in the nipple or have a second that appears to be completely separate from the Paget disease.

In literature, the rate of associated underlying carcinoma of the breast ranges from 82 to 100 %, and in nearly 60 %, the carcinoma is a unifocal disease [1, 2].

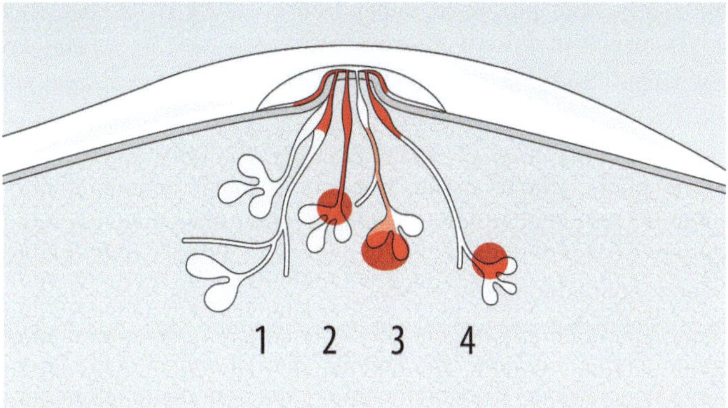


**Fig. 14.3** Clinical patterns of mammary Paget disease based on accepted concepts of pathogenesis. *1* Paget cells, derived from epithelium of the main ducts, have an extension into epidermis of overlying nipple; no mass is found in about half of cases. *2* Epidermotropic lesion with detectable mass and spread of the tumour toward the surface and the depth (about one-third of cases). *3* BC with occasional histological finding of Pagetoid cells with minimal epidermotropic diffusion and usually without skin involvement (few cases). *4* Coexistence of typical PD with detached distant tumour (rare)

A schematic diagram of clinical patterns of mammary Paget disease based on accepted concepts of pathogenesis is showed in Fig. 14.3.

*Primary treatment* of PD is still surgical. However, due to conflicting theories of how PD develops, there is much controversy with regard to radical versus conservative surgical treatment. If the epidermotropic ductal theory is correct, lumpectomy or mastectomy are the treatments of choice. If the in situ theory is correct, a wide skin excision alone would be the most appropriate therapy in case of a disease involving a limited area.

Mastectomy has been considered as the standard treatment procedure for these patients for many years (Ashikari R) (Chaudary MA) (Yim JH). However, it is reasonable to consider breast-conserving surgery since similar long-term survival rates to mastectomy have been reported [3]. Several studies have already shown that breast conservation with radiation therapy is an oncologically safe option [4].

In patients with only nipple or areolar complex involvement, some experts recommend skin excision with consideration of adjunct radiation therapy. There have been some reports of using radiation therapy alone, with varying results. At present, radiation therapy alone is not considered a standard method of treatment.

Breast-conserving surgery that includes removal of the nipple and areola followed by whole-breast radiation therapy is a safe option for people with PD assessed as localized with some radiological changes in the retroareolar area (microcalcifications or suspicious opacities), without an underlying distant invasive cancer.

Mastectomy, associated with oncoplastic repair techniques to maximize cosmesis, is the treatment of choice in patients with distant or multicentric masses or with an extensive intraductal component or in those with relapses after conservative treatment.

Sentinel lymph node biopsy should be performed to evaluate the axilla when invasive BC is present [2, 5] and in any case of mastectomy given the possibility of an unrecognized invasive component. In a study, the frequency of positive sentinel lymph node biopsy was reported to be 11 % patients [6].

Adjuvant therapy and prognosis depend on a variety of factors, including the presence or absence of invasive cancer and, if an invasive component is present, on its stage. For patients with PD alone, as for DCIS, preventive treatment with tamoxifen could be discussed with the patient.

*Prognosis.* As treatment, prognosis depends on the presence or absence of palpable masses or axillary nodes and underlying invasive carcinoma. One half (50 %) of patients with PD presenting with a palpable breast mass have associated axillary lymph node metastasis. Two-thirds of patients with axillary node metastasis were reported to have a palpable breast mass.

Even in patients with mammary PD and no underlying tumour, 30 % may develop an invasive carcinoma at a later date, and 20 % of patients already have an associated in situ carcinoma of the breast. However, other reports indicate that no axillary metastases were detected in patients without a palpable breast mass.

Patients with an identifiable associated underlying breast tumour have a survival rate of 38–40 % at 5 years and a survival rate of 22–33 % at 10 years. Mortality for metastatic breast carcinoma in patients with mammary PD and underlying cancer is 61.3 %, with a 10-year cumulative survival rate of 33 %.

The reported survival rate of patients with PD without a palpable breast tumour (prior to surgery) ranges from 92 to 94 % at 5 years and from 82 to 91 % at 10 years [7].

## 14.2 Inflammatory Breast Cancer

**Clinical Practice Points**

- Inflammatory breast cancer (IBC) is a rare disease that typically presents with a rapidly enlarging erythematous breast, a *peau d'orange* appearance and/or abnormal breast warmth, often with no detectable breast mass.
- In the presence of IBC, defining the presence or absence of ipsilateral and contralateral disease in the nodal region, and defining the presence or absence of distant metastatic disease, is mandatory.
- Treatment for IBC is usually more aggressive than treatment for most other BC. Preoperative systemic chemotherapy is the standard of care. The aggressive biology of IBC should encourage enrolling patients in clinical trials that are testing new treatments.
- On note, a dimpled appearance of the skin, but without extensive redness, may be due to massive axillary node involvement in some advanced non-inflammatory BC.

*Incidence.* This uncommon type of invasive BC accounts for about 1–3 % of all BCs. IBC has rapid and deceitful onset, often in a matter of weeks but also few months, and often lymph nodes are involved, as well as one or more distant sites.

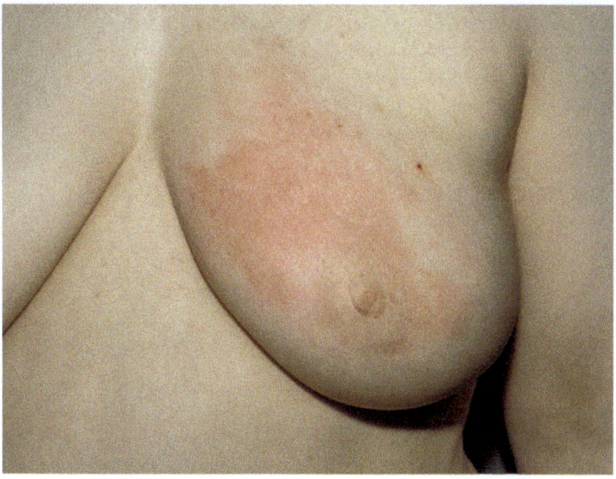

**Fig. 14.4** In IBC, redness involves more than one-third of the breast, and the skin is usually thickened

Compared with noninflammatory types of BC, IBC tends to be diagnosed at younger ages with a mean age of 50–58 years. However, there are no validated risk factors that might aid in raising suspicion for IBC. Like other types of BC, inflammatory can occur in men, but usually at an older age than in women, with a median age at diagnosis of 66.5 years. IBC is also more common in obese women than in women of normal weight and in black than in white women.

The aggressive course of IBC, together with accumulating data on its unique molecular and epidemiological characteristics, lends support to the hypothesis that IBC may in fact be a distinct biological entity rather than a subtype on the spectrum of locally advanced breast cancers (LABC). To this end, it is important to distinguish two distinct clinical varieties of IBC that are commonly cited in the literature. The term *primary IBC* is used to describe the de novo development of IBC in a previously normal breast. In contrast, *secondary IBC* describes the development of inflammatory skin changes that mimic primary IBC either in a breast that already had cancer or on the chest wall after a mastectomy for non-IBC [8].

*Clinical presentation.* Diagnosis of IBC is mainly clinical. Patients with IBC usually present with a complaint of colour change in one breast, usually pink (Fig. 14.4) that evolves into a darker red (purple) and spreads over the entire breast. The patient might describe a sensation of heat in the breast, and the breast itself enlarges rapidly over a period of only a few weeks. Patients usually do not experience fever neither leucocytosis. The typical *peau d'orange* appearance of IBC stems from lymphatic oedema around deepened hair follicles.

Of note, a pitted appearance of the skin with *peau d'orange*, but without extensive redness, may be due to massive axillary node involvement in some advanced noninflammatory BC (Fig. 14.5). Some cases of moderate severity involving only a part of the breast are rather *pseudo IBC*. Peritumoral and cutaneous oedema is more often to be found beyond the limits of the tumour, even though at times, it is difficult to precise its limits. The enlarged lymph nodes are sometimes matted together and attached to the tumour by an indurated cord of *neoplastic lymphangitis*.

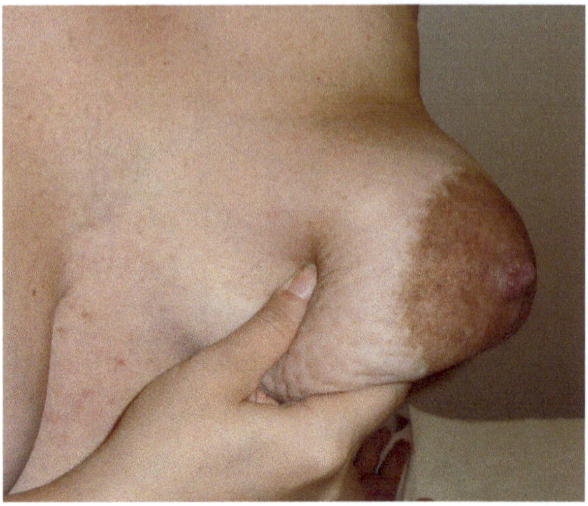

**Fig. 14.5** A pitted appearance of the skin, with *peau d'orange* but without extensive redness, may be due to massive axillary node involvement, as in this 58-year-old woman. This case should not be considered as IBC

American Joint Committee on Cancer (AJCC) provides the current gold standard definition for this form of BC, describing it as a clinic-pathologic entity that is characterized by diffuse erythema and oedema (*peau d'orange*), often without an underlying palpable mass. The clinical presentation of IBC is due to tumour emboli within dermal lymphatic vessels, which may or may not be present on skin biopsy. Therefore, the AJCC relies on the clinical features of IBC and considers the pathologic features to be supportive of, but not necessary for, diagnosis.

Recently, minimum diagnostic criteria have been set forth by an international expert panel [9], which include:

- History of rapid onset of breast erythema, oedema and/or peau d'orange and/or warm breast, with or without an underlying palpable mass.
- History of flattening, crusting or retraction of the nipple may be present.
- Patients may have a history of being diagnosed with mastitis not responding to at least 1 week of antibiotics.
- Duration of history of no more than 6 months.
- Clinical examination revealing erythema occupying at least one-third of the breast.
- Clinical examination may reveal underlying palpable mass with or without palpable locoregional lymph nodes with or without nipple abnormalities.

*Assessment*. The key roles of imaging in IBC are to identify a primary breast tumour and facilitate image-guided diagnostic biopsy, stage locoregional disease, diagnose distant metastases and evaluate tumour response to neoadjuvant therapy [8]. So all women with a suspected IBC should undergo a mammography and an ultrasound of the breast and regional lymph nodes. Probability of axillary nodal involvement is 90 %.

Most women diagnosed with IBC have dense breast tissue, and a lump or mass is rarely seen in mammograms that show an increase in the thickness or density of breast tissue. MRI might be sometimes recommended in instances where breast parenchymal lesions are not detected by mammography or breast ultrasound [9]. However, biopsy of the skin is mandatory any time a clinical suspicion of IBC is raised, regardless of imaging.

Pathological findings frequently show poorly differentiated cells. IBC, classically, presents dermal lymphatic invasion, with or without lymphatic invasion.

A complete staging workup is recommended including bone scans, chest X-ray scans and abdominal ultrasound scans, with more focused tests if there are any additional symptoms. Data on PET or PET/CT are not sufficient to recommend its routine use in women with IBC [9] but can be considered especially within study protocols.

*Treatment.* IBC is treated with a multimodal approach: first with systemic chemotherapy, then with surgery followed by radiation therapy. Studies have found that women with IBC who are treated with a multimodal approach have better responses to therapy and longer survival. Since there are no data to indicate a different biology or a different prognosis in young women, the management of IBC should be the same as in the older population [9].

Owing to the skin involvement of IBC, the risk of locoregional and distant recurrence is too high to justify immediate mastectomy. Primary chemotherapy represents the upfront treatment. Surgery should be delayed after preoperative chemotherapy and usually consists in a modified radical mastectomy. Current data also indicate that sentinel lymph node biopsy is not a reliable method of assessing axillary lymph nodes among women with IBC [10]. Postmastectomy radiation therapy to the chest wall is a standard part of multimodal therapy. Because of the high probability of involvement of locoregional lymph nodes, it is recommended to provide radiation therapy including the supraclavicular region and internal mammary lymph nodes [8, 9]. In most of the patients with IBC, immediate breast reconstruction is delayed at the end of the whole treatment planning.

Postoperative adjuvant systemic therapy may be given after surgery to reduce the chance of cancer recurrence. This therapy may include additional chemotherapy, hormonal therapy, targeted therapy if indicated or some combination of these treatments [9].

*Prognosis.* When compared with other patients presenting at the same stage, women with IBC have worse prognoses if untreated. Moreover, 25–50 % of all patients develop contralateral BC, usually in the setting of metastatic disease.

Median overall survival for IBC patients is about 3–4 years, with lower survival rates among black women and those with negative ER status. These survival rates have not changed significantly over the past 30 years, emphasizing the aggressive nature of the disease [2, 11].

## 14.3 Occult Primary Breast Carcinoma

**Clinical Practice Points**

- As for all carcinomas of unknown primary site, a staging by CT scans of the thorax, abdomen and pelvis must be performed to exclude non-breast metastases.
- A core needle or excisional biopsy should be performed as the initial diagnostic test to differentiate more common axillary mass due to lymphoma or metastatic breast.
- If mammogram and ultrasound give no evidence of suspicious lesions, especially in radio-dense breast, MRI is strongly indicated.
- Axillary dissection with breast conservation and ipsilateral breast radiotherapy seems to be a good therapeutic option.
- Most published cases series of OPBC patients have demonstrated outcome superior to those of non-occult node-positive patients.

Occult primary breast carcinoma (OPBC) is a subgroup of cancer of unknown primary site (CUP), a non-common but larger group of clinical entities marked by the presence of metastatic cancer with an undetectable primary site at the time of presentation.

OPBC affects women (rarely men) who have metastatic poorly differentiated carcinoma in the axillary lymph nodes without evident primary breast lesion. Commonly, after completion of the routine staging evaluation, no distant disease spread is established. Although the exact incidence of OPBC is difficult to ascertain, occult accounts for about 1 % of all cancer diagnoses [12].

*Assessment.* The onset of the OPBC is the unexpected finding of an axillary nodal mass without any breast symptom.

Magnetic resonance imaging (MRI) and/or positron emission tomography (PET) have been successful in challenging cases with negative mammograms, particularly in women with radio-dense breasts. There is also evidence that breast scintimammography may be a useful, inexpensive and practical diagnostic tool in the evaluation of the patient with OPBC, but experience with this modality is still limited.

MRI sensitivity for OPBC is high, and MRI findings may have an impact on the type of treatments patients with OPBC ultimately receive. However, OPBC incidence has not definitively decreased since the introduction of MRI, and the relatively modest specificity of MRI may lead that many women will undergo unnecessary procedures based on false-positive results [13].

A core biopsy can be performed as the initial diagnostic test. A negative result does not exclude a malignancy, and, therefore, an excisional biopsy may be necessary. Axillary mass could correspond to lymphoma or metastatic breast, lung and melanoma. If pathology shows carcinoma, immunostains may be helpful to differentiate breast from lung primary [14].

*Care plan.* OPBC is certainly an orphan disease within breast oncology. As with other rare diseases, evidence-based approaches to OPBC diagnosis and treatment would benefit from initiation of a prospectively accrued international patient registry. Anyway, if a breast primary is identified, the woman should be treated like any other stage II patient, including chemotherapy. Even in cases where a breast primary is not identified, such patients are potentially managed according to standard guidelines for stage II.

*Surgery.* Axillary lymph node dissection is the main treatment for these cases. Because the metastatic node could be due to small foci of breast tissue in the axilla, most women in the past and also to date have undergone mastectomy. No primary lesions were found in about 30 % of mastectomy specimens. Large lumpectomy of suspicious or doubtful mammographic findings followed by RT or RT alone seems to give the same results.

Data from larger studies eventually revealed an unacceptable outcome in patients who only received a "wait-and-see" therapeutic approach. Also a blind upper outer resection failed to lead to a better outcome.

Literature does not clearly support the overwhelming use of one or the other [13]. However, with whole-breast radiation, the breast is preserved, and the survival rates would surely support its use as an alternative to mastectomy [15].

In conclusion, in absence of detected foci, there is no proven benefit of mastectomy over the conservative surgery (or no surgery). So axillary dissection with breast conservation and ipsilateral breast radiotherapy seems to be a good therapeutic option and can be recommended to improve local control in addition to aesthetic results.

*Prognosis.* OPBC presenting with axillary lymphadenopathy has been thought to have a similar natural history and biological profile (e.g. histology, receptor status) to non-occult node-positive BCs [14]. Furthermore, most published case series of OPBC patients have demonstrated outcomes superior to those of non-occult node-positive patients, with a 5-year survival rate of about 85 % [16].

On the whole, it appears that OPBC patients may actually have a better prognosis than non-occult node-positive breast cancer patients, and this difference in outcomes may be related to the paucity or absence of macroscopic intramammary disease [15].

## 14.4 Other Breast Malignancies

**Clinical Practice Points**

- In phyllodes tumour, treatment is essential to achieve wide negative margins, and often other adjuvant treatments after surgery are not recommended.
- Primary angiosarcoma of the breast is a rare malignancy affecting young women, with a poor prognosis even after complete resection.
- Primary breast lymphoma is a rare form of non-Hodgkin lymphoma that does not have a well-defined treatment strategy.

### 14.4.1 Phyllodes Tumour

The phyllodes tumour (also known as *phylloides tumour* or *cystosarcoma phyllodes*), as previously described in Sect. 9.3, is a rare fibroepithelial tumour of the breast which has some resemblance to a fibroadenoma [17]. Clinically, it is usually a large, fast-growing mass that forms from the periductal and intralobular stroma of the breast [18].

Pathological presentation of phyllodes tumour ranges from grade I (benign) to malignant phyllodes tumours (grade III) where the stromal component clearly exhibits a sarcoma pattern. Reports suggest that about 85–90 % of phyllodes tumours are benign and that approximately 10–15 % are malignant. Fine-needle aspiration is inaccurate, and even core biopsy has moderate sensitivity due to tumour heterogeneity causing inadequate sampling [19]. For this reason, malignancy can be occasionally found in removed masses.

The first goal of treatment is to achieve negative margins. While removing the tumour along with a limited margin of normal breast tissue treats benign phyllodes tumour, a malignant phyllodes tumour should be treated with a wider margin of normal tissue or by mastectomy [20]. Surgery is often the only treatment, and other adjuvant treatments are usually not recommended.

After a wide local excision, local recurrence is relatively frequent (up to 25 %), and up to 10 % can metastasize to distant organs [21]. Treatment of metastases is according to the clinical practice guidelines in use for soft tissue sarcoma.

### 14.4.2 Angiosarcoma

Angiosarcoma is a tumour of the inner lining of blood vessels, and it can occur in any area of the body. In approximately 8 % of cases, angiosarcoma is found in breast tissue.

In most cases, the cause of a sarcoma is unknown (primary angiosarcoma). Secondary angiosarcoma has its most widely known cause in chronic long-lasting lymphoedema, or in radiation exposure, as in the case of patients previously treated with radiation therapy. This is an extremely rare complication of breast radiation therapy that can develop about 5–10 years after radiation [22].

Angiosarcoma has different ways of presentation. It can look like a skin infection, a bruise or a lesion that does not heal. It may have a violet colour, and one should be particularly concerned if such an area arises in a site of prior radiation therapy. It might also present as a soft lump that can be felt or seen.

Diagnosis usually begins with a physical exam and may include imaging studies such as an X-ray, CT scan, MRI or PET scan. A definite diagnosis is made with a biopsy procedure. Most angiosarcomas are high-grade tumours that are aggressive and fast growing, while very few are low-grade tumours.

Surgery is the primary method of treatment. Axillary surgery is usually not performed for the very low probability of lymph nodes metastases. Only in aggressive cases, chemotherapy and/or radiation therapy can be an important part of the treatment plan [23]. Studies suggest that better outcomes are achieved for patients who have smaller tumours that are removed with clear margins [23, 24]. Low-grade angiosarcoma of the breast is also reported as having a better prognosis.

### 14.4.3 Primary Breast Lymphoma

Primary breast lymphoma is a malignant lymphoma primarily occurring in the breast in the absence of previously detected lymphoma localizations [25]. Breast lymphoma is a rare disease, accounting for only 0.4–0.5 % of all breast malignancies, 0.4–0.7 % of all non-Hodgkin lymphomas and about 2 % of extranodal non-Hodgkin lymphomas. The median age of patients with diagnosed breast lymphoma ranges from 60 to 65 years. The disease occurs almost exclusively in women [26].

Bilateral breast involvement accounts from 5 to 11 of all breast lymphomas [27]. This rare situation is especially observed during pregnancy or postpartum, suggesting that tumour growth is influenced by hormonal stimulation.

Breast lymphoid cells probably originate in mucosa-associated lymphoid tissue (MALT) or from lymphatic tissue adjacent to ducts and lobules or from intramammary lymph nodes. A painless mass is the most common presenting sign in primary breast lymphoma occurring in approximately 61 % of cases, especially (48 %) in the external superior quadrant. Other symptoms and signs are the following: local pain, local inflammation, palpable lymph nodes and incidental mammography finding [26].

Mammographic findings are nonspecific. Most of the lesions are oval-shaped and high-density masses. The masses revealed by ultrasound examination are usually hypoechoic. No masses have spiculated margins or calcifications. Fine-needle aspiration, core biopsy and excisional biopsy are effective techniques used in the evaluation of breast nodules and axillary lymph nodes. However, histological, immunohistochemical and, sometimes, genetic studies are necessary for establishing the diagnosis [26].

The behaviour of primary lymphoma of the breast is thought to be similar to that of lymphomas of the same histological types and stages arising at other sites, with a similar stage-for-stage clinical outcome. The method chosen for treating breast lymphoma using radiation therapy and/or chemotherapy also varies in the literature. Currently, the use of combined therapy is considered to be a more useful treatment even in the early stages of the illness. Mastectomy is not recommended because it offers no benefit as regards survival or recurrence risk [26].

## References

1. Morrogh M, Morris EA, Liberman L, et al. MRI identifies otherwise occult disease in select patients with Paget disease of the nipple. J Am Coll Surg. 2008;206:316–21.
2. Caliskan M, Gatti G, Sosnovskikh I, et al. Paget's disease of the breast: the experience of the European Institute of Oncology and review of the literature. Breast Cancer Res Treat. 2008;112:513–21.

3. Chen CY, Sun LM, Anderson BO. Paget disease of the breast: changing patterns of incidence, clinical presentation, and treatment in the U.S. Cancer. 2006;107:1448–58.
4. Joseph KA, Ditkoff BA, Estabrook A, et al. Therapeutic options for Paget's disease: a single institution long-term follow- up study. Breast J. 2007;13:110–1.
5. Laronga C, Nasson D, Hoover S, et al. Paget's disease in the era of sentinel lymph node biopsy. Am J Surg. 2006;192:481–3.
6. Sukumvanich P, Bentrem DJ, Cody HS, et al. The role of sentinel lymph node biopsy in Paget's disease of the breast. Ann Surg Oncol. 2007;14:1020–3.
7. Osteen R. Paget's disease of the nipple. In: Harris J, Hellman S, Henderson JC, editors. Breast diseases. 2nd ed. Philadelphia: Lippincott; 1991.
8. Robertson FM, Bondy M, Yang W, et al. Inflammatory breast cancer: the disease, the biology, the treatment. CA Cancer J Clin. 2010;60:351–75.
9. Dawood S, Merajver SD, Viens P, et al. International expert panel on inflammatory breast cancer: consensus statement for standardized diagnosis and treatment. Ann Oncol. 2011;22:515–23.
10. Stearns V, Ewing CA, Slack R, et al. Sentinel lymphadenectomy after neoadjuvant chemotherapy for breast cancer may reliably represent the axilla except for inflammatory breast cancer. Ann Surg Oncol. 2002;9:235–42.
11. Hance KW, Anderson WF, Devesa SS, Young HA, Levine PH. Trends in inflammatory breast carcinoma incidence and survival: the surveillance, epidemiology, and end results program at the National Cancer Institute. J Natl Cancer Inst. 2005;97:966–75.
12. Montagna E, Bagnardi V, Rotmensz N, et al. Immunohistochemically defined subtypes and outcome in occult breast carcinoma with axillary presentation. Breast Cancer Res Treat. 2011;129:867–75.
13. Fayanju OM, Stoll CRT, Fowler S, et al. Geographic and temporal trends in the management of occult primary breast cancer: a systematic review and meta-analysis. Ann Surg Oncol. 2013;20:3308–16.
14. Pavlidis N, Pentheroudakis G. Cancer of unknown primary site. Lancet. 2012;379:1428–35.
15. Barton SR, Smith IE, Kirby AM, Ashley S, Walsh G, Parton M. The role of ipsilateral breast radiotherapy in management of occult primary breast cancer presenting as axillary lymphadenopathy. Eur J Cancer. 2011;47:2099–106.
16. Kaklamani V, Gradishar WJ. Axillary node metastases with occult primary breast cancer. http://www.uptodate.com. Accessed 15 Aug 2013.
17. Yohe S, Yeh IT. 'Missed' diagnoses of phyllodes tumor on breast biopsy: pathologic clues to its recognition. Int J Surg Pathol. 2008;16:137–42.
18. Parker SJ, Harries SA. Phyllodes tumours. Postgrad Med J. 2001;77:428–35.
19. Yasir S, Gamez R, Jenkins S, Visscher DW, Nassar A. Significant histologic features differentiating cellular fibroadenoma from phyllodes tumor on core needle biopsy specimens. Am J Clin Pathol. 2014;142:362–9.
20. Pezner RD, Schultheiss TE, Paz IB, Pezner R. Malignant phyllodes tumor of the breast: local control rates with surgery alone. Int J Radiat Oncol Biol Phys. 2008;71:710–3.
21. Wei J, Tan YT, Cai YC, et al. Predictive factors for the local recurrence and distant metastasis of phyllodes tumors of the breast: a retrospective analysis of 192 cases at a single center. Chin J Cancer. 2014;33:492–500.
22. Seinen JM, Styring E, Verstappen V, et al. Radiation-associated angiosarcoma after breast cancer: high recurrence rate and poor survival despite surgical treatment with R0 resection. Ann Surg Oncol. 2012;19:2700–6.
23. Depla AL, Scharloo-Karels CH, de Jong MA, et al. Treatment and prognostic factors of radiation-associated angiosarcoma (RAAS) after primary breast cancer: a systematic review. Eur J Cancer. 2014;50:1779–88.
24. Torres KE, Ravi V, Kin K, et al. Long-term outcomes in patients with radiation-associated angiosarcomas of the breast following surgery and radiotherapy for breast cancer. Ann Surg Oncol. 2013;20:1267–74.

25. Jeanneret-Sozzi W, Taghian A, Epelbaum R, et al. Primary breast lymphoma: patient profile, outcome and prognostic factors. A multicentre Rare Cancer Network study. BMC Cancer. 2008;8:86.
26. Joks M, Mysliviec K, Lewandowski K. Primary breast lymphoma – a review of the literature and report of three cases. Arch Med Sci. 2011;7:27–33.
27. Ganjoo K, Advani R, Mariappan MR, McMillan A, Horning S. Non-Hodgkin lymphoma of the breast. Cancer. 2007;110:25–30.

## Further Reading

Matro JM, Li T, Cristofanilli M, Hughes ME, Ottesen RA, Weeks JC, Wong YN. Inflammatory breast cancer management in the national comprehensive network: the disease, recurrence pattern, and outcome. Clin Breast Cancer. 2015;15:1–7.

Mituś J, Reinfuss M, Mituś JW, et al. Malignant phyllodes tumor of the breast: treatment and prognosis. Breast J. 2014;20:639–44.

Rueth NM, Black DM, Limmer AR, et al. Breast conservation in the setting of contemporary multimodality treatment provides excellent outcomes for patients with occult primary breast cancer. Ann Surg Oncol. 2015;22:90–5.

Sandoval-Leon AC, Drews-Elger K, Gomez-Fernandez CR, Yepes MM, Lippman ME. Paget's disease of the nipple. Breast Cancer Res Treat. 2013;141:1–12.

**Websites in Appendix**: *Paget*, A-4.16.

# Breast Cancer in General Population 15

Oreste D. Gentilini and Maria Virginia Thomazini

## Contents



**Abstract**

• American Joint Committee on Cancer (AJCC) proposes the term *multiple* BCs rather than multifocal or multicentric BC. • The incidence of pregnancy-associated BC is the same as expected in general population, and also the ultimate comparison of prognosis, stage-for-stage and age-matched, may be similar. • Treatment of BC in young women is not substantially different from other age groups, and also systemic therapy is mainly linked to the biology of the tumor. However, in appropriate situations, it may also be important to evaluate very

O.D. Gentilini (✉) • M.V. Thomazini
Division of Breast Surgery, European Institute of Oncology (IEO), Milano, Italy
e-mail: oreste.gentilini@ieo.it



A.M. Pluchinotta (ed.), *The Outpatient Breast Clinic: Aiming at Best Practice*,
DOI 10.1007/978-3-319-15907-2_15

young women separately. • Management of BC in the elderly vulnerable and frail women could be a major challenge for oncologists and geriatricians alike. Dedicated oncologists are needed.

*Future Directions.* Many preconceptions about women are far from being cleared. Besides those related to individual variability, those related to age/biological age, fertility, and quality of life in complex contexts are equally important. There should be room for special situations such as a customized treatment for very young or elderly women.

## 15.1 Multiple Ipsilateral and Bilateral Breast Cancers

**Clinical Practice Points**

- In multifocal and multicentric BC, establishing whether separate foci are polyclonal or monoclonal in origin is challenging and a matter of debate.
- Because the incidence of BC is increasing and prognosis is improving, a growing number of women with BC are at risk of developing bilateral disease.
- There are important differences in the incidence trends and prognostic outcome between synchronous and metachronous bilateral BC diagnosed at different ages.
- Adjuvant chemotherapy has a dual effect on metachronous cancer: it reduces the risk of a second disease, while it seems to worsen the prognosis whenever it occurs.
- Women with multiple BC have an increased risk of developing a subsequent non-breast cancer.

### 15.1.1 Overview

Multiple cancers are defined as two or more primary cancers occurring in an individual that are not an extension, recurrence, or metastasis.

Multiple ipsilateral BCs are categorized as multifocal (MF) or multicentric (MC) based on the location of presentation. Multiple BCs in both breasts (bilateral BC) are categorized as synchronous or metachronous based on the chronology of presentation.

For most authors, multifocal breast carcinoma refers to the presence of more than one distinct tumor within the same quadrant of the breast, while multicentric mammary carcinoma describes the presence of a clinically or mammographically evident tumor in a different breast quadrant from the index lesion [1].

New molecular studies suggest some inconsistencies in this common attitude to categorize multiple BCs. The above usual nomenclature is established on multiple tumors diagnosed clinically on physical examination and on breast imaging studies including mammogram, ultrasound, and magnetic resonance imaging (MRI).

Nevertheless, multiple breast carcinomas, especially when occurring in an ipsilateral breast, are a challenge for pathologists in terms of the identification of their cellular origins.

Because in situ carcinoma is a precursor of invasive carcinoma, the presence of in situ disease in multiple separate cancer foci has led investigators to consider such foci as polyclonal tumors versus those of monoclonal origin. However, unless clonal analysis is performed on each cancer focus, the polyclonal or monoclonal origin cannot be assessed by spatial presentation alone [1, 2].

Moreover in TNM classification, multicentric invasive cancers are staged using the largest primary carcinoma to designate the T stage. Tumor sizes are not added together, and a designation to identify the carcinoma as multicentric is added to allow separate analysis of this group of tumors. There is some evidence to suggest that this staging system may not accurately reflect outcomes in multicentric carcinoma. When the diameter of the largest of the multicentric tumors was used to determine tumor size, patients with multicentric tumors had significantly more nodal metastases for T1 and T2 tumors than those with unicentric cancers.

## 15.1.2 Multiple Ipsilateral BCs

*Definition*. MF/MC BC is a debated subject with no international consensus on its definition or recommended methods of assessment. The classic studies conducted by Holland demonstrated that the majority of breast carcinomas are multifocal and extensive [3]. The reported prevalence of multicentric cancer has ranged from 13 to 75 %. This discrepancy can be explained by two reasons: first, many studies are based on a traditional morphologic workup that focuses on macroscopically visible dominant masses that typically include a low proportion of multifocal cases, and second, there is a lack of significant differences between unifocal and multifocal cancers [4].

Generally, multifocality is defined as the presence of two or more malignant lesions in the same quadrant separated by normal breast tissue, while a multicentric lesion refers to two or more malignant lesions also separated by normal breast tissue but located in different quadrants [5]. Katz et al. [6] defined multifocality as foci separated by less than 4 cm or located in the same quadrant and multicentricity as foci separated by at least 4 cm or in different quadrants; foci were identified mammographically or on gross pathologic examination.

Middleton et al. instead defined multicentric mammary carcinoma as an evident focus in a quadrant outside that of the primary tumor but considered patients with different foci in the same quadrant that were microscopic only as having a unicentric tumor; multifocality was defined as more than one distinct tumor in the same quadrant [1, 6].

*Incidence*. The incidence of multicentric BC is variously reported as ranging approximately from 5 to 65 % of cases. Likewise, multifocal BC may occur in as many as 60 % of cases. In addition to this, about 3–5 % of patients with BC will have bilateral disease at the time of presentation.

Pathology studies using standard clinical techniques of examining breast tissue which include gross inspection of the specimen and a limited number of random sections of grossly normal breast have also identified multicentric carcinoma in about 5–13 % of cases. Also, in the presence of ductal carcinoma in situ (DCIS), discontinuous growth was more frequent in well-differentiated DCIS (70 %) than in poorly differentiated DCIS (10 %). These findings suggest that true multicentricity is uncommon in DCIS, but multifocal growth within a ductal system is common in low-grade lesions [1].

*Diagnosis.* The sensitivity of mammography for detection of multifocal and multicentric tumors ranges between 15 and 45 % [7]. Ultrasonography (US) has been shown to be useful as a complement to mammography for detecting additional (about 20 %) occult tumor.

Numerous studies have shown that MRI detects multifocal and/or multicentric disease with greater accuracy than conventional imaging. Houssami et al. [8] published a meta-analysis examining the accuracy of MRI for detecting multifocal and/or multicentric cancer. Data from these studies showed that MRI found additional disease in the affected breast in 16 % of women with BC. However, MRI has a disappointing false-positive rate. In this meta-analysis, MRI had a positive predictive value of 66 % and a true-positive to false-positive ratio of 1:9.

Histologic subtype of invasive carcinoma does not appear to be predictive of multicentricity. Older studies have suggested that infiltrating lobular carcinoma is more likely to be a multicentric process, but when lobular carcinoma in situ is excluded from consideration, multicentricity is not so frequent with invasive lobular carcinoma. In contrast, several small studies suggest that multicentricity is more frequent in micropapillary DCIS than in other histologic types of intraductal carcinoma.

*Treatment.* The conservative surgical approach to MF/MC BC is still debated: no consensus has been reached. According to some reports, the local recurrence rate in MF/MC BC after breast conservative therapy (BCT) was significantly higher than that of a single tumor. This conclusion leads many physicians to continue to perform mastectomy for MF/MC BC. Fowble et al. [9] performed a pathologic review of the mastectomy specimens and revealed extensive residual disease in three or four quadrants of the breast after excisional biopsy in 50 % of the patients with MF/MC BC. However, recently in a large retrospective series, Gentilini et al. [10] found that breast-conserving surgery was safe for patients with MF/MC BC, when the disease was adequately excised.

Several authors have shown a correlation between lymph node involvement and multifocality, which is a surrogate factor for predicting recurrence and survival; they have shown a positive association between multifocality and the presence of lymph node metastases. By combining these studies, we might estimate an approximately 20 % increase in risk of lymph node involvement in the presence of multifocality. Interestingly, this increased risk seems also to be present for small tumors [11] as well.

This higher risk of lymph node metastasis seen with multifocal tumors may result from greater tumor volume or potential for dissemination. In fact, multifocal invasive BCs occur in younger patients and have aggressive characteristics that have been previously reported (higher histoprognostic grade, higher proliferation, more Her-2 expression); therefore, secondary foci may be metastases from a tumor with an elevated metastatic potential.

In multifocal BC, axillary lymph node dissection is the standard, and the sentinel node biopsy procedure remains in question. Several authors have reported that the rate of false negatives (FN) differed depending on the study, ranging from 0 to 21 % [12].

*Prognosis*. The prognostic significance of multifocality in invasive BCs remains unclear. Yerushalmi et al. [13] evaluated prospectively whether patients with MF/MC BC have different outcomes compared to unifocal disease in terms of survival and the development of contralateral BC (CBC) disease. The author reported that the 5-year cumulative incidence of CBC in the unifocal versus MF/MF group was 2.3 % [(95 % CI 2.1–2.5)] versus 2.4 % [(95 % CI 1.6–3.4) ($p=0.349$)]. Breast cancer-specific survival rate revealed a slightly worse outcome with MF/MC disease, RR = 1.174 [(95 % CI 1.004–1.372)]. There is no clear evidence that patients with multifocal BC have a worse clinical outcome than those with unicentric BC who have been treated in a similar way.

### 15.1.3 Bilateral BC

*Definition*. Bilateral BCs are divided into synchronous (when cancers in both breasts develop simultaneously) and metachronous (when cancers in each breast develop at different times). Synchronous bilateral cancers can be further subdivided into two groups. The first group consists of cancers with signs or symptoms present in both breasts, and the second group consists of contralateral cancers that are not palpable and are diagnosed only as a result of imaging studies precipitated by the initial diagnosis. In general, the incidence of synchronous bilateral BC is varying from 1 to 3 %, whereas the incidence of metachronous is around 0.3–0.8 % *per annum*.

*Risk factors*. The risk factors for contralateral BCs are: early age at diagnosis, family history of cancer (10-year risk 10–15 %), BRCA1/2 mutation (10-year risk 25–30 %), and CHEK2 mutation (10-year risk 10–20 %) [14, 15]. In addition, there is a concordance between increasing incidence and lobular carcinoma. In a cohort study, 2,855 patients with unilateral BC were followed up for a median of 7 years. The cumulative risk of contralateral BC was estimated to be 20.9 % after invasive lobular cancer, compared to 11.2 % after invasive ductal cancer [16].

The findings of some studies suggest that the risk of contralateral BC is greater for women whose first cancer is ER-negative than it is for women with ER-positive cancers. However, most ER-positive cancers are treated with tamoxifen, and most ER-negative cancers are not. So that tamoxifen treatment greatly reduces the risk of contralateral cancer, it is not possible to interpret these results without adjustment for hormonal therapies, and it has not been yet established that ER-negative status is an independent risk factor for contralateral BC [17].

*Treatment*. In the past, clinicians have approached bilateral disease more aggressively than unilateral disease, and studies have shown a disproportionately higher incidence of bilateral mastectomies performed in patients with bilateral cancer. A number of studies have demonstrated that bilateral breast conservation treatment is feasible and is not associated with an increased risk in the outcome [18].

Patients with a genetic mutation are at a significantly increased risk for the development of new primary cancers, and this should be considered in the decision-making process.

Both tamoxifen and aromatase inhibitors substantially reduce the risk of contralateral BC. A standard course of tamoxifen is associated with a reduction of approximately 50 % in the risk of contralateral BC, and the decrease in risk lasts for at least 15 years [19].

*Prognosis*. The 10-year survival of women with synchronous bilateral BC is inferior to that of women with unilateral BC (45 % vs. 33 %, respectively, $P<0.001$). In detail, women diagnosed with metachronous cancer within *more than 5 years* have a four times higher mortality rate compared to women with unilateral BC after adjustment for age at diagnosis.

In contrast, women with metachronous cancers diagnosed *more than 10 years* after initial diagnosis had a prognosis similar to that of women with unilateral cancer. Among women with metachronous BC, the lowest mortality from BC is seen for those with the longest time interval between the first and the second cancer. After 10 years of follow-up, the cumulative BC-specific mortality is around 50 % among women with bilateral cancer diagnosed within 5 years and around 35 % among those diagnosed with bilateral cancer more than 10 years after their first primary [20].

### 15.1.4 BC and Risk of Associated Non-breast Cancer

*Unilateral BC*. Besides an elevated risk of contralateral BC, several studies revealed that women with a primary BC have an increased risk of developing a subsequent non-BC. Increased risks are most consistently found for tumors of the ovary, endometrium, soft tissue, and for leukemia. Though less consistently, also excess risks of melanoma of the skin and cancer of the bone, esophagus, kidney, and lung have also been reported.

The risk of subsequent non-BC appears to be associated with genetic and other risk factors that are common for both cancers. Moreover, BC patients with primary BC experienced an increased risk of lung cancer and soft tissue sarcomas that could be attributed to radiation. Increased risks of melanoma of the skin, uterine cancer, and leukemia are found to be associated with the use of chemotherapy for patients older than 50 years, whereas the increased risk of endometrial cancer was related to endocrine therapy. At the same time, chemotherapy is associated with a reduced risk of colon and lung cancer for women younger than 50 years.

*Bilateral BC*. Information about the risk of third cancer of non-breast origin after synchronous or metachronous invasive bilateral BC is lacking. Patients with bilateral BC may have been exposed to more carcinogenic or carcino-protective cancer treatment. Moreover, a higher risk could be expected for genetic, reproductive, or lifestyle-related cancers.

Women with bilateral BC have a 1.5 times higher risk of all non-BCs combined. Young women have a 2.8 times higher risk of all non-breast tumors combined and a tenfold higher risk of ovarian cancer, compared with the general population, which is probably related to genetic factors. Chemotherapy is associated with a decreased risk of all non-breast tumors combined, whereas radiotherapy and endocrine therapy are associated with an increased risk.

## 15.2 Breast Cancer During Pregnancy

**Clinical Practice Points**

- Pregnancy-associated BC (PABC) is a purely arbitrary definition of cancer diagnosed during pregnancy or within 1 year of delivery.
- Ultrasonography of the breast and regional lymph nodes is used to assess the extent of disease and also to guide biopsy. Core needle biopsy is preferred for histological diagnosis and biomarker analysis.
- The general philosophy of treatment today is to treat the cancer and allow the pregnancy to proceed.
- Significant emotional issues surround care of women with pregnancy-associated BC, and multiple specialties are involved in patient management and in an essential psychological support.
- Pregnancy after BC should not in principle be discouraged, and retrospective available data report no detrimental effect of a subsequent pregnancy on BC outcome.

Pregnancy-associated breast cancer (BCDP) is defined as BC diagnosed during pregnancy or within the year after delivery, but the real challenging clinical scenario is represented by BC diagnosed during pregnancy. The exact incidence is unknown; however, it is estimated to constitute around 10 % of BC cases diagnosed below the age of 40 in Western nations. Statistical analysis proves that the incidence of PABC is 1 out of 3,000 deliveries [21, 22].

Some studies have found that BCDP is more commonly diagnosed at an advanced stage with larger tumor size and with lymph nodes metastases. Delay in diagnosis is typical because tumor masses can be masked by breast engorgement owing to lactation, and inflammatory changes may be mistaken for mastitis, but also because of increased breast density, making clinical examinations and mammography more difficult to interpret. [23]

*Risk factors*. No specific risk factors for BC in pregnancy are known. Genetic or environmental risk factors are similar to those for age-adjusted BC in the general population. Individuals with *BRCA1* or *BRCA2* mutations might be at increased risk, but they do not have an increased incidence of BC in pregnancy [24].

*Clinical presentations and diagnosis*. BC in pregnancy typically presents as a painless lump palpated by the woman. Physiological breast changes associated with pregnancy, such as breast enlargement, hypertrophy, and nipple discharge obscure detection for patient and physician, and this implies a delay in diagnosis, leading to more advanced stages at diagnosis than in the general population. As a consequence, BC in pregnancy is associated with more metastases and subsequently poorer outcomes [25].

Breast ultrasonography is the first diagnostic instrument used by clinicians when a breast mass and the axillary area need to be assessed in a pregnant woman with high sensitivity and specificity. Mammography is not particularly useful, since the radiodensity of the breast tissue in pregnant and lactating women significantly decreases the sensitivity of this examination. Nevertheless, it can be used, with proper shielding, to rule out diffuse microcalcifications.

MRI with contrast agents is possible during pregnancy but should only be used when it will alter clinical decision-making and when ultrasonography is inadequate. The reason of this caution is because some studies have underline that gadolinium-based MRI contrast agents pass through the placental barrier and enter fetal circulation [26, 27].

The standard examination to obtain a histological diagnosis is a core biopsy, which can be safely done during pregnancy. The major risks of infection and milk fistula can be minimized if the woman ceases breastfeeding at least 48 h prior to biopsy [28]. Fine needle aspiration (FNA) is not recommended because hormonal changes during pregnancy could lead to false positive or false negative.

*Pathology.* The histopathological and immunohistochemical findings of BC in pregnancy are similar to those in nonpregnant women who are younger than 35 years. Most pregnant patients are diagnosed with infiltrating ductal adenocarcinomas (71–100 %), which are often associated with aggressive behavior: high incidence of grade 3 tumors (40–95 %), lymph vascular invasion, and a high rate of estrogen-receptor negativity [29].

Gestational BC is associated with larger tumors and a higher incidence of nodal involvement (53–71 %) than in nonpregnant patient. Most PABC is estrogen-receptor and progesterone-receptor (ER/PR) negative, whereas HER2 positivity has been reported in 42 % of cases [30].

*Treatment.* Therapeutic strategies are determined by tumor biology, tumor stage, gestational stage, and the patient's and her family's wishes and should involve a multidisciplinary team.

Pregnancy termination, once routinely advocated because of fear that the hormonal and immunologic milieu would adversely affect the patient's survival, is now rare. Patients should be informed that abortion does not improve prognosis of the disease and that effective treatments can be safely performed during pregnancy.

Surgery can be done safely during any stage of pregnancy, and most anesthetic agents seem to be safe for the fetus [31]. The mother should be strictly monitored to avoid hypoxia, hypotension, hypoglycemia, fever, pain, infections, or thrombosis. The choice of BC surgery during pregnancy should follow the same guidelines as for nonpregnant women; however, breast conservation performed during a very early gestational age is associated with a long delay in postoperative radiotherapy [32]. Clinicians can safely use sentinel lymph node staging during pregnancy because estimated absorbed doses are largely below the 0.1–0.2 Gy fetal threshold absorbed dose [33].

Chemotherapy can be adjuvant or neoadjuvant and should be administered after the first trimester. For fetal protection, chemotherapy is contraindicated until

12–14 weeks gestation. The regimens of chemotherapy (see Sect. 18.3) recommended to pregnant BC patients are the same as the ones recommended to non-pregnant counterparts. Chemotherapy can be safely administrated to pregnant BC patients using standard anthracycline-based regimens (e.g., FEC, FAC, EC, AC). These regimens should be followed by a taxane whenever indicated. The taxane can also be administered during pregnancy, although there are less available data. Trastuzumab and endocrine therapy must not be prescribed during pregnancy but must be postponed until after delivery [34].

Hormonal agents such as selective estrogen-receptor modulators can disturb the hormonal environment, and so such treatments should be delayed until after delivery. Tamoxifen has the potential to induce fetal harm during pregnancy and is associated with birth defects including craniofacial malformations, ambiguous genitalia, and fetal death [35].

Radiation therapy is impracticable during pregnancy because even with abdominal shielding, the fetal dose is high.

*Prognosis*. Pregnant women are less likely to be diagnosed with stage 1 but two and a half times more likely to be diagnosed with advanced disease than nonpregnant women. The discussion about prognosis remains open for BC during pregnancy: while few studies have pointed to poor prognosis of patients diagnosed during pregnancy, others did not reproduce the same results. A recent meta-analysis of 30 retrospective cohort studies showed worse prognosis of PABCs, even after adjustment for age and stage, and that PABC is independently associated with poor survival particularly those diagnosed shortly postpartum. This underscores a possible impact of the pregnant breast microenvironment on the biology and consequently the prognosis of these tumors. Apparently, it is not possible to establish definitions about the prognosis, because the available studies have important methodological limitations, with many confounding variables.

*PREGNANCY AFTER BREAST CANCER* – Due to rising trend to delay pregnancy at a later age, more women are diagnosed with BC before completing their families. Therefore, inquiry into the feasibility and safety of pregnancy following BC diagnosis is steadily growing. Available evidence suggests that women with a history of BC are frequently advised against future conception for fear that pregnancy could adversely affect their outcome. Pregnancy after BC should not in principle be discouraged. Retrospective available data report no detrimental effect of a subsequent pregnancy on BC outcome [36]. Nonetheless, a thorough staging should be performed before trying for conception, depending on the individual risk of relapse, and patients should be informed about the possibility of BC recurrence even many years after diagnosis [37].

There is no definitive evidence to recommend a fixed time frame from diagnosis to pregnancy [38]. Despite absence of supporting evidence, some experts recommend avoiding early pregnancy (within 2 years from diagnosis) in patients of higher risk of early relapse. In addition, potential disadvantages of early stopping of ongoing recommended anticancer treatments must be discussed and balanced with the risk of infertility due to aging and iatrogenic effects of cancer treatment. Delaying pregnancy should be discussed on an individual basis in order to allow for continuation/completion of adjuvant therapy. The discussion should take into account the half-life of administered treatment (to prevent detrimental effects on the fetus), the detection of early relapse in high-risk disease, and/or overcoming early treatment-related side effects.

In general, an interval of at least 4–6 months from the end of chemotherapy and the attempt to conceive is recommended [39]. Data on endocrine treatment are less conclusive: as a practical advice, an interval of at least 3 months from the end/interruption of therapy is recommended due to the half-life of tamoxifen. Women should be fully informed about the risk of stopping tamoxifen treatment prematurely. If a woman prematurely stops endocrine treatment to achieve a pregnancy, resuming tamoxifen after breastfeeding completion can be considered, and an ongoing worldwide clinical trial is addressing this issue. Limited data on the efficacy and safety of ovarian stimulation after treatment of BC are available. Caution and individualized decision-making are recommended.

Data about pregnancy and fetal outcome after BC treatment are reassuring. No increased fetal malformation rates have been reported after completion of chemotherapy or endocrine treatment, but some population-based data report an increased risk of delivery complications, caesarean section, very preterm birth (<32 weeks), and low birth weight (<1,500 g), highlighting the need for careful pregnancy surveillance and management in this population.

Breastfeeding after BC is not contraindicated and should be supported with adequate information and counseling [4]. Milk production after breast-conserving surgery and radiotherapy is reduced, but breastfeeding from the other breast is feasible and safe for the mother and the child, provided the patient is not taking any medications that may be harmful for the child.

## 15.3 Breast Cancer in Young Woman

**Clinical Practice Points**

- Approximately 1 in 40 women diagnosed with early BC is very young (under 35 years). Age has been shown to be an independent adverse prognostic factor for women with a diagnosis of BC.
- Intrinsic difficulties in diagnosis of BC in young women are dense breast tissue, lack of previous routine breast screening, and shorter tumor doubling times. By the time a mass can be felt, the cancer may be advanced.
- Genetic counseling is indicated for all young patients, since 10–15 % of patients diagnosed under the age of 35 present with a gene mutation.
- Multidisciplinary management and care is strongly recommended to avoid an opinionated standard of practice and the risk of overtreatment.
- Medical treatment of BC in young women is not substantially different from other age groups, since therapy is mainly linked to the biology of the tumor. However, in appropriate situations, it may also be important to evaluate very young women separately.

The European Society of Breast Cancer Specialists (EUSOMA) working group decided to define "young women" as women under the age of 40. Since both biology and endocrine milieu are a continuum, that age group definition will always be arbitrary. However, women under the age of 40 have specific issues related to fertility preservation, pregnancy, and lactation that deserve a different approach and management from slightly older pre- and perimenopausal women.

The care of young women with BC has become a more recent focus with improvements in diagnosis, treatment, and survivorship. This population, usually defined as women diagnosed under the age of 40, requires individualized treatment plans. Given the differences in epidemiology and management options, as well as the unique issues surrounding fertility, sexuality, and pregnancy, the multidisciplinary approach to treatment for these women frequently may also incorporate other areas of expertise.

### 15.3.1 Epidemiology and Risk Factors

Around 5–7 % of BCs are diagnosed in women younger than 40, making it the most commonly diagnosed female cancer in the 25- to 39-year-old age group [22, 40]. In patients younger than 40 years specifically, African American females have the highest relative incidence of BC. Young women tend to present at more advanced stages and their tumors tend to be higher grade and hormone-receptor negative and have increased HER2/Neu overexpression and more lymphovascular invasion [41]. An analysis from EORTC and NSABP indicated a higher risk of local recurrence in patients younger than 35 years [42, 43].

BC at a young age is associated with an increased risk for contralateral BC (CBC). Overall, patients younger than 50 years have a risk of CBC of 0.1 % annually or approximately 13 % cumulative risk in a 10-year period. Diagnosis before the age of 45 doubles the risk of having a CBC [44]. A review from by Gnerlich et al. indicated young patients with stage 1 or 2 BC had a higher disease-specific mortality rate when adjusted for other factors; this seems to be due to the aggressive phenotype of these tumors or more advanced stages at presentation [45].

### 15.3.2 Clinical Presentation and Diagnosis

Young women are more likely to present with a mass or symptom due to the lack of screening programs and to inadequate imaging for their frequently dense breasts. Women presenting with breast symptoms and a strong suspicion of BC should be evaluated by triple assessment in order to exclude or confirm a diagnosis of cancer.

As in older women, a lesion considered malignant following clinical examination, imaging, or cytology alone should, where possible, have a histopathological confirmation of malignancy before any surgical procedure takes place.

Ultrasound (US) and magnetic resonance (MRI) are often used to delineate the extent of disease given dense breasts in young women. However, there is no evidence to recommend routine preoperative MRI in young women with BC. Magnetic resonance imaging (MRI) should be performed in the second week of the menstrual cycle (day 6–13 counting from the first day of bleeding) and should follow the usual recommended technical requirements. It should also be noted that imaging is not influenced by hormonal contraception [46, 47]; in addition, young women presenting with BC are at risk to have a genetic syndrome (Li-Fraumeni o Cowden syndrome) [48].

### 15.3.3 Treatment of BC in Young Woman

Because of a lack of patient numbers or difficulty of randomization due to very personal issues, clinical trials encompassing the specificities of BC in very young women are difficult to plan. However, the research community should make all efforts globally, to develop research programs, which needs are not yet met.

*Early BC*. Breast-conserving surgery (BCS) followed by radiotherapy (RT) provides the same long-term survival benefit as modified radical mastectomy in women with stage I–II BC, despite a significantly higher rate of local recurrences [49]. Esthetic outcomes, body image changes, and the impact on sexuality may be more relevant in young women: when mastectomy is indicated, skin- and nipple-sparing techniques with immediate breast reconstruction, when feasible, or other oncoplastic techniques can provide adequate oncological control while also addressing the cosmetic needs. Indication for SLNB and surgical management of patients with SLN involvement should be the same as in older patients.

After breast-conserving surgery, whole breast radiotherapy (WBR) should be given. An additional radiation dose to the tumor bed (boost) should be considered, as well an enrollment into an appropriate prospective clinical boost trial. Because young patients have a risk factor of increased local relapse after mastectomy and involvement of the internal mammary chain, the possibility of postmastectomy radiotherapy and IMC irradiation should be discussed on an individualized basis [50]. Partial breast irradiation (PBI), such as intraoperative radiotherapy (IORT) or other techniques, is not recommended [51].

The indications for and the choice of type of adjuvant systemic treatment for invasive BC should be driven, as for women in other age categories, by the biological characteristics of the tumor (including, but not limiting to, HR and HER-2 receptors, proliferation markers (e.g., Ki-67), and grade), the tumor stage, patient's comorbidities, and menopausal status.

Young women with invasive hormone-receptor positive (HR+) BC should be considered for adjuvant tamoxifen regardless of age, lymph node status, or chemotherapy administration [52]. The optimal duration of ET for high-risk premenopausal women has not been adequately studied. Studies reported that extending adjuvant tamoxifen treatment for a total of 10 years, compared to stopping at 5 years, reduced BC mortality by about one third in the first 10 years following diagnosis and by a half subsequently [53].

The HERA trial has demonstrated that the benefit of adjuvant trastuzumab appears independent of age [54].

*Advanced BC* in young women is defined as metastatic disease diagnosed <40 years old. Whenever feasible, the metastatic lesion should be biopsied and tested for confirmation of diagnosis, histology, and biology, especially in case of late relapse. Therapeutic recommendations should not differ from those for older women with the same disease characteristics and extent.

Endocrine therapy is the preferred option for HR+ disease, unless there is concern or proof of endocrine resistance or need for rapid disease and/or symptom control. A meta-analysis comparing GnRH analogs + tamoxifen showed that the outcomes were significantly improved in patients who received the combination. Recommendations regarding chemotherapy should not differ from those for older women with the same disease characteristics [55].

In patient with BRCA 1/2 mutation, bilateral risk-reducing mastectomy may be considered. Therapeutic decisions should reflect a balance between the risk of recurrence of the diagnosed BC and the potential benefit of preventing an additional primary tumor. In addition, prophylactic salpingo-oophorectomy should be discussed from the age of 35 provided that the woman has completed family planning and should preferably be done before 40, always respecting the patient's preferences and considering family history [56, 57].

### 15.3.4 Social Life and Sexual Issues

*SOCIAL LIFE*

*Premature menopause*. High cumulative doses of alkylating agents after the age of 35 years are associated with a high probability of premature menopause. Menopausal symptoms can be particularly bothersome in young patients with iatrogenic ovarian exhaustion. Hot flashes can be reduced with nonhormonal treatments such as selective serotonin reuptake inhibitors (SSRI). Other available nonhormonal treatments against hot flashes include gabapentin, clonidine, and acupuncture [58]. Fatigue, a common complaint in BC patients, may be worsened by menopausal symptoms, insomnia and restlessness, and be of special concern in young patients who have to cope with multiple tasks linked to a young family, work, and career.

*Infertility*. Fertility and family planning are major concerns for young women with BC.

Even women with regular menses after chemotherapy have a reduced ovarian reserve and experience impaired fertility and an earlier menopause. This is mainly due to the direct toxicity of chemotherapy on the oocyte pool, which physiologically diminishes with age and is significantly reduced after chemotherapy. Chemotherapy might also damage ovarian granulosa cells. The risk of genetic fetal anomalies, when pregnancy occurs during chemotherapy, should enable a thorough discussion about contraception before this treatment is initiated in order to evaluate possible options of fertility preservation.

*Contraception*. Pregnancy must be discouraged during active treatment of BC, so effective contraception is recommended. Exogenous hormonal contraception is generally contraindicated in BC survivors, and alternative strategies (i.e., barrier methods such as condoms, cervical diaphragm, and copper IUDs) should be considered. For women asking for permanent contraception, laparoscopic tubal ligation or hysteroscopic tubal plugging can be used. In case of a steady male partner, vasectomy is an option which might be taken into consideration [59].

*SEXUAL ISSUES*. Sexuality encompasses three major dimensions: sexual identity, sexual function, and sexual relationship, which may be variably wounded in young women with BC.

*Sexual identity* and body image are more vulnerable in younger women, the breast being a prominent sign of femininity and beauty. If mastectomy is required, attention to immediate reconstruction techniques may positively improve the psychosexual outcome in terms of body image and sexual identity [60].

*Sexual function*. Young women with BC are at particular risk for sexual dysfunction, which is being increasingly reported during and after treatment. For vaginal dryness and dyspareunia, nonhormonal methods, including moisturizing and lubricating agents, are preferred. Local estrogens with low/minimal (<1 %) systemic absorption like promestriene could be helpful, yet few safety data in women with BC are available. In women with estrogen-receptor negative BC, twice a week vaginal estradiol or estriol that have low systemic absorption and stronger efficacy on the vaginal mucosa and ecosystem can be considered in cases with severe symptoms [61]. If loss of desire and central arousal difficulties persist after correction of physical symptoms and depression, psychological support should be offered.

*Sexual relationship*. BC diagnosis and treatment may dramatically impair the quality of the couple's relationship. Data indicate that the emotional intimacy, the sense of bonding, affection, and commitment may be improved in the majority of couples (60–70 %), while the physical, erotic intimacy may be variably affected. The longer the time is between surgery and having intercourse again, the higher the probability of sexual dysfunction.

Patients and their partners should be reassured that there is no medical contraindication to sexual intimacy including touching the operated breast during BC therapy and afterwards. These issues should be addressed promptly, as sexual prognosis improves if effective management/treatment is implemented early [61].

## 15.4 Breast Cancer in the Elderly Woman

**Clinical Practice Points**

- Aging is the single greatest risk factor for developing BC. The 5-year relative survival for women with BC increases with age until the age of 75 years and more.
- When facing an individual elderly patient with BC, her chronologic age should be secondary, and her physiologic age should be examined.
- More favorable biological characteristics were found in elderly woman compared with younger postmenopausal ones.
- The age itself may be a risk factor of not receiving adequate therapies or not standard therapies. The treatment of BC in frail women should be managed by dedicated oncologists.

Recommendations for management of BC in older individuals are limited by a lack of evidence. Treatment is largely based on limited retrospective subgroup analyses, and extrapolation of study results from younger patients [62]. Age alone should not dictate any aspect of management for older individuals with BC. All decisions should consider physiological age, estimated life expectancy, risks, benefits, treatment tolerance, patient preference, and potential treatment barriers.

### 15.4.1 Epidemiology and Risk Factors

Incidence of BC for women 70 years or older diagnosed between 200 and 2004 varied from 100 to 350 per 100,000 per year. Compared with younger women, older women are more likely to have BC with estrogen-receptor (ER) and progesterone-receptor expression. ER-positive cancers increase from greater than 60 % among women aged 30–34 years to 85 % among women 80–84 years. HER2-positive tumors decrease from 22 % among women younger than 40 years to 10 % in women 70 years or older [63].

Tumor size and nodal involvement increase with age, at least partly explained by delayed diagnosis in older women. Five-year and ten-year relative survival of patients 70 years or older are lower than those of patients aged 40–70 years. Undertreatment, socioeconomic differences, and unequal access to health care contribute to poorer prognosis [64].

Many older patients with operable BC die of noncancer-related causes. In fact, in a study of more than 900 women with early BC, women with at least three of seven selected morbid conditions were 20 times more likely to die from causes other than BC [65]. In addition the age itself may be a risk factor of not receiving adequate treatment or not standard therapies [62]. This is true in particular for 75-year-old patients or over, when BC is more frequent. Factors contributing to receiving non-adequate therapies are:

- Reluctance of physician in treating a cancer apparently less aggressive than in younger counterparts and the fear of important toxicities
- Comorbidity, including cognitive status, depression, and anxiety
- Polypharmacy
- Level of dependence and social support
- Nutritional assessment
- Physical barriers like sensory impairment and poor mobility, ethnic origin, socioeconomic status, and sociocultural environment

### 15.4.2 Geriatric Assessment

Estimation of life expectancy and ability to undergo treatment might be improved by collaborative geriatric and oncology management and a multidomain geriatric assessment [66, 67].

The comprehensive geriatric assessment (CGA) is a structured evaluation of elderly patients, developed by geriatricians, based on multiple levels including physical and functional status, comorbidities, nutritional status, and geriatric syndromes such as dementia or depression. It is useful to identify and manage age-related problems, allowing clinicians to select patients more appropriately for therapy and avoiding futile therapies and overtreatment as well as undertreatment [67].

According to the CGA results, patients can be divided into three groups:

- *Fit* patients
- *Vulnerable* patients
- *Frail* patients

Patients in the first group are fit to treatments as well as their younger counterparts. Patients of the last group are fit only for the best supportive care. For the patients in the second group, which is the biggest, individualized approaches and specific trials are recommended.

The most important strategy to assess geriatric patients is to define the physical function and the expectancy of life. Functional status includes patients' ability to perform daily tasks such as dressing themselves, walking, cooking meals, and other daily activities. Comorbidities are very important in the evaluation because they affect the tolerance to cancer treatment, in particular to systemic treatment and to radiotherapy. Nutrition is an important issue: where present, a loss of muscle mass is associated with a poor function and a shorter survival.

### 15.4.3 Treatment of BC in Elderly Woman

*Surgery*. Standard of care for operable BC is BCS plus whole breast radiotherapy (WBRT) or mastectomy followed by postoperative radiotherapy in selected patients. Management of the axilla is the same as in younger counterparts with sentinel node biopsy being the standard in patients with a negative axilla. For patients with clinically positive or highly suspected nodes, axillary lymph node dissection (ALND) is recommended [68, 69].

*Radiotherapy*. Most randomized trials assessing whole breast radiotherapy excluded patients older than 70 years. Breast irradiation should be recommended to older women with a life expectancy >5 years, particularly those with large tumors, positive lymph nodes, or negative hormone receptors. Quality of life is an important additional endpoint to consider with radiotherapy in older patients [70]. The option of radiotherapy should be balanced with the logistics of daily travel and individual preference regarding the potential of local relapse. PBI could be a choice to take into account: the TARGIT 1 trial, in which older patients were well represented, compared post-BCS TARGIT (single intraoperative 20 Gy fraction) with WBRT. At 4-year follow-up, LRRs were 1.2 and 0.95 %, respectively [71].

*Endocrine treatment*. Primary endocrine therapy refers to systemic endocrine treatment as sole treatment for early-stage ER-positive BC. Primary endocrine therapy (tamoxifen or aromatase inhibitors) should only be offered to elderly individuals with ER-positive tumors who have a short estimated life expectancy (<2–3 years), who are considered unfit for surgery after optimization of medical conditions, or who refuse surgery.

A Cochrane review showed a decrease in local progression with surgery plus endocrine treatment compared with primary endocrine therapy alone; however, no difference was observed in overall survival. For optimum local control, surgery (with or without radiotherapy) plus adjuvant endocrine therapy is better than primary endocrine therapy [72].

Tamoxifen can reduce BC mortality by 31 % in postmenopausal women, regardless of age, and the side effects (vasomotor symptoms, endometrial cancer, thromboembolic disease) are infrequent and do not significantly contribute to the likelihood of dying of non-BC causes.

Aromatase inhibitors are slightly better than tamoxifen, improving disease-free survival by 3–5 %. The major complication of these medications is musculoskeletal complications, including osteoporotic fractures. These women should undergo baseline and every 1–2 years bone densitometry [73].

*Adjuvant chemotherapy*. Chemotherapy is feasible in most patients 70 years or older who are selected for adjuvant chemotherapy, but increasing age, lower function, and comorbidity are associated with dose reductions and treatment breaks. Regimes should be individualized based on life expectancy and comorbidities. Myelosuppression and neutropenic infections increase with age. Age is a known risk factor for anthracycline-associated cardiac toxicity, and age is associated with higher rates of cardiomyopathy in women treated with chemotherapy. An increased mortality rate secondary to chemotherapy has been reported in older women, which may offset some of the benefit [74, 75].

## References

1. Middleton LP, Vlastos G, Mirza NQ, Eva S, Sahin AA. Multicentric mammary carcinoma: evidence of monoclonal proliferation. Cancer. 2002;94:1910–6.
2. Coombs NJ, Boyages J. Multifocal and multicentric breast cancer: does each focus matter? J Clin Oncol. 2005;23:7497–502.
3. Holland R, Veling SH, Mravunac M, Hendriks JH. Histologic multifocality of Tis, T1-2 breast carcinomas. Implications for clinical trials of breast-conserving surgery. Cancer. 1985;56: 979–90.
4. Tressera F, Rodriguez I, Garcia-Yuste M, Grases PJ, Ara C, Fabregas R. Tumor size and lymph node status in multifocal breast cancer. Breast J. 2007;13:68–71.
5. Andea AA, Bouwman D, Wallis T, Visscher DW. Correlation of tumor volume and surface area with lymph node status in patients with multifocal/multicentric breast carcinoma. Cancer. 2006;200:20–7.
6. Katz A, Strom EA, Buchholz TA, Theriault R, Singletary SE, McNeese MD. The influence of pathologic tumor characteristics on locoregional recurrence rates following mastectomy. Int J Radiat Oncol Biol Phys. 2001;50:735–42.
7. Zonderland HM, Coerkamp EG, Hermans J, van de Vijver MJ, van Voorthuisen AE. Diagnosis of breast cancer: contribution of US as an adjunct to mammography. Radiology. 1999;213: 413–22.

8. Houssami N, Ciatto S, Macaskill P, et al. Accuracy and surgical impact of magnetic resonance imaging in breast cancer staging: systematic review and meta-analysis in detection of multifocal and multicentric cancer. J Clin Oncol. 2008;26:3248–58.
9. Fowble B, Yeh IT, Schultz DJ, et al. The role of mastectomy in patients with stage I-II breast cancer presenting with gross multifocal or multicentric disease or diffuse microcalcifications. Int J Radiat Oncol Biol Phys. 1993;27:567–73.
10. Gentilini O, Botteri E, Rotmensz N, Da Lima L, Caliskan M, Garcia-Etienne CA, et al. Conservative surgery in patients with multifocal/multicentric breast cancer. Breast Cancer Res Treat. 2009;113:577–83.
11. Tot T. Clinical relevance of the distribution of the lesions in 500 consecutive breast cancer cases documented in large-format histologic sections. Cancer. 2007;110:2551–60.
12. Kim HJ, Lee JS, Park EH, et al. Sentinel node biopsy in patients with multiple breast cancer. Breast Cancer Res Treat. 2008;109:503–6.
13. Yerushalmi R, Kennecke H, Woods R, Olivotto IA, Speers C, Gelmon KA. Does multicentric/multifocal breast cancer differ from unifocal breast cancer? An analysis of survival and contralateral breast cancer incidence. Breast Cancer Res Treat. 2009;117:365–70.
14. Mavaddat N, Peock S, Frost D, et al. Cancer risks for BRCA1 and BRCA2 mutation carriers: results from prospective analysis of EMBRACE. J Natl Cancer Inst. 2013;105:812–22.
15. Reiner AS, John EM, Brooks JD, et al. Risk of asynchronous contralateral breast cancer in noncarriers of BRCA1 and BRCA2 mutations with a family history of breast cancer: a report from the Women's Environmental Cancer and Radiation Epidemiology Study. J Clin Oncol. 2013;31:433–9.
16. Arpino G, Bardou VJ, Clark GM, Elledge RM. Infiltrating lobular carcinoma of the breast: tumor characteristics and clinical outcome. Breast Cancer Res. 2004;6:R149–56.
17. Saltzman BS, Malone KE, McDougall JA, Daling JR, Li CI. Estrogen receptor, progesterone receptor, and HER2-neu expression in first primary breast cancers and risk of second primary contralateral breast cancer. Breast Cancer Res Treat. 2012;135:849–55.
18. Barry M, Sacchini V. When is contralateral mastectomy warranted in unilateral breast cancer? Expert Rev Anticancer Ther. 2011;11:1209–14.
19. Vogel VG, Costantino JP, Wickerhan DL, et al. Update of the National Surgical Adjuvant Breast and Bowel Project Study of Tamoxifen and Raloxifene (STAR) P-2 trial: preventing breast cancer. Cancer Prev Res. 2010;3:696–706.
20. Hartman M, Czene K, Reilly M, et al. Incidence and prognosis of synchronous and metachronous bilateral breast cancer. J Clin Oncol. 2007;25:4210–6.
21. Psyrri A, Burtness B. Pregnancy-associated breast cancer. Cancer J. 2005;11:83–95.
22. Anders CK, Johnson R, Litton J, Phillips M, Bleyer A. Breast cancer before age 40 years. Semin Oncol. 2009;36:237–49.
23. Anderson BO, Petrek JA, Byrd DR, Senie RT, Borgen PI. Pregnancy influences breast cancer stage at diagnosis in women 30 years of age and younger. Ann Surg Oncol. 1996;3:204–11.
24. Wohlfahrt J, Olsen JH, Melby M. Breast cancer risk after childbirth in young women with family history (Denmark). Cancer Causes Control. 2002;13:169–74.
25. Ulery M, Carter L, McFarlin BL, Giurgescu C. Pregnancy-associated breast cancer: significance of early detection. J Midwifery Womens Health. 2009;54:357–63.
26. Oto A, Ernst R, Jesse MK, Chaljub G, Saade G. Magnetic resonance imaging of the chest, abdomen, and pelvis in the evaluation of pregnant patients with neoplasms. Am J Perinatol. 2007;24:243–50.
27. Kanal E, Barkovich AJ, Bell C, et al. ACR guidance document for safe MR practices. AJR Am J Roentgenol. 2007;188:1447–74.
28. Shannon J, Douglas-Jones AG, Dallimore NS. Conversion to core biopsy in preoperative diagnosis of breast lesions: is it justified by results? J Clin Pathol. 2001;54:762–5.
29. Loibl S, von Minckwitz G, Gwyn K, et al. Breast carcinoma during pregnancy. International recommendations from an expert meeting. Cancer. 2006;106:237–46.
30. Halaska MJ, Pentheroudakis G, Strnad P, et al. Presentation, management and outcome of 32 patients with pregnancy-associated breast cancer: a matched controlled study. Breast J. 2009;15:461–7.

31. Moran BJ, Yano H, Al Zahir N, Farquharson M. Conflicting priorities in surgical intervention for cancer in pregnancy. Lancet Oncol. 2007;8:536–44.
32. Toesca A, Gentilini O, Peccatori F, Azim H, Amant F. Locoregional treatment of breast cancer during pregnancy. Gynecol Surg. 2014;11:279–84.
33. Gentilini O, Cremonesi M, Toesca A, et al. Sentinel lymph node biopsy in pregnant patients with breast cancer. Eur J Nucl Med Mol Imaging. 2010;37:78–83.
34. Peccatori FA, Azim Jr HA, Scarfone G, et al. Weekly epirubicin in the treatment of gestational breast cancer (GBC). Breast Cancer Res Treat. 2009;115:591–4.
35. Isaacs RJ, Hunter W, Clark K. Tamoxifen as systemic treatment of advanced breast cancer during pregnancy—case report and literature review. Gynecol Oncol. 2001;80:405–8.
36. Azim Jr HA, Santoro L, Pavlidis N, et al. Safety of pregnancy following breast cancer diagnosis: a meta-analysis of 14 studies. Eur J Cancer. 2011;47:74–83.
37. Cardoso F, Loibl S, Pagani O, et al. The European Society of Breast Cancer Specialists recommendations for the management of young women with breast cancer. Eur J Cancer. 2012; 48:3355–77.
38. Amant F, Deckers S, Van Calsteren K, et al. Breast cancer in pregnancy: recommendations of an international consensus meeting. Eur J Cancer. 2010;46(18):3158–68.
39. Azim Jr HA, Bellettini G, Liptrott SJ, et al. Breastfeeding in breast cancer survivors: pattern, behaviour and effect on breast cancer outcome. Breast. 2010;19:527–31.
40. Gabriel CA, Domchek SM. Breast cancer in young women. Breast Cancer Res. 2010;12:212.
41. Assi HA, Khoury KE, Dbouk H, Khalil LE, Mouhieddine TH, El Saghir NS. Epidemiology and prognosis of breast cancer in young women. J Thorac Dis. 2013;5:S2–8.
42. de Bock GH, van der Hage JA, Putter H, Bonnema J, Bartelink H, van de Velde CJ. Isolated loco-regional recurrence of breast cancer is more common in young patients and following breast conserving therapy: long-term results of European Organisation for Research and Treatment of Cancer studies. Eur J Cancer. 2006;42:351–6.
43. Wapnir IL, Anderson SJ, Mamounas EP, et al. Prognosis after ipsilateral breast tumor recurrence and locoregional recurrences in five National Surgical Adjuvant Breast and Bowel Project node-positive adjuvant breast cancer trials. J Clin Oncol. 2006;24:2028–37.
44. Hartman M, Czene K, Reilly M, et al. Genetic implications of bilateral breast cancer: a population based cohort study. Lancet Oncol. 2005;6:377–82.
45. Gnerlich JL, Deshpande AD, Jeffe DB, Sweet A, White N, Margenthaler JA. Elevated breast cancer mortality in women younger than age 40 years compared with older women is attributed to poorer survival in early-stage disease. J Am Coll Surg. 2009;208:341–7.
46. Morrow M, Waters J, Morris E. MRI for breast cancer screening, diagnosis, and treatment. Lancet. 2011;378(9805):1804–11.
47. Golshan M, Miron A, Nixon AJ, et al. The prevalence of germline BRCA1 and BRCA2 mutations in young women with breast cancer undergoing breast-conservation therapy. Am J Surg. 2006;192:58–62.
48. Mester JL, Moore RA, Eng C. PTEN germline mutations in patients initially tested for other hereditary cancer syndromes: would use of risk assessment tools reduce genetic testing? Oncologist. 2013;18:1083–90.
49. Fisher B, Anderson S, Bryant J, et al. Twenty-year follow-up of a randomized trial comparing total mastectomy, lumpectomy, and lumpectomy plus irradiation for the treatment of invasive breast cancer. N Engl J Med. 2002;347:1233–41.
50. Poortmans PM, Collette L, Bartelink H, et al. The addition of a boost dose on the primary tumour bed after lumpectomy in breast conserving treatment for breast cancer. A summary of the results of EORTC 22881–10882 "boost versus no boost" trial. Cancer Radiother. 2008;12:565–70.
51. Shah C, Khan AJ, Arthur D, Fernandez E, Martinez AA, Vicini F. Intraoperative radiation therapy in breast cancer: not ready for prime time. Ann Surg Oncol. 2014;21:351–3.
52. Davies C, Godwin J, Gray R, et al. Relevance of breast cancer hormone receptors and other factors to the efficacy of adjuvant tamoxifen: patient-level meta-analysis of randomised trials. Lancet. 2011;378(9793):771–84.

53. Davies C, Pan H, Godwin J, et al. Long-term effects of continuing adjuvant tamoxifen to 10 years versus stopping at 5 years after diagnosis of oestrogen receptor-positive breast cancer: ATLAS, a randomised trial. Lancet. 2013;381:805–16.
54. Partridge AH, Gelber S, Piccart-Gebhart MJ, et al. Effect of age on breast cancer outcomes in women with human epidermal growth factor receptor 2-positive breast cancer: results from a herceptin adjuvant trial. J Clin Oncol. 2013;31:2692–8.
55. Michaud LB, Jones KL, Buzdar AU. Combination endocrine therapy in the management of breast cancer. Oncologist. 2001;6:538–46.
56. Bernstein JL, Thomas DC, Shore RE, et al. Contralateral breast cancer after radiotherapy among BRCA1 and BRCA2 mutation carriers: a WECARE study report. Eur J Cancer. 2013;49(14):2979–85.
57. Domchek SM, Friebel TM, Singer CF, et al. Association of risk-reducing surgery in BRCA1 or BRCA2 mutation carriers with cancer risk and mortality. JAMA. 2010;304:967–75.
58. Loren AW, Mangu PB, Beck LN, et al. Fertility preservation for patients with cancer: American Society of Clinical Oncology clinical practice guideline update. J Clin Oncol. 2013;31:2500–10.
59. Blanc B, Lazard A, Estrade JP, Agostini A, Gurriet B. Contraceptive methods after gynecological and breast cancer. Bull Acad Natl Med. 2010;194:521–7.
60. Lee MC, Bhati RS, von Rottenthaler EE, et al. Therapy choices and quality of life in young breast cancer survivors: a short-term follow-up. Am J Surg. 2013;206:625–31.
61. Broeckel JA, Thors CL, Jacobsen PB, Small M, Cox CE. Sexual functioning in long-term breast cancer survivors treated with adjuvant chemotherapy. Breast Cancer Res Treat. 2002;75:241–8.
62. Bouchardy C, Rapiti E, Fioretta G, et al. Undertreatment strongly decreases prognosis of breast cancer in elderly women. J Clin Oncol. 2003;21:3580–7.
63. Schonberg MA, Marcantonio ER, Li D, Silliman RA, Ngo L, McCarthy EP. Breast cancer among the oldest old: tumor characteristics, treatment choices, and survival. J Clin Oncol. 2010;28:2038–45.
64. Rosso S, Gondos A, Zanetti R, et al. Up-to-date estimates of breast cancer survival for the years 2000–2004 in 11 European countries: the role of screening and a comparison with data from the United States. Eur J Cancer. 2010;46:3351–7.
65. Satariano WA, Ragland DR. The effect of comorbidity on 3-year survival of women with primary breast cancer. Ann Intern Med. 1994;120:104–10.
66. Stotter A, Tahir M, Pretorius R, Robinson T. Experiences of a multidisciplinary elderly breast cancer clinic: using the right specialists, in the same place, with time. In: Reed M, Audisio R, editors. Management of breast cancer in older women. London: Springer; 2010.
67. Pallis AG, Fortpied C, Wedding U, et al. EORTC elderly task force position paper: approach to the older cancer patient. Eur J Cancer. 2010;46:1502–13.
68. Martelli G, Boracchi P, De Palo M, et al. A randomized trial comparing axillary dissection to no axillary dissection in older patients with T1N0 breast cancer: results after 5 years of follow-up. Ann Surg. 2005;242:1–6.
69. Rudenstam CM, Zahrieh D, Forbes JF, et al. Randomized trial comparing axillary clearance versus no axillary clearance in older patients with breast cancer: first results of International Breast Cancer Study Group Trial 10–93. J Clin Oncol. 2006;24:337–44.
70. Hughes KS, Schnaper LA, Berry D, et al. Lumpectomy plus tamoxifen with or without irradiation in women 70 years of age or older with early breast cancer. N Engl J Med. 2004;351:971–7.
71. Vaidya JS, Joseph DJ, Tobias JS, et al. Targeted intraoperative radiotherapy versus whole breast radiotherapy for breast cancer (TARGIT-A trial): an international, prospective, randomised, non-inferiority phase 3 trial. Lancet. 2010;376:91–102.
72. Hind D, Wyld L, Reed MW. Surgery, with or without tamoxifen, vs tamoxifen alone for older women with operable breast cancer: Cochrane review. Br J Cancer. 2007;96:1025–9.
73. Biganzoli L, Licitra S, Claudino W, et al. Clinical decision making in breast cancer: TAM and aromatase inhibitors for older patients—a jungle? Eur J Cancer. 2007;43:2270–8.

74. Garg P, Rana F, Gupta R, Buzaianu EM, Guthrie TH. Predictors of toxicity and toxicity profile of adjuvant chemotherapy in elderly breast cancer patients. Breast J. 2009;15:40.
75. Loibl S, von Minckwitz G, Harbeck N, et al. Clinical feasibility of (neo)adjuvant taxane-based chemotherapy in older patients: analysis of >4,500 patients from four German randomized breast cancer trials. Breast Cancer Res. 2008;10:R77.


## Further Reading


Azim Jr HA, Del Mastro L, Scarfone G, et al. Treatment of breast cancer during pregnancy: regimen selection, pregnancy, monitoring and more. Breast. 2011;20:1–6.

Biganzoli L, Wildiers H, Oakman C, et al. Management of elderly patients with breast cancer: updated recommendations of the International Society of Geriatric Oncology (SIOG) and European Society of Breast Cancer Specialists (EUSOMA). Lancet Oncol. 2012;13:148–60.

Cardonick E, Dougherty R, Grana G, et al. Breast cancer during pregnancy: maternal and fetal outcomes. Cancer J. 2010;16:76–82.

Cardoso F, Loibl S, Pagani O, et al. The European Society of Breast Cancer Specialists recommendations for the management of young women with breast cancer. Eur J Cancer. 2012;48:3355–77.

Garcia-Manero M, Royo MP, Espinos J, et al. Pregnancy associated breast cancer. Eur J Surg Oncol. 2009;35:215–8.

Kell MR, Morrow M. Multifocal, multicentric and bilateral breast cancer. In: Hudis CA, Norton L, Winchester DJ, Winchester DP, editors. Breast cancer. Hamilton: BC Decker; 2006.

Le Saux O, Ripamonti B, Bruyas A, et al. Optimal management of breast cancer in the elderly patient: current perspectives. Clin Interv Aging. 2015;6(10):157–74.

Li Z, Sergent F, Bolla M, Zhou Y, Gabelle-Flandin I. Prognostic factors of second primary contralateral breast cancer in early-stage breast cancer. Oncol Lett. 2015;9:245–51.

Méry B, Avi Assouline A, Rivoirard R, et al. Portrait, treatment choices and management of breast cancer in nonagenarians: an ongoing challenge. Breast. 2014;23:221–5.

Mustacchi G, Scanni A, Capasso I, Farris A, Pluchinotta A, Isola G. Update of the Phase III trial 'GRETA' of surgery and tamoxifen versus tamoxifen alone for early breast cancer in elderly women. Future Oncol. 2014;10:1–9.

Ogunbiyi SO, Lee S, Mathew J, Cheung KL. Primary breast cancer in the elderly: a systematic literature review on histological type and clinical outcome. Future Oncol. 2015;11:259–65.

Partridge AH, Pagani O, Abulkhair O, et al. First international consensus guidelines for breast cancer in young women (BCY1). Breast. 2014;23:209–20.

Senkus E. Synchronous and metachronous metastatic breast cancer – two incarnations of the same beast? Breast. 2014;23:1.

Shaikh T, Tam TY, Li T, et al. Multifocal and multicentric breast cancer is associated with increased local recurrence regardless of surgery type. Breast J. 2015. doi:10.1186/1471-2407-13-361.

Tomasi-Cont N, Lambertini M, Hulsbosch S, Peccatori AF, Amant F. Strategies for fertility preservation in young early breast cancer patients. Breast. 2014;23:503–10.


**Websites in Appendix**: *Fertility*, A-4.9; *Young Women*, A-4.23.

# The Role of Surgery on Breast Cancer

# 16

Virgilio S. Sacchini, Alfonso M. Pluchinotta,
and Vincenzo Vindigni

## Contents



V.S. Sacchini (✉)
Breast Service, Department of Surgery, Memorial Sloan-Kettering
Cancer Center (MSKCC), New York, NY, USA
e-mail: sacchinv@mskcc.org

A.M. Pluchinotta
Breast Surgery, Policlinic of Abano Terme, Padova, Italy
e-mail: pluchinotta.alfonso@gmail.com

V. Vindigni
Plastic Surgery Clinic, University of Padova, Padova, Italy
e-mail: vincenzo.vindigni@unipd.it



A.M. Pluchinotta (ed.), *The Outpatient Breast Clinic: Aiming at Best Practice*,
DOI 10.1007/978-3-319-15907-2_16

**Abstract**

• Women with invasive BC who are undergoing breast surgery should be offered the choice of either breast conservation surgery or mastectomy. • The choice of surgery must be tailored to the individual patient or, at least, must reassure the patient that the choice of surgery has been tailored to her as much as possible. • Surgery for BC must be carried out or directly supervised by a fully trained surgeon, specialised in breast surgery. • All patients with invasive BC who are operable should have surgical management of the axilla. • All patients with unusual presentations of BC should be discussed within the multidisciplinary team before any decision is made.

*Future Directions.* Improved outcomes of surgery, with significantly less morbidity, have been facilitated by a multitude of factors, including improvements in technology and screening, better quality and more widely used adjuvant therapies. This scenario should also properly consider the variety of technologies now available for nonsurgical ablation, with techniques such as cryoablation, radiofrequency ablation and high-intensity focused ultrasonography (HI FU), each with its own advantages and disadvantages.

## 16.1 Overview

**Clinical Practice Points**

- For patients with single small BCs, survival outcomes from breast-conserving treatment are equivalent to that of mastectomy.
- The surgeon should be fully involved in the assessment of the patient and should always see and examine her before accepting her for surgery.
- Therapeutic surgery needs to carry out treatments with the least possible number of intervention. Oncoplastic surgery should be performed more than once to achieve the best possible cosmetic outcome.
- Every measure should be taken to minimise anxiety and to achieve the best possible cosmetic result.
- Non-standard treatment should be reserved to unifocal large BC in order to reduce the size, to inflammatory BC and to BRCA carriers.

### 16.1.1 Basis of Surgical Treatment

1. *Breast-conserving surgery vs. mastectomy.* Meta-analysis of six randomised controlled trials (RCTs) found that breast-conserving surgery (BCS) and radiotherapy to the breast (the two therapies together are called breast-conserving treatment, or BCT) resulted in similar long-term mortality rates compared with mastectomy in patients with operable invasive BC. Only one trial showed that mastectomy significantly reduced mortality. In four of the six trials, mastectomy significantly reduced the risk of locoregional recurrence compared to BCS.
2. *Breast-conserving surgery as first choice.* Breast conservation (wide local excision and RT) is the local treatment of choice in the majority of patients with invasive cancer. In some circumstances, mastectomy may still be carried out because of tumour size (relative to breast size), tumour multicentricity, prior radiation to the chest wall or breast or patient choice.
3. *Tumour-free margins are crucial.* The aim of surgery in invasive BC is to achieve tumour-free margins with the least possible mutilation, in accordance with the needs of the well-informed patient. To reach this goal, optimal preoperative imaging should be carried out depending on the clinical problem. The results of imaging should be available in the operating theatre.
4. *Information is not optional.* The surgeon must have seen the patient before any surgery in order to completely inform her about the clinical situation and the surgical treatment options available to her. When appropriate, patients should be given an informed choice between BCS and mastectomy. If a choice of BCS is not offered, the reasons should be documented in the patient's case notes.
5. *Oncoplastic surgery.* All patients with primary operable BC, for whom mastectomy is advised or preferred by the patient, should have access to breast reconstruction surgery, have the opportunity to discuss their breast reconstruction options and have immediate breast reconstruction if appropriate. If breast reconstruction is not offered, the reasons should be documented in the patient's case notes.
6. *Preoperative diagnosis.* The preoperative histological or cytological diagnosis of malignant lesions improves the quality and completeness of therapeutic excisional biopsies (lumpectomies). In cases of clinically occult lesions or doubts of the location of the tumour, preoperative localisation guided by ultrasound or stereotactic mammography equipment is mandatory. Bracketing wires facilitate the completeness of excision of microcalcifications. Tissue biopsy with core needle sampling should provide conclusive proof of malignancy. Additionally, CNB reduces unnecessary surgery besides avoiding scars that may complicate the placement of the subsequent lumpectomy incision.
7. *Cosmetic outcome.* In BCS incisions are placed to ensure best possible cosmetic result, and the possibility of mastectomy should be taken into account. Closure of breast tissue, use of drains and closure of skin depend on local anatomy, width of excision and location of the tumour in the breast.

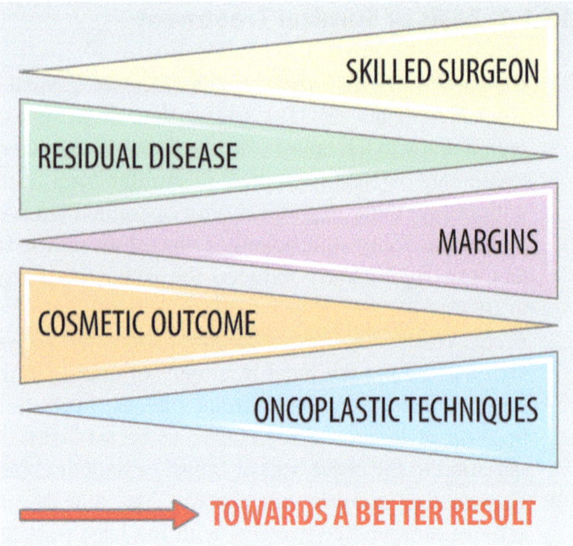


**Fig. 16.1** Factors influencing adequate surgical margins and acceptable cosmetic results in BCS. Without regard to free and safe margins, expertise of operating surgeon and observance of oncoplastic techniques are considered equally critical in order to achieve better results

Since cosmetic results are evenly important, a thorough consideration should be given to the following factors (Fig. 16.1):

- *Operating surgeon*, in some circumstances, may represent a prognostic factor, as believed in the past and now scientifically and statistically accepted.
- Acceptable *cosmetic outcome* is directly related to potential *residual disease* and inversely related to extension of adequate surgical *margins*.
- *Oncoplastic techniques*, for some selected groups of patients (e.g. too large or small breast), could strikingly improve the overall results.

8. *One en bloc specimen*. The surgeon should aim to perform excision in one complete specimen and mark the specimen for the pathologist. Margin assessment by so-called touch prep-imprint cytology or random shave biopsies from the cavity might be helpful, but has not proven to be superior over a complete careful assessment of the wide local excision specimen.
9. *Staging of axilla*. In the case of proven axillary lymph node disease, axillary lymph node clearance should be undertaken; if there is no proven disease, the optimal axillary procedure is a sentinel lymph node biopsy, or, if not available, axillary node sampling is an alternative.
10. *Multidisciplinary group*. Breast surgeons who act alone are an anomaly that should be eliminated. The best treatment is the one that comes out after a discussion among several people about several options has been carried out.

The surgeon is a member of the MDT and should participate in regular multidisciplinary reviews for case management and audit purposes. MDT is now involved mainly in primary therapy, and it is hoped that, in future, MDT will more involved also in the diagnostic phase. Preoperative MDT discussion is not mandatory but preferable:

- To select optimal treatment based on guidelines and clinical criteria
- To select patients for non-standard treatment based on individual patient needs and tumour-related factors (e.g. older patients with low-risk BC)
- To document proposed treatments (medicolegal issues)
- To select patients for clinical trials
- To treat rare histological cases, associated diseases and their individual characteristics

*NON-STANDARD TREATMENTS* may be required for the following three groups and should be identified and properly well thought out.

- *Unifocal operable tumours too large* for BCS for which downsizing with neoadjuvant systemic therapy could be considered (see Sect. 18.4). However, systemic therapy for histologically confirmed invasive BC too large for BCT should be carefully monitored. In fact, a reasonable possibility is that neoadjuvant therapy may efficiently eliminate highly differentiated tumour cells and less so poorly differentiated ones that may be in a dormant state and reactivate under specific circumstances.
- *Inflammatory BC*, where neoadjuvant chemotherapy is the standard of care (see Sect. 15.2). In other locally advanced BC (e.g. with massive nodal involvement), results are still debatable except for some molecular BC subtypes like triple-negative, HER2-positive and some luminal B subsets (Sect. 18.4).
- *BRCA carriers*. In healthy BRCA mutation carriers, risk- reducing surgery, such as bilateral mastectomy and oophorectomy, needs to be discussed as part of the initial assessment (see Sect. 2.3).

In this last particular case of BRCA mutation carriers with diagnosed BC the oncological safety of BCT is still debated. Based on current evidence, BCT can be considered a reasonable option since it does not seem to increase the risk for IBTR in BRCA-mutation carriers versus non-carriers. However, several aspects should be taken into account before the final decision-making, including therapeutic and cosmetic outcomes of bilateral mastectomy.

The same applies to the high risk patients with a strong family history of BC. What is more, in very young patients with BC, rapid BRCA testing is indicated if knowledge of the mutation status would impact the BC treatment plan. Nevertheless, if the patient needs more time to decide on any possible prophylactic surgery or if a rapid test is not available, stage-adapted treatment of BC should be performed while postponing any potential prophylactic procedure to a second stage.

Lastly, outside of the genetic or familiar risk, a woman with a personal history of BC has a 3 to 4-fold increased risk of developing a new cancer in the other breast or in another part of the same breast. However, that is not a sufficient reason for implementing prophylactic measures as contralateral surgery, unless in certain special situations as pluricentric lobular carcinoma or atypical hyperplasia.

### 16.1.2 Quality Indicators in Breast Surgery

Almost all guidelines highlight operative measures aimed at obtaining best oncological results without neglecting some minor aspects of quality assurance [1, 2].

*Unnecessary surgery*. To minimise unnecessary surgery, i.e. open surgical diagnostic biopsies that prove to be malignant, invasive BCs should have a nonoperative pathological diagnosis in at least 90 % of cases. For non-invasive BC, the minimum standard for a nonoperative pathological diagnosis is 85 %.

*Cosmesis*. To minimise the cosmetic impairment of diagnostic open biopsy, the fresh weight of tissue removed for all cases where a diagnostic open biopsy is performed should be recorded. It is recommended that more than 90 % of open surgical biopsies carried out for diagnosis, which prove to be benign, should weigh less than 20 g.

*Anxiety*. To minimise patient anxiety regarding a diagnostic operation which is required to confirm or exclude malignancy and the date for an operation, patients should be admitted for a diagnostic operation within 2 weeks in more than 90 % of cases.

*Delay*. To minimise the delay between referral for investigation and first BC treatment, 100 % of patients diagnosed with BC should receive their first treatment within 62 days of an urgent referral with suspected BC or recall from the screening programme. This is valid whether surgery is the first treatment or neoadjuvant systemic therapy is planned.

*Timing*. To minimise patient anxiety regarding a therapeutic operation, which is required for cancer and the date of the actual operation, 100 % of patients should receive their first treatment within 31 days of the *decision to treat*. This is valid whether surgery is the first treatment or neoadjuvant systemic therapy is planned.

*Preoperative investigations*. Finally, to minimise unnecessary investigations prior to BC treatment, nonoperative staging investigations for metastatic disease should not be routinely performed.

*Minimal number of operations*. The proportion of patients (invasive cancer only) who receive a single (breast) operation for the primary tumour (excluding reconstruction) should be a minimum of 70 %.

## 16.2 Breast-Conserving Surgery

**Clinical Practice Points**

- The goals of BCT are to provide a survival equivalent to mastectomy, a cosmetically acceptable breast and a low rate of recurrence in the treated breast.
- Breast-conserving therapy (BCT) is a combination of breast-conserving surgery (BCS) aimed at microscopically free margins and radiotherapy (RT) of the breast.
- The patient should be fully informed that breast irradiation is required following conservation and that further surgery may be required if the margins are not clear of tumour.
- In BCS the radial tumour margins must be clear (>1 mm) in order to keep the breast relapse rate of invasive cancer lower than 1–1.5 % per follow-up annum (less than 10 % at 10 years).
- While a slight asymmetry may be tolerated, a deformity is to be avoided. Wide margins do not appear to achieve better local control rates and may impair cosmetic results.
- Patients who have had BCS and have a poor cosmetic outcome can be offered partial breast reconstruction to improve results.

### 16.2.1 Introduction

For patients with single small BCs, survival outcomes from breast-conserving treatment (BCT) are equivalent to that of mastectomy. That is true only in the absence of local recurrence which should be avoided. Although in the past it was thought that local therapy had little influence on overall survival, it is becoming clear that local failure is responsible, at least in part, for some patients developing metastatic disease [3].

Completeness of excision is the major surgical factor influencing local recurrence. The size of the lesion and the size of the excision are related to the size of the breast. No upper size limit for breast-conserving surgery (BCS) for invasive cancer can be given.

The appropriate selection of patients is crucial to the success of BCS, which it is not applicable to all patients. Mastectomy is mandatory for tumour control for some subgroups of patients with BC, and it may provide more satisfactory outcomes in others.

*Contraindications* for BCS, and consequently absolute indication for mastectomy, are:

- Multicentric disease with two or more primary tumours in separate quadrants of the breast such that they cannot be encompassed in a single excision.

- Diffuse malignant microcalcifications on mammography.
- A history of prior therapeutic RT that would result in an excessively high total radiation dose to the chest wall.
- Extensive skin changes, a clinical diagnosis of inflammatory BC and dermal lymphatic involvement.
- In pregnancy, however, it may be possible to perform breast-conserving surgery in the third trimester, deferring breast irradiation until after delivery.
- Persistently positive resection margins after multiple attempts at re-excision.

*Individual patient's preference*. The appropriate selection starts from individual patient needs and expectations that should be accurately assessed. There are many issues to consider regarding this decision: benefits and risks of mastectomy compared to BCS in regard to specific concerns, possibility and consequence of local recurrence with either treatment, impact on cosmetic outcome and psychosocial adjustment.

### 16.2.2 Selection Criteria for BCT

*Preoperative assessment*. Imaging typically includes a combination of bilateral mammographic evaluation, with appropriate magnification views if needed, and ultrasound. The size of the tumour should be included in the mammographic report, as well as documentation of associated microcalcifications, and the extent of the calcifications within and outside the mass. Some surgeons incorporate breast MRI in the workup of patients considering BCT; however, the use of MRI in this setting is not routinely indicated.

MRI for the preoperative assessment of disease in newly diagnosed BC is indicated:

- For a clinical presentation of disease that is larger than what is appreciated by mammography, particularly in the setting of dense breasts which lower the sensitivity of mammography
- For invasive cancers that are contiguous to the chest wall and not completely included on mammographic projections
- For patients with axillary nodal metastases and a clinically and mammographically occult primary tumour
- For women with Paget disease of the breast who have a negative physical examination and mammogram
- In women with locally advanced BC who are being considered for neoadjuvant systemic therapy to assess tumour response to therapy
- For women with very high risk for contralateral disease because of an inherited predisposing condition or prior chest wall irradiation

Women should be informed of the risks and benefits of preoperative breast MRI (see Sect. 5.3). The limits of the accuracy of MRI should be discussed with patients, so that they understand the need for biopsy of MRI-detected lesions before definitive surgery. Breast MRI should be performed with a dedicated breast coil by expert breast imaging radiologists in institutions that have the capability to perform MRI-guided needle biopsy and/or wire localisation of the findings.

Surgical decisions should not be based on MRI findings alone. All suspicious findings on MRI require pathologic confirmation. MRI findings alone should not be used to change surgical plans and to shift from breast conservation to mastectomy.

*Age* is not a contraindication to BCT in very young as well as in older women. Younger patients (<40 years of age) have an increased risk of local recurrence after BCS as well as after a mastectomy, but there is no evidence to suggest that wider than no ink surgical margins on the tumour reduces the local recurrence risk in this population (see Sect. 15.1). For older women, the primary determinants of local therapy should be physiologic age and presence of comorbid conditions (see Sect. 15.4).

*Family history of BC* is not a contraindication to BCT; however, women with a strong family history suggestive of a genetic predisposition should be informed about their increased risk of a second primary cancer.

*Dense breast tissue* is not, in itself, a contraindication for BCS. If patients with dense breasts are more likely to be treated with an initial mastectomy, this may reflect the surgeon's or the patient's bias rather than an inability to meet the criteria for BCS. In fact, breast density is not associated with higher positive margins, and preoperative MRI does not decrease the risk of positive margins [4].

*Tumour location* should not influence the choice of treatment. Tumours in a superficial subareolar location may require resection of the nipple-areolar complex to achieve negative margins. In that case only cosmetic, no oncologic, outcomes will be affected. If anything, it is important to establish that the tumour is unicentric and clearly localised.

*Tumour size* – Tumour size in itself is not an absolute contraindication to BCS. A large tumour in a small breast is a relative contraindication, since an adequate resection would result in significant cosmetic alteration. In patients with unifocal operable tumours too large for BCS, downsizing with neoadjuvant systemic therapy should be considered in order to reduce tumour size and allow for breast conservation with acceptable rates of local recurrence. Metallic clip placement in the tumour bed under ultrasound guidance should be accomplished before or soon after neoadjuvant treatment begins in order to properly identify the location in case there is a complete response to chemotherapy.

There is no role for preoperative chemotherapy in patients with invasive BC who are already candidates for BCS or have dispersed microcalcifications and multifocal diseases. At this moment neither the optimal combination nor duration of chemotherapy has been clearly evaluated; thus, preoperative chemotherapy to downsize the tumour in order to facilitate BCT should be applied with caution.

*Lymph node metastases* are a marker of worse prognosis, but positive lymph nodes are not a contraindication for BCS, as BCT and mastectomy have equivalent outcomes independent of nodal metastases. In general, patients with aggressive biological factors do not benefit from wider margins.

*Retraction* of the skin, nipple or breast parenchyma is not necessarily a sign of locally advanced BC and does not contraindicate BCS. Only cosmetic implications of a larger resection should be factored into the decision to proceed with BCS.

*Histologic subtypes* other than invasive ductal carcinoma (e.g. invasive lobular cancer) are not associated with an increased risk of BC recurrence; these women are candidates for BCT if the tumour distribution is not dispersed and it can be excised with negative margins.

*Extensive intraductal* component (EIC), if present, is an indicator that disease extent may be greater than clinically suspected. EIC is not a contraindication for BCS, providing negative margins are achieved. There is no evidence to support a wider margin than no ink on tumour when all suspicious microcalcifications identified on the mammogram in the vicinity of the cancer have been resected. If residual microcalcifications are present, a wider excision should be attempted.

*Connective tissue disease* – Some patients with a history of connective tissue disease tolerate irradiation poorly, and so the use of RT as a component of BCT must be weighed against the possible complications. However, large studies noted that patients with scleroderma and systemic lupus erythematosus (SLE), but not rheumatoid arthritis, are at a significantly increased risk of late toxicities. As a result, many radiation oncologists consider only scleroderma and active SLE to be relative contraindications to BCT.

### 16.2.3 Techniques of BCS

*Wire localisation* – For resection of non-palpable lesions, preoperative wire localisation by the radiologist allows accurate identification of the area requiring resection (see Sect. 6.4.2). Multiple bracketing wires may be helpful for the delineation of the boundaries of the resection, but do not ensure clear histologic margins of resection.

*Incision* – The type and location of the incision can be critical to the quality of cosmesis for several reasons. First, any patient who undergoes lumpectomy may ultimately require a mastectomy, and incisions should be planned with possible mastectomy incisions in mind. Moreover, the incision should be placed close to the tumour to avoid extensive tunnelling that could impair tumour bed boost radiotherapy.

In the upper part of the breast, incisions should be curvilinear or transverse and follow the natural skin creases (Langer's lines). Radial incisions in the upper half of the breast may displace the ipsilateral nipple-areola complex due to scar contracture. In the lower part of the breast, the choice of a curvilinear or radial incision is dependent upon the contour of the breast, the distance from the skin to the tumour and the amount of breast tissue to be resected. Generally, skin removal with a curvilinear incision in the inferior part of the breast distorts the breast contour and may displace the nipple-areolar complex downward. At 3 and 9 o'clock position and in the lower breast, a radial or curvilinear incision provides a better result, particularly if skin removal is necessary (Fig. 16.2).

The incision should be over the tumour and of adequate size to allow the tumour to be removed in one piece. In the upper inner aspect of the breast, some retraction of the skin may be necessary to avoid an incision that may be visible with clothing.

In deeper lesions, it is not necessary to remove the skin. Preservation of the subcutaneous fat and avoidance of thin skin flaps are important in maintaining a normal

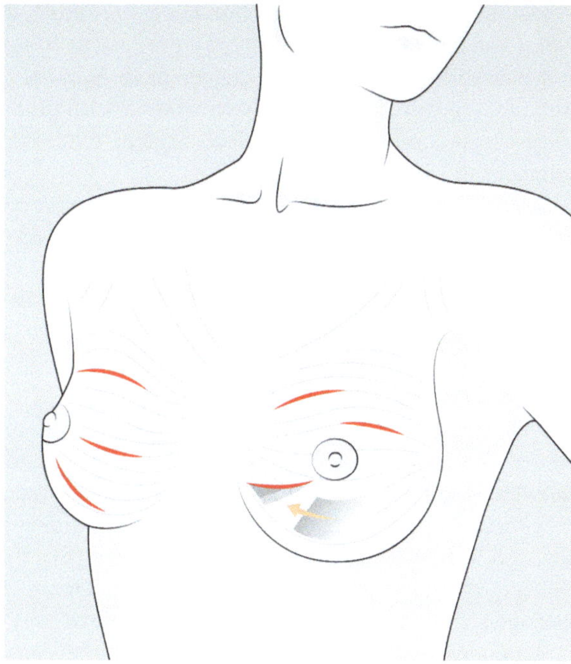

**Fig. 16.2** In the upper part of the breast, curvilinear skin incisions following Langer's lines generally achieve the best cosmetic result. Only in the lower part of the breast, a radial or oblique incision may provide a good result. Particularly in the lower pole locations, the effective mobilisation of the gland, as shown here, is a key in achieving a natural breast shape

posttreatment breast contour. If the tumour is superficial, it may be necessary to remove the overlying skin and, if it is deep, the underlying fascia. For both conditions, resection should provide a reasonable distance of 5–10 mm. Finally, needle track from CNB or FNS does not need to be removed.

*Glandular resection* – Cosmetic outcomes can be improved with oncoplastic techniques; however re-approximation of the breast tissue without tissue advancement is best avoided since it can result in distortion of the breast contour, which may not be apparent with the patient supine on the operating table.

Facing small non-palpable BC without a definite preoperative diagnosis of cancer, the surgeon may be tempted to perform biopsies wider than necessary in the hope that the surgery can be both diagnostic and curative. This is risky if it is negative and is associated with an undesirable aesthetic outcome, and if positive, the excision turns out to be inadequate. In both cases, the doors are open to litigation. All this confirms the necessity to have a definitive preoperative diagnosis.

*Margins of resection* – The optimal amount of normal tissue that should surround the tumour to minimise the risk of a local recurrence is still controversial. The appropriate macroscopic margin of normal breast tissue to resect around the tumour for women should be 0.5–1.0 cm of grossly normal breast tissue, which will usually result in histologically negative margins (>1 mm distance between tumour and ink) in the majority of patients. There is no evidence that a wider margin of normal tissue than no ink on the tumour decreases the rate of local recurrence in the clinical setting of multimodality treatment. Factors independently associated with positive resection margins included mammographic microcalcifications, tumour size, presence of EIC, grade 2/3 and caudal location of the lesion.

Obtaining tumour-free resection margins is more challenging for non-palpable breast cancer. Models to predict margins status in patients undergoing BCS for non-palpable invasive breast cancer have been developed, which are moderately able to differentiate between women with high versus low risk of positive margins, and may be useful for surgical planning and preoperative patient counselling [5].

Several approaches can be used for intraoperative margin assessment, including frozen section, cytological touch prep analysis, shaved margin analysis and intraoperative ultrasound. There is no prevailing standard of care for intraoperative margin assessment, and practices vary widely. The use of these techniques may assist in obtaining negative margins, but does not guarantee the absence of microscopic tumours on permanent sections. Patients should be advised that additional surgery to obtain clean margins may be necessary.

*Specimen orientation* – The specimen should be removed as a single piece of tissue. The lesion should be well centred with equidistant margins of resection (Fig. 16.3). Sometimes gross inspection of the specimen in the operating room, with or without frozen section analysis, permits identification of positive or close margins and immediate re-excision, if appropriate [6]. This will decrease the need to return to the operating room for re-excision. The operating surgeon to orient the specimen uses sutures, clips and/or multicoloured inks.

An alternative to removing the entire tumour and margins as a single specimen is to remove the lesion intact and then to resect (to *shave*) individual margins of normal-appearing tissue that completely encompasses the primary cancer site [7]. Each margin is labelled and oriented in relationship to the primary cancer.

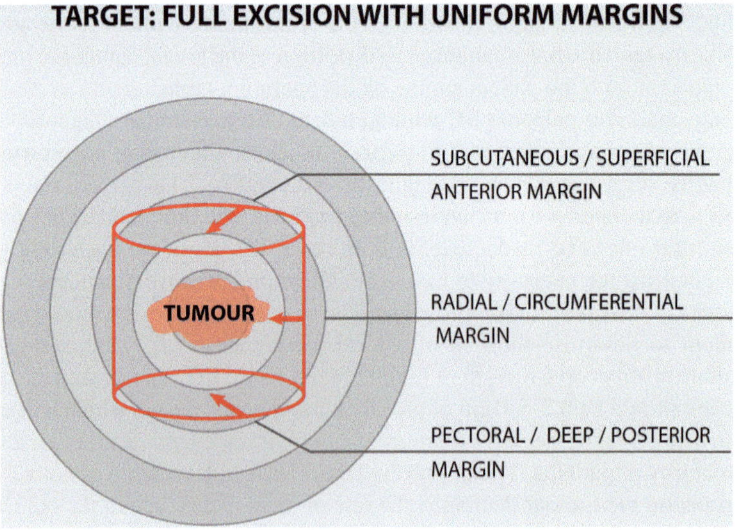


**Fig. 16.3** Tumour in the specimen should be well centred with uniform margin of resection

*Specimen radiography* – Specimen radiography should be performed during the surgical procedure to confirm excision of the targeted lesion when the lesion was not palpable. Additional oriented margins can be resected prior to closure when radiography suggests inadequate resection, which may eliminate the need for a delayed re-excision.

### 16.2.4 Outcomes of BCS

*Pathological results* – The first aim of BCS is to obtain radial clear tumour margins (>1 mm) in order to keep the breast relapse rate of invasive cancer lower than 1–1.5 % per follow-up annum (<10 % at 10 years). If pathological results prove a higher risk for breast relapse (incompletely excised infiltrating or in situ cancer, impossibility to deliver an adequate dose of radiation therapy), a re-excision (when cosmetically feasible) or mastectomy must be considered. To minimise the number of therapeutic operations in women undergoing conservation surgery for an invasive cancer, all patients (or at least 95 %) should have less than three operations.

*Cosmetic outcome* – Another aim of BCS is to result in an acceptable cosmetic appearance in the majority of women. There is a direct correlation between cosmetic outcome after BCS and psychological morbidity. Better cosmetic outcomes reduce the levels of psychological morbidity, with less anxiety and depression and improved body image, sexuality and self-esteem, compared with mastectomy [8]. An all-inclusive good result should be achieved considering both oncological procedures and aesthetic details (Table 16.1).

Excellent or good cosmetic result from a patient's point of view should be at least 80 % at 3 years. Many surgical factors will play a role in the ultimate cosmetic

**Table 16.1** Oncological procedures and aesthetic (but important) details to allow a safe BCS and a satisfactory cosmetic outcome

| *Oncological procedures* | *Aesthetic details* |
|---|---|
| Increasing tumour size does not associate with increasing local recurrence rates. So that limiting BCS to cancer below a certain size is illogical | Incision that follows the lines of maximum resting skin tension produces the most cosmetically acceptable scar |
| Patients having BCS are adequate treated by wide local excision and do not require either a segmental or quadrantic excision | Routine excision of skin when performing an excision cannot be justified in most cases |
| Factors independently associated with positive resection margins include mammographic microcalcifications, tumour size, presence of DCIS, grade 3 and caudal location of the lesion | Effective mobilisation of the gland is a key component in achieving a natural breast shape. Drains and approximation sutures should be avoided or kept to a *minimum* |
| Full-thickness excision ensures free anterior and posterior margins, leaving only the lateral margins in question | Skin staples and interrupted suture do not produce satisfactory results and are not an acceptable method of wound closure in the breast |

appearance of the breast. These include the size and placement of the incision, management of the lumpectomy cavity and the extent of axillary dissection if necessary. The surgeon has control over several of these issues, and careful attention to detail will improve the aesthetic results. Although treatment-related changes in the breast stabilise at approximately 3 years, other factors that affect the untreated breast, such as change in size because of weight gain or the normal ptosis seen with aging, continue to affect breast symmetry.

To help assess the cosmetic outcome after BCT, a scoring system to standardise the grading of cosmetic outcome has been recommended in order to define results as: *excellent*, the treated and untreated breast are almost identical; *good*, minimal differences between the treated and untreated breasts; *fair*, obvious differences between the treated and untreated breasts; and *poor*, major aesthetic sequelae in the treated breast.

While a slight asymmetry may be tolerated, a deformity is to be avoided. Wide margins do not appear to achieve better local control rates and may impair cosmetic results [9]. Avoiding deformity should be the objective parameter of quality of cosmesis and breast deformities recorded in the chart as follow:

- *Grade I* – Patient has a treated breast with a normal appearance, but there is asymmetry between the two breasts.
- *Grade II* – Patient has a deformity of the treated breast. This deformity can be corrected by partial breast reconstruction and breast conservation, with the irradiated breast tissue being spared in the reconstruction.
- *Grade III* – Patient has a major distortion of the treated breast or diffuse painful fibrosis. These sequelae are so severe that only a mastectomy can be considered.

The most important factor influencing cosmetic outcome after BCS is the percentage of volume of breast excised. Removing more than 20 % of breast volume results in the majority of women having a poor cosmetic outcome. In a trial from the National Cancer Institute of Milan that compared quadrantectomy to gross tumour excision (lumpectomy), women undergoing quadrantectomy had significantly greater discrepancies in the inferior profile of the breasts and greater distance from the midline to the nipple and were more likely to have more than a 3 cm difference in height between the nipples (21 % versus 7 %) than those treated with lumpectomy [10].

Similar data were noted in other series, as in one large study by the Breast Health Center of Boston that correlated cosmetic outcome to the volume of breast tissue resected (estimated by multiplying the dimensions of the resected breast specimens). For women with <35 $cm^3$ resected tissue, excellent and excellent or good scores were reported by 85 and 96 %, respectively. In a later series, cosmetic results declined over the first 3 years and then stabilised; they were still judged by clinicians to be excellent in 77 %, good in 9, fair in 9 and poor in 5 % of cases [11].

## 16.2.5 Nonsurgical Options for a Breast-Conserving Treatment

Accessibility and diffusion of BC screening, together with improvement of new technologies, have led to the detection of smaller and earlier-stage BCs, where lumpectomy still remains the absolute standard of care for the local treatment.

However, given a trend towards less aggressive treatment of small BCs and the ability to target non-palpable lesions, the development of less invasive alternatives seems a more logical alternative than surgery with promising effectiveness and less morbidity [12]. Therefore, the next inevitable step in the evolution of BC therapy could be the replacement of lumpectomy with nonsurgical methods for destroying the tumour, at least for a select group of patients, as those older than 70 years or with comorbidities that make surgery a difficult and unpleasant treatment.

Minimally invasive ablation techniques have been studied in early-stage small tumours with the goal of attaining efficacy similar to that of breast conservation therapy. These techniques have several potential advantages, including lower cost of care and simplifying treatment, increased patient comfort and superior cosmetic results with less scarring, better preservation of breast tissue and faster recovery time.

There are five types of thermal ablations that have been or currently are in research clinical trials: cryoablation, radiofrequency, laser, microwave and high-intensity focused ultrasound (HI FU) ablation. The first 4 methods destroy cancers using percutaneous image-guided probe placement.

With HI FU, the operator, rather than creating an incision to remove the tumour, uses magnetic resonance imaging (MRI) or ultrasound guidance to identify the tumour and to direct a focused beam of acoustic energy through the skin into the tumour. This beam heats and destroys the tumour without damaging nearby structures or tissues. A follow-up MRI can determine whether the entire tumour has been ablated/destroyed, and if necessary, focused ultrasound can be repeated [13].

However, as for other thermal ablations, because there is no surgical removal of tissue involved, there are some potential drawbacks to focused ultrasound treatment:

- It does not allow for laboratory verification of complete removal of the tumour.
- It does not produce extensive samples to enable analysis of the tumour, so that adjuvant therapy will be planned only on basis of previous NCB.

## 16.3 Mastectomy

**Clinical Practice Points**

- Mastectomy is indicated for patients who are not candidates for BCT, patients who prefer mastectomy and for prophylactic purposes to reduce the risk of BC.
- Some indications to mastectomy are still uncertain, but extensive microcalcifications on the preoperative mammogram are a risk factor for local recurrence after conservation surgery.
- As for BCS, the aim of mastectomy is to achieve tumour-free margins. This result may be difficult to obtain in presence of skin or muscle involvement, vascular invasion and extensive modal involvement.
- Reconstructive surgery should be available in all cases of mastectomy, and the technique of mastectomy should be appropriate to the method of reconstruction.

### 16.3.1 Introduction

A mastectomy is the en bloc removal of all breast parenchyma, usually including parts of overlying skin with the nipple-areola complex. Several indications for mastectomy are considered.

*Patient not eligible for BCS* – Mastectomy remains a reasonable option to achieve local control in invasive BC for patients who are not eligible for BCT (see Sect. 16.2) and in case of patient's preference. The patient should be informed about this option, including the possibility of immediate breast reconstruction. Breast reconstruction can be offered, but may not delay or hamper locoregional treatment.

*Patient's choice* – Some patients may choose to have a mastectomy rather than BCS for various reasons, including a desire to avoid the need for postoperative radiation, further screening or biopsies, as well as to reduce the risk of local recurrence. Patients should be presented with the advantages and disadvantages of the two approaches when both BCS and mastectomy are clinically and oncologically acceptable. This should include discussion of cosmetic concerns, because BCS may result in unacceptable cosmetic results if the patient has a small amount of breast tissue.

*Risk-reducing measure* – For patients with hereditary breast and ovarian syndromes and patients with mutations of the BC type 1 and 2 susceptibility genes (BRCA1 and BRCA2), a prophylactic mastectomy reduces the risk of developing BC by more than 90 %. Skin-sparing mastectomy with or without preservation of the nipple-areolar complex and immediate reconstruction provides superior cosmetic results for these patients without oncologic compromise. A contralateral mastectomy may be indicated for patients who have been diagnosed with unilateral BC and carry a deleterious BRCA1 or BRCA2 mutation. Otherwise, there is little survival benefit for a prophylactic contralateral mastectomy (see Sect. 2.3).

*Locally advanced BC* – In extensive disease (either clinically or after histological workup of the excisional specimen), mastectomy may not result in sufficient local control. Factors associated with a high risk for local recurrence after mastectomy are:

- Invasive tumour >5 cm (measured by pathologist)
- Vascular invasion
- Skin or muscle involvement
- Involved or close (<1 mm) surgical margins
- Extensive nodal involvement (4 or more positive nodes)

*Management of the axilla* – The management of the axilla is performed following the same workup of all other procedures. For patients with a clinically positive ALN (including ultrasound identified suspicious nodes), the standard of care is a complete axillary dissection, performed at the time of mastectomy.

For patients undergoing a SLN dissection (i.e. clinically negative disease) with node-negative disease or micrometastatic disease (≤2 mm disease), no further axillary dissection is necessary. For patients with a positive SLN, the management of the axilla is evolving, although most surgeons typically would perform a complete

ALND at the time of the mastectomy, while other oncologists prefer to plan administration of radiation to the chest wall and axilla. However, trends are changing based upon data extrapolated from management of the axilla in patients treated with BCS.

### 16.3.2 Techniques for Mastectomy

*Radical mastectomy*. A radical mastectomy (Halsted mastectomy) consists of en bloc removal of the breast, the overlying skin, the pectoralis major and minor muscles and the entire axillary contents (level I, II and III nodes). The curative potential of this operation remains limited, and the attempts to further expand the field of resection by including the internal mammary nodes failed to improve survival. Radical mastectomy is rarely used unless the tumour has invaded the pectoral muscle.

*Modified radical mastectomy*. A modified radical mastectomy (MRM) consists of the complete removal of the breast and the underlying fascia of the pectoralis major muscle along with the removal of the level I and II axillary lymph nodes. Survival rates are equivalent to radical mastectomy but with less morbidity.

*Simple* (or *total*) *mastectomy*. A simple mastectomy is the removal of the entire breast, with preservation of the pectoral muscles and the axillary contents. With the emergence of sentinel node biopsy, simple mastectomy is performed more frequently than a modified radical mastectomy.

*Skin-sparing mastectomy*. In the skin-sparing mastectomy, the majority of the natural breast skin envelope is not resected. Preservation of the skin of the breast and the inframammary fold provides the reconstructed breast with a more natural shape and contour. This procedure is an oncologically safe and acceptable option for the surgical management of patients with non-invasive and invasive BC. It is also an acceptable option for high-risk women who prefer a mastectomy as risk-reducing procedure. SSM is contraindicated for women with inflammatory BC (IBC), because of cancer cell invasion of the dermal lymphatics (see Sect. 14.2).

Nipple-areolar-sparing mastectomy. A nipple-areolar-sparing mastectomy (NSM) preserves the dermis and epidermis of the nipple but removes the major ducts from within the nipple lumen. This approach is an option for carefully selected patients, particularly those who are having surgery for prophylactic purposes and are having immediate reconstruction.

NSM for the treatment of BC is becoming more widely accepted with time. Because this technique results in large flaps, it is primarily useful for women with small- to moderate-sized breasts with minimal ptosis. The candidate criteria exclude only patients with a distance between tumour and nipple-areolar complex (NAC) of <1 cm, clinical involvement of NAC, Paget disease, bloody ductal discharge and/or inflammatory carcinoma.

An intraoperative biopsy of the retroareolar margin must be histologically negative for malignancy. A precise measurement of a negative margin has not been defined. However, these biopsies of the areola and nipple are not completely reliable in predicting occult involvement in patients with BC. NAC necrosis or skin desquamation rate is about 15–20 %, with a risk slightly more evident in smokers.

*The choice of mastectomy* depends on the clinical situation, on planning of immediate reconstruction and sometimes on the patient's choice. Of the patients who are not having immediate reconstruction, when a modified radical (that includes axillary dissection) or simple mastectomy with sentinel node biopsy is indicated, the latter is performed more commonly.

For patients having immediate reconstruction, a skin-sparing mastectomy preserves the skin of the breast and the inframammary fold resulting in a superior cosmetic result.

For patients having mastectomy for prophylactic purposes, or with a unifocal tumour less than 2 cm in diameter and distant greater than 2 cm from the nipple, a skin-sparing or nipple-sparing mastectomy will provide the best cosmetic result.

*Technical consideration for mastectomy.* The most frequent complication of mastectomy is redundant tissue, which causes difficulty with bra fitting and often rubs uncomfortably on the prosthesis, arm or bra. To avoid this inconvenience, prior to surgery the patient should be examined sitting up to assess lateral tissue and plan the lateral end of scar.

The incision should be low enough to be hidden in low neckline clothes. The scar should be also made with the method of delayed reconstruction in mind. A lower scar, if practical, is desirable because it allows a flap-based reconstruction to be set at the inframammary fold.

A contralateral breast reduction can be a simple and very effective option to enable woman with heavy breasts to wear a lighter prosthesis and feel less unbalanced.

### 16.3.3 Outcomes of Mastectomy

*Restoring body profile.* Patients not undergoing immediate breast reconstruction should be provided with breast external prostheses. Breast prostheses should be freely available to patients treated with mastectomy together with easy access to a fitting service.

*Post-mastectomy pain.* Burning, aching and tight constriction of the axilla, upper arm and chest wall, with superimposed lancinations and scar sensitivity, are characteristic of post-mastectomy pain. Chronic pain, paresthesias and phantom sensations in up to one-half of cases are also related to radiation therapy and/or chemotherapy, which are sometimes needed in addition to surgery. Although available data are scant, at least one long-term follow-up study suggests that approximately one-half of cases resolve over time, while the remainder persists long term.

*Phantom breast syndrome.* Patients may describe a change in chest wall sensation after mastectomy, sometimes described as *phantom breast syndrome*. The sensation of residual breast tissue can persist for years after surgery. The most common complaint is pain, but itching, nipple sensation, erotic sensations and premenstrual-type breast soreness are also described. Although the cause is unknown, psychological factors related to mastectomy have been implicated.

Patient education before mastectomy, outlining the possible changes in chest wall sensation and the possibility of phantom breast syndrome, may help to relieve patient anxiety if symptoms develop and may even reduce the frequency of this syndrome.

*Arm morbidity*. Arm morbidity is common after mastectomy and can include arm swelling, arm pain, arm numbness, arm stiffness, shoulder stiffness, shoulder pain or nerve injury. Post-mastectomy radiation also contributes to arm morbidity and shoulder dysfunction. After BC surgery, particularly after extensive node dissection, patients should be provided with rehabilitation services as needed and informed about methods to improve shoulder function and reduce the risk of lymphoedema (see Sect. 21.3).

*Recurrences rate*. The chest wall relapse rate after mastectomy for invasive BC should be less than 10 % after 10 years. Therefore, in the presence of high-risk factors for local relapse after mastectomy (as in presence of tumour invasion of underlying fascia or subcutaneous fat), almost all patients (at least 90 %) should have a consultation with a radiation oncologist to inform them about the possibility of adjuvant radiation therapy of the chest wall and regional lymph node area.

## 16.4 Surgery of the Axilla

**Clinical Practice Points**

- Regional lymph nodes are harbingers of systemic diseases and not barriers to tumour spread. Removal of lymph nodes at surgery does not affect the frequency of recurrence, the development of distant metastases or survival rates.
- Patients with palpable axillary lymph nodes should undergo axillary ultrasound and ultrasound-guided FNA o CNB to confirm or not metastases.
- Sentinel lymph node biopsy (SLNB), rather than full axillary nodal clearance, is the standard of care, unless axillary node involvement is proven preoperatively.
- It is also recommended to excise also any suspicious nodes regardless of whether they take up the tracer or the dye.
- Permanent section is the most accurate pathologic method of assessment of lymph node status.
- Micrometastases (defined as those measuring 0.2–2 mm) are classified as node positive, while isolated tumour cells (defined as those measuring <0.2 mm) are classified as node negative.

### 16.4.1 Introduction

Metastatic disease to axillary nodes is the most significant prognostic indicator for BC and one of the major determinants of appropriate systemic adjuvant therapy; thus, axillary surgery is necessary for adequate staging and guiding treatment [14].

Approximately 30–40 % of symptomatic patients with early BC have axillary nodal involvement. The likelihood of axillary nodal involvement is directly related to the size of the tumour, the higher histological grade and the presence of lymphovascular invasion.

Sentinel lymph node biopsy (SLNB) is the preferred technique for most cases, validated in large cohort studies, as well as randomised controlled trials which demonstrated that the false-negative rate is low and that survival is no different for node-negative patients who undergo sentinel node biopsy compared with axillary node dissection [15]. Sentinel node biopsy is a safe, accurate and minimally invasive mean of staging the axilla in patients with BC. Moreover, sentinel node biopsy allows quality of life, as well as functional outcomes, significantly better than ALND [16].

Minimal surgery, rather than lymph node clearance, should be performed to stage the axilla for patients with early invasive BC and no evidence of lymph node involvement.

In order to reach this aim, preoperative ultrasound evaluation of the axilla should be performed for all patients being investigated for early invasive BC, and if morphologically abnormal lymph nodes are identified, ultrasound-guided needle sampling should be offered. Up to 50 % of patients with axillary metastatic disease can be diagnosed using this method, avoiding the need for sentinel node biopsy in women with pathologically proven nodal involvement [17].

Axillary lymph node dissection (ALND) remains standard treatment for patients with macrometastases identified on SLNB. Also, in clinical positive nodes, ALND is the most widely used technique because it gives additional staging information. When ALND is indicated, a level I/II anatomical dissection is the preferred operation. ALND substantially reduces the risk of axillary recurrence, although the evidence of its impact on survival remains insufficient, and, as it is well known, there is significant morbidity associated with ALND, compared to SLNB.

Micrometastases (defined as those measuring 0.2–2 mm) are classified as node positive, while isolated tumour cells (defined as those measuring <0.2 mm) are classified as node negative. The prognostic difference between these two groups remains somewhat controversial [18].

### 16.4.2 Techniques of SLNB

*Lymphatic mapping* is based upon the concept that one or more nodes are the first to be involved with metastatic disease within a given lymph node basin. If these sentinel lymph nodes are not involved, the entire basin should be free of tumour.

Sentinel lymph node mapping is a technique used to identify the lymph drainage basin, determine the number of sentinel nodes, differentiate sentinel nodes from subsequent nodes, locate the sentinel node in an unexpected location and mark the sentinel node biopsy.

Sentinel lymph node biopsy (SLNB) can be applied to those patients in whom the axillary lymph node status is negative on preoperative evaluation or is unknown prior to surgery. In these cases minimal surgery should be performed to stage the axilla. Moreover, no sampling is indicated in most cases of non-invasive BC after BCS or in few low-grade tumours in elderly women [19].

*Radioactive colloid* – SLN identification shows a significantly higher proportion of successful mappings in studies using radioactive colloid rather than blue dye alone. Usually technetium-labelled human serum albumin is used. The radioactive material may be injected peritumourally, intradermally or into the subareolar plexus; there is ongoing debate about the best site for injection. Intradermal injection of radiocolloid appears to be superior to subdermal injection in almost all cases. If internal mammary node visualisation is needed, injections into the dermis and subareolar area are associated with a lower potential for this imaging.

A sensitive hand-held gamma probe is used to systematically survey the axilla and identify the hot spots. Subsequently in the operating room, a small skin incision is made over the hot spot, and the hand-held gamma probe is used to guide the surgeon to the labelled LN(s). For SLN identification with radioactivity, the *10%* rule has been proposed as a guideline and refers to removal of all SLN with counts over 10 % of the most radioactive node. Because this technique is easier to learn, proficiency is attained sooner than with blue dye.

*Blue dye* – The surgeon injects a small amount of blue dye (Patent Blue V) around the tumour periphery, at the palpable edge of the biopsy cavity or into the subareolar plexus. It is important not to inject the dye into the tumour itself (because the lymphatics can be occluded by the tumour) or into the seroma cavity following breast biopsy (as the seroma itself does not contain lymphatic channels). These errors in technique are likely to lead to a failure of mapping. Breast massage is then carried out for about 5 min to dilate breast lymphatics.

Successful SLN identification by blue dye is defined as the identification of any blue node or any non-blue node with a blue afferent lymphatic (Fig. 16.4).

*Dual tracer*. Dual tracer has been shown to be superior to injection of either radioactive tracer or blue dye alone in terms of sentinel node identification rate and false-negative rates and is the technique of choice to identify sentinel nodes [20].

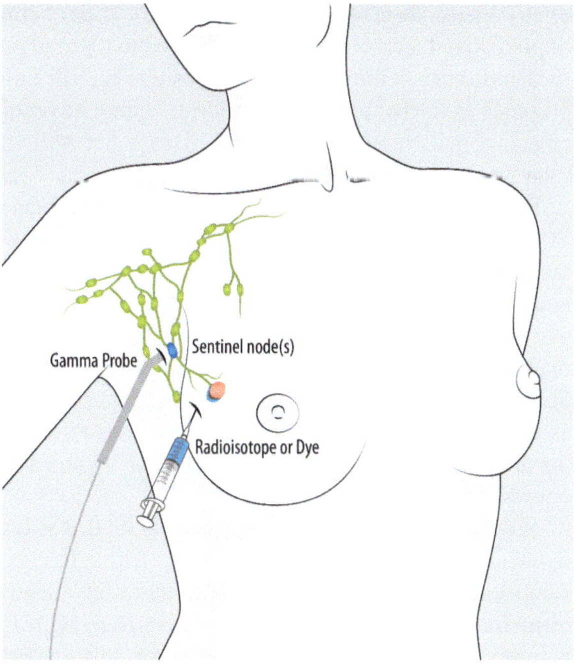


**Fig. 16.4** A radiotracer (the day before) or a blue dye (few minutes before) or both are injected near the tumour to locate the position of sentinel lymph node(s). The radiotracer and/or the dye move down the lymphatics to the draining node(s), while valves allow fluid to flow in one direction only. The surgeon then uses a gamma probe that detects radioactivity to find the increased radiotracer uptake, and/or follows the thin blue track in the tissue, to find the stained sentinel lymph node(s)

*Sampling*. Some studies have shown that four-node axillary sampling provides accurate prognostic information. Both four-node axillary sampling and SLNB have been shown to reduce the incidence rate of complications, especially of lymphoedema.

*Blue dye-directed sampling*. Some centres familiar with the procedure practise blue dye-directed axillary sampling.

*Importance of surgeon's experience*. A major issue in the use of SLNB is the amount of experience necessary to master the procedure. Proper performance requires significant training, and results vary according to a surgeon's skill and experience. The number of cases that should be performed to establish an individual surgeon's false-negative rate is unclear. One report estimated that a surgeon must perform about 20 procedures to attain competency, while others recommend 30–60 procedures. One-on-one training with an experienced surgeon most rapidly improves the learning of the technique.

*Intraoperative evaluation* with frozen section and/or touch imprint cytology has a high specificity (99 %); the sensitivity of frozen section is better than that of touch imprint cytology. The use of routine intraoperative evaluation is now under question, and many no longer use it. Intraoperative evaluation of the SLN will not identify all patients with positive nodes because of sampling limitations and may also yield a false-positive result. Permanent section is the most accurate method of assessment. Performing immunohistochemistry on routine SLNB is not recommended.

*Treatment of patients with a positive SLNB*. The management of the axilla after a positive sentinel lymph node biopsy is a controversial and an evolving area of clinical practice. Axillary metastases are limited to the sentinel node in 40–60 % of cases with the remainder of the axillary nodes being clear of tumour. A variety of predictive factors have been employed to try to identify those patients who have further disease in the axilla after a positive SLNB. Since no one is reliable and the presence of further axillary metastases cannot be predicted with certainty, axillary clearance will remove all further disease but will show no further evidence of lymph node disease in up to 60 % of patients.

Regional radiotherapy has been used as an alternative in patients with a positive SLNB. Results are pending from the AMAROS trial, which is evaluating the use of radiotherapy as an alternative to axillary dissection in women with involved lymph nodes after SLNB. In this trial, patients with positive sentinel lymph nodes (any number and any tumour size), including those undergoing conservation surgery or mastectomy, are being randomised to have either axillary clearance or radiotherapy. Studies are needed to determine effectiveness of local control and overall survival, as well as side effects and quality of life, cost effectiveness, and whether the additional information on the total number of involved nodes obtained by ALND is relevant for optimum management.

*SLNB after neoadjuvant chemotherapy*. SNLB is feasible after neoadjuvant chemotherapy; however, its accuracy in this setting has been questioned, and this is the subject of ongoing randomised controlled trials. Sentinel lymph node biopsy may be performed before neoadjuvant chemotherapy with a plan for ALND if the patient is node positive. The disadvantages of this approach are the need for two

**Table 16.2** Techniques of axillary sampling

| Techniques | Procedure | Notes |
|---|---|---|
| No sampling | No sampling is obtained | Indicated in most cases of non-invasive BC after BCS |
| | | May be indicated in few low-grade tumours in elderly women |
| Sentinel lymph node biopsy (SLNB) with isotope | Selective removal of the first tumour-draining node(s) | The more validated standard technique |
| Sentinel lymph node biopsy (SLNB) with blue dye alone | Selective removal of the first tumour-draining node(s) | More reliable for lateral than medial quadrants |
| | | Some nodes may be disregarded |
| Axillary sampling | Picks out a minimum of four individual lymph nodes from the axillary fat | More reliable if blue dye directed |
| Axillary lymph node dissection (ALND) | Block dissection of the axillary contents, usually level 1 (up to the lateral border of *pectoralis minor*) and level 2 (up to the medial border of *pectoralis minor*), rarely level 3 (up to the apex of the axilla) | At least 10 nodes should be retrieved in more than 90 % of cases |
| | | Gives more information in clinically positive lymph nodes |
| | | Its impact on survival remains insufficient |
| | | Has a significant morbidity if compared to SLNB |

procedures, and the possibility that ALND will be performed when all disease has been eradicated by chemotherapy.

If the sentinel lymph node biopsy contains tumour, further treatment to the axilla, either axillary lymph node dissection or radiotherapy, should be given. Patients undergoing breast conservation surgery and radiotherapy for T1/T2 and clinically node-negative BC and who have one or two positive nodes at sentinel lymph node biopsy may be considered for no further treatment to the axilla.

*SLNB in multiple cancers.* A subareolar injection technique is suggested for sentinel node biopsy in patients with multifocal and multicentric BC.

*SLNB in recurrences.* In the case of in-breast recurrence after BCS, lymphoscintigraphy has limited utility for most cases of sentinel node mapping; however, this technique may be useful in identifying alternative drainage pathways.

Techniques of axillary sampling are outlined in Table 16.2.

### 16.4.3 Quality Indicators on Axillary Staging

To increase the nonoperative diagnosis of axillary node metastases, all patients diagnosed with invasive BC undergoing surgical treatment should have a preoperative axillary ultrasound scan, and, if appropriate, FNA or core biopsy should be carried out.

To ensure adequate surgical treatment of involved axillary lymph nodes, if a positive nonoperative diagnosis of axillary nodal metastasis is made in a patient undergoing surgery for BC, the patient should normally proceed to an axillary clearance.

To minimise morbidity from axillary surgery to obtain staging information, SLNB using the combined blue dye/radioisotope technique is a recommended axillary staging procedure for the majority of patients with early invasive BC.

Patients with positive (macro- or micrometastases) axillary staging procedures should proceed to subsequent treatment for axillary disease. This may take the form of full axillary clearance, axillary radiotherapy or entry into an appropriate clinical trial. This should be discussed at the MDT meeting according to local guidelines, and the reasons should be documented in the patient's medical record.

When axillary node clearance is carried out, the level of anatomical dissection should be specified, and at least 10 nodes should be retrieved in more than 90 % of cases. When axillary node sampling is carried out, at least 4 nodes should be retrieved.

Axillary recurrence should be minimised by effective staging and treatment where appropriate. Axillary recurrence at 5 years should occur in 5 % or less of cases, with a gold standard at 5 years of 3 % or less.

## 16.5 Oncoplastic Surgery of the Breast

**Clinical Practice Points**

- Cosmesis in BCS and breast reconstruction following mastectomy complement oncologic interventions and play a significant role in the woman's physical, emotional and psychological recovery from BC.
- Training in breast surgery should include essential training in oncoplastic surgery, at least for level I oncoplastic techniques, while specific training is required for level II techniques.
- Due to the variable needs of individual patients, the reconstructive surgeon must be able to provide the full range of reconstructive options, irrespective of whether they are all locally available.
- The use of acellular dermal matrices (ADM), as well as new meshes, in tissue expander/implant-based breast reconstruction represents one of the promising advances in implant reconstruction.
- Autologous reconstructions have aesthetic results superior to those of implant-based reconstruction due to their versatility, more natural appearance, consistency and durability.
- Improvement in fat grafting techniques has the potential to improve on all existing form of breast reconstruction and may revolutionise the approach to breast reconstruction as a whole.
- Even the best reconstruction will not be able to replace the natural breast that has been lost.

### 16.5.1 Introduction

Over the past 30 years, several studies have documented the psychological, social, emotional and functional benefits of breast reconstruction, including improved psychological health, self-esteem, sexuality, body image and reduced concern for cancer recurrence. The literature provides support for offering post-mastectomy reconstruction, as this is an important determinant of long-term health and wellbeing for BC patients.

The role of oncoplastic therapeutic mammoplasty compared with BCS for invasive and pre-invasive (DCIS) BC remains to be fully defined, and randomised clinical trials have not yet been reported. Retrospective case series of patients treated with a variety of oncoplastic techniques, and which have included patients with tumours larger than have been treated previously with conservation surgery, have indicated tumour local recurrence rates of 0–7 %. However, it is not possible to make associations because of the great variability of the techniques and the diversity of situations, including the volume of the tumour and the proper location of the margins to irradiate.

The low rates of breast reconstruction are in part due to a low referral rate to plastic surgeons. A survey of patients diagnosed with BC reported that the desire to avoid additional surgery was the most common reason given for not pursuing reconstruction. Inadequate education about reconstructive options also plays a role.

Approximately 40 % of all patients undergoing a mastectomy also undergo breast reconstruction. Implant-based reconstruction has been increasing at a rate of 10 % per year, while the rate of autologous reconstruction has remained unchanged. Despite improvement of social care, breast reconstruction remains an underutilised option. The underlying reasons seem to be multifactorial and related to socioeconomic factors, including access to care, insurance coverage, education and race/ethnicity, as well as geographic location, age and personal choice.

Oncoplastic procedures can achieve better cosmetic outcomes, especially in patients with large breasts, with a less favourable tumour/breast size ratio or with a cosmetically difficult location of the tumour in the breast.

Coaching in breast surgery should include training in oncoplastic surgery. Commonly level I and level II oncoplastic techniques are considered (Table 16.3). Specific training is required to be able to perform level II techniques, while all surgeons doing breast surgery should be able to perform level I oncoplastic surgical techniques.

### 16.5.2 Oncoplasty in Breast-Conserving Surgery

The type of breast-sparing reconstruction selected will be determined by the site and extent of resection and by the patient's size, morphology and personal preference. The first element affecting cosmesis is excision volume, which is the single most predictive factor for satisfying surgical outcome and potential for breast

**Table 16.3** Levels of oncoplastic breast surgery

| Level | Kind of surgery | Procedure/result |
|---|---|---|
| Level I | BCS: excision volume ratio <20 % | Skin incision: allows wide access for excision and reshaping |
| | | Skin undermining: facilitates wide excision and glandular mobilisation for reshaping |
| | | NAC undermining: avoids displacement of nipple towards excision defect |
| | | Full-thickness excision: prevents anterior and posterior margin involvement |
| | | Glandular approximation: late-occurring deformity is avoided |
| | | De-epithelialisation and NAC repositioning: recentres NAC on new breast mound |
| | Mastectomy: expander/implant | Expander implant is a temporary device that may be placed by breast surgeon immediately following the mastectomy |
| Level II | BCS: excision volume ratio 20–50 % | Large breast volume excision will require excision of excess skin to reshape the breast, usually based upon mammoplasty techniques. Contralateral breast need to be reshaped |
| | Mastectomy: breast implants autologous flap, reshaping | Specific training is required |

deformity. Resection of more than 20 % of breast volume, particularly from central, medial or inferior locations, significantly increases the likelihood of a significant and unsightly local deformity, which results in psychological morbidity [21].

Reshaping of the breast is required after any tumour excision in order to recreate a normal breast shape in one operative procedure. In most cases this can be achieved with a simple unilateral approach, mobilising glandular flaps to close the defect or by recentralising the NAC. In other cases, a bilateral approach incorporating a bilateral mammoplasty will be the only way to perform a wide excision with no deformity [22].

In BCS some slight asymmetries may be tolerated, but deformities following wide local excision even for large cancers are to be avoided. Defects can be avoided by breast-sparing reconstruction using volume replacement or volume displacement.

*Volume displacement* is most suitable for patients with medium or large breasts who are willing to undergo breast reduction (often bilateral), avoiding more major reconstructive surgery. Volume displacement allows large-volume resection of tissue without cosmetic consequence [23].

*Volume replacement* is most suitable for patients with small- or medium-sized breasts who wish to avoid contralateral surgery. It can also be used for the correction of deformities following previous BCS. The use of a *latissimus dorsi* muscular miniflap to replace the volume loss after major breast sector resection is an option [9].

*Lipofilling*, performed at the same time as wide local excision, is a new technique currently being evaluated to improve cosmetic outcomes in patients with smaller breasts where excision of even a small cancer would produce a poor cosmetic outcome [24].

### 16.5.3 Oncoplasty in Reconstructive Surgery

A productive, caring relationship is crucial to the patient's satisfaction with the reconstructive process and must be established early. The patient with newly diagnosed BC may have feelings of grief and anger as well as unrealistic expectations that may be directed at her health care team. If possible, the patient's family should be included in the consultation. Educational literature, including preoperative and postoperative photographs, is helpful for the patient at the initial consultation to facilitate her decision-making process. Peer-reviewed Internet sites and the opportunity to speak with other women who have undergone breast reconstruction may also be worthwhile [25].

*History*. A thorough history and physical examination should focus on the following factors: disease status and oncologic history, future treatment plans, past surgical history/comorbid health problems, volume and shape of the contralateral breast, body habitus and patient preference. A past history of RT or current disease extent for which RT is mandated may impact the patient's reconstructive options.

Comorbidities such as obesity, insulin-dependent diabetes mellitus, chronic obstructive pulmonary disease, smoking and connective tissue disease may also influence reconstructive options. Likewise, past surgical histories, that include open cholecystectomy and abdominoplasty, may limit reconstructive choices because of their potential adverse effects on the blood supply to autogenous tissues at donor sites.

Smokers are at a significantly greater risk of developing surgical complications, particularly from autogenous tissue reconstructions. Breast reconstruction in overweight and obese patients also presents a difficult challenge for plastic surgeons. Previous studies have reported higher complication rates and disappointing aesthetic results in this population compared with normal weight women. Higher body mass index (BMI) was associated with a greater likelihood of postoperative complications. Free flap breast reconstruction in obese patients is associated with a high risk of total flap loss, major postoperative complications and delayed abdominal wound healing. Although patient satisfaction with post mastectomy reconstruction remains high in obese patients, these patients should be counselled preoperatively regarding their higher complication rates.

*Physical examination*. The breasts are evaluated for volume, ptosis, asymmetry and scars, and the axilla examined for palpably abnormal lymph nodes. If RT has been administered previously, the quality of the breast and chest wall soft tissues must be assessed. The abdomen, back and buttocks are evaluated as possible donor sites, taking note of scars, overall fat content and abdominal wall strength.

Potential asymmetry between the native contralateral breast and the newly reconstructed breast must be addressed. The contralateral breast may require a reconstructive procedure, such as mastopexy, reduction or even augmentation, in order to obtain symmetry. The patient's personal distribution of excess skin and fat are also considered, because they dictate whether a given reconstructive choice can provide enough tissue volume to recreate the breast. Finally, the patient's wishes regarding scar location, tissue sacrifice, postoperative recovery and aesthetic outcome are also important in guiding the reconstructive surgeon.

*Immediate versus delayed reconstruction.* Breast reconstruction can be carried out at the time of the mastectomy (immediate) or during a subsequent operation (delayed). Immediate reconstruction can be offered to most patients. However, patients should be informed that if the skin flaps have compromised perfusion following mastectomy, delayed reconstruction would be necessary [26].

*Immediate reconstruction.* Initially, delayed procedures were favoured because it was assumed that the time between mastectomy and reconstruction provided women with the opportunity to psychologically adjust to the loss of a breast, therefore allowing for a greater appreciation for their reconstruction. This assumption was found to be faulty when several studies revealed that women undergoing immediate reconstruction experienced significant psychosocial benefits.

*Delayed reconstruction* is more appropriate for patients who will need post-mastectomy radiation for locally advanced BC or inflammatory BC. Comparison of advantages and disadvantages between immediate and delayed breast reconstruction is summarised Table 16.4.

**Table 16.4** Comparison of advantages and disadvantages between immediate and delayed breast reconstructions

| Reconstruction | Advantages | Disadvantages | Contraindications |
|---|---|---|---|
| *Immediate* | Removal of BC and reconstruction are streamlined (and less expensive) | Women with immediate reconstruction had a higher rate of complications | Advanced disease (stage III or higher) |
| | Normal perceptions of body image provide substantial psychosocial benefits | Necrosis of the mastectomy skin flaps can adversely affect the aesthetic result of the reconstruction | Need for postoperative RT |
| | Normal breast landmarks (such as the inframammary fold) are preserved yielding a more natural-appearing breast | Some conditions may necessitate postoperative RT, which can adversely affect the reconstruction | Medical comorbidities such as active smoking, obesity, poorly controlled diabetes mellitus |
| *Delayed* | Assurance of clear margins prior to definitive reconstruction | Need for subsequent surgery | Medical comorbidities such as active smoking, obesity, poorly controlled diabetes mellitus |
| | Minimise the effect of poorly perfused mastectomy skin flaps | Limited reconstructive options following radiation therapy | Limited mobility cannot meet the patient's expectancies |
| | Allows completion of all adjuvant treatment | Lesser aesthetic quality compared with immediate reconstruction | |

### 16.5.4 Techniques of Breast Reconstruction

There are three general types of reconstructive options:

- Prosthetic devices (e.g. saline implants, silicone implants, tissue expanders)
- Autologous tissue reconstructions with tissue flaps that are transferred from adjoining or distant donor sites to the anterior chest wall
- Autologous tissue reconstructions with adipose tissue grafts

In order of incidence, the most common surgical techniques are tissue expansion, *latissimus dorsi* musculocutaneous flap with or without implant, lower abdominal tissue and other free tissue transfers and adipose tissue graft.

IMPLANTS – Implant-based techniques require limited surgery initially but have some limitations and are not always quick and trouble-free. The quality of the long-term result is directly related to the tolerance of breast implants but may be disappointing unless performed after bilateral mastectomy. Moreover, further procedures may be required for complications and maintenance. Asymmetry may reoccur due to the effects of gravity on the contralateral breast and fluctuations in body weight.

*Advantages and disadvantages.* The advantages of implant reconstruction are surgical simplicity, the use of cosmetically similar adjacent tissue for coverage of the implant, the lack of donor site morbidity, reduced operative time and more rapid postoperative recovery as compared with purely autologous reconstructions. For older patients, those with significant medical comorbidity and women with minimal tissue at the various potential donor sites (abdomen, buttock, back and thigh), expander/implant techniques may be the preferred option.

The main disadvantages are that tissue expansion requires frequent clinic visits for expansion (usually every 1–2 weeks for 1–2 months) and a second surgery to place the reconstructive implant.

*Patient selection.* As with any type of reconstruction, patients need to be carefully selected and counselled prior to undertaking reconstruction with expander/implant techniques. Women with smaller, minimally ptotic breasts are good candidates for primary implant reconstruction, while those with large, ptotic breasts may require more skin excision during the mastectomy and therefore need more expansion. Such women may require a contralateral breast procedure in order to achieve acceptable symmetry. Moreover, for women who require post-mastectomy chest wall RT, tissue expansion could be a difficult, complication-prone endeavour. In these cases, autogenous tissue (flap) reconstruction is generally preferred.

*One-stage implant reconstruction.* Women with small, non-ptotic breasts can occasionally be reconstructed in a single stage. This type of reconstruction is usually performed as an immediate procedure, provided the mastectomy flaps are non-traumatised and well perfused. Single-stage reconstruction may also be possible in patients who have been previously augmented, because the skin and soft tissues are pre-expanded, and the contralateral augmented breast is usually well matched with an implant. One-stage reconstruction has been increasing in popularity as reconstructive techniques have improved and patients prefer fewer operative procedures.

Single-stage implant reconstruction remains relatively less frequent than the two-stage techniques because most women require additional skin for implant coverage and the two-stage implant reconstruction allows for the opportunity to revise the reconstruction more often. However, advancements with skin-sparing and nipple-areolar-sparing mastectomy allow the surgeon to take the one-stage implant option into consideration, although revision procedures are sometimes necessary.

*Two-stage implant reconstruction* – The most common technique used for expander/implant placement consists of initially positioning the tissue expander in a pocket deep into the pectoralis major muscle and overlying breast skin (Fig. 16.5b). For immediate tissue expander reconstructions, the serratus anterior muscle may be used to provide additional muscle coverage for the expander. Overall the pocket size should match the size of the expander. It is important to not alter or undermine the inframammary fold or to undermine to the contralateral breast, as these lower and medial borders are critical landmarks for the aesthetic appearance of the breast. If there is concern that the mastectomy flaps have compromised vascular supply, expander placement should be delayed.

*Acellular dermal matrices and other mesh implants*. The use of acellular dermal matrices (ADM) has expanded the indications for prosthetic reconstruction following mastectomy. The ADM is supplied as a sheet of decellularised material consisting primarily of collagen and elastin. ADM is claimed to serve as biologic scaffolding for fibroblast and angioblast ingrowth and is replaced by host connective tissue at varying rates. The principal benefit of ADM in breast reconstruction is to provide adequate tissue support to the lower mastectomy and to stabilise the position of the pectoralis major muscle in order to prevent upward migration of the muscle (Fig. 16.5c). ADM can be used for both one- and two-stage prosthetic reconstruction [27].

Other devices for single-stage implant-based breast reconstruction are the titanium-coated polypropylene mesh, the silk-derived biological scaffold and other meshes that have a good biocompatibility and can be used in a similar way as ADM.

*Tissue expanders* – A tissue expander is a silicone shell that is incrementally filled with saline through either an integrated or remote port. Modern expanders are shaped anatomically to preferentially expand in the lower pole of the breast. One to three weeks after the expander is placed, the expansion begins in the outpatient clinic. For expanders with integrated ports, a magnetic finder (compass) is used to locate the proper injection site under the skin. A needle is then inserted into the skin through the port, and sterile saline is infused into the expander (Fig. 16.5d). This procedure is repeated every 1–2 weeks, until the desired volume of expansion is achieved. Tissue expansion should be fulfilled before the start of radiotherapy and should not be attempted during or after the treatment [28].

Several months after the last expansion (to allow for maximal skin growth), the patient is returned to the operating room for the second stage of the reconstruction. The expander is removed, and the reconstructive implant is placed. The implant

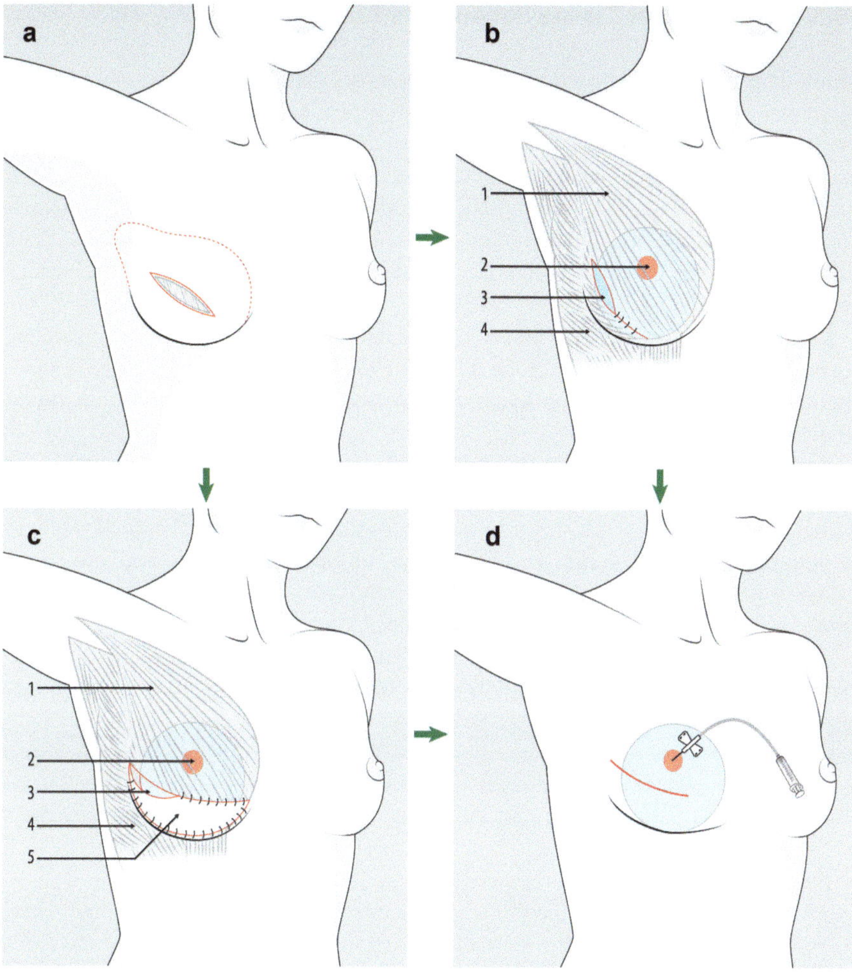


**Fig. 16.5** Placement of expander or definitive implant in post-mastectomy reconstruction. (**a**) In the immediate reconstruction, a larger part of the skin is spared, consistently with the location of the tumour. (**b**) A temporary tissue expander (*3*) with a built-in valve (*2*) is placed in a pocket created deep to the *pectoralis major* (*1*) and the *serratus anterior* (*4*). (**c**) With the use of an acellular dermal matrix (ADM) or other mesh implants (*5*), a higher volume of saline expander or also a definitive implant could be placed. (**d**) If an expander has been placed, through a butterfly needle the implant is partially filled with saline to stretch the chest muscle

(a silicone shell) may be filled with silicone or saline. In addition, necessary revisions are performed at this time, while the nipple may be reconstructed immediately or after a few months. Patients should be offered nipple-areola reconstruction as an integral part of their reconstruction. It completes the reconstructed breast and leads to increased satisfaction with the reconstruction, a sense of completeness and an enhanced sense of attractiveness, especially when the patient is unclothed.

### 16.5.5 Autologous Tissue Reconstruction

Autologous tissue reconstructions have aesthetic results superior to those of implant-based reconstruction due to their more natural appearance, consistency and durability. The autologous flap is highly versatile, has acceptable donor site morbidity and, moreover, can better withstand radiotherapy [29].

The skin and fat of the lower abdomen are ideal for autologous breast reconstruction, but donor- site morbidity is being increasingly appreciated. Muscle-sparing techniques preserve abdominal wall function at the cost of a more complex procedure.

Further surgery is often necessary following reconstruction to the reconstructed breast, the contralateral breast or the donor site of the breast reconstruction. Nipple-areola complex reconstruction leads to increased patient satisfaction with breast reconstruction.

Autogenous reconstruction may be the only available reconstructive option for patients who have large soft tissue deficits or chest wall skin that is unsuitable for tissue expansion due to scar tissue or radiation-induced changes. The disadvantages of autologous reconstruction include longer surgical procedures and prolonged recovery time as compared with prosthetic reconstruction. The risk of total flap failure is usually less than 3 % with experienced surgeons.

*KINDS OF FLAPS* – The development of musculocutaneous flaps and microsurgical tissue transplantation paved the way for modern autogenous tissue breast reconstruction. Three kinds of flaps are considered:

- *Pedicle flap*. Musculocutaneous flaps consist of a segment of vascularised muscle with the overlying skin and fat, which are perfused by perforating vessels from the underlying muscle. These flaps may be transposed into position with their vascular origin intact (pedicled flaps).
- *Free flaps*. Alternatively, the flap and its vascular supply can be completely harvested and transferred to the mastectomy site, requiring anastomosis of the flap's artery and vein to local vessels at the recipient site, usually the internal mammary or thoracodorsal vessels.
- *Perforator free flap*. Although these microvascular free flaps have traditionally included a segment of underlying muscle, perforator free flap harvests only the vascular supply (artery and vein) and the overlying skin and fat, without muscle fibres.

FLAP RECONSTRUCTION PROCEDURES – Pedicle *latissimus* flap. Reconstruction with the *latissimus dorsi* myocutaneous flap produces a breast with ptosis and projection while maintaining the natural consistency and feel of normal tissue. This flap provides ample bulk for reconstruction due to the large surface of the muscle. In many patients, the flap can be used without the use of an implant, restoring volumes of up to 1.5 L in large patients or with the use of modified techniques. It restores the anterior chest wall with healthy tissue, particularly of benefit in patients who previously have undergone irradiation. The latissimus muscle flap is an anchor flap for salvage of failed expander/implant reconstructions. The flap also provides trophic stimulation to the surrounding tissues without increased disease morbidity or interference with mammographic evaluation.

Recently, because of the increased use of the TRAM flap, the *latissimus dorsi* flap often is reserved for patients in whom TRAM reconstruction is contraindicated. This subset of patients includes extremely thin patients in whom the infraumbilical soft tissues are limited and patients who previously have undergone abdominoplasty or other abdominal operations or who have abdominal scars that may entail compromise of the *rectus abdominis* pedicle. Relative to TRAM reconstruction, the *latissimus dorsi* is more resistant to the effects of impaired wound healing posed by smoking and diabetes. Additionally, *latissimus dorsi* reconstruction does not compromise the abdominal wall, which may be of issue in patients desiring future pregnancy.

*Pedicled TRAM flap*. One of the most commonly used autogenous tissue reconstructions is the TRAM (transverse *rectus abdominis* myocutaneous). This procedure is sometimes necessary to allow chest wall radiation; however, it can also be performed at the time of mastectomy to provide immediate reconstruction. Either the contralateral or ipsilateral *rectus abdominis* muscle can be utilised.

Free TRAM flap reconstruction after skin-sparing mastectomy. The free TRAM flap completely detaches and directly transfers the lower abdominal tissue to the mastectomy site. The deep inferior epigastric artery and vein, which provide the vascular supply for the free flap, are anastomosed to local recipient vessels, using either the internal mammary or thoracodorsal vessels.

*Perforator DIEP flap*. The most commonly used perforator flap for breast reconstruction is the deep inferior epigastric perforator (DIEP) flap. The DIEP uses the lower abdominal island of skin and fat and spares the *rectus abdominis* muscle. Although the underlying muscle must be split to dissect out the perforating vessels, the muscle itself is not included in the transfer. The deep inferior epigastric artery and vein, which provide the vascular supply for the free flap, are anastomosed to local recipient vessels, using either the internal mammary or thoracodorsal vessels.

Other perforator flaps – For patients who do not have sufficient lower abdominal fat for reconstructive flaps, but who prefer the use of autologous tissue, a more viable donor site may be the buttock area. For this free flap, perforating vessels from either the superior gluteal artery (SGAP flap) or the inferior gluteal artery (IGAP flap) can be used as the vascular supply for the transferred tissue. For the SGAP flap, the upper buttock tissue is used, resulting in a donor site scar that is concealable under most swimwear. If an IGAP flap is performed, the donor site scar lies within the lower buttock crease. The transverse upper *gracilis* (TUG) flap is based on the proximal *gracilis* muscle and its vascular pedicle, the ascending branch of the medial circumflex femoral artery. This flap utilises tissue from the posterior upper thigh/lower buttock and provides another choice for women with insufficient lower abdominal fat for breast reconstruction.

*AUTOLOGOUS FAT GRAFT*. Autologous fat grafts have as main objective: (1) total breast reconstruction that need several surgical session of adipose tissue grafts and (2) secondary refinements of the shape of reconstructed breasts.

Today it is considered an essential tool for additional breast shaping because of its relative ease of use, low morbidity and longevity. There are, however, few controlled studies of the effectiveness and oncological safety of autologous fat graft and its longer-term aesthetic outcomes, and so it is preferable to follow national guidelines for its use.

### 16.5.6 Outcomes of Reconstructive Surgery

Aiming at symmetry. Once reconstruction of the affected breast has begun, the challenge of creating symmetry with the contralateral breast is undertaken. Contralateral breast surgery can be performed at the time of the initial reconstruction or during the second stage. Mastopexy, reduction, augmentation or a combination of procedures can be used both for aesthetic improvement and improved symmetry. As an example, in a woman with very large breasts who undergoes a mastectomy with reconstruction, a contralateral reduction will decrease the size discrepancy, resulting in improved patient comfort and increased symmetry.

*Reconstruction of the nipple-areola complex.* The final component of breast reconstruction is the creation of the nipple and areola. This is typically performed during the second stage of breast reconstruction but can also be performed in an outpatient setting. The goal of nipple and areolar reconstruction is to achieve symmetry of position of the nipple-areolar complex in the contralateral breast with comparable appearance and colour.

There are multiple techniques of local tissue rearrangement for creation of a new nipple. Some are based on skin grafts, while others utilise donor sites that are closed primarily. Nipple projection varies among the different techniques, but adequate results can be achieved with most. Symmetry of position on the breast mound is the most important goal of nipple reconstruction, as even small discrepancies are obvious. Once the projecting papilla has been created, the appearance of the entire nipple-areola complex can be enhanced by the use of tattooing.

*Surgical results.* The final cosmetic result of the reconstructed breast following mastectomy should give women complete satisfaction in at least 75 % of cases.

Complications following reconstructive surgery appear higher than with standard BCS, and up to 6 % of patients experience delays in receiving adjuvant treatment due to these complications. In some case immediate or delayed surgery may be required for complications of the reconstruction or for oncological reasons. Minor complications as infection, persistent pain and limited skin necrosis should be expected in less than 10 % of cases. Asymmetry of the breast with modification in shape and consistency should occur in less than 20 % of cases.

*Safety of implants.* After some controversies in the past, the Food and Drug Administration (FDA) confirmed there was no convincing evidence linking silicone implants with connective tissue disease and recommended that all women with silicone implants undergo regular MRI screening throughout their lifetimes to assess for leakage (silent rupture), starting 3 years after the first implant surgery and every 2 years thereafter. However, there is little evidence to support a recommendation for regular MRI screening, which is expensive and may lead to anxiety and false-positive results, resulting in unnecessary surgery. Therefore, most experts agree that breast MRI should be used as a confirmatory diagnostic test and not be used to screen asymptomatic women for implant rupture.

*Capsular contracture*. A rather common complication of reconstructive implants is capsular contracture, in which a scar forms around the implant and contracts, resulting in pain and loss of breast contour. Capsular contracture is a consequence of the immune system defending the patient's bodily integrity and health. It may reoccur even after the requisite corrective surgery for the initial incidence. The degree of incidence of postimplant capsular contracture is classified using the four-grade *Baker's classification*:

- *Grade I* – the breast is normally soft and appears natural in size and shape.
- *Grade II* – the breast is a little firm but appears normal.
- *Grade III* – the breast is firm and appears abnormal.
- *Grade IV* – the breast is hard and painful to the touch and appears abnormal.

Incidence of capsular contracture may be lessened by the use of implants with a textured shell rather than a smooth shell or by the use of polyurethane-coated implants, by placement of the implant in a full covering submuscular placement and by avoiding the use of this technique in women who need RT. Grades I and II should be obtained in less than 10 % of cases.

*Risk of lymphoma*. There are a few reports of a very rare *anaplastic large cell lymphoma* arising in the breast, in the scar capsule adjacent to a silicone or saline-filled breast implant. Thus, the overall risk of breast lymphoma among women who have breast implants is extremely low, and a causal relationship is far from proven [30]. The usual clinical presentation is of a periprosthetic mass or fluid collection. Whether there is any link between the reports of autoimmune disease or chronic immune stimulation and the discovery of ALCL in some of these patients is unclear.

*Physical functioning after autogenous flaps*. The variability in the degree of muscle that is sacrificed, denervated or injured in creating abdominal wall flaps for breast reconstruction makes the comparison of abdominal wall function after abdominal flaps challenging. Several studies have evaluated abdominal function using basic physical functioning tests such as getting out of bed and the ability to perform sit-ups, although more sensitive testing of muscle function, such as isokinetic dynamometry, which measure the maximum strength a muscle can reach, may be necessary for accurate comparison.

Physical functioning following free pedicled flap reconstructive surgery depends on whether the reconstruction was unilateral or bilateral, whether the motor innervation to the *rectus abdominis* muscles was sacrificed or preserved and the degree of postoperative fibrosis occurring within the remaining muscle. In general, for most women who require unilateral reconstruction, breast reconstruction with a perforator pedicle TRAM flap will not have a significant impact on the activities of daily living. However, for women who need bilateral reconstruction, perforator or muscle-sparing flaps may confer an advantage in physical function.

*Patient satisfaction* – As a key measure of quality of care and outcomes, patient satisfaction is being used as a basis for policy formulation and quality improvement programmes and to direct the patient-clinician decision-making process. Moreover patient satisfaction surveys provide consumer feedback about the structure, process and outcomes of care.

In general, breast reconstruction is associated with high levels of patient satisfaction, but the type of reconstructive procedure appears to affect postoperative patient satisfaction with regard to aesthetic result (softness, symmetry) and general satisfaction with the process and outcome of care. At 1 year following surgery, women with pedicled TRAM flaps, free TRAM flaps and expander/implants had similar levels of general satisfaction. Autogenous tissue reconstructions were associated with greater aesthetic satisfaction than expander/implant techniques. At 2 years, these procedural differences had diminished, but patients continued to be more aesthetically satisfied with autogenous tissue compared to expander/implant reconstructions.

## References

1. Rutgers EJTH. Quality control in the locoregional treatment of breast cancer. (EUSOMA Group). Eur J Cancer. 2001;37:447–53.
2. Association of Breast Surgery at BASO. Surgical guidelines for the management of breast cancer, 2009. Eur J Surg Oncol. 2009;35 Suppl 1:1–22.
3. Fortin A, Larochelle M, et al. Local failure is responsible for the decrease in survival for patients with breast cancer treated with conservative surgery and postoperative radiotherapy. J Clin Oncol. 1999;17:101–9.
4. Kapoor NS, Eaton A, King TA, et al. Should breast density influence patient selection for breast conserving surgery? Ann Surg Oncol. 2013;20:600–6.
5. Barentsz MW, Postma EL, van Dalen T, et al. Prediction of positive resection margins in patients with non-palpable breast cancer. Eur J Surg Oncol. 2015;41:106–12.
6. Coopey S, Smith BL, Hanson S, et al. The safety of multiple re-excisions after lumpectomy for breast cancer. Ann Surg Oncol. 2011;18:3797–801.
7. Roughton MC, Shenaq D, Jaskowiak N, et al. Optimizing delivery of breast conservation therapy: a multidisciplinary approach to oncoplastic surgery. Ann Plast Surg. 2012;69:250–5.
8. Al-Ghazal SK, Fallowfield L, Blarney RW. Comparison of psychological aspects and patient satisfaction following breast conserving surgery, simple mastectomy and breast reconstruction. Eur J Cancer. 2000;36:1938–43.
9. Rainsbury RM, Clough KB, Kaufman GJ, Nos C, Dixon JM. Oncoplastic procedures to allow breast conservation and a satisfactory cosmetic outcome. In: Dixon JM, editor. Breast surgery. London: Elsevier; 2014.
10. Veronesi U, Luini A, Galimberti V, Zurrida S. Conservation approaches for the management of stage I/II carcinoma of the breast: Milan Cancer Institute trials. World J Surg. 1994;18:70–5.
11. Harris JR, Levene MB, Svensson G, Hellman S. Analysis of cosmetic results following primary radiation therapy for stages I and II carcinoma of the breast. Int J Radiat Oncol Biol Phys. 1979;5:257–61.
12. Sabel MS. Non surgical ablation of breast cancer: future options for small breast tumors. Surg Oncol Clin N Am. 2014;23:593–608.
13. Cavallo Marincola B, Pediconi F, Anzidei M, et al. High-intensity focused ultrasound in breast pathology: non-invasive treatment of benign and malignant lesions. Expert Rev Med Devices. 2015;12:191–9.
14. Sanghani M, Balk EM, Cady B. Impact of axillary lymph node dissection on breast cancer outcome in clinically node negative patients: a systematic review and meta-analysis. Cancer. 2009;115:1613–20.

15. Chagpar AB. The axilla: current management including sentinel node and lymph edema. In: Dixon JM, editor. Breast surgery. London: Elsevier; 2014.
16. Land SR, Kopec JA, Julian TB, et al. Patient-reported outcomes in sentinel node-negative adjuvant breast cancer patients receiving sentinel-node biopsy or axillary dissection: National Surgical Adjuvant Breast and Bowel Project phase III protocol B-32. J Clin Oncol. 2010;28:3929–36.
17. Berg WA, Zhang Z, Lehrer D, et al. Detection of breast cancer with addition of annual screening ultrasound or a single screening MRI to mammography in women with elevated breast cancer risk. JAMA. 2012;307(13):1394–404.
18. Carlson GW, Wood WC. Management of axillary lymph node metastasis in breast cancer: making progress. JAMA. 2011;305:606–7.
19. Chagpar AB, McMasters KM, Edwards MJ. North American Fareston Tamoxifen Adjuvant Trial. Can sentinel node biopsy be avoided in some elderly breast cancer patients? Ann Surg. 2009;249:455–60.
20. Rodier JF, Velten M, Wilt M, et al. Prospective multicentric randomized study comparing periareolar and peritumoral injection of radiotracer and blue dye for the detection of sentinel lymph node in breast sparing procedures: FRANSENODE trial. J Clin Oncol. 2007;25:3664–9.
21. Cochrane RA, Valasiadou P, Wilson AR, et al. Cosmesis and satisfaction after breast-conserving surgery correlates with the percentage of breast volume excised. Br J Surg. 2003;90:1505–9.
22. Clough KB, Kroll SS, Audretsch W. An approach to the repair of partial mastectomy defects. Plast Reconstr Surg. 1999;104:409–20.
23. Clough KB, Kaufman GJ, Nos C, Buccimazza I, Sarfati IM. Improving breast cancer surgery: a classification and quadrant per quadrant atlas of oncoplastic surgery. Ann Surg Oncol. 2010;17:1375–91.
24. Gainer SM, Lucci A. Oncoplastics: techniques for reconstruction of partial breast defects based on tumor location. J Surg Oncol. 2011;103:341–7.
25. Cho BC, McCready DR. Oncologic principles in breast reconstruction. Clin Plast Surg. 2007;34:1–13.
26. Metcalfe KA, Semple J, Quan ML, et al. Changes in psychosocial functioning 1 year after mastectomy alone, delayed breast reconstruction, or immediate breast reconstruction. Ann Surg Oncol. 2012;19:233–41.
27. Colwell AS, Damjanovic B, Zahedi B, et al. Retrospective review of 331 consecutive immediate single-stage implant reconstructions with acellular dermal matrix: indications, complications, trends, and costs. Plast Reconstr Surg. 2011;128:1170–8.
28. Eriksson M, Anveden L, Celebioglu F, et al. Radiotherapy in implant-based immediate breast reconstruction: risk factors, surgical outcomes, and patient-reported outcome measures in a large Swedish multicenter cohort. Breast Cancer Res Treat. 2013;142:591–601.
29. Gart MS, Smetona JT, Hanwright PJ, et al. Autologous options for postmastectomy breast reconstruction: a comparison of outcomes based on the American College of Surgeons National Surgical Quality Improvement Program. J Am Coll Surg. 2013;216:229–38.
30. Kim B, Roth C, Chung KC, et al. Anaplastic large cell lymphoma and breast implants: a systematic review. Plast Reconstr Surg. 2011;127:2141–50.

## Further Reading

Agostinho JL, Zhao X, Sun W, et al. Prediction of positive margins following breast conserving surgery. Breast. 2015;24:46–50.

Association of Breast Surgery. Oncoplastic breast surgery – a guide to good practice. www.associationofbreastsurgery.org.uk/media/4525/oncoplastic_breast_surgery_-_a_guide_to_good_practice.pdf. Accessed 30 Jan 2015.

Atalay C. New concepts in axillary management of breast cancer. World J Clin Oncol. 2014;5:895–900.

Bundred NJ, Barnes NL, Rutgers E, Donker M. Is axillary lymph node clearance required in node-positive breast cancer? Nat Rev Clin Oncol. 2015;12:55–61.

Edge SB. Advances in breast surgery, 2002-2012. J Natl Compr Canc Netw. 2013;11:53–9.

Fernandez-Delgado J, Lopez-Pedraza MJ, Blasco JA, et al. Satisfaction with and psychological impact of immediate and deferred breast reconstruction. Ann Oncol. 2008;19:1430–4.

Galimberti V, Cole BF, Zurrida S, et al. Axillary dissection versus no axillary dissection in patients with sentinel-node micrometastases (IBCSG 23-01): a phase 3 randomised controlled trial. Lancet Oncol. 2013;14:297–305.

Giuliano AE, Hunt KK, Ballman KV, et al. Axillary dissection vs no axillary dissection in women with invasive breast cancer and sentinel node metastasis. JAMA. 2011;305:569–75.

Laronga C, Smith P. Nipple-sparing mastectomy. Surg Oncol Clin N Am. 2014;23:549–66.

Lyman GH, Temin S, Edge SB, et al. Sentinel lymph node biopsy for patients with early-stage breast cancer: American Society of Clinical Oncology clinical practice guideline update. J Clin Oncol. 2014;32:1365–83.

Murthy V, Chamberlain RS. Defining a place for nipple sparing mastectomy in modern breast care: an evidence based review. Breast J. 2013;19:571–81.

Valachis A, Nearchou AD, Lind P. Surgical management of breast cancer in BRCA-mutation carriers: a systematic review and meta-analysis. Breast Cancer Res Treat. 2014;144:443–55.

**Websites in Appendix**: *Surgery*, A-4.21; *Breast Forms/Implants*, A-4.4.

# The Role of Adjuvant Radiation Therapy in BC

# 17

Alfonso M. Pluchinotta, Maria Cristina Leonardi, and Ornella Lora

## Contents



**Abstract**

• Postoperative RT is strongly recommended after breast-conserving surgery (BCS). Boost irradiation gives a further risk reduction and is usually indicated for most of the patients regardless of risk factors. • Shorter fractionation schemes have been validated in large prospective studies. Currently, the ideal candidates are considered being at least 50 years old with unicentric, unifocal, node-negative, small non-lobular BC, without extensive intraductal component or lymphovascular invasion • Postmastectomy RT is recommended for patients at a high risk of local recurrence, including those with four or more positive axillary lymph nodes or involved resection margins. • Postmastectomy RT should be also considered for patients at an intermediate risk of local recurrence, including

A.M. Pluchinotta (✉)
Breast Surgery, Policlinic of Abano Terme, Padova, Italy
e-mail: pluchinotta.alfonso@gmail.com

M.C. Leonardi
Division of Radiotherapy, European Institute of Oncology (IEO), Milano, Italy

O. Lora
Division of Radiotherapy, Istituto Oncologico Veneto (IOV), Padova, Italy



A.M. Pluchinotta (ed.), *The Outpatient Breast Clinic: Aiming at Best Practice*,
DOI 10.1007/978-3-319-15907-2_17

those with one to three lymph nodes involved, lymphovascular invasion, grade 3 and ER-negative tumours.

*Future directions*. Given its greater convenience and perceived better associated quality of life, accelerated partial-breast radiation (APBI) is becoming an increasingly popular alternative to conventional whole-breast irradiation (WBI) among women with early-stage breast cancer. Published data on APBI are still limited, while prospectively collected phase II trials have shown high rates of local control in appropriately selected patients.

## 17.1 Indications of Adjuvant Radiation Therapy

**Clinical Practice Points**

- Postoperative RT is strongly recommended after BCS. Boost irradiation gives a further 50 % risk reduction and is indicated for patients with unfavourable risk factors for local control.
- Postmastectomy RT is recommended for patients with four or more positive axillary nodes and/or with T3-T4 tumours and should be considered for patients with one to three positive axillary lymph nodes, especially in the presence of additional risk factors.
- Partial-breast irradiation may be considered an acceptable treatment option in patients older than 50 years with unicentric, unifocal, node-negative, non-lobular BC up to 3 cm in size with negative margins of at least 1 mm.
- Shorter fractionation schemes have been validated in large prospective studies and are generally recommended in selected groups of patients.

The objective of adjuvant radiation therapy (RT) is to eradicate any tumour deposits following surgery for patients treated by either breast-conserving surgery (BCS) or mastectomy. The indications for adjuvant breast radiation therapy (RT) are broad and listed in Table 17.1

### 17.1.1 Patients Treated with Breast-Conserving Surgery

Most patients treated with BCS are candidates for breast RT. Efforts to identify groups for whom radiation is not indicated because their prognosis is highly favourable or for whom RT is not effective have not been successful. One exception to this includes older women (≥70 years) with node-negative, stage I BC who are treated with endocrine therapy. For these women, the risk of an in-breast recurrence is quite low for them to derive much of a benefit from RT.

For almost all women treated with BCS external beam, whole-breast radiation therapy (WBRT) is indicated. Especially for women deemed to be at a relatively

**Table. 17.1** More common indications for radiation therapy after breast surgery

| Indications | Notes |
|---|---|
| After breast-conserving surgery | Should be performed in almost all subsets |
| | No subsets are identified which can safely avoid RT |
| | Benefit is minimal in older women with T1 N0 RE+ BC |
| After mastectomy for large or deep tumours | All T4 |
| | All T3 if resection margins are positive or with more risk factors |
| | All T with tumour involvement at deep margin (fascia or muscle) |
| After mastectomy in the presence of lymph nodes involvement | Recommended in patients with four or more positive axillary lymph nodes at a high risk of local recurrence |
| | Considered for patients with one to three lymph nodes involved at an intermediate risk of local recurrence |
| After mastectomy in the presence of DCIS | Patients with DCIS identified at the surgically excised margins on final pathologic analysis as the sole indication for postmastectomy RT |
| After mastectomy following neoadjuvant chemotherapy | The role of RT has not been conclusively demonstrated but is suggested in any pre-chemotherapy stage III and in the presence of residual disease in the breast or in the nodes |
| After mastectomy triple-negative BC, also in the absence of nodal involvement | The role of RT has not been conclusively demonstrated, but its benefits are suggested from the presence of more negative prognostic factors |

higher risk of local recurrence, a radiation therapy (RT) boost is added to the tumour bed to further reduce the risk of an in-breast tumour recurrence [1].

*Whole-breast radiation therapy* (*WBRT*). The benefit of WBRT is supported by large meta-analysis studies, which result that WBRT gives:

- A significant reduction in the 10-year risk of recurrence by nearly half of BCS patients, if compared with BCS alone
- A significant reduction in the 15-year risk of BC death

These data suggest that about one death from BC is avoided for every four recurrences avoided. Moreover, the benefits of RT were seen in women regardless of whether or not there was evidence of pathologically involved regional nodes [2].

In addition to the survival advantages seen with RT, meta-analysis also reported that first recurrence patterns differ depending on whether or not RT is administered. For women treated with surgery alone, the majority of first recurrences were locoregional and not distant (25 versus 10 %). In contrast, for women treated with adjuvant RT after surgery, the first recurrence is more commonly distant because the disease is well controlled locally.

Conventionally dosed WBRT is delivered to the entire field (including the whole breast and regional nodes as indicated) in 1.8–2 Gy daily fractions over 4–5 weeks to a total dose of 45–50 Gy.

A shorter fractionation scheme, which reduces the duration of treatment, may be reasonable for properly selected patients. In general, a shorter fractionation scheme delivers 39–41.6 Gy in approximately 3 weeks with or without a boost. In 2011 the ASTRO panellists [3] stated that whole-breast hypofractionated radiotherapy is appropriated for selected women, such as those:

- Aged 50 years or older
- With pT1-2 N0 BC
- With oestrogen-receptor (ER)-positive disease treated primarily with adjuvant hormonal therapy

Compared with conventional regimen, shorter fractionation resulted in:

- No difference in the risk of an ipsilateral local recurrence at 10 years – no significant difference in overall survival
- A significant decrease in acute and/or late radiation toxicity

Other studies confirm shorter fractionation schedules are safe and effective, and there is no difference in the loco-regional relapse rate (considering distant relapses as well as disease-free survival and overall survival) with shorter fractionation scheme 39–41.6 Gy. At 10 years, treatment to 39 Gy resulted in a significantly less rate of breast induration compared with treatment at 41.6 or 50 Gy, while it resulted in a lower incidence of telangiectasia and breast oedema [4].

The data from these two trials were compiled in a meta-analysis which showed there was no significant difference between the shorter fractionation and conventionally dosed RT schedules, and this was irrespective of age, type of primary surgery, axillary node status, tumour grade, administration of adjuvant chemotherapy or the use of a tumour-bed boost RT. Despite these results, several caveats apply:

- Additional studies are needed to more fully evaluate both efficacy and toxicity in particular subgroups, particularly in women with large breasts and/or more advanced tumours as those larger than 5 cm or with positive lymph nodes.
- There are insufficient data to evaluate the tolerability of shorter fractionation with other therapies (e.g. chemotherapy or monoclonal antibodies) [5].

*Radiation therapy boost to the tumour bed.* While RT to the tumour bed following BCS and WBRT is recommended in younger women, its routine use in older women is less clear. RT boost following WBRT is strongly indicated especially if patients have high-risk factors for recurrence as age <50 years old, pathologically involved axillary nodes, lymphovascular invasion and/or close or positive resection margins [6].

Whether to include a tumour-bed boost for patients who undergo shorter fractionation WBRT is controversial and is left to the discretion of the treating physician.

If an RT boost is administered, 10–16 Gy in either 2 Gy or 2.5 Gy fractions is usually administered. Two trials that evaluated the impact of an RT boost suggest that it results in a lower rate of recurrences and, as a result, a lower rate of subsequent mastectomies; however, there is no appreciable benefit in overall survival. Other data support the role of an RT boost and underscore the importance of discussing the role of an additional dose with younger women treated with WBRT, especially if they are deemed to be at high risk of a local recurrence.

*Accelerated partial-breast irradiation (APBI).* Accelerated partial-breast irradiation refers to the use of limited, focused RT as an alternative to conventional WBRT for women with early BC following BCS. Compared with WBRT, APBI delivers a higher dose of RT per day to a limited volume of tissue over a shorter period of time. Although APBI is a promising alternative to WBRT, there are still limited data to support the role of APBI as an alternative to conventional WBRT. Several sets of published guidelines are mainly focused on which patients should be considered reasonable candidates for treatment with APBI [7, 8]. Partial-breast irradiation may be considered an acceptable treatment option in patients older than 50 years with unicentric, unifocal, node-negative BC up to 3 cm in size and with negative margins of at least 1 mm. Lobular-type BC and the presence of an extensive intraductal component or lymphovascular invasion are still on debate.

Different techniques of APBI are external beam radiation therapy, conformal external beam radiotherapy, intensity-modulated radiotherapy, brachytherapy and intraoperative radiation therapy. The last two techniques are areas of particular attention [9].

*Brachytherapy***.** Brachytherapy for BC involves the temporary placement of radioactive material into body tissues for local radiation treatment. Brachytherapy can be delivered with interstitial or intracavitary delivery systems (Fig. 17.1).

For *interstitial brachytherapy* (Fig. 17.1a), several small hollow catheters are placed into the breast surrounding the lumpectomy site. Potential disadvantages of this approach include the risk of infection and poor cosmesis with scarring due to the multiple catheters, although these have been seen in older studies.

For *intracavitary brachytherapy* (Fig. 17.1b), a radiation delivery device is placed into the partial mastectomy site. Single-lumen and multi-lumen balloon catheter and non-balloon devices have all been used successfully. The presumed advantage of the multi-lumen devices as compared with single-lumen catheters is more precise dosimetric planning and safer treatment delivery, avoiding skin and other organ damage. The device can be placed at the time of lumpectomy (*open* technique) or several days later under ultrasound guidance (*closed* technique). The closed technique is preferable because, if the device is placed during surgery, final pathology results may require the device to be removed due to involved margins or positive lymph nodes.

*Intraoperative radiation therapy (IORT)***.** Ongoing research is aimed at exploring other modalities of RT that will minimize toxicity without reducing effectiveness. An example of this is intraoperative radiation therapy (IORT), which condenses the entire therapeutic dose into a single fraction, permitting surgery and radiation to be completed in 1 day. At this time, however, IORT should not be administered out of a clinical trial because the available data suggest that IORT is associated with a higher risk of in-breast tumour recurrences (IBTR). For patients in whom the duration of therapy required for standard WBRT is a concern, shorter fractionation schedules are a viable option.

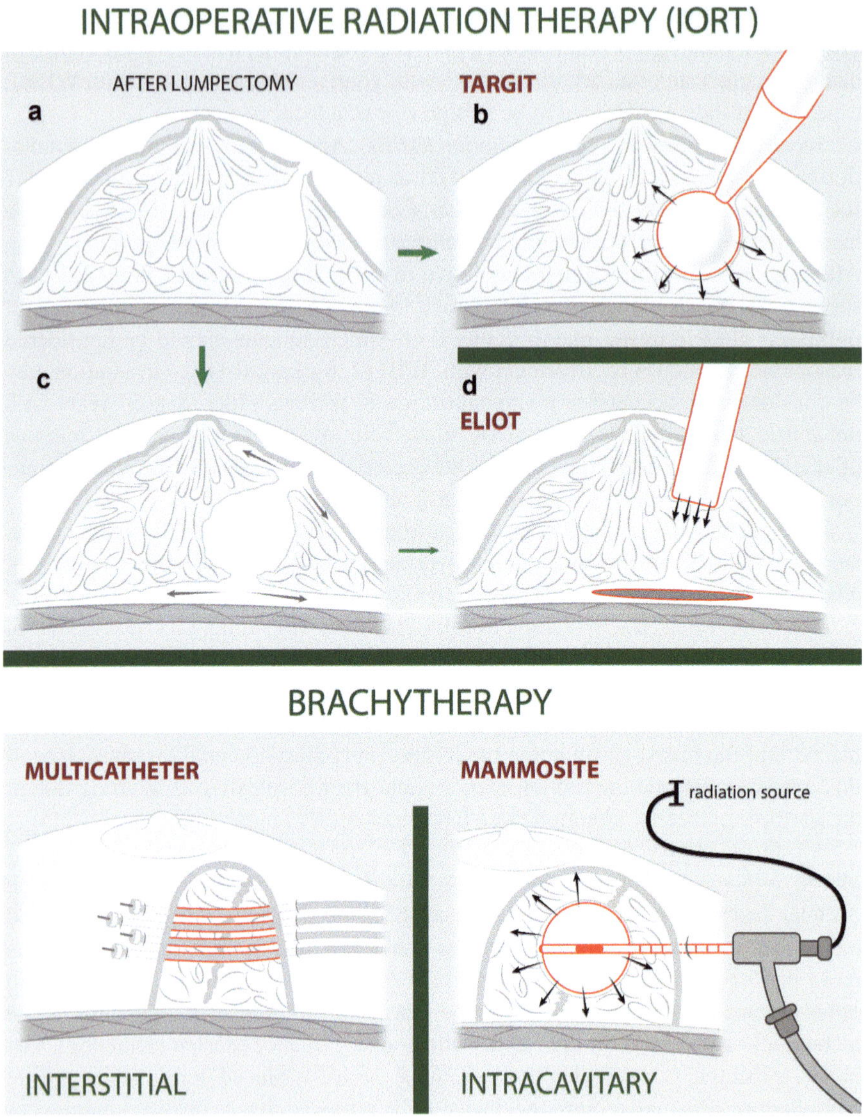


**Fig. 17.1** Thumbnails of different types of accelerated partial-breast irradiation (APBI). On the top, intraoperative radiation therapy (*IORT*) following lumpectomy (**a**): with low-energy photons (50 kV) from a miniaturized x-ray generator (INTRABEAM) (**b**), with electrons from a dedicated linear accelerator after a dual-plane glandular undermining (**c**) on closely spaced margins (**d**), with a lead shield placed on the pectoralis fascia to protect the lung. On the bottom, brachytherapy, interstitial via multicatheter (**e**) or intracavitary, as with MammoSite balloon (**f**)

Several devices have been used for intraoperative radiation. A portable radiation-generating device is placed into the lumpectomy cavity (Fig. 17.1c) just after specimen resection, and purse-string sutures are placed within the breast to ensure that the breast tissue is in contact with the applicator surface. Treatment is then delivered with low-energy x-rays, for a dose of approximately 20 Gy at the applicator surface and 5 Gy at a depth of 1 cm over 20–45 min, depending upon the size of the cavity and the device.

With another technique (ELIOT, Fig. 17.1d), dedicated mobile linear accelerator is used to deliver electrons at a dose of 21 Gy in one fraction intraoperatively, with a lead shield placed on the *pectoralis fascia* to protect the lung.

The results of the trials suggest that IORT may be associated with an unacceptably increased risk of IBTR compared with WBRT in women with high-risk BC as grade 3, ER negative or triple negative [10]. Although the absolute magnitude of any differences between these randomized groups appears to be small, more extensive follow-up (at 10–15 years) is required to evaluate whether these differences become clinically relevant. Until then, IORT may be indicated in patients with early BC enrolled in clinical trials.

### 17.1.2 Patients Treated with Mastectomy

For women treated with mastectomy, a postmastectomy radiation therapy (PMRT) to the chest wall and supraclavicular/apex of axilla region (SNC-RT) is appropriate in patients at high risk of recurrence based on the presence of unfavourable tumour features such as large tumour size (T3 or greater), positive axillary nodes, grade 3, lymphovascular invasion, young age and positive deep margins at final pathologic analysis [11].

While for patients with >3 positive axillary nodes, SCN-RT as part of regional node irradiation is mandatory on the basis of recent data, it should also be strongly considered in the case of those with 1–3 nodes. In fact, the recent EBCTCG meta-analysis pointed out that patients with 1–3 involved lymph nodes showed the same survival benefit from PMRT as patients with >3 involved lymph nodes. The update showed that in women with axillary dissection and any positive nodes, radiotherapy reduced loco-regional recurrence, overall recurrence and BC mortality, even in the presence of systemic therapy [12].

For patients with one to three positive nodes, the unirradiated women had an absolute 10-year risk of overall recurrence of 45.7 %, which was reduced to 34.2 % by radiotherapy, so their absolute gain was 11.5 %. For this subgroup, the 20-year risk of BC mortality was reduced by radiotherapy from 50.2 to 42.3 %, achieving an absolute gain from radiotherapy of 7.9 %.

In women with four or more positive nodes, the absolute 10-year risk of overall recurrence was reduced from 75.1 to 66.3 % by adding radiotherapy, with an absolute gain of 8.8 %. For this subgroup, the 20-year risk of BC mortality was reduced by radiotherapy from 80 to 70.7 %, so the absolute gain was 9.3 %.

Radiotherapy to the internal mammary chain is being revised in light of new evidence from recent randomized trials and meta-analysis. In particular, the decision-making for IMN irradiation in the context of regional node treatment should take into consideration the medial tumour location and axillary positive nodes. Intermediate/long-term follow-up of 10 years did not show any increased cardiovascular disease or severe complications [13].

*Timing of radiation therapy*. There is only low-quality evidence to inform the optimal timing of RT. Therefore, the administration of RT in relation to systemic therapy is based on institutional standards of practice. A reasonable approach takes into account the type of systemic therapy being administered.

For patients who have been recommended to receive adjuvant chemotherapy, RT is usually administered following the completion of chemotherapy. The concomitant treatment could also be considered according to the chemotherapy schedule: some antineoplastic agents have been proven to be safe when combined with radiotherapy [14].

For those patients with ER-positive disease who were recommended to have endocrine therapy, the optimal sequencing of TAM and radiotherapy (RT) after breast-conserving surgery has not been stated in lack of randomized trials, and currently the concomitant or sequential approach is based upon institutional preference [15]. For patients with BCs that overexpress HER2 receptor, RT can be administered concomitantly with adjuvant trastuzumab [16].

## 17.2 Special Issues of Adjuvant Radiotherapy

*Neoadjuvant therapy*. Patients treated with chemotherapy prior to breast surgery should undergo adjuvant RT. Some data suggest that postoperative RT improves local control even for women without nodal involvement who have an in-breast pathologic complete response (pCR) to neoadjuvant chemotherapy [17].

As known, the factors that have been associated with an increased risk for a loco-regional recurrence are mainly:

- Tumour size before neoadjuvant chemotherapy >5 cm
- Clinical node involvement before neoadjuvant chemotherapy
- Presence of residual cancer in the breast or the lymph nodes after neoadjuvant chemotherapy

The response to neoadjuvant therapy can be a useful predictor of the risk for a loco-regional recurrence following neoadjuvant chemotherapy. In the same way, it could potentially be used to identify appropriate patients for adjuvant RT. However, data regarding RT advantages came out from retrospective analyses of prospective trials studying the effect of different chemotherapy regimens, and the use of RT was at the discretion of the treating oncologist. Therefore, higher-quality evidence is needed to be given as strong recommendation for RT [18].

*Triple-negative BC*. Women with triple-negative BC (TNBC) have an aggressive clinical course compared with women with other BC subtypes. This is characterized by early relapse, a higher incidence of visceral and brain metastases and a relatively poor prognosis. Because of these differences, women with TNBC who underwent a mastectomy should meet with a radiation oncologist to discuss the risks and benefits of adjuvant RT.

*Older women with ER-positive BC.* It may be reasonable to avoid RT in selected older women with oestrogen-receptor (ER)-positive BC. Specifically, this includes women aged 70 years or older with clinically node-negative, small (T size <2 cm) BC who are willing to initiate adjuvant endocrine therapy. Patients should understand that the rate of in-breast recurrence may be higher over time and that there are some data to show that the risk of subsequently requiring a mastectomy is higher in women who are not treated with adjuvant RT. Therefore, such patients should be referred to a radiation oncologist to discuss the pros and cons of endocrine therapy alone versus endocrine therapy plus RT. Ultimately, the decision to omit RT should take into account potential comorbidities that could affect long-term survival. Some studies with longer follow-up show that while RT significantly reduces the risk of a loco-regional recurrence, there is no appreciable impact on overall survival in this low-risk elderly population [19]. In regard to the impact of adjuvant RT on the need for a subsequent mastectomy, only inconclusive data are still available.

*Women with a BRCA gene mutation.* Women with a BRCA1 or BRCA2 gene mutation who undergo surgery for BC and are otherwise candidates for RT should proceed with RT if it is clinically indicated. Although preclinical studies suggest that women with BC and a BRCA1 or BRCA2 gene mutation might be sensitive to the toxicity of RT, there is no clinical evidence of an increased toxicity risk in these patients [20].

*Women with a connective tissue autoimmune disorder.* Although there are only low-quality data available, women with BC and active systemic discoid lupus erythematosus or scleroderma appear to be at an increased risk of radiation-related toxicities, especially late toxicities. These concerns should be considered when deciding whether to deliver RT for these patients. The severity of collagen vascular disease should be taken into account to help determine the relative benefits and risks of RT to treat their BC [21].

In addition, intraoperative RT (IORT) may be an effective and safer method to deliver RT. However, it remains investigational at present.

## 17.3 Side Effects of Radiation Therapy

External beam radiation therapy is a non-invasive treatment with some short-term and some longer-term side effects. Patients undergoing a few weeks of treatment usually experience fatigue caused by the healthy tissue repairing itself, and aside from this, there can be no side effects at all. However, many BC patients develop a suntan-like change in skin colour in the exact area being treated. As with a suntan, this darkening of the skin usually returns to normal in 1–2 months after treatment. In some cases, permanent changes in the colour and texture of the skin are experienced. Other side effects sometimes experienced with radiation can include muscle stiffness, mild swelling, tenderness in the area and lymphoedema.

After surgery, radiation and other treatments have been completed, many patients notice the affected breast seems smaller or seems to have shrunk. The use of adjuvant radiation has potentially negative effects if the patient has to later undergo breast reconstruction surgery. Fibrosis of chest wall skin from radiation negatively affects skin elasticity and makes tissue expansion techniques difficult. Traditionally, most patients are advised to defer immediate breast reconstruction when adjuvant radiation is planned and are most often recommended surgery involving autologous tissue reconstruction rather than breast implants. Clinically significant lung changes and heart problems are rare, thanks to the improvement of radiotherapy treatment planning [22].

## References


1. Jones HA, Antonini N, Hart AA, et al. Impact of pathological characteristics on local relapse after breast-conserving therapy: a subgroup analysis of the EORTC boost versus no boost trial. J Clin Oncol. 2009;27:4939–47.
2. Darby S, McGale P, Correa C, et al. on behalf of the Early Breast Cancer Trialists' Collaborative Group (EBCTCG). Effect of radiotherapy after breast-conserving surgery on 10-year recurrence and 15-year breast cancer death: meta-analysis of individual patient data for 10,801 women in 17 randomised trials. Lancet. 2011;378:1707–16.
3. Smith BD, Bentzen SM, Correa CR, et al. Fractionation for whole breast irradiation: an American Society for Radiation Oncology (ASTRO) evidence-based guideline. Int J Radiat Oncol Biol Phys. 2011;81:59–68.
4. Eblan MJ, Vanderwalde NA, Zeman EM, Jones E. Hypofractionation for breast cancer: lessons learned from our neighbors to the north and across the pond. Oncology. 2014;28:536–46.
5. James ML, Lehman M, Hider PN, Jeffery M, Francis DP, Hickey BE. Fraction size in radiation treatment for breast conservation in early breast cancer. Cochrane Database Syst Rev. 2008;(3):CD003860.
6. Bartelink H, Maingon P, Poortmans P, et al. on behalf of the European Organisation for Research and Treatment of Cancer Radiation Oncology and Breast Cancer Groups. Whole-breast irradiation with or without a boost for patients treated with breast-conserving surgery for early breast cancer: 20-year follow-up of a randomised phase 3 trial. Lancet Oncol. 2014; S1470-2045(14):71156–8.
7. Smith BD, Arthur DW, Buchholz TA, et al. Accelerated partial breast irradiation consensus statement from the American Society for Radiation Oncology (ASTRO). Int J Radiat Oncol Biol Phys. 2009;15(74):987–1001.
8. Polgár C, Van Limbergen E, Pötter R, et al. on behalf of the GEC-ESTRO breast cancer working group. Patient selection for accelerated partial-breast irradiation (APBI) after breast-conserving surgery: recommendations of the Groupe Euroṕeen de Curiethérapie-European Society for Therapeutic Radiology and Oncology (GEC-ESTRO) breast cancer working group based on clinical evidence (2009). Radiother Oncol. 2010;94:264–73.
9. Cox JA, Swanson TA. Current modalities of accelerated partial breast irradiation. Nat Rev Clin Oncol. 2013;10:344–56.
10. Veronesi U, Orecchia R, Maisonneuve P, et al. Intraoperative radiotherapy versus external radiotherapy for early breast cancer (ELIOT): a randomised controlled equivalence trial. Lancet Oncol. 2013;14:1269–77.
11. Rowell NP. Radiotherapy to the chest wall following mastectomy for node-negative breast cancer: a systematic review. Radiother Oncol. 2009;91:23–32.
12. McGale P, Taylor C, Correa C, et al. on behalf of the Early Breast Cancer Trialists' Collaborative Group (EBCTCG). Effect of radiotherapy after mastectomy and axillary surgery on 10-year

recurrence and 20-year breast cancer mortality: meta-analysis of individual patient data for 8135 women in 22 randomised trials. Lancet. 2014;383:2127–35.
13. Budach W, Kammers K, Boelke E, Matuschek C. Adjuvant radiotherapy of regional lymph nodes in breast cancer – a meta-analysis of randomized trials. Radiat Oncol. 2013;8:267.
14. Arcangeli G, Pinnarò P, Rambone R, Giannarelli D, Benassi M. A phase III randomized study on the sequencing of radiotherapy and chemotherapy in the conservative management of early-stage breast cancer. Int J Radiat Oncol Biol Phys. 2006;64:161–7.
15. Pierce LJ, Hutchins LF, Green SR, et al. Sequencing of tamoxifen and radiotherapy after breast-conserving surgery in early-stage breast cancer. J Clin Oncol. 2005;23:24–9.
16. Shaffer R, Tyldesley S, Rolles M, Chia S, Mohamed I. Acute cardiotoxicity with concurrent trastuzumab and radiotherapy including internal mammary chain nodes: a retrospective single-institution study. Radiother Oncol. 2009;90(1):122–6.
17. Buchholz TA, Lehman CD, Harris JR, et al. Statement of the science concerning locoregional treatments after preoperative chemotherapy for breast cancer: a National Cancer Institute conference. J Clin Oncol. 2008;26(5):791–7.
18. Mamounas EP, Anderson SJ, Dignam JJ, et al. Predictors of locoregional recurrence after neoadjuvant chemotherapy: results from combined analysis of National Surgical Adjuvant Breast and Bowel Project B-18 and B-27. J Clin Oncol. 2012;30:3960–6.
19. Hughes KS, Schnaper LA, Bellon JR, et al. Lumpectomy plus tamoxifen with or without irradiation in women age 70 years or older with early breast cancer: long-term follow-up of CALGB 9343. J Clin Oncol. 2013;31:2382–7.
20. Haffty BG, Lannin D. Is breast-conserving therapy in the genetically predisposed breast cancer patient a reasonable and appropriate option? Eur J Cancer. 2004;40:1105–8.
21. Lin A, Abu-Isa E, Griffith KA, Ben-Josef E. Toxicity of radiotherapy in patients with collagen vascular disease. Cancer. 2008;113:648–53.
22. Darby SC, McGale P, Taylor CW, Peto R. Long-term mortality from heart disease and lung cancer after radiotherapy for early breast cancer: prospective cohort study of about 300,000 women in US SEER cancer registries. Lancet Oncol. 2005;6:557–65.

## Further Reading

American Society for Radiation Oncology. Guidelines. www.astro.org/Clinical-Practice/Guidelines/Active-Guidelines.aspx. Accessed 30 Jan 2015.

Corradini S, Niemoeller OM, Niyazi M, et al. Timing of radiotherapy following breast-conserving surgery: outcome of 1393 patients at a single institution. Strahlenther Onkol. 2014;190:352–7.

Hickey BE, Francis DP, Lehman M. Sequencing of chemotherapy and radiotherapy for early breast cancer. Cochrane Database Syst Rev. 2013;4:CD005212. doi:10.1002/14651858.CD005212.pub3.

Kurtz J. The curative role of radiotherapy in the treatment of operable breast cancer. Eur J Cancer. 2002;38:1961–74.

Moran MS, Schnitt SJ, Giuliano AE. Society of Surgical Oncology-American Society for Radiation Oncology consensus guideline on margins for breast-conserving surgery with whole-breast irradiation in stages I and II invasive breast cancer. Ann Surg Oncol. 2014;21:704–16.

Mukesh MB, Duke S, Parashar D, Wishart G, Coles CE, Wilson C. The Cambridge post-mastectomy radiotherapy (C-PMRT) index: a practical tool for patient selection. Radiother Oncol. 2014;110:461–6.

Sheitelman SF, Kim LH. Accelerated partial-breast irradiation: the current state of our knowledge. Oncology. 2013;27:329–42.

Vaidya JS, Frederik Wenz F, Bulsara M, et al. Risk-adapted targeted intraoperative radiotherapy versus whole-breast radiotherapy for breast cancer: 5-year results for local control and overall survival from the TARGIT-A randomised trial. Lancet. 2014;383:603–13.

**Websites in Appendix**: *Adjuvant Radiotherapy*, A-4.2.

# The Role of Adjuvant Systemic Therapy 18

Alfonso M. Pluchinotta, Cristina Ghiotto, and Zora Baretta

## Contents



A.M. Pluchinotta (✉)
Breast Surgery, Policlinic of Abano Terme, Padova, Italy
e-mail: pluchinotta.alfonso@gmail.com

C. Ghiotto • Z. Baretta
Division of Oncology, Istituto Oncologico Veneto (IOV), Padova, Italy
e-mail: cristina.ghiotto@ioveneto.it; zora.baretta@gmail.com



A.M. Pluchinotta (ed.), *The Outpatient Breast Clinic: Aiming at Best Practice*,
DOI 10.1007/978-3-319-15907-2_18

**Abstract**

• Theoretically if the tumour has not yet disseminated metastases to tissues that are biologically vital, it is curable with local therapy only. • Approximately half of women with operable breast BC who do not receive any systemic therapy will die from metastatic disease. • Randomised trials have shown that adjuvant treatment (endocrine therapy, chemotherapy or molecular-targeted agents) significantly improves survival. • Adjuvant systemic therapies, including chemotherapy, should be considered for all patients with BC when benefit outweighs risks.

*Future directions*. The response to neoadjuvant chemotherapy in vivo could provide a useful prediction of prognosis and helps define strategies for an individual patient's future treatment with alternative chemotherapy regimens or molecular-targeting agents. Furthermore, the discovery of predictive markers for tumour response to neoadjuvant chemotherapy may also help facilitate individualised chemotherapy, particularly in patients, as those with triple-negative BC, with a poor prognosis.

## 18.1 Overview

**Clinical Practice Points**

- Before deciding whether to use adjuvant systemic therapy, the prognosis without adjuvant therapy should be estimated.
- Several guidelines have been published in order to reach an agreement on the principles of the treatment of BC. Nevertheless, disparities and differences in availability of therapeutic options are still observed across countries.
- A patient's risk for recurrence can be categorised as low, intermediate or high on the basis of extension of the tumour (e.g. tumour size and nodal status) and the cancer phenotype essentially determined by oestrogen receptor (ER), progesterone receptor (PR) status and HER2 expression.
- Additional factors such as histological grade, proliferative index (Ki67) and lymphovascular invasion can also affect the management of BC patients.

### 18.1.1 Introduction

Over the last years, there have been important developments in the management of BC including new types of drugs and multigene test such as Onco*type* DX. The aim of clinical guidelines is to make the treatment of BC equal worldwide. However, a quite big difference in the management of BC patients is seen across the countries because of disparities and differences in availability of therapeutic options. This book is designed to outline the essentials of the breast outpatient practice, and the discussion of the trials and multiple studies inspecting the treatment of BC is far beyond its scope.

First of all, there are single factors that can help select patients who are most likely to benefit from adjuvant therapy. These factors should be categorised as prognostic or predictive. Prognostic and predictive factors are universally utilised in the management of BC and can be used to stratify patients into two groups:

- Those who are expected to derive the most benefit from adjuvant systemic therapy
- Those for whom the risks and costs of adjuvant therapy outweigh the expected benefits

*Prognostic factors* are correlated with the clinical outcome at the time of diagnosis, independently of therapy. Factors, such as tumour size and lymph node status, are important because they can help to determine the absolute benefit of chemotherapy. So that, if an agent can reduce the chance of dying from BC by 25 %, it is important to know how bigger is the chance of dying from BC in each patient. If the chance of dying is only 4 %, then the absolute benefit of the drug is only 1 % (meaning 100 women need to be treated for 1 woman to survive), while if the chance of dying is 40 %, the absolute benefit is 10 % (10 women need to be treated for 1 woman to survive).

*Predictive factors* are associated with the response to therapy. These factors are usually the target of the therapy or related to the pathway where the drug is active.

Some factors are both prognostic and predictive (Table 18.1). For example, HER2 status is a prognostic factor because HER2-positive women have worse outcomes than patients who are HER2 negative, regardless of treatment. Moreover only HER2-positive BC women showed benefit from molecular-targeted agents as trastuzumab (Herceptin®). Same considerations regard ER/PR status.

**Table 18.1** Prognostic and predictive factors in BC

| | |
|---|---|
| Prognostic factors | Patient age |
| | Axillary lymph node status |
| | Histological subtypes (e.g. tubular, mucinous, papillary) |
| | Tumour size |
| | Histological grade |
| | Lymphatic/vascular invasion |
| | HER2 gene amplification and/or overexpression |
| | Oestrogen receptor/progesterone receptor status |
| | Response to neoadjuvant therapy |
| Predictive factors | Oestrogen receptor (RE) and progesterone receptor (PR) status |
| | HER2 gene amplification and/or overexpression |
| Additional factors (potentially prognostic and/or predictive) | Multigene expression profile (e.g. Onco*type* DX) |
| | BRCA1/2 gene mutation |
| | Bone marrow micrometastases |
| | p53 gene analysis |
| | Cathepsin D level |

*Lymph node involvement* is the most important single prognostic factor in BC, as discussed in Sect. 13.2. The vast majority of patients with lymph node metastases are candidates to adjuvant systemic therapy. However, determining which lymph node-negative patients should receive adjuvant therapy is challenging, particularly because the majority are cured by local treatment (surgery +/– radiotherapy). The benefit from adjuvant treatment for patients who are at risk of relapse may be minimal, with significant costs and toxicities. Thus, additional prognostic and predictive factors should be used to decide which lymph node-negative patients may benefit from adjuvant treatment.

*Tumour size* is a well-recognised independent prognostic factor and predictor of axillary node involvement, being a large tumour associated with higher probability of lymph node involvement and worse prognosis.

All cases of invasive BC are evaluated for ER and PR status that, as already underlined, have both predictive and prognostic value. In fact, ER and/or PR positivity is associated with reduced mortality compared to women with ER- and/or PR-negative disease; the presence of hormone receptors is a powerful predictive factor for the likelihood of benefit from adjuvant hormonal therapy. A tumour is defined positive for ER/PR when the percentage of tumour cells stained positively by immunohistochemistry is >1 %.

*HER2 oncogene* is amplified and/or overexpressed in approximately 20 % of BC and is a strong predictor of relapse and worse overall survival, particularly in node-positive patients. Moreover HER2 positivity predicts response to trastuzumab. Amplification and/or overexpression of the HER2 is routinely evaluated, using immunohistochemistry and/or fluorescence in situ hybridisation (FISH), respectively, even if variability across the laboratories involved in this determination remains a major issue with both methodologies (see Sect. 13.2).

*Additional established prognostic factors* include patient's age, tumour grade, and lymphovascular invasion. Certain histological subtypes of BC are generally associated with a favourable prognosis, such as tubular, mucinous and papillary carcinoma. The proliferation rate of the tumour as determined by the mitotic count is also an important prognostic factor, but this information is usually used to determine the tumour grade. The prognostic relevance of proliferative index expressed by Ki67 value is controversial, and its determination is problematic because of absence of standardised method of evaluation and interpretation.

*Oncotype Dx* is a diagnostic test that estimates the *likelihood* of disease recurrence in women with newly diagnosed, early-stage, lymph node-negative, ER-positive BC by analysis of a panel of 21 genes. Moreover, this test helps define whether chemotherapy should or should not be added to hormonal therapy (see Sect. 13.3).

The Onco*type* DX gene panel was validated in a large, independent, multicenter clinical trial of adjuvant tamoxifen treatment (NSABP B-14 study). In this study, patients with low or intermediate risk had a significant benefit from the use of adjuvant tamoxifen, whereas the high-risk group did not. Moreover, in a retrospective subset analysis of the NSABP B-20 study (a randomised trial of adjuvant chemotherapy with CMF-like regimens), patients in the high-risk recurrence score strata significantly benefited from adjuvant chemotherapy, whereas the intermediate- and low-risk groups did not achieve statistical significance.

On*cotype* DX has also been evaluated in a pilot retrospective study in patients with lymph node-positive, ER-positive disease. Similar to observations in lymph node-negative disease, the pilot study indicated little (if any) benefit from anthracycline-based (but not containing a taxane) adjuvant chemotherapy for patients with low risk of recurrence, whereas patients with high risk of recurrence had a significant impact from adjuvant therapy.

*Response to neoadjuvant* chemo- and hormonal therapy has been shown to be a strong prognostic factor and has the added benefit of providing a short-term endpoint for the rapid evaluation of treatment protocols. Determining patient response to neoadjuvant therapy is best achieved using pathological evaluation of the post-treatment specimen.

*Factors not routinely used* in clinical practice, although may have prognostic impact, are detection of bone marrow micrometastases at the time of diagnosis, p53 gene analysis, markers of invasion (e.g. levels of the proteolytic enzyme cathepsin D), markers of angiogenesis (e.g. microvessel density as detected by immunohistochemistry) and so on.

*DECISION-MAKING PROCESS* (See also Sect. 13.3). As known, adjuvant treatment of BC is designed to treat micrometastatic disease or BC cells that have escaped the breast and regional lymph nodes but have not yet developed identifiable metastases. The decision to administer adjuvant systemic therapy must take into account not only the individual patient's risk of relapse but also the absolute benefits of treatment, the potential short-term and long-term complications and the patient's comorbidities and life expectancy. Depending on the model of risk reduction, adjuvant systemic therapy has been estimated to reduce the mortality rate by 35–70 %.

Not all factors have similar influence on the decision-making process, for their different prognostic/predictive value, as well as the potential overlap of some with others. It is therefore appropriate to divide them into essential and additional factors. Indications and choice of type of adjuvant systemic treatment for invasive BC should be driven by:

- The histological characteristics of the tumour, including *essential factors* such as tumour size (pT) and nodal involvement (pN) and *additional factors* such as grade and peritumoural lymphovascular invasion (LVI)
- The biological characteristics of the tumour, including *essential factors* such as ER/PR status and HER2 expression and *additional factors* such as Ki67 and multigene test (On*cotype* DX and others), if available

In Table 18.2 are summarised factors that help to decide which kind of adjuvant therapy should be considered. Special groups of general population like young (<40 years old) and very young (<35 years old) women (see Section 15.3) or elderly woman (see Section 15.4) have few different options.

*PARAMETERS USED TO CHOOSE ADJUVANT THERAPY*. The St. Gallen International Consensus Conference gathers a worldwide group of BC experts to provide updates on adjuvant therapy recommendations based on low, intermediate and high risk [1]. They recommend adjuvant chemotherapy for patients with

**Table 18.2** Factors involved in decision-making process for adjuvant treatment of BC patients

| | Relative indications for chemotherapy with/without endocrine therapy | Factors not useful for decision | Relative indications for endocrine therapy alone |
|---|---|---|---|
| *Biological factors* | | | |
| ER and PR status | Lower ER and PR level | | Higher ER and PR level |
| Ki67 | High (>30 %) | Intermediate (16–30 %) | Low (<15 %) |
| HER2 expression | 3+ by IHC or FISH positive | | |
| Multigene test (if available) | High score | Intermediate score | Low score |
| *Histological factors* | | | |
| pT | >5 cm | 2.1–5 cm | <2 cm |
| Grade | Grade 3 | Grade 2 | Grade 1 |
| LVI | Present | | Absent |
| pN | 4 or more involved nodes | 1–3 involved nodes | Node negative (pN0) |
| *Patient's characteristics* | | | |
| Patient preference | Choice of all available treatments | | Avoid chemotherapy-related side effects |
| Patient comorbidity | | | Intolerance to chemotherapy |

*Abbreviations*: *ER* oestrogen receptor, *PR* progesterone receptor, *IHC* immunohistochemistry, *FISH* fluorescence in situ hybridisation, *pT* pathological tumour size of invasive component, *LVI* peritumoural lymphovascular invasion

hormone receptor-positive, high-risk disease or hormone receptor-negative, intermediate- or high-risk disease. They also recommend consideration of chemotherapy for patients with hormone receptor-positive, intermediate-risk disease. High-risk disease is defined as four or more positive nodes with any HER2 status or one to three positive nodes and HER2 positive. Low-risk group includes patients with age greater than 35, tumour size less than or equal to 2 cm, grade 1, no lymphovascular invasion and HER2-negative status (Table 18.3).

The National Comprehensive Cancer Network (NCCN) gathers experts to create practice guidelines in oncology, which are available to all practitioners [2]. The NCCN guidelines consider some factor like grading and Ki67 as non-important factors to decide adjuvant treatment of BC patients and state that ER and PR status should be evaluated on every BC to guide the decision to use hormonal therapy, whereas HER2 overexpression should be evaluated on every BC to select patients who have to be treated with trastuzumab. NCCN guidelines recommend adjuvant chemotherapy for patients with lymph node involvement, hormone receptor-negative BC and tumour size greater than 1 cm and for those with hormone receptor and HER2-positive disease and tumour size greater than 1 cm.

In some cases, St. Gallen guidelines differ slightly from NCCN recommendations, being slightly more conservative, and sometime contrasting, for example, a

**Table 18.3** St. Gallen systemic adjuvant therapy recommendations

| Risk category | Associated features | Adjuvant therapy options |
|---|---|---|
| *Low risk* | Node negative, ER/PR positive, T <1 cm, grade 1, no LVI, HER2 negative, age >35 (*all listed factors*) | None |
| | | Endocrine only |
| | | Consider multigene test (Onco*type* DX) |
| *Intermediate risk* | Node negative *and at least one of the following*: T>2 cm, grade >1, LVI, age<35, HER2 positive | Endocrine only (ER/PR+) |
| | | CT followed by endocrine (ER/PR+) |
| | Node positive (one to three nodes) and HER2 negative | Consider multigene test (if node negative and ER/PR+) |
| | | CT (ER/PR-) |
| *High risk* | Node positive (one to three nodes) and HER2 positive | CT followed by endocrine (ER/PR+) |
| | | CT |
| | Node positive (> four nodes) | |

woman with a 1.5-cm, node-negative, grade 1 tumour. ER positive, HER2 negative has an approximate 15 % 10-year risk of recurrence without systemic therapy. The NCCN guidelines would recommend considering adjuvant chemotherapy in addition to hormonal therapy, whereas the St. Gallen guidelines would recommend hormonal therapy only.

*MULTIDISCIPLINARY TEAM (MDT).* Diagnosis and treatment should be carried out in specialised institutions (Breast Units) caring for a high volume of BC patients, and the care of BC patients should be assigned to a MDT including at least a surgeon, a radiation oncologist, a medical oncologist, a radiologist and a pathologist—all specialised in BC. Patients should be provided with full, preferably written, information about their disease and treatment.

*TIMING.* It is recommended to start adjuvant chemo- or endocrine therapy (or radiotherapy), within 8 weeks from surgery.

## 18.2 Adjuvant Endocrine Therapy

**Clinical Practice Points**

- Premenopausal women with ER-positive BC should be treated with tamoxifen (TAM) for at least 5 years, to a total of 10 years, unless there are contraindications or side effects.
- Postmenopausal women with ER-positive BC should be considered rather for treatment with aromatase inhibitors (AI) as an alternative to TAM, either upfront AI for 5 years or switch to an AI after 3–3 years of TAM for a total of 5 years.
- Postmenopausal women who have completed 5 years of TAM may be considered for extended (5 years) treatment with an AI.
- The choice and sequence of adjuvant endocrine agents should consider benefit and side effects of treatment.

### 18.2.1 Agents

Hormone therapy decreases oestrogens level avoiding growth of dormant cancer cells. In ER-positive early-stage BC, hormone therapy plays a main role in adjuvant treatment, either alone or in combination with chemotherapy. Approved endocrine therapies for adjuvant treatment of BC include tamoxifen and aromatase inhibitors (anastrozole, letrozole, exemestane). Gonadotropin-releasing hormones (GnRH) analogue is an additional agent for premenopausal women (Table 18.4).

*TAMOXIFEN (TAM)* is a selective oestrogen receptor modulator that binds to and inhibits oestrogen receptor signalling in the breast [3]. As a receptor antagonist in BC, it is effective in all age groups, both in premenopausal and postmenopausal women. TAM acts also as agonist in other tissues, including bone (resulting in preservation of bone density) and endometrium (leading to an increased risk of endometrial cancer).

*Beneficial effects* of TAM are greater when taken for at least 5 years. There is little but important evidence that TAM is of additional benefit if taken for more than 5 years. Effects of TAM on outcomes are the following:

1. Increases 10-year survival from about 70 to 80 % among women without lymph node involvement with an absolute gain of 15.6 %
2. Increases 10-year survival from about 50 to 60 % among women with lymph node involvement with an absolute gain of 15.5 %
3. Almost halves the risk of development of cancer in the contralateral breast

Of note, up to 7 % of the white and black populations are *poor metabolisers* of tamoxifen. Poor metabolisers have been shown in several retrospective studies to have lower disease-free survival and higher recurrence rates than extensive metabolisers. Poor metabolisers also seem to tolerate tamoxifen better, with less severe hot flashes and endocrine-related toxicities.

**Table 18.4** Hormone agents used in BC

| | | |
|---|---|---|
| *Premenopausal* | Tamoxifen | 20 mg PO every day |
| | +/– GnRH analogue: | |
| | Leuprorelin or Triptorelin | 3.75 mg IM/SC depot q1mo/11.25 mg IM/SC q3mo |
| | Goserelin | 3.6 mg SC depot q1mo/10.8 mg SC q3mo |
| *Postmenopausal* | Tamoxifen | 20 mg PO every day |
| | Aromatase inhibitor: | |
| | Anastrozole | 1 mg PO every day |
| | Letrozole | 2.5 mg PO every day |
| | Exemestane | 25 mg PO every day |

*AROMATASE INHIBITORS (AIs).* AIs, in contrast to TAM, act via inhibition of oestrogen synthesis. There are two classes of AIs: nonsteroidal, as anastrozole and letrozole, and *steroidal*, as exemestane. As AIs have no effect on ovarian oestrogen production, they are effective only in postmenopausal women and should not be used in premenopausal women. Beneficial effects of AIs are the improvement of disease-free and metastatic-free survival rate which appears to be higher than with tamoxifen in postmenopausal women [4].

*Beneficial effects* of AIs on outcomes are the following.

- Absolute gain at 8 years in risk of relapse of 3.9 % if administered upfront.
- Absolute gain at 6 years in risk of relapse of 3.6 % if administered for 2–3 years after 2–3 years of TAM (switch strategy).
- Reduction in risk of recurrence when used as extended adjuvant therapy after 5 years of TAM as well as improved overall survival in the lymph node-positive BC patients.
- Reduction in risk of contralateral BC by a further 40–50 % when given instead of or after TAM.
- AIs may be more effective than TAM in HER2-positive BC.
- None of the head-to-head comparison trials between AIs and TAM has yielded an improvement in overall survival.

### 18.2.2 Schemes of Endocrine Therapy

The choice of treatment should be made after discussion between clinician and patient about the risks and benefits of each option. Factors to consider when making the choice include whether the woman has received TAM before, the side-effect profiles of the individual drugs and the recurrence score (Table 18.5).

In *premenopausal women*, TAM is offered for an initial duration of 5 years. After 5 years, ASCO suggests women not at low risk should receive additional therapy based on reassessment of the menopausal status. If women are pre- or perimenopausal or if menopausal status is unknown or cannot be determined, they should be offered continued TAM for a total duration of 10 years [5]. If women have become definitively postmenopausal, they should be offered continued TAM for a total duration of 10 years or switching to up to 5 years of an AI for a total duration of up to 10 years of adjuvant endocrine therapy [6]. Adjuvant ovarian ablation/suppression can be offered in addition to TAM to premenopausal women with ER-positive early invasive BC. The benefit of ovarian suppression is not clear, and this treatment represents a therapeutic option mainly in young premenopausal women [7].

In *postmenopausal women*, AIs represent the first therapeutic choice, both upfront and for 2–3 years after 2–3 years of TAM (switch strategy). TAM should be considered when therapy with AIs is contraindicated. Extended therapy with AIs after 5 years of TAM represents a therapeutic option mainly in high-risk BC patients.

**Table 18.5** Adjuvant endocrine therapy for women with hormone receptor-positive BC

| |
|---|
| *Pre- or perimenopausal* |
| TAM for an initial duration of 5 years |
| Adjuvant ovarian ablation/suppression in addition to TAM may be offered to women with ER-positive early invasive BC |
| After 5 years, women could receive additional therapy based on menopausal status |
| If women are pre- or perimenopausal or if menopausal status is unknown or cannot be determined, they should be offered continued TAM for a total duration of 10 years (in selected cases) |
| If women have become definitively postmenopausal, they should be offered to switch to 5-year treatment with an AI |
| *Postmenopausal* |
| AIs for a duration of 5 years (no data available for a greater duration) |
| TAM for an initial duration of 5 years, then switch to an AI for up to 5 years, for a total duration of up to 10 year |
| TAM for a duration of 2–3 years and switch to an AI for up to 5 years |
| Tamoxifen for a duration of 10 years (in selected cases) |
| *Appropriate sequence of endocrine therapy* |
| *Intolerance* – women who are postmenopausal and are intolerant of either TAM or an AI should be offered the alternative type of adjuvant endocrine therapy |
| *If women have received an AI* but discontinued treatment at less than 5 years, they may be offered *TAM* for a total of 5 years |
| *If women have received TAM* for 2–3 years, they should be offered switching to an AI for up to 5–10 years |

### 18.2.3 Side Effects of Endocrine Therapy

Table 18.6 presents a review of hormonal agents with their mechanism of action, side effect and main risks.

*SIDE EFFECTS OF TAM.* TAM is the most widely used hormonal agent and is not without risks and side effects. TAM is associated with an increased incidence of hot flashes, vaginal discharge and night sweats. Sexual dysfunction is not a common complaint, although it may correlate with vaginal dryness. In addition to menopause symptoms, there is an increased risk of tamoxifen inducing menopause in premenopausal women, although this is restricted to women 45 years or older and is in part related to the normal aging process. Several studies have shown that despite these symptoms, the quality of life of women undergoing therapy with TAM is not significantly worse than women receiving a placebo.

One of the most significant and deleterious side effects of treatment with TAM appears to be its proliferative effect on the endometrium. Overall endometrial pathologies, including hyperplasia, polyps, carcinoma and sarcoma, have been identified in up to 36 % of postmenopausal BC patients treated with TAM. However, monitoring of endometrium changes during treatment with TAM is simple and feasible using transvaginal ultrasonography. Moreover, the incidence of endometrial cancer is rare.

*Endometrial hyperplasia* is more commonly diagnosed in TAM-treated patients as compared to nontreated patients and among postmenopausal BC TAM-treated

**Table 18.6** Mechanism of action, side effects and specific toxicity of hormonal agents used for the treatment of BC, with their mechanism of action, side effects and main risks

| Agent | Mechanism | Side effects | Risks |
|---|---|---|---|
| *Oestrogen receptor modulator or suppressor* | | | |
| *Tamoxifen* (TAM) (Nolvadex®) | Selective oestrogen receptor modulator (SERM) | Fatigue, hot flashes, vaginal discharge, rapid change in mood, headache, skin rash, nausea and fluid retention/weight gain | Thromboembolic events, uterine cancer and cataracts |
| *Aromatase inhibitors (AIs)* | | | |
| *Letrozole* (Femara®) *Anastrozole* (Arimidex®) | *Nonsteroidal*: inhibits the synthesis of oestrogen via vreversible competition for the aromatase enzyme | Joint stiffness, bone and joint pain, nausea, headache and fluid retention/weight gain | Osteoporosis |
| *Exemestane* (Aromasin®) | *Steroidal*: forms a permanent and deactivating bond with the aromatase enzyme | | |
| *GnRH analogues* | | | |
| *Goserelin* (Zoladex®) *Triptorelin* (Decapeptyl®) *Leuprorelin* | Blocks ovarian production of oestrogen | Hot flashes and menopause symptoms | |

patients with vaginal bleeding as compared to patients without this symptom. The occurrence has been observed in 4–30 % of TAM-treated patients, with a higher rate in patients with symptoms of vaginal bleeding.

*Endometrial polyps* represent the most common endometrial pathology associated with postmenopausal TAM exposure, with a rate of 8–36 %. Some risk factors have been identified for endometrial polyps in postmenopausal BC TAM-treated patients:

- Older age at menopause
- Longer duration of BC
- Higher body weight
- Thicker endometrial thickness, measured by transvaginal ultrasound, compared with similar patients without endometrial polyps

*Malignant Endometrial Polyps*. A high rate of malignant transformation with a high grade of malignancy was reported in endometrial polyps recovered from postmenopausal BC TAM-treated patients. In particular:

- Malignant transformation was reported in 3–10 % of endometrial polyps recovered.
- Vaginal bleeding was associated with only 50 % of the cases.
- No correlation between malignant polyps and polyp size or treatment duration.

*Endometrial Cancer*. The most significant risk of tamoxifen appears to be that of uterine cancer.

Longer duration of TAM use was associated with an increased risk (2–3/1,000 per year) of endometrial cancer, when compared to nontreated patient. Risk does not decrease after cessation of TAM treatment, as the effect of TAM can last several years beyond discontinuation of exposure. Moreover, endometrial cancer mortality rate among TAM-treated patients was significantly higher compared to nontreated patients (33.3 % vs. 2.6 %). The more unfavourable histology and the advanced stage at diagnosis are related with increasing exposure to TAM. Routine screening with transvaginal ultrasound or endometrial biopsy is weakly useful and thus not recommended in all guidelines. Instead, women should be counselled about the need to alert their physician for abnormal vaginal bleeding and undergo regular gynaecologic evaluations.

*Ocular Toxicity*. Tamoxifen has also been associated with ocular toxicities, specifically corneal changes and retinopathy. For this reason, it has been recommended that women consider a baseline ophthalmic evaluation during the 1st year of initiating tamoxifen and have appropriate follow-up.

*Thromboembolic disease* is a worrisome risk of tamoxifen because it can lead to fatal consequences. This appears to affect less than 1 % of patients and is more common in women over the age of 50.

Studies about the use of tamoxifen in BC prevention revealed that women treated with TAM had an approximately 2.3× increased risk of thromboembolic disease than those treated with placebo.

*SIDE EFFECTS OF AIS*. Common side effects of AIs include hot flashes (from 10 to 35 % of cases), arthralgia/arthritis (about 15–20 %), headache (about 10 %), vaginal dryness (2–3 %) and mood changes (about 20 %).

*Osteoporosis*. Since AIs reduce circulating oestrogen levels, a decrease in bone mineral density can be anticipated, leading to osteopenia and low-intermediate osteoporosis. Thus, AIs are associated with higher rate of fracture than TAM. Because anastrozole, letrozole and exemestane have different structures and pharmacokinetic profiles, it cannot be assumed they will all have the same safety profiles. However, long-term data is available only for anastrozole, and head-to-head comparisons have not been performed. Women with osteoporosis or at risk of osteoporosis should have their bone mineral density formally assessed by bone densitometry at the beginning of treatment and at regular intervals thereafter. Treatment or prophylaxis for osteoporosis should be initiated as appropriate and patients treated with AIs should be carefully monitored.

*Gynaecological events*, a problem for TAM, do not appear to be as much of a problem for AIs. In the ATAC trial, anastrozole was associated with significantly fewer effects on the endometrium, a lower number of endometrial cancers and reductions in hot flashes, vaginal bleeding and vaginal discharge compared with TAM. Similar findings were reported with exemestane and letrozole from those studies, although not all were significant.

*Thromboembolic Disease*. Another major concern of TAM is the risk of thromboembolic disease. Again, AIs seem to have a lower risk compared to TAM, and in the ATAC trial, there was a significant reduction of ischemic cerebrovascular and thromboembolic events with anastrozole.

*Lipid Profile.* While TAM has been shown to improve lipid profiles, AIs have a different mode of action and do not possess the oestrogen-agonistic effects of TAM. At present, available data suggest that the different AIs have different effects on lipid profiles. Some studies show anastrozole as generally having little effect on lipids, while others have indicated adverse effects on lipid profiles increasing cholesterolaemia. Letrozole has been associated with adverse effects on lipid profiles in some studies, but short-term data from randomised trials do not show increased cardiovascular morbidity. In general, the changes are likely to be of little relevance in women with advanced BC, but if these agents are widely used in early BC, their impact on lipid profiles may become more important.

*Cardiac Risk.* A meta-analysis of seven randomised controlled trials comparing the use of AIs with TAM in nearly 30,000 postmenopausal women with early-stage BC has shown that AIs are associated with a statistically significant 26 % increased risk of cardiovascular disease.

*SIDE EFFECTS OF GNRH ANALOGUES.* Common side effects of GnRH analogues include hot flashes, increased sweating, night sweats, tiredness, headache, acne, joint/muscle aches, trouble sleeping, reduced sexual interest, vaginal discomfort/dryness, vaginal bleeding, swelling of the ankles/feet, increased urination at night and dizziness.

## 18.3 Adjuvant Chemotherapy and Targeted Therapy

**Clinical Practice Points**

- Chemotherapy should be offered to all premenopausal women (less than 50 years of age) with stage II BC and to almost all postmenopausal women (50 years of age or older) with ER-negative BC.
- Combination of 2–3 drugs is the standard in the adjuvant setting. Anthracycline-based chemotherapy is superior to non-anthracycline-based regimens. Sequential use of anthracyclines and taxanes is superior to anthracycline-based chemotherapy.
- Cardiac toxicity, neuropathy and chemotherapy-induced second cancers are long-term effects of chemotherapy.
- Adjuvant trastuzumab should be considered in all patients with HER2-positive BC who receive adjuvant chemotherapy because it reduces by 50 % the recurrence risk and improves overall survival, compared with chemotherapy alone.
- Trastuzumab should be used with caution in patients with significant cardiac comorbidity. The benefits of adjuvant chemotherapy with or without trastuzumab may be outweighed by the potential harms in these patients.

### 18.3.1 Introduction

Adjuvant chemotherapy is usually prescribed in BC patients with high risk of relapse. In fact aims of chemotherapy are to kill residual tumour cells (micrometastases, dormant cells) and to improve outcomes (disease-free survival, DFS, and overall survival, OS) of BC patients. The benefit from chemotherapy is more pronounced in ER-negative tumours. In ER-positive tumours, chemotherapy at least partially exerts its effect by induction of ovarian failure.

Early Breast Cancer Trialists' Collaborative Group (EBCTCG) meta-analysis showed that women who receive chemotherapy have an absolute 10-year gain of 8–10 % in DFS, of 5 % in OS and of 6 % in BC-specific survival (BCSS) compared with those who do not receive chemotherapy [8]. According to this meta-analysis, anthracycline-based chemotherapy is better than non-anthracycline-based chemotherapy, and sequential anthracycline-taxane regimens represent the best therapeutic option in terms of benefit. The decision to prescribe chemotherapy must to be made based on benefit that the patient can derive from the treatment and the side effects and toxicities related with chemotherapy. Prognostic and predictive factors involved in the decision-making process have been previously described.

*Kinetics*. The first principle is that chemotherapy works by first-order kinetics. This means that the drugs kill a fixed fraction of cells with each cycle and not a fixed number of cells (referred to as log-kill hypothesis). Thus, a single dose could potentially be effective. However, because the drugs kill only a fraction of cells, repetitive cycles are necessary.

*Effectiveness*. The efficacy of adjuvant therapy is related to how efficacious is the drug (how large is the fraction of cells killed), how many cycles are used and how quickly the remaining cells grow between cycles.

*Resistance*. One barrier to the efficacy of adjuvant chemotherapy is resistance. Some cancer cells are inherently resistant to particular agents; others will gain resistance via mutation. One way to avoid resistance is the use of combination chemotherapy rather than single agents. In general, using agents in combination is more effective and the more common approach when there is a curative intent, as in the adjuvant setting.

*Overlapping*. The best combinations include agents that act synergistically, which are most likely to occur when they have different mechanisms of action and resistance. When combining chemotherapy, however, potential overlapping effects, as well as side effects, should be properly considered to avoid excessive toxicity.

### 18.3.2 Regimens of Chemotherapy

ESMO Guidelines for chemotherapy of primary BC include also evidence and grades of recommendations applied using the system shown in Sect. 1.3 [9]. Most frequently used regimens contain anthracyclines and/or taxanes, although in selected patients CMF may still be used. Four cycles of AC (doxorubicin, cyclophosphamide) are considered equal to six cycles of CMF, whereas six cycles of three-drug anthracycline-based regimens are superior (LoE IA). The addition of taxanes improves the efficacy of chemotherapy, independently of age, nodal status, tumour size or grade, steroid receptor expression or tamoxifen use, but at the cost of increased non-cardiotoxicity (LoE IA). Sequential rather than the concomitant use of anthracyclines and taxanes is superior (LoE IB). Non-anthracycline, taxane-based regimens (such as four cycles of TC) may in selected patients (such as those at risk of cardiac complications) be used as an alternative to four cycles of anthracycline-based chemotherapy (LoE IA).

The treatment should start preferably within 2–8 weeks after surgery; data show an important decrease in systemic therapy efficacy when administered more than 12 weeks after surgery. Chemotherapy is usually administered for 12–24 weeks (four to eight cycles), depending on the individual recurrence risk and the selected regimen. The use of dose-dense schedules [with granulocyte colony-stimulating factor (G-CSF) support] should be considered, in particular in highly proliferative tumours (LoE IB).

Triple-negative tumours benefit from adjuvant chemotherapy, with the possible exception of low-risk 'special' histological subtypes such as medullary or adenoid cystic carcinomas (LoE IA). HER2-positive BCs, apart from selected cases with very low risk such as Tla NO, are treated with chemotherapy plus trastuzumab (LoE IA). Trastuzumab may routinely be combined with non-anthracycline-based chemotherapy (LoE IA), while concomitant use with anthracyclines is not routinely recommended outside of clinical trials. For most patients, the use of a sequential anthracycline-based followed by taxane-trastuzumab-based regimen is the preferred choice.

*Trastuzumab*. This molecular-targeted agent is recommended for patients with HER2-positive BC for 1 year because it significantly improves both DFS and OS among women with HER2-positive BC. Based on the results of four phase III clinical trials in HER2-positive patients, trastuzumab and chemotherapy approximately halve the recurrence risk compared with chemotherapy alone [10]. Addition of trastuzumab to chemotherapy leads to an absolute gain of 12 % in 4 years in DFS and 7.4 % in 4 years in OS (LoE IA). Trastuzumab is approved in patients with node-positive disease and in N0 patients with tumours >1 cm, although it should also be considered in N0 patients with tumour <1 cm with high risk of relapse such as ER-negative BC cases (LoE IVB).

Trastuzumab is usually well tolerated, although a usually reversible cardiac dysfunction may occur. Selection of patients based on the baseline cardiac function (expressed by the left ventricular ejection fraction) and periodic monitoring during treatment are necessary. Due to its cardiotoxicity, trastuzumab should not be routinely administered concomitantly with anthracyclines (LoE IB). Combination with taxanes is safe and has been demonstrated to be more effective than sequential treatment (LoE IA). Trastuzumab may also be safely combined with RT and endocrine therapy. Adjuvant chemotherapy regimens are listed in Table 18.7.

*Radiotherapy During Chemotherapy*. RT may be delivered safely during non-anthracycline-based chemotherapy with or without trastuzumab (LoE III B). If chemotherapy and RT are to be used separately, chemotherapy usually precedes RT. In general, chemotherapy should not be used concomitantly with endocrine therapy (LoE IID).

**Table 18.7** Adjuvant chemotherapy regimens for BC

| Regimen | Drugs | Dose |
|---|---|---|
| FEC | 5-Fluorouracil<br>Epirubicin<br>Cyclophosphamide<br>*every 21 days for 6 cycles* | 500 mg/m$^2$ IV day 1<br>75–100 mg/m$^2$ IV day 1<br>500 mg/m$^2$ IV day 1 |
| FAC | 5-Fluorouracil<br>Adriamycin<br>Cyclophosphamide<br>*every 21 days for 6 cycles* | 600 mg/m$^2$ IV day 1<br>60 mg/m$^2$ IV day 1<br>600 mg/m$^2$ IV day 1 |
| TAC | Docetaxel<br>Doxorubicin<br>Cyclophosphamide<br>*every 21 days for 6 cycles* | 75 mg/m$^2$ IV day 1<br>50 mg/m$^2$ IV day 1<br>500 mg/m$^2$ IV day 1 |
| AC/EC → paclitaxel | Adriamycin/epirubicin<br>Cyclophosphamide | 60 mg/m$^2$ IV day 1<br>600 mg/m$^2$ IV day 1 |
| | *every 21 days for 4 cycles, followed by* | |
| | Paclitaxel<br>*every 7 days for 12 cycles* | 80 mg/m$^2$ IV day 1 |
| Dose-dense AC → paclitaxel | Adriamycin<br>Cyclophosphamide | 60 mg/m$^2$ IV day 1<br>600 mg/m$^2$ IV day 1 |
| | *every 14 days for 4 cycles with G-CSF, followed by* | |
| | Paclitaxel<br>*every 7 days for 12 cycles* | 60–80 mg/m$^2$ IV day 1 |
| FEC → docetaxel | 5-Fluorouracil<br>Epirubicin<br>Cyclophosphamide | 500 mg/m$^2$ IV day 1<br>75–100 mg/m$^2$ IV day 1<br>500 mg/m$^2$ IV day 1 |
| | *every 21 days for 3 cycles, followed by* | |
| | Docetaxel<br>*every 21 days for 3 cycles* | 100 mg/mq |
| CMF (Bonadonna regimen) | Cyclophosphamide<br>Methotrexate<br>5-Fluorouracil<br>*every 28 days for 6 cycles* | 100 mg/m$^2$ PO days 1–14<br>40 mg/m$^2$ IV days 1 and 8<br>600 mg/m$^2$ IV days 1 and 8 |
| CMF | Cyclophosphamide<br>Methotrexate<br>5-Fluorouracil<br>*every 28 days for 6 cycles* | 600 mg/m$^2$ IV days 1 and 8<br>40 mg/m$^2$ IV days 1 and 8<br>600 mg/m$^2$ IV days 1 and 8 |
| TC | Docetaxel<br>Cyclophosphamide<br>*every 21 days for 4 cycles* | 75 mg/m$^2$ IV day 1<br>600 mg/m$^2$ IV day 1 |
| AC/<br>EC → paclitaxel + trastuzumab | Adriamycin/epirubicin<br>Cyclophosphamide | 60 mg/m$^2$ (A), 90 mg/m$^2$ (E) IV day 1<br>600 mg/m$^2$ IV day 1 |
| | *every 21 days for 4 cycles*, followed by | |
| | Paclitaxel | 80 mg/m$^2$ IV day 1 |
| | *weekly for 12 cycles* | |
| | Trastuzumab | 4 mg/kg IV first dose, then 2 mg/kg weekly with paclitaxel, then 6 mg/kg IV *every 21 days until 1 year* |

**Table 18.7** (continued)

| | | |
|---|---|---|
| TCH | Docetaxel<br>Carboplatin<br>*every 21 days for 6 cycles*<br>Trastuzumab | 75 mg/m² IV day 1<br>AUC6 IV day 1<br>8 mg/kg first dose, then 6 mg/kg<br>*every 21 days for 1 year* |
| TC+H (for small HER2-positive N0) | Docetaxel<br>Cyclophosphamide<br>*every 21 days for 4 cycles*<br>Trastuzumab | 75 mg/m²<br>600 mg/m²<br>8 mg/kg then 6 mg/mq *every 21 days for 1 year* |
| Paclitaxel+H | Paclitaxel<br>Trastuzumab | 80 mg/m² IV weekly for 12 cycles<br>4 mg/kg first dose, then 2 mg/kg concomitant with paclitaxel then 6 mg/kg *every 21 days until 1 year* |

### 18.3.3 Side Effects of Chemotherapy

*SHORT-TERM SIDE EFFECTS.* More frequent short-term toxicity side effects of chemotherapeutic agents are hair loss, nausea and vomiting, myelosuppression, neurologic toxicity and fatigue.

*Hair loss (alopecia)* is the most common side effect of chemotherapy for BC. Alopecia is almost 100 % with regimens including anthracyclines or taxanes. Alopecia does not always occur with CMF, with an incidence between 40 and 65 %.

*Nausea and vomiting* during chemotherapy are primarily caused by serotonin release from the gastrointestinal mucosa, which leads to stimulation of the emesis centre of the medulla. The availability of new antiemetic agents has decreased the severity of this side. Aprepitant (Emend®) and palonosetron (Aloxi®) are highly effective in avoiding vomiting derived from anthracycline-based chemotherapy. Other antiemetic medications include 5-hydroxy-triptamine 3 (5-HT3) serotonin antagonists, dexamethasone, metoclopramide or prochlorperazine.

*Myelosuppression* is a common side effect of chemotherapy, and thus patients are carefully monitored for the development of neutropenia, anaemia or thrombocytopenia. It typically occurs within 5–15 days after the infusion of chemotherapy.

The management of neutropenia depends on the severity. Mild neutropenia is defined as an absolute neutrophil count of less than 1,500/mm³, but greater than 1,000/mm³ does not require treatment. It may be prudent to decrease the dose of chemotherapy. Patients with moderate (500–1,000) or severe (<500) neutropenia are at an increased risk of infection and must be instructed to report any fevers. Fevers should be thoroughly worked up and antibiotics initiated, even if no source is found. Granulocyte colony-stimulating factors should be considered for any patient who had neutropenic fever with prolonged neutropenia or prophylactically when neutropenia is expected (such as with dose-dense regimens). Anaemia is treated with blood transfusion. Patients with thrombocytopenia may require platelet transfusion.

*Neurologic Toxicity*. The addition of taxanes (paclitaxel, docetaxel) to adjuvant chemotherapy carries with it several neurologic toxicities. These can take the form of both motor and sensory neuropathies. The severity is dose and schedule dependent, and symptoms can be improved by early recognition with subsequent dose reduction. Within 72 h of receiving paclitaxel, myalgias and arthralgias may develop, which can be relieved by either nonsteroidal anti-inflammatory drugs (NSAIDs) or a short course of glucocorticoids.

*Fatigue* is one of the most common complaints during chemotherapy. The reasons are multifactorial. Anaemia should be ruled out, as should other potentially reversible factors, such as sleep disturbance, uncontrolled pain, depression or poor nutrition. However, in most cases a specific cause is not identified. During chemotherapy symptomatic relief may be provided by initiating an exercise regime, changing the diet or using stimulants or antidepressants.

*LONG-TERM SIDE EFFECTS*. Long-term effects must be considered in addition to the acute toxicity. The most frequent manifestations are cognitive dysfunction, ovarian failure, cardiac toxicity as well as leukaemia and myelodysplastic syndromes.

*Cognitive Dysfunction*. A considerable amount of data is now coming out on the long-term effect of chemotherapy on cognition. As many as one third of patients who receive adjuvant chemotherapy may develop some dysfunction in memory or the ability to concentrate, although for many patients, this will eventually return to baseline. There may be a relationship between the intensity of the adjuvant therapy and the incidence of cognitive impairment. Further research is necessary to better clarify the impairment and identify ways to avoid or reverse it.

*Ovarian Failure*. Premature termination of ovarian function is a significant concern for younger women receiving adjuvant chemotherapy for BC. On one hand, the induction of premature menopause may be beneficial. In fact chemotherapy-induced amenorrhea improves DFS and OS in women with ER-positive BC. However, many young women being treated for BC would like to maintain reproductive function, hoping to have children after completing therapy. Even in women who no longer desire to have children, premature ovarian failure can affect quality of life by heralding menopausal symptoms (hot flashes, vaginal dryness, dyspareunia, depression, sleep disturbance) and result in significant bone loss. Premature ovarian failure can occur in any woman, but the major risk factors are older age, a longer duration of treatment and alkylant-based regimens. Women receiving taxanes have a lower incidence of ovarian failure. Using GnRH agonists during chemotherapy reduces the rate of chemotherapy-induced amenorrhea. In women who experience ovarian failure, supplemental calcium, vitamin D and regular exercise should be used to mitigate bone loss, while bisphosphonates are used to treat osteoporosis in women with premature menopause.

*Cardiac Toxicity*. Women treated with anthracyclines or with trastuzumab are at an increased risk of cardiac toxicity that is higher in women who receive radiation therapy for left-sided BC. Anthracyclines directly damage the myocardium and lead to cardiomyopathy. The risk of cardiac failure increases with a cumulative dose of doxorubicin >450 mg/m$^2$.

The risk of cardiac dysfunction appears to be related to age, baseline left ventricular ejection fraction (LVEF) and use of concomitant antihypertensive medications. Candidates for treatment with anthracycline or trastuzumab should undergo thorough baseline cardiac assessment, including history and physical examination and assessment of LVEF by echocardiogram or radionuclide scan. Monitoring may not identify all patients who will develop cardiac dysfunction. Caution should be exercised in treating patients with pre-existing cardiac dysfunction. Discontinuation of trastuzumab treatment should be strongly considered in patients who develop a clinically significant decrease in LVEF.

*Leukaemia and Myelodysplastic Syndromes.* Although chemotherapy can lead to the development of leukaemias and myelodysplastic syndromes, the incidence appears low for regimens used to treat BC, being less than 1 %. This may be slightly higher among women who receive radiation therapy or with the administration of G-CSF, although the data is not clear. Two distinct types of treatment-related leukemic syndromes can occur. The first is typically associated with alkylating agents and takes 3–7 years to develop, often preceded by myelodysplastic syndrome. The second is associated with topoisomerase II inhibitors and has more rapid onset, within 2–3 years of therapy. Unfortunately the treatment-related leukaemias have a poor prognosis and are more refractory to conventional antileukaemic therapies.

## 18.4 Neoadjuvant Systemic Therapy

**Clinical Practice Points**

- Neoadjuvant systemic therapy should be considered for patients with inoperable BC, as locally advanced or inflammatory BC.
- For patients candidate to mastectomy but suitable to conservative surgery after downsizing of tumour, neoadjuvant chemotherapy safely allows for a more limited operative approach, including sentinel lymph node dissection, without an increase in local-regional recurrence rates in selected patients.
- All modalities (chemotherapy, endocrine therapy and targeted therapy) used in adjuvant treatment may also be used preoperatively.
- Combination of anthracyclines and taxanes should be considered for all patients receiving neoadjuvant chemotherapy, and patients with HER2-positive BC should receive anti-HER2 agents.
- Neoadjuvant endocrine therapy for women with ER-positive BC is usually not used in young women outside clinical trials, but is frequent in elderly women to enable BCS.
- Response to neoadjuvant systemic therapy and molecular subtype holds important implications for prognosis and individualised patient outcomes.

### 18.4.1 Introduction

Neoadjuvant systemic therapy, or primary systemic therapy, should be considered for patients with inoperable BC or for those that are candidate for mastectomy but can be suitable candidates for conservative surgery after downsizing of tumour.

The *potential objectives* of neoadjuvant chemotherapy are the following:

- To make operable an inoperable BC
- To allow for breast conservative surgery in women who would otherwise require a mastectomy
- To improve the aesthetic outcomes of lumpectomy by decreasing the volume of tissue needing to be resected
- To allow the assessment of chemosensitivity of the tumour
- To improve outcomes of BC patients

*Contraindications* to neoadjuvant chemotherapy are the following:

- Women for whom the use of chemotherapy is not indicated based on clinical staging
- Women with diffuse in situ component
- Women who cannot undergo radiotherapy and therefore are not candidates for breast conservation

*PRETREATMENT EVALUATION*. Tumour size should be documented prior to treatment. In most cases, ultrasound of the breast is sufficient to document tumour size. However, breast magnetic resonance imaging (MRI) may be helpful to evaluate disease extent, including assessing for the presence of multicentric disease or invasion of the underlying chest wall. Before starting neoadjuvant chemotherapy, radiopaque clips should be placed in the tumour. Because the aim of neoadjuvant therapy is to shrink the primary tumour, the clip will aid in planning locoregional treatment (surgery and radiation therapy) and the subsequent pathological assessment of the surgical specimen.

Because neoadjuvant therapy is expected to impact pathological findings at surgery, the status of regional lymph nodes should be determined at baseline. This information will influence decisions about radiation therapy after surgery. For patients with palpable axillary nodes, an ultrasound-guided fine-needle aspiration (FNA) and/or core-needle biopsy of one or more suspicious nodes before neoadjuvant treatment is recommended to determine if the axillary nodes are pathologically involved. If the FNA is negative, a sentinel lymph node biopsy (SLNB) is advised in order to stage the axilla prior to treatment. If the FNA is positive, no further evaluation is required.

As with all patients presenting with a new diagnosis of BC, histopathological confirmation and evaluation of ER, PR and HER2 statuses must be obtained before initiating treatment. Patients should undergo an appropriate initial staging workup prior to neoadjuvant systemic therapy that may include imaging studies to rule out detectable metastatic disease.

*SURGERY*. After neoadjuvant therapy, surgery is accomplished as usual. Sentinel node biopsy is feasible after neoadjuvant chemotherapy; however, its accuracy in this setting has been questioned, and this is under investigation of ongoing randomised controlled trials. Advantages and disadvantages of sentinel lymph node biopsy before and after neoadjuvant systemic therapy are listed in Table 18.8.

### 18.4.2 Neoadjuvant Endocrine Therapy

Luminal BC subtype, mainly luminal A (ER-positive/HER2-negative BC with low proliferative index), shows low response to neoadjuvant chemotherapy, and endocrine therapy represents an alternative option in these patients. In clinical practice, neoadjuvant endocrine therapy is usually not used in young women outside clinical trials, but is frequent in elderly women to enable BCS. However, a complete pathological response (pCR) is rare with endocrine therapy, and some studies have recently demonstrated that the decrease of Ki67 can be an indicator of response to endocrine treatment in neoadjuvant setting [11].

For postmenopausal women who are candidates for neoadjuvant endocrine therapy, AIs rather than TAM are recommended, based on evidence of higher response rates with AIs, all equally active.

For patients undergoing neoadjuvant endocrine therapy, treatment should be continued for at least three to 4 months. In fact, a response to endocrine therapy may not be evident for at least 3–4 months, and maximal response may not be achieved until much later. If the tumour is amenable to surgery after 3–4 months, definitive surgical treatment can be carried out. However, if the tumour is responding to endocrine therapy, extending treatment to 6 months or longer with clinical monitoring of response may permit a higher percentage of patients to undergo breast conservative surgery. Thus, the duration of endocrine treatment before surgery must be individualised based on the patient's clinical status and the clinical response. If at any time there is evidence of progression or nonresponse, surgery is recommended.

**Table 18.8** Advantages and disadvantages of sentinel lymph node biopsy before and after neoadjuvant systemic therapy

| | Advantages | Disadvantages |
|---|---|---|
| *Before therapy* | Higher identification rate | Requires an additional surgery |
| | Likely lower false-negative rate<br>Accurate pre-therapy nodal staging | Delays the beginning of chemotherapy |
| | | May subject patients converted to node negative to an unnecessary axillary lymph node dissection |
| *After therapy* | No need for surgery before chemotherapy | Slightly lower identification rate |
| | No axillary lymph node dissection performed on patients who become node negative | Higher false-negative rate |
| | | Will mislabel some patients who were initially node positive as node negative |

### 18.4.3 Neoadjuvant Chemotherapy

Neoadjuvant chemotherapy is as effective as adjuvant chemotherapy in prolonging survival for patients with locally advanced BC. In operable cases, the timing of treatment (pre- vs. postoperative) has no effect on long-term outcomes (LoE IIC). After neoadjuvant systemic treatment, the amount of residual disease is an important prognostic factor, but no uniform guidelines exist for the evaluation of response to neoadjuvant treatment. The pCR should be defined as the disappearance of microscopic evidence of all invasive disease at both the primary site and the axilla. However, some studies used a different definition of pCR, considering CR in patients without tumour in the breast but with residual disease in lymph nodes.

Recently it has been showed that the absence of disease in both breast and lymph nodes better predicts outcomes compared with the absence of tumour only in the breast. Moreover, in patients with ER-negative or HER2-positive tumours, the pCR rate is >20 % and predicts clinical outcomes better than in other BC phenotypes [12]. Recent data in the neoadjuvant setting suggest that young women have a bigger benefit from combination of anthracyclines and taxanes (LoE III).

As told before, ER-positive, HER2-negative carcinomas (luminal phenotype) benefit from primary endocrine therapy, while they are generally less responsive to primary chemotherapy than ER-negative and HER2-positive BC. The chemotherapy regimens to be used in the neoadjuvant setting are the same ones used in the adjuvant setting. Regimen of sequential anthracyclines and taxanes should be used (LoE IB). As in the adjuvant setting, trastuzumab should be administered in addition to chemotherapy in HER2-positive BC to increase the probability of achieving pCR. Recent studies have shown that double block of HER2 pathway (e.g. pertuzumab + trastuzumab or lapatinib + trastuzumab) improves the pCR rate compared with trastuzumab alone [13].

## 18.5 Treatment of Metastatic BC

**Clinical Practice Points**

- In the setting of advanced disease, the goal of treatment is to prolong survival while maintaining a good quality of life.
- Treatment should be chosen based on factors including number and type of metastases, symptoms as well as comorbidity.
- For hormone receptor-positive patients, endocrine treatment represents the first therapeutic choice.
- Upfront chemotherapy is reserved to the patient with life-threatening disease and/or severe symptoms that require quick relief. Single agent or combination of two agents represents both valid therapeutic options.
- The best candidates for resection or ablation of distant metastases are the patients with oligo-metastatic disease, favourable prognostic factors and long DFS.

### 18.5.1 Introduction

In the setting of advanced disease, the goal of treatment is to prolong survival while maintaining a good quality of life. Hormone receptor and HER2 statuses are the most important factors to choose type of treatment of patients with metastatic BC. Change in these factors occurs in 10–15 % of cases with important consequences in management of disease; therefore, biopsy of metastatic sites could be required in some cases to better understand the characteristics of present disease [14].

For patients who have hormone receptor (ER and/or PR)-positive disease without a life-threatening component (e.g. massive liver metastases) or systemic symptoms requiring immediate palliation, hormone treatment is the first therapeutic choice. On the contrary, hormone receptor-negative patients have to be treated with chemotherapy. Patients with HER2-positive and hormone receptor-positive BC should be treated with endocrine therapy and anti-HER2 drugs, trastuzumab or lapatinib (Tykerb®), while those with hormone receptor-negative BC with chemotherapy and anti-HER2 drugs.

*ENDOCRINE THERAPY.* In *premenopausal* young patients with hormone receptor-positive or hormone receptor unknown metastatic BC, TAM in combination with ovarian suppression with GnRH agonist is the first-line endocrine therapy of choice (LoE IA). AIs together with ovarian suppression can be considered after progression on TAM and ovarian suppression (LoE IIB). Fulvestrant has not yet been studied in premenopausal women and specific studies are needed.

In *postmenopausal patients*, AIs and fulvestrant represent both valid therapeutic options. Recent studies have shown that in patients who relapsed after treatment with nonsteroidal AIs (letrozole or anastrozole), the addition of everolimus (Afinitor®) to exemestane improves progression-free survival (PFS) compared with exemestane alone.

In the setting of combined endocrine therapy alone, there are data suggesting that zoledronic acid improves disease-free survival and maintains bone mineral density in premenopausal women.

*CHEMOTHERAPY.* Chemotherapy is the first therapeutic option in metastatic setting for patients with hormone receptor-positive BC but life-threatening disease and for patients with hormone receptor-negative BC. According to ESMO Guidelines, the sequential use of single cytotoxic agents is the standard [13], while ASCO panel considers that choice between sequential single agents or combination chemotherapy should be done on the basis of a balance of the efficacy, toxicity and patient's preference [15]. Concerning the duration of chemotherapy, a meta-analysis showed that prolonged chemotherapy is associated with increased OS compared with shorter chemotherapy. Continuation of chemotherapy beyond third line is appropriate in patients with response to previous chemotherapy.

Choice of chemotherapy depends from disease-related factors (DFS, previous therapies and response, tumour burden, biology, need for rapid disease control) and patient's-related factors (patient's preference, age, menopausal status, comorbidities, performance status).

Treatments with single agent include the anthracyclines (doxorubicin, epirubicin, pegylated liposomal doxorubicin), the taxanes (paclitaxel, docetaxel, albumin-bound paclitaxel), the anti-metabolites (capecitabine and gemcitabine) and the non-taxane microtubule inhibitors (eribulin and vinorelbine). Combination regimens are the same used in adjuvant setting (FEC, FAC, CMF, etc.). Platinum-based regimens seem to be particularly active in triple-negative BC, even if clinical data derive from retrospective clinical series. Ongoing clinical trials are evaluating this type of chemotherapy in triple-negative BC patients.

Bevacizumab (Avastin®), an anti-angiogenetic drug, has been tested in addition to chemotherapy in first and second line, showing an increase in PFS compared with chemotherapy alone.

In HER2-positive BC patients, the addition of trastuzumab to chemotherapy has shown to increase both PFS and OS compared with chemotherapy alone. Trastuzumab can be administered in association with taxanes, vinorelbine and capecitabine. Recently, the regimen including trastuzumab, pertuzumab (Perjeta®) and docetaxel has been demonstrated to increase PFS and OS in first line compared with trastuzumab alone and docetaxel. Thus, based on these results, the standard first-line chemotherapy for HER2-positive metastatic BC is represented by trastuzumab, pertuzumab and docetaxel, except for patients with early distant relapse (<6 months) after adjuvant trastuzumab for whom the best option is trastuzumab emtansine (T-DM1). T-DM1 can be prescribed also in second or further lines, while pertuzumab can be administered only in first line.

### 18.5.2 Local Treatment of Specific Sites

A small but important subset of patients with metastatic BC has limited systemic tumour burden and biologically indolent disease. They represent less than 5 % of patients with newly diagnosed metastatic BC. However, for such patients, an intensified multidisciplinary approach combining systemic therapies with surgery, radiation and regional chemotherapy may offer therapeutic benefit and prolong OS.

However, it is not clear from the available evidence if the local therapy is responsible for long-term survival or if these highly selected patients would have done well anyway. Although there is more evidence in favour of surgical resection, alternative approaches such as radiofrequency ablation and stereotactic body radiation therapy are valid therapeutic options.

Patients selected for surgery are younger, with less disseminated disease and less visceral metastases. Patients with significant comorbidities are not recommended for intensive therapies, whereas patients selected for surgery are often those who have good prognostic features and indolent biologic behaviour.

*SELECTION OF PATIENTS.* The factors that have to be evaluated for selecting patients suitable of local treatment are the following:

- *Performance status and comorbidity*: performance status and medical comorbidity should be considered carefully for local treatment, especially surgery, to evaluate postoperative morbidity and mortality. Patients evaluated for lung resection should have a complete pulmonary evaluation, while those being considered for liver resection should have relatively preserved liver function.

- *Extension of metastatic disease*: only patients with limited metastatic disease, i.e. solitary or few detectable lesions (oligo-metastatic disease) and limited to a single organ, are more likely to benefit from local therapy than those with multiple metastases.
- *Disease-free interval (DFI)*: a long disease-free interval is associated with a better outcome with local therapy. The specific cutoff value of DFI that best discriminates between favourable and an unfavourable outcome is unclear.
- *Probability of complete resection*: careful preoperative evaluation is necessary to determine the likelihood of complete resection of the metastatic disease.

#### 18.5.2.1 Treatment of Specific Sites

*Lung Metastases*. Isolated lung metastases occur in 10–25 % of patients with metastatic BC. Pulmonary resection or metastasectomy offers an opportunity for long-term survival in highly selected patients with metastatic BC, with cases series demonstrating 5-year overall survival ranging from 30 to 80 % and median survival duration ranging from 40 to 100 months. Patients most likely to experience long-term survival after metastasectomy are those with solitary metastases and a disease-free interval greater than 36 months. Pulmonary resection may be diagnostic as well as therapeutic in BC patients, since a significant number of solitary pulmonary nodules in patients with a history of BC are not BC metastases.

*Liver Metastases*. Hepatic metastases occur in over half of patients with metastatic BC. They are most commonly a late development, associated with disseminated disease and a poorer prognosis than bone or soft tissue metastases. Only 5–12 % of patients have isolated liver involvement. Hepatic resection for BC metastases may be associated with long-term survival in appropriately selected patients. In a systematic review of 19 studies involving 535 patients who underwent hepatectomy for metastatic BC, the median OS was 40 months (range, 23–77 months) with 5-year survival after resection of 40 % (range, 21–80 %). Postoperative mortality ranged from 0 to 6 % and the complication rate ranged from 0 to 44 %.

Prognostic factors after hepatic resection were positive margins and hormone-refractory disease. Bilobar disease and location close to the *porta hepatis* are typically considered a contraindication to resection. Initial laparoscopic exploration may spare unresectable patients the morbidity of a laparotomy, since up to one-half of patients considered for resection is discovered to have diffuse liver lesions or peritoneal dissemination at the time of laparotomy. Hepatic resection is appropriate for highly selected patients, but alternative local therapies are being increasingly used to treat liver metastases. Liver-directed therapy includes radiofrequency ablation (RFA), stereotactic body RT (SBRT), selective internal RT (SIRT), percutaneous ethanol injection, cryotherapy, hepatic arterial infusion chemotherapy, trans-hepatic arterial chemoembolisation (TACE) and interstitial laser therapy.

*Brain Metastases*. As patients with metastatic BC live longer, the incidence of brain metastases appears to be increasing. The mainstream therapy for brain metastasis is surgery, in selected cases, or radiation therapy that includes whole-brain RT and stereotactic radiosurgery.

*Bone Metastases*. Bone is the most common site of metastatic involvement in BC and can be associated with significant morbidity and mortality. Surgery, RT and RFA can provide effective pain relief and prevent fracture. Surgery and RT are also used for the palliative treatment of epidural spinal cord or nerve compression. Bone-confined metastatic BC is usually characterised by an indolent course and good response to systemic therapy. There is a limited role for resection as a curative option for the majority of bone metastases, except for selected patients with isolated spine or sternal involvement.

Sternal metastases may remain solitary for a long time, possibly because there is no communication with the paravertebral venous plexus through which cancer cells can spread to other bones. In other cases, isolated sternal involvement represents locoregional recurrence (i.e. direct extension from an internal mammary nodal recurrence) rather than true metastatic disease. Surgical resection of BC confined to the sternum may improve quality of life and prolong survival. Bisphosphonates (Zometa®) and denosumab (Prolia®) have been shown to reduce the morbidity of metastatic bone disease, in particular skeletal-related events, which include fracture, need for surgery or radiation to bone, spinal cord compression and hypercalcaemia.

*Abdominal and pelvic metastases*. Limited data suggest that ovarian BC metastases can appear many years following the initial diagnosis of BC and tend to be hormone receptor positive. Surgical evaluation of an ovarian mass may be required to discriminate metastatic BC from a primary ovarian cancer.

## References

1. Goldhirsch A, Winer EP, Coates AS, et al. Personalizing the treatment of women with early breast cancer: highlights of the St Gallen International Expert Consensus on the Primary Therapy of Early Breast Cancer 2013. Ann Oncol. 2013;24:2206–23.
2. NCCN guidelines 2014. www.nccn.org. Accessed 20 June 2014.
3. Davies C, Godwin J, Gray R, et al. on behalf of the Early Breast Cancer Trialists' Collaborative Group (EBCTCG). Relevance of breast cancer hormone receptors and other factors to the efficacy of adjuvant tamoxifen: patient-level meta-analysis of randomised trials. Lancet. 2011;378:771–84.
4. Eisen A, Trudeau M, Shelley W, Messersmith H, Pritchard KI. Aromatase inhibitors in adjuvant therapy for hormone receptor positive breast cancer: a systematic review. Cancer Treat Rev. 2008;34:157–74.
5. Davies C, Pan H, Godwin J, et al. on behalf of the Adjuvant Tamoxifen: Longer Against Shorter (ATLAS) Collaborative Group. Long-term effects of continuing adjuvant tamoxifen to 10 years versus stopping at 5 years after diagnosis of oestrogen receptor-positive breast cancer: ATLAS, a randomised trial. Lancet. 2013;381:805–16.
6. Goss PE, Ingle JN, Pater JL, et al. Late extended adjuvant treatment with letrozole improves outcome in women with early-stage breast cancer who complete 5 years of tamoxifen. J Clin Oncol. 2008;26(12):1948–55.

7. Goel S, Sharma R, Hamilton A, Beith J. LHRH agonists for adjuvant therapy of early breast cancer in premenopausal women. Cochrane Database Syst Rev. 2009;(4):CD004562.
8. Peto R, Davies C, Godwin J, et al. on behalf of the Early Breast Cancer Trialists' Collaborative Group (EBCTCG). Comparisons between different polychemotherapy regimens for early breast cancer: meta-analyses of long-term outcome among 100,000 women in 123 randomised trials. Lancet. 2012;379(9814):432–44.
9. Senkus E, Kyriakides S, Penault-Llorca F, et al. Primary breast cancer: ESMO Clinical Practice Guidelines for diagnosis, treatment and follow-up. Ann Oncol. 2013;24 Suppl 6:vi7–23.
10. Gianni L, Eiermann W, Semiglazov V, et al. Neoadjuvant and adjuvant trastuzumab in patients with HER2-positive locally advanced breast cancer (NOAH): follow-up of a randomised controlled superiority trial with a parallel HER2-negative cohort. Lancet Oncol. 2014;15:640–7.
11. Mauri D, Pavlidis N, Ioannidis JPA. Neoadjuvant versus adjuvant systemic treatment in breast cancer: a meta-analysis. J Natl Cancer Inst. 2005;97:188–94.
12. Cortazar P, Zhang L, Untch M, et al. Pathological complete response and long-term clinical benefit in breast cancer: the CTNeoBC pooled analysis. Lancet. 2014;384(9938):164–72.
13. Gianni L, Pienkowski T, Im YH, et al. Efficacy and safety of neoadjuvant pertuzumab and trastuzumab in women with locally advanced, inflammatory, or early HER2-positive breast cancer (NeoSphere): a randomised multicentre, open-label, phase 2 trial. Lancet Oncol. 2012;13:25–32.
14. Cardoso F, Costa A, Norton L, et al. ESO-ESMO 2nd international consensus guidelines for advanced breast cancer (ABC2). Breast. 2014;23:489–502.
15. Partridge AH, Rumble BR, Carey LA, et al. Chemo- and targeted therapy for women with HER2 negative (or unknown) advanced breast cancer: American Society of Clinical Oncology Clinical Practice Guideline. http://jco.ascopubs.org/content/32/29/3307.full.pdf+html.

## Further Reading

Amir E, Seruga B, Niraula S, et al. Toxicity of adjuvant endocrine therapy in postmenopausal breast cancer patients: a systematic review and meta-analysis. J Natl Cancer Inst. 2011;103:1299–309.

Burstein HJ, Temin S, Anderson H, et al. Adjuvant endocrine therapy for women with hormone receptor-positive breast cancer: American Society of Clinical Oncology Clinical Practice Guideline Focused Update. http://jco.ascopubs.org/cgi/doi/10.1200/JCO.2013.54.2258. Accessed 30 Jan 2015.

De Melo GD, Gonzalez-Angulo A, Lei X, et al. Clinical impact of delaying initiation of adjuvant chemotherapy in patients with breast cancer. J Clin Oncol. 2014;32:735–44.

Dhesy-Thind SK. Screening for osteoporosis in postmenopausal women with breast cancer receiving aromatase inhibitors: less is more? J Clin Oncol. 2012;30:1408–10.

Smith IE, Dowsett M, Yap YS, et al. Adjuvant aromatase inhibitors for early breast cancer after chemotherapy-induced amenorrhoea: caution and suggested guidelines. J Clin Oncol. 2006;24:2444–7.

Untch M, Konecny GE, Paepke S, von Minckwitz G. Current and future role of neoadjuvant therapy for breast cancer. Breast. 2014;23:526–37.

**Websites in Appendix**: *Advanced BC* A-4.1; *Adjuvant Systemic Therapy*, A-4.2; *Clinical Trials*, A-4.6; *Fatigue*, A-4.8.

# Male Breast Diseases

# 19

Oreste D. Gentilini and Chiara Boccardo

## Contents




**Abstract**

• No cause is found in 25 % of patients who develop gynaecomastia. • After persistent pubertal gynaecomastia, medication use and substance use are the most common causes of non-physiologic gynaecomastia. • In adult males gynaecomastia is often multifactorial, due to increased aromatisation of testosterone to oestradiol and the gradual decrease of testosterone production. • In men symptomatic or at high risk, the presence of gynaecomastia or obesity may mask early symptoms of MBC. • Core biopsy should be performed following imaging in those patients with uncertain or suspicious clinical or radiological findings. FNA is not recommended.

*Future directions*. Treatment for men with BC is the same as for women with the disease, but, according to new research, differences have been found that may change the way men will be treated in the future. Superficially, both genders



O.D. Gentilini (✉) • C. Boccardo
Division of Breast Surgery, European Institute of Oncology (IEO), Milano, Italy
e-mail: oreste.gentilini@ieo.it







A.M. Pluchinotta (ed.), *The Outpatient Breast Clinic: Aiming at Best Practice*,
DOI 10.1007/978-3-319-15907-2_19

appeared similar, but using more detailed analysis, subtle variations were observed specifically in relation to the hormone receptors, which influence the growth of most BCs. These findings highlight the need to understand more about how anti-hormone treatments can be optimised.

## 19.1 Gynaecomastia

**Clinical Practice Points**

- Some patients with gynaecomastia may present with breast pain, embarrassment, or cancer phobia. Understanding the patient's concerns can help how direct the treatment.
- In other patients, gynaecomastia is discovered on routine physical examination, and only the patient's perception of an undesirable size makes the condition clinically significant.
- Asymptomatic, stable gynaecomastia is often self-limiting and needs minimal workup.
- The assessment of physiologic gynaecomastia must be carried out in case of hormonal onset rapidly evolving and sore, especially if bilateral.
- Only gynaecomastia that causes severe pain, disfigurement, or social embarrassment should be treated medically or surgically.
- Surgical treatment needs careful consideration and should take into account the causes. Most true gynaecomastia and all pseudo-gynaecomastia should be treated by a plastic surgeon.

### 19.1.1 Overview

Gynaecomastia is defined as generalised enlargement of male breast tissue, with the presence of a rubbery or firm mass extending concentrically and symmetrically from the nipple, accompanied by histopathologically benign proliferation of glandular male breast tissue [1–3].

*True gynaecomastia* should be differentiated from *pseudo-gynaecomastia* (lipomastia), which is characterised by a concentric enlargement due to excess adipose tissue usually present at the periphery of the breast (fatty breast) with no increase in stromal or ductal tissue (Fig. 19.1). In *mixed gynaecomastia* both types can present together. Physical examination method to distinguish gynaecomastia from pseudo-gynaecomastia is discussed in Fig. 19.2.

*Epidemiology*. Gynaecomastia is the most common breast disorder in more than 70–80 % of male breast disorders. The prevalence of gynaecomastia was reported to be between 32 and 65 % [2]. Usually there is a trimodal age distribution [4]: the first peak occurs during infancy, but this condition tends to regress within 3 weeks from the delivery [5]; the second peak occurs during puberty and has a prevalence

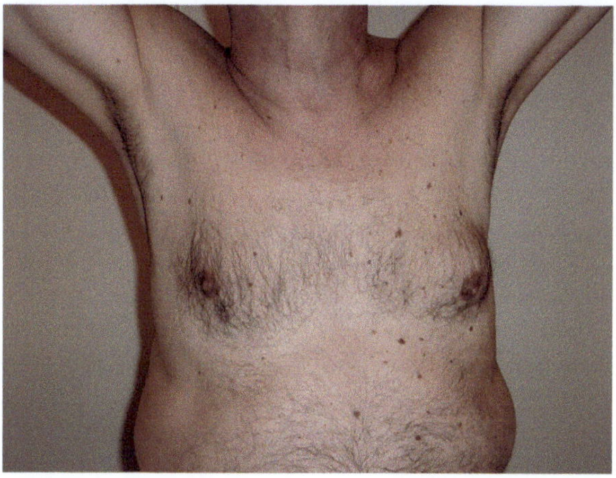

**Fig. 19.1** True even though asymmetrical gynaecomastia in a 62-year-old man

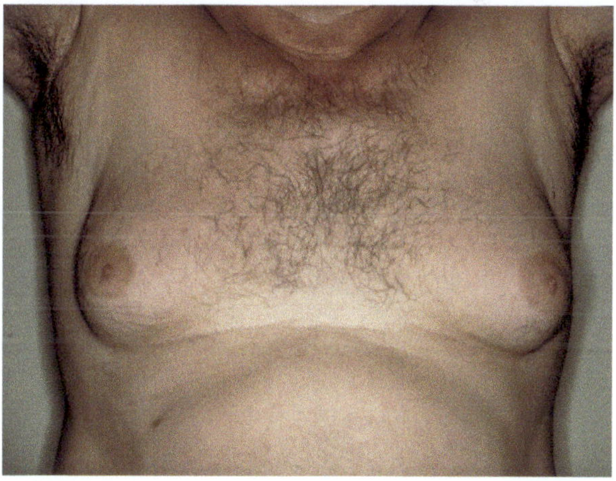

**Fig. 19.2** Pseudo-gynecomastia (lipomastia) in a 50-year-old man, characterised by fat deposition without glandular proliferation

of 4–69 % [2, 5]; it begins between 12 and 14 years old and usually regresses in 18 months [4]. The last peak occurs in senile age (50–80 years old) and seems to be due to increase adiposity typical of this age [5].

*Pathophysiology*. Gynaecomastia results from an altered oestrogen-androgen balance, in favour of oestrogen, or also from increased breast sensitivity to a normal circulating oestrogen level. The imbalance is between the stimulatory effect of oestrogens and the inhibitory effect of androgens [2, 5]. Oestrogens induce ductal epithelial hyperplasia, ductal elongation and branching, proliferation of the periductal fibroblasts, and an increased vascularity.

Oestrogen production in males results mainly from the peripheral conversion of androgens (testosterone and androstenedione) to oestradiol and oestrone, which occurs through the action of the aromatase enzyme. Increased oestrogen production from peripheral conversion due to increased activity of aromatase is observed in chronic liver disease, malnutrition, hyperthyroidism, adrenal tumours, and in rare familial gynaecomastia [6].

Less frequently, an increased substrate can occur at the testicular level due to testicular tumours or to ectopic production of human chorionic gonadotropin (hCG), as is reported with carcinoma of the lung, kidney, gastrointestinal tract, and extragonadal germ cell tumours [6]. Rarely, hyperprolactinaemia may lead to gynaecomastia through its effects on the hypothalamus causing central hypogonadism. Prolactin has also been reported to decrease androgen receptors and increase oestrogen and progesterone receptors in breast cells, which can lead to male gynaecomastia [5].

*Aetiology*. Gynaecomastia can occur as a result of a relative or absolute excess of oestrogens or a relative or absolute decrease in the levels of androgens or their action. An absolute excess of oestrogens might be attributable to administration of exogenous oestrogens or to endogenous overproduction of oestrogens in males. Oestrogens directly stimulate the proliferation of breast tissue, suppress LH secretion (causing hypogonadotropic hypogonadism), and increase serum levels of sex hormone-binding globulin (decreasing levels of free testosterone). Below are briefly described the most frequent causes of gynaecomastia.

- *Altered serum androgen to oestrogen ratio* gather the most common expression of gynaecomastia.

*Puberty*. Gynaecomastia during puberty is extremely common: up to 70 % of all boys might have breast enlargement during puberty. During early puberty, the testes might secrete more oestradiol than they do after puberty, resulting in a relative oestrogen excess. The marked increase in IGF1 levels during puberty could also contribute to the development of pubertal gynaecomastia [9].

*Senile age*. The age-related decline in serum levels of testosterone, increasing adiposity (with resultant raised serum levels of leptin and increased aromatisation of androgens to oestrogens), and rising serum levels of SHBG with a consequent decrease in free testosterone levels all contribute to the relative oestrogen excess in ageing men. In addition older men have multiple co-morbidities and take medications that can contribute to the development of gynaecomastia [8].

*Refeeding gynaecomastia*. Starvation and substantial weight loss cause secondary hypogonadism; return to a normal diet can lead to a 'second puberty' with a transient imbalance in the secretion of oestrogen and androgen, which causes transient gynaecomastia.

*Renal failure and dialysis*. Dialysis-associated gynaecomastia is probably attributable to refeeding of the chronically ill and malnourished patients with renal failure when they are able to expand their diet and their appetite improves after initiating dialysis treatment. Men with chronic kidney disease frequently have low levels of testosterone that are related to both decreased production and increased metabolism of testosterone, and raised serum levels of prolactin are often seen in patients with chronic kidney disease, as a result of decreased renal clearance and increased production of prolactin.

*Hepatic cirrhosis*. Men with alcoholic liver cirrhosis have increased serum levels of androstenedione (with resulting increased aromatisation to oestrone), raised levels of SHBG (with reduced free testosterone levels), and increased serum levels of progesterone, all of which might contribute to the development of gynaecomastia. In addition hypogonadism and testicular atrophy are common in men with alcoholic liver cirrhosis.

*Hyperthyroidism*. Increased serum levels of SHBG and progesterone, as well as increased aromatisation of androgens to oestrogens, might contribute to gynaecomastia.

- *Absolute excess of oestrogens*:
  - Administration of exogenous oestrogens
  - Intentional therapeutic use: therapeutic oestrogens used in prostate cancer treatment and to initiate breast development in male-to-female transgender patients [7]
  - Unintentional exposure to oestrogens: occupational; dietary (phytoestrogens), alcoholic beverages; dietary supplements (dong quai, supplements contaminated with oestrogens); other factors such as transdermal absorption, anti-balding lotions and partner's vaginal lubricants
- *Increased endogenous oestrogen production*:
  - Increased secretion of oestrogens: from the testes (Leydig cell tumours, Sertoli cell tumours, stimulation of normal Leydig cells by human chorionic gonadotropin or luteinising hormone) and from the adrenal glands (feminising adrenocortical tumours)
  - Increased aromatisation of androgens to oestrogens: aromatase excess syndrome, drugs (e.g. androgens and ethanol), alcoholic cirrhosis of the liver, ageing, obesity, hyperthyroidism, human chorionic gonadotropin-secreting tumours, and dietary supplements (contaminated with androgens) [8, 9]
- *Absolute deficiency of androgens* (hypogonadism):
  - Primary hypogonadism:
  - Klinefelter syndrome is the most common chromosomal anomaly in men that leads to primary hypogonadism, gynaecomastia, and infertility.
  - Testicular trauma or testicular radiation.
  - Cancer chemotherapeutic agents.
    Infections (e.g. mumps orchitis, leprosy).
  - Disorders in enzymes of testosterone biosynthesis: drugs (e.g. ketoconazole, spironolactone, metronidazole) and inherited defects in androgen biosynthesis.
  - Secondary hypogonadism (pituitary and/or hypothalamic damage from disease, surgery, or radiation).
- *Decreased androgen action*:
  - Androgen receptor defects
  - Absent or defective androgen receptors
  - Expansion of CAG repeats in the androgen receptor gene
- *Medications or abuse of drugs* [8, 10]:
  - Increased serum levels of oestrogens or oestrogen-like activity
  - Exposure to exogenous oestrogens (intentional or unintentional)
  - Increased aromatisation of androgens to oestrogens (androgens, ethanol abuse)
  - Oestrogen agonist activity (digitoxin)

- *Decreased serum testosterone levels*:
  - Hypogonadotropic hypogonadism (caused by gonadotropin-releasing hormone agonists/antagonists and possibly HAART therapy for HIV)
  - Hypergonadotropic hypogonadism (possible causes: destruction or inhibition of Leydig cells by chemotherapeutic/cytotoxic agents (e.g. alkylating agents, vincristine, methotrexate, nitrosoureas, cisplatin, imatinib) or inhibition of testosterone or DHT biosynthesis by ketoconazole, metronidazole, high doses of spironolactone, or finasteride and dutasteride)
- *Androgen receptor blockade*:
  - Flutamide, bicalutamide, and enzalutamide
  - Cimetidine
  - Marijuana
  - Spironolactone
- *Increased serum prolactin levels*:
  - Antipsychotic agents
  - Metoclopramide
  - Possibly calcium channel blockers
- *Less known causes*:
  - Isoniazid
  - Digoxin
  - Effective HAART therapy for HIV infection
  - Human growth hormone
  - Amiodarone
  - Calcium channel blockers (e.g. nifedipine, verapamil, diltiazem)
  - Amphetamines
  - Diazepam
  - Antidepressants (tricyclic and selective serotonin reuptake inhibitors)

### 19.1.2 Clinical Assessment and Diagnosis

*Clinical history* should include the following: [5, 6]

- Age of onset and duration of the condition
- Any recent changes in nipple size and any pain or discharge from the nipples
- History of parotitis, testicular trauma, and alcohol or drug use
- Family history of gynaecomastia
- History of sexual dysfunction, infertility, or hypogonadism

*Physical examination* should include the following [5, 6]:

- Examination of the breasts, with attention to volume, area, tissue consistency, surrounding skin redundancy, and areolar size.

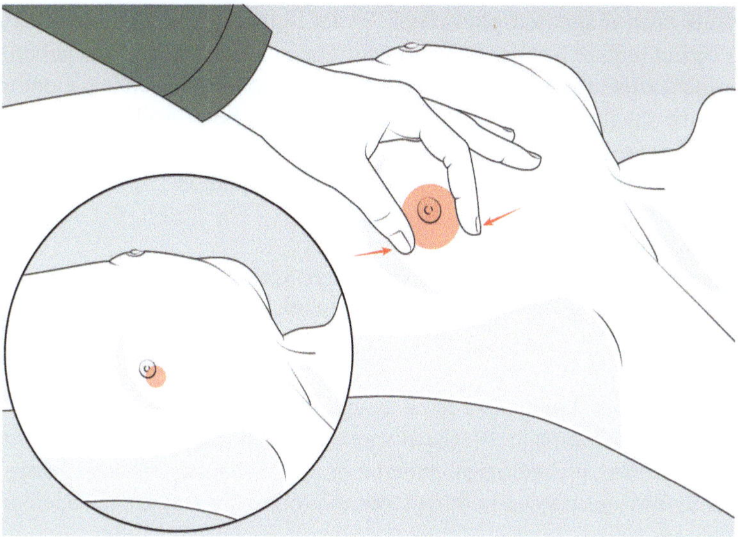

**Fig. 19.3** Examination for gynaecomastia. Physical examination method to distinguish gynaecomastia, due to enlargement of the glandular tissue, from pseudo-gynaecomastia, due to excessive adipose tissue. The thumb and forefinger are placed on opposite sides of the enlarged breast and slowly brought together towards the areolar-nipple complex. Gynaecomastia is appreciated as a concentric, rubbery-to-firm disc of tissue, often mobile, located directly beneath the areolar area. Pseudo-gynaecomastia presents no discrete mass. Note that other masses due to disorders such as cancer tend to be eccentrically positioned (insert)

- Firm (glandular) and soft (fatty) tissue may require testing to differentiate between true gynaecomastia and pseudo-gynaecomastia.
- Assessment of any nipple discharge.
- The chest wall should be observed for obvious signs of deformity.
- The axilla should also be examined for the presence or absence of pathological lymph nodes.

In general, palpable, firm glandular tissue in a concentric mass around the nipple-areolar complex is most consistent with gynaecomastia (Fig. 19.3). Increase in subareolar fat is more likely pseudo-gynaecomastia, whereas hard, immobile masses should be considered breast carcinoma until proven otherwise. Similarly, masses associated with skin changes, nipple retraction, nipple discharge, or enlarged lymph nodes should raise concern for malignancy.

In some cases diagnosis should be extended throughout:

- Examination of the testes, with attention to size and consistency, as well as nodules or asymmetry
- Observation of any signs of feminisation
- Checking for any signs of chronic liver disease, thyroid disease, or renal disease

Patients with diagnosed physiologic gynaecomastia or pseudo-gynaecomastia usually do not require further evaluation. Similarly, asymptomatic and pubertal gynaecomastia do not require further tests and should be re-evaluated in 6 months. Only rare prepubertal (premature) gynaecomastia should be considered for additional testing or close re-evaluation.

Further evaluation is necessary in the following situations:

- Breast size greater than 5 cm (*macromastia*)
- A lump that is tender, of recent onset, progressive, or of unknown duration
- Suspicious signs of malignancy (hard or non-concentric lump, positive lymph node findings)

*Laboratory tests* should be ordered using a stepwise approach guided by history and physical examination [5, 6]. Usually tests are not indicated in patients with fatty breast enlargement, physiological pubertal or senile changes, identified drug cause, or clinically obvious cancer. In other cases the following may be considered:

- Serum chemistry panel in hepatic and renal failure
- Thyroid-stimulating hormone (TSH) and free thyroxin levels in hyperthyroidism
- Serum concentrations of hCG, luteinising hormone, oestradiol, and free testosterone to differentiate pathologic causes if gynaecomastia is of recent onset, painful, or tender, without liver, adrenal, or testicular abnormalities

*Imaging*. Mammography is the primary imaging method. It accurately distinguishes between malignant and benign male breast diseases and can differentiate true gynaecomastia from a mass that requires tissue sampling to exclude malignancy, reducing the need for biopsies. In cases of pseudo-gynaecomastia, breast tissue is filled with radiolucent adipose tissue [2, 6]. Breast ultrasound is widely used in the diagnosis of gynaecomastia cases and is more comfortable for male patients. Scrotal USG and abdominal computerised tomography (CT) can also be used to rule out other causes of the disease [3]. If it is not possible to differentiate between gynaecomastia and breast with physical and imaging findings, a percutaneous biopsy should be taken although the number of cells taken in a gynaecomastia biopsy is often insufficient, because gynaecomastia is a predominantly fibrous lesion and this can cause false negative.

### 19.1.3 Treatment

Before beginning treatment, the patient should be informed that gynaecomastia is often self-limiting. Over time fibrotic tissue replaces the symptomatic proliferation of glandular tissue, meaning that the pain and tenderness will resolve. In pubertal males, 85–90 % of cases regress between 6 m and 2 years, and continuation after the age of 17 is rare.

If a reversible cause of gynaecomastia is suspected (e.g. medications, recreational drugs, occupational exposure to oestrogens, or hyperthyroidism), the medication or source of gynaecomastia should be withdrawn or avoided, respectively, if at all possible. Treatment might be considered in males with symptomatic gynaecomastia or for cosmetic reasons (as breast enlargement can cause considerable social anxiety in many young men).

*Nonsurgical treatment.* Patient and parent reassurance of the transient and benign nature is often all that is required in the management of most cases of idiopathic gynaecomastia. If the patient has pain or tenderness or experiences embarrassment or distress, a trial of medical therapy should be offered.

In most cases medical management benefits from a high success rate and avoids further surgery. It should be considered that the evidence for the commonly prescribed drugs, tamoxifen and danazol, is based on small non-randomised trials and does not include recurrence rates, optimum dose, length of treatment, or associated long-term risks.

As gynaecomastia is usually the result of an imbalance of androgens and oestrogens, medical therapy for gynaecomastia is based on decreasing oestrogen production (using aromatase inhibitors), or action (with antioestrogens), and/or increasing the levels of androgens (with the use of systemic or topical androgens). Medical therapy of gynaecomastia will probably be most effective if used in patients with recent (within 2 years) onset of breast enlargement [5].

Antioestrogens such as tamoxifen and raloxifene block oestrogen action in breast tissue but might have an oestrogen agonist action at other tissues. Tamoxifen doses of 10–20 mg daily used for 3–9 months have shown efficacy of up to 90 % for the resolution of gynaecomastia [11, 12].

Aromatase inhibitors (anastrozole) might have an important role in selected patients with increased aromatisation of androgens to oestrogens. Testosterone therapy usually improves gynaecomastia in men with hypogonadism [13].

Danazol might be considered in a short 6-week course, with 100 mg twice a day for the first week followed by 100 mg three times a day from the second to sixth weeks; the response will be assessed at the eighth week. Repeat courses may be required.

Prophylactic breast radiation has been successfully used in older men (mostly >50 years of age) with prostate cancer to prevent or decrease new-onset gynaecomastia or breast pain and tenderness after starting antiandrogen therapy.

*Surgical treatment.* In men with long-standing, symptomatic gynaecomastia, medical therapy will probably be ineffective, and surgery can be considered. Surgery might also be considered if a patient does not respond to medical therapy, is unable to tolerate it or declines treatment, or if the patient prefers surgery for cosmetic reasons or wants immediate correction of gynaecomastia. The classic surgical approach with semicircular periareolar incision was the standard operation for excision of gynaecomastia.

However, the surgical management of gynaecomastia has undergone significant changes over the past decades, from a predominantly open approach to a mini-invasive involving liposuction [14, 15].

Several classifications of gynaecomastia can be used in order to plan surgery, but a classification system that is qualitative or descriptive is to be preferred to a quantitative or specific one, in terms of grammes of tissue removed. The American Society of Plastic Surgeons' classification, for instance, lists four grades of gynaecomastia:

- Grade I. Small breast enlargement with localised button of tissue around the areola
- Grade II. Moderate breast enlargement exceeding areola boundaries with edges that are indistinct from the chest
- Grade III. Moderate breast enlargement exceeding areola boundaries with edges that are distinct from the chest with skin redundancy
- Grade IV. Marked breast enlargement with skin redundancy and feminisation of the breast

Potential candidates for surgery are patients rated as Grade II, III, or IV after systemic conditions have been ruled out. Various surgical techniques can be used; the technique used depends on the consistency of the tissue and the amount of redundant skin. Tissue may be removed by direct excision or liposuction or a combination of both.

This is particularly recommended for pseudo-gynaecomastia that, because of its skin redundancy, should be better treated by a plastic surgeon. Fatty tissue, usually present in the periphery of the chest, is amenable to liposuction through a periareolar or an inframammary crease approach. Fibrous, glandular tissue resides deep to the areola and may require direct excision through a periareolar incision.

## 19.2 Other Male Breast Disorders

Excluding gynaecomastia, any other disease of the male breast is uncommon, even if most diseases of the breast that affect women have also been reported in men. Although there is no lobular activity in the male, extremely rare lesions can have their origin in lobular tissue, chiefly in XXY phenotypes and in patients with long-standing raised oestrogen levels.

*Fibroadenomas* require oestrogen stimulation so it is not surprising that most examples recorded in males have mainly occurred in patients receiving oestrogen treatment for prostatic cancer, especially when the doses used have been in excess of those normally recommended. Most recorded cases of male fibroadenomas are associated with gynaecomastia, and some phyllodes tumours have also been described in men with gynaecomastia.

*Ductal ectasia* is a rare clinical entity, mainly involving one or few ducts, with possibility of periductal mastitis. Nevertheless nipple discharge due to duct ectasia is very uncommon. The incidence of duct ectasia is increased in HIV-positive males who have a susceptibility to develop subareolar abscesses.

*Nipple discharge and papilloma.* An array of proliferative lesions of the ducts, ranging from papillary hyperplasia in gynaecomastia to papilloma and invasive papillary carcinoma, has been observed, in most cases associated to gynaecomastia or nodular lesions, less frequently associated with nipple discharge (Fig. 19.4).

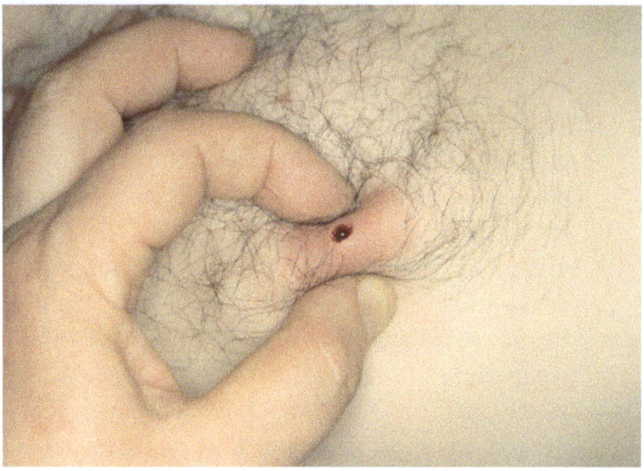

**Fig. 19.4** Bloody nipple discharge as a clinical sign of a male intraductal papilloma

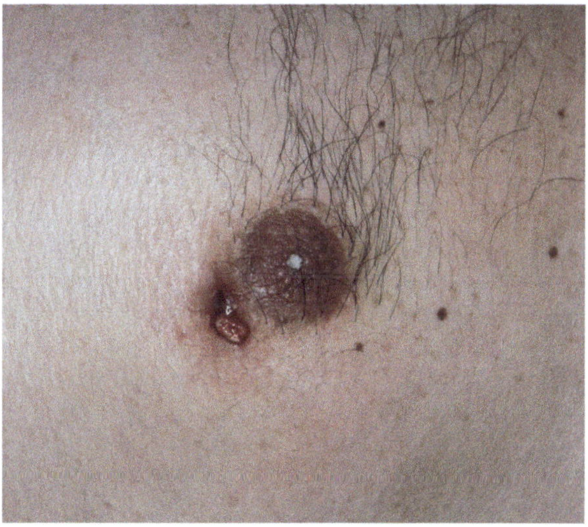

**Fig. 19.5** Subareolar recurrent breast abscess in a 50-year-old man

*Infections* and abscesses are being seen more commonly in HIV-positive and otherwise immunocompromised males, so any infective episodes should raise the possibility of HIV infection. Not all periareolar infections in men are due to duct ectasia (Fig. 19.5). More commonly, inflammatory masses around the nipple in men are due to retention cysts or infection in adjacent skin structures.

*Lymphoma* of the breast tissue is another disease observed in HIV-positive male, associated with gynaecomastia secondary to retroviral drugs.

*Others*. Lipoma gives a soft asymmetric lobulated breast enlargement. A sebaceous cyst is a lump close to the skin than a part of deeper tissue, characterised by a drainage of pus from the site. Fat necrosis, haematoma, or postsurgical changes may appear in men who have a history of trauma or surgery.

## 19.3 Male Breast Cancer

**Clinical Practice Points**

- Although MBC is not treated significantly different to female BC, it should be considered a rare and unique disease, rather than being considered as an analogous to postmenopausal female.
- The impression that MBC has a worse prognosis may derive from the tendency for later diagnosis. Back to front high tumour grade and ER- and PR-negative expressions are less frequent.
- Up to 20 % of MBC patients report a family history of BC, and about one in six men with MBC will have a prostate cancer in their lifetime. Moreover having prostate cancer may increase a man's risk of developing BC.

### 19.3.1 Risk Factors

Male breast cancer (MBC) accounts for less than 1 % of all cancers in men and less than 1 % of BCs. About 10 % of BCs in men are in situ disease. Median age at the diagnosis is 65 years old, approximately 5 years older than the mean age of female BC [16].

*Genetics*. Men with Klinefelter syndrome have a risk of developing BC 20–50 times higher. Studies had estimated that 3–7. 5 % of men with BC have this syndrome. A family history of breast or ovarian cancer is reported in approximately 15–20 % of MBC and confers a relative risk of 2.5.

It is estimated that approximately 10 % of MBC have a genetic predisposition, BRCA 2 being the most prevalent gene mutation. It is estimated that these mutations contribute to 4–40 % of hereditary BC in men, compared to 5–10 % of female BC. The American Society of Clinical Oncology (ASCO) recommends that men with BC should be considered for genetic counselling and testing [17]. MBC has also been associated with PTEN, p53, and CHEK2 mutations. Germ-line mutations in the androgen receptor have been identified in few cases of MBC and have been speculated as a risk factor for this disease due to changes in androgen-oestrogen balance.

*Endocrine*. The endocrine influence in terms of oestrogen excess and lack of androgens contributes to several conditions associated to the risk of MBC [18]. Men with liver disease are also at risk due to increased production of androstenedione from the adrenal glands and subsequent aromatisation to oestrone, finally converted to oestradiol [19]. The association of obesity and MBC is biologically explained by the increased peripheral aromatisation of oestrogen is documented.

Testicular abnormalities as undescended testis, congenital inguinal hernia, orchiectomy, mumps orchitis (older than 20 years), testicular injury, and infertility have been associated with MBC risk, which is possibly related to the reduction of testosterone levels associated to these conditions [20]. Finally case reports of MBC in men with hyperprolactinaemia due to pituitary adenomas are described [21].

*Race*. Black men have a higher incidence of BC compared to white men, with incidence of 1.8 per 100, 000 and 1.1 per 100, 000, respectively. They also present with more aggressive disease, higher grade, larger tumour size, and higher rate of nodal involvement [22].

*Other risk factors*. Sasco et al. [23] reported an increased risk of 1.6–1.9 for the use of radiotherapy to treat unilateral gynaecomastia and thymic enlargement. A slight increase in the risk was seen with alcohol consumption and cigarette smoking, but no dose-response relationship was found, possibly related to small numbers. The association of gynaecomastia with MBC is also not clear, as the incidence of this abnormality in this disease reported in epidemiologic studies is similar to the general population.

### 19.3.2 Clinical Features and Diagnosis

Male breast tumours are usually found by palpation. The most common presentation is a painless subareolar mass. Other clinical features include nipple retraction (10–51 %), local pain (4–20 %), nipple ulceration (4–17 %), nipple discharge (1–12 %), and nipple bleeding (1–9 %) [24]. Bilateral MBC is a rare form of presentation (less than 2 %). Clinically suspected axillary nodes are identified in half of patients at the time of diagnosis.

The SEER data evaluating 2,524 cases of female BC has shown that men are significantly older at diagnosis ($P<0.0001$), are more likely to present with later-stage disease ($P<0.0001$), and have larger tumours ($P<0.0001$), nodal involvement ($P<0.0001$), ductal histology ($P<0.0001$), and ER-positive tumours ($P<0.0001$) [16].

*Imaging*. Mammographic and sonographic findings are usually present at the time of diagnosis, but microcalcifications are less common in male than in female BC. The sensitivity and specificity of mammography in this setting are 92 and 90 %, respectively [25]. The main differential diagnosis of a breast mass in a man is gynaecomastia. Others include breast abscess, metastases to the breast, and other non-BC primary tumours. Diagnosis and pathologic evaluation are the same as in women.

*Histopathology and biomarkers*. The majority of MBC are invasive ductal type (85–95 %), followed by ductal carcinoma in situ (10 %). This is explained by the low differentiation of male breast tissue to lobule formation, unless hyperoestrogenism occurs. Other tumour types such as invasive papilloma and medullary carcinoma are rare, but papillary carcinoma is most frequent in men (2–4 %) than in women. The frequency of oestrogen receptor positivity in MBC is higher than in female BC with more than 90 % of tumours being positive for both oestrogen and progesterone receptors [26].

The data on over-expression of the HER2 have been inconsistent. The studies included a small number of patients, and no standardised methodology to access HER2 is reported. Recent series revealed 2–15 % of HER2 positivity in MBC [19]. Expression of androgen receptor has been reported, but its prognostic factor is still uncertain.

### 19.3.3 Treatment and Prognosis

*Surgery*. Literature describes rates of modified radical mastectomy in MBC as approximately 70 %, radical mastectomy 8–30 %, total mastectomy 5–14 %, and lumpectomy with or without radiation 1–13 % [27].

Axillary dissection has been usually performed in invasive BC for sampling or clearance. Lymph node involvement is present in approximately 50 % of men, and in 40 % more than three nodes are affected by the disease [16, 27]. Sentinel node biopsy has been proven to be feasible in men [28] and should be performed whenever axillary nodes are negative at clinical and imaging assessment.

*Radiation therapy*. The indications for adjuvant radiation therapy for MBC should follow the accepted guidelines for female BC [27, 29].

*Systemic treatment*. Hormonal therapy has been the mainstay of treatment for metastatic MBC, and in the past the first treatment strategy in this setting was bilateral orchiectomy and adrenalectomy. Tamoxifen is the most extensively studied drug in MBC and is recommended in adjuvant setting for hormonal receptor-positive tumours for 5 years. Retrospective data provides outcomes of MBC treated with tamoxifen versus no hormonal treatment. In Giordano's study 92 % of patients received tamoxifen, which was associated with decreased recurrence and improved overall survival [30]. Tamoxifen is worse tolerated by men than women: side effects include decreased libido (29 %), weight gain (25 %), hot flashes (21 %), mood alteration (21 %), depression (17 %), insomnia (12 %), and thrombosis (4 %). These discomforts were severe enough to lead to treatment interruption in about 21 % of cases.

Tamoxifen has response rates over 80 %, whereas the role of aromatase inhibitors (AIs) in advanced MBC is still unclear because only small case series are available [31]. Data on adjuvant chemotherapy for MBC come from small and non-randomised studies but consistently suggest a reduction in the risk of recurrence and death and should therefore be considered for men with intermediate or high-risk early BC, especially those with hormone-receptor-negative disease.

The larger data on adjuvant chemotherapy comes from a study performed by Giordano et al. [24] analysing a 14-year follow-up of 135 cases of MBC, where 25 % of patients received chemotherapy alone and 37 % received chemotherapy and hormonal therapy. The use of chemotherapy was associated with a nonsignificant lower risk of death (hazard ratio = 0.78).

Chemotherapy for metastatic MBC has been used as second- or third-line treatment after endocrine therapy failure as response is more favourable to endocrine treatment in this setting or in oestrogen receptor-negative patients or in cases of life-threatening lesions. There are no data on the benefit of adjuvant trastuzumab in MBC because HER2 amplification in these patients is rare (2–15 %).

*Prognosis and survival*. Estimates for overall 5-year survival are around 36–66 % [16]. The most important prognostic indicators are stage at diagnosis and lymph nodal status. Five-year survival has been reported as 75–100 % for stage I disease, 50–80 % for stage II disease, and 30–60 % for stage III disease [25]. Studies suggest a worse survival for men with BC compared to women, but this is most probably related to the fact that men are diagnosed with more advanced disease and at an older age.

## References


1. Braunstein GD. Clinical practise. Gynecomastia. N Engl J Med. 2007;20(357):1229–37.
2. Rahmani S, Turton P, Shaaban A, Dall B. Overview of gynecomastia in the modern era and the Leeds Gynaecomastia Investigation algorithm. Breast J. 2011;17:246–55.
3. Handschin AE, Bietry D, Hüsler R, Banic A, Constantinescu M. Surgical management of gynecomastia- a 10 year analysis. World J Surg. 2008;32:38–44.
4. Gikas P, Mokbel K. Management of gynaecomastia: an update. Int J Clin Pract. 2007;61:1209–15.
5. Carlson HE. Approach to the patient with gynecomastia. J Clin Endocrinol Metab. 2011;96:15–21.
6. Johnson RE, Murad MH. Gynecomastia: pathophysiology, evaluation, and management. Mayo Clin Proc. 2009;84:1010–5.
7. Dobs A, Darkes MJ. Incidence and management of gynecomastia in men treated for prostate cancer. J Urol. 2005;174:1737–42.
8. Deepinder F, Braunstein GD. Drug-induced gynecomastia: an evidence-based review. Expert Opin Drug Saf. 2012;11:779–95.
9. Mieritz MG, Sorensen K, Aksglaede L, et al. Elevated serum IGFI, but unaltered sex steroid levels, in healthy boys with pubertal gynaecomastia. Clin Endocrinol (Oxf). 2014;80:691–8.
10. Bowman JD, Kim H, Bustamante JJ. Drug-induced gynecomastia. Pharmacotherapy. 2012;32:1123–40.
11. Boccardo F, et al. Evaluation of tamoxifen and anastrozole in the prevention of gynecomastia and breast pain induced by bicalutamide monotherapy of prostate cancer. J Clin Oncol. 2005;23:808–15.
12. Perdonà S, et al. Efficacy of tamoxifen and radiotherapy for prevention and treatment of gynaecomastia and breast pain caused by bicalutamide in prostate cancer: a randomised controlled trial. Lancet Oncol. 2005;6:295–300.
13. Plourde PV, Reiter EO, Jou HC, et al. Safety and efficacy of anastrozole for the treatment of pubertal gynecomastia: a randomized, double-blind, placebo-controlled trial. J Clin Endocrinol Metab. 2004;89:4428–33.
14. Petty PM, Solomon M, Buchel EW, et al. Gynecomastia: evolving paradigm of management and comparison of techniques. Plast Reconstr Surg. 2010;125:1301–8.
15. Cordova A, Moschella F. Algorithm for clinical evaluation and surgical treatment of gynaecomastia. J Plast Reconstr Aesthet Surg. 2008;61:41–9.
16. Giordano SH, Cohen DS, Buzdar AU, Perkins G, Hortobagyi GN. Breast carcinoma in men: a population-based study. Cancer. 2004;101:51–7.
17. Korde LA, Zujewski JA, Kamin L, et al. Multidisciplinary meeting on male breast cancer: summary and research recommendations. J Clin Oncol. 2010;28:2114–22.
18. Thomas DB, Jimenez LM, McTiernan A, et al. Breast cancer in men: risk factors with hormonal implications. Am J Epidemiol. 1992;135:734–8.
19. Gómez-Raposo C, Zambrana-Tévar F, Sereno-Moyano M, López-Gómez M, Casado E. Male breast cancer. Cancer Treat Rev. 2010;36:451–7.
20. D'Avanzo B, LaVecchia C. Risk factors for male breast cancer. Br J Cancer. 1995;71:1359–62.
21. Okada K, Kajiwara S, Tanaka H, Sakamoto G. Synchronous bilateral non- invasive ductal carcinoma of the male breast: a case report. Breast Cancer. 2003;10:163–6.
22. Anderson WF, Jatoi I, Tse J, Rosenberg PS. Male breast cancer: a population-based comparison with female breast cancer. J Clin Oncol. 2009;28:232–9.
23. Sasco AJ, Lowenfels AB, Pasker-deJong J. Review article: epidemiology of male breast cancer. A meta-analysis of published case-control studies and discussion of selected etiological factors. Int J Cancer. 1993;53:538–49.
24. Giordano SH, Valero V, Buzdar AU, Hortobagyi GN. Efficacy of anastrozole in male breast cancer. Am J Clin Oncol. 2002;25:235–7.
25. Fentiman IS, Fourquet A, Hortobagyi GN. Male breast cancer. Lancet. 2006;367:595–604.

26. Shaaban AM, et al. A comparative biomarker study of 514 matched cases of male and female breast cancer reveals gender-specific biological differences. Breast Cancer Res Treat. 2012;133:949–95.
27. Cutuli B. Strategies in treating male breast cancer. Expert Opin Pharmacother. 2007;8: 193–202.
28. Gentilini O, Chagas E, Zurrida S, et al. Sentinel lymph node biopsy in male patients with early breast cancer. Oncologist. 2007;12:512.
29. Katz A, Buchholz TA, Thames H, et al. Recursive partitioning analysis of locoregional recurrence patterns following mastectomy: implications for adjuvant irradiation. Int J Radiat Oncol Biol Phys. 2001;50:397–403.
30. Giordano SH, Perkins GH, Broglio K, et al. Adjuvant systemic therapy for male breast carcinoma. Cancer. 2005;104:2359–64.
31. Doyen J, Italiano A, Largillier R, Ferrero JM, Fontana X, Thyss A. Aromatase inhibition in male breast cancer patients: biological and clinical implications. Ann Oncol. 2010;21: 1243–5.

## Further Reading

ASPS. Gynecomastia, Practice Parameters. www.plasticsurgery.org/Documents/Gynecomastia-PP.pdf. Accessed 30 Jan 2015.

Cloyd JM, Hernandez-Boussard T, Wapnir IL. Outcomes of partial mastectomy in male breast cancer patients: analysis of SEER, 1983-2009. Ann Surg Oncol. 2013;20:1545–50.

Doyen J, Italiano A, Largillier R, et al. Aromatase inhibition in male breast cancer patients: biological and clinical implications. Ann Oncol. 2010;21:1243–5.

Giordano SH, Hortobagyi GN. Leuprolide acetate plus aromatase inhibition for male breast cancer. J Clin Oncol. 2006;24:e42–3.

Greif JM, Pezzi CM, Klimberg VS. Gender differences in breast cancer: analysis of 13,000 breast cancers in men from the National Cancer Data Base. Ann Surg Oncol. 2012;19:3199–204.

Hurwitz DJ. Boomerang pattern correction of gynaecomastia. Plast Reconstr Surg. 2015;135: 433–6.

Ruddy KJ, Winer EP. Male breast cancer: risk factors, biology, diagnosis, treatment and survivorship. Ann Oncol. 2013;24:1434–43.

**Websites in Appendix**: *Male BC*, A-4.14.

# 20 Loco-regional Breast Cancer Recurrences

Oreste D. Gentilini and Chiara Boccardo

## Contents



**Abstract**

• A minority of patients treated both by breast conservation and mastectomy will develop a local recurrence, which remains one of the greatest concerns of primary BC treatment. • In contrast with past studies that showed an incidence of local recurrence around 10–20 %, in the present time a very low incidence of local recurrences has been described, with a cumulative incidence of 1.1 % at 5 years. • Local recurrence can be considered a marker of tumour aggressiveness as it is linked to an increased risk of distant metastases and death. Therefore, all patients with local recurrence should undergo workup to rule out concurrent distant metastases. On the other hand, patients with isolated local or regional recurrence, without synchronous distant localisations, can be successfully treated. • Principal risk factors involved in local recurrence are tumour size, nodal status, tumour biology, age, margins and histopathological characteristics. • Mastectomy is considered

O.D. Gentilini (✉) • C. Boccardo
Division of Breast Surgery, European Institute of Oncology (IEO), Milano, Italy
e-mail: oreste.gentilini@ieo.it



A.M. Pluchinotta (ed.), *The Outpatient Breast Clinic: Aiming at Best Practice*,
DOI 10.1007/978-3-319-15907-2_20

the current standard of care for ipsilateral recurrence of BC; however, some retrospective analyses showed that second conservative treatments for local relapse were feasible and gave results comparable to standard mastectomy.

*Future Directions*. Further studies are needed to delineate optimal management of recurrences. Novel treatments, including cryotherapy, radiofrequency ablation and photodynamic and microwave therapy, will continue to be explored to move toward less aggressive but more effective local management of local recurrences. However, important impulses are expected from the potential utility of genomic profiles in estimating the usefulness of more tailored approaches to systemic therapy including recognition and use of newer biological agents.

## 20.1 Characteristics of Recurrence Patterns

**Clinical Practice Points**

- The clinical significance of an isolated local recurrence as a first event after treatment of early-stage invasive BC and its impact on survival remain controversial.
- The clinical features of recurrent BC together with their therapeutic implications could be highly influenced by some previous treatments.
- True ipsilateral breast recurrence (IBTR) of the original tumour in some cases is difficult to differentiate from a new primary tumour.
- The presence of a palpable mass in the axilla or in the supraclavicular fossa should be considered a tumour recurrence until otherwise proven.
- For a woman, learning that she has a recurrent BC may be harder than dealing with the initial diagnosis.

### 20.1.1 Introduction

Survival of early-stage breast cancer patients after breast-conserving surgery and breast radiotherapy is equivalent to survival after mastectomy [1, 2], and today breast conservation is the treatment of choice for early-stage breast cancer worldwide. A minority of patients treated both by breast conservation and mastectomy will develop a local or loco-regional recurrence, which remains one of the greatest concerns of primary breast cancer treatment [3–5].

*Definitions*. Recurrence is a reappearance of a treated BC in a patient previously considered no evidence of disease. BC can recur at any time (or not at all), but most recurrences, even many years after treatment. Types of recurrence are many and the terms to define them are:

- *Local recurrence*, when recurrence occurs in the residual breast after breast-conserving treatment (BCT), which includes BCS and RT, or in the soft tissues of the anterior chest after mastectomy

- *Ipsilateral breast tumour recurrence* (*IBTR*), when recurs after lumpectomy and breast irradiation in either the skin or parenchyma of the ipsilateral breast without clinical-radiologic evidence of regional or distant disease
- *Loco-regional recurrence* (*LRR*), when relapse occurs in the ipsilateral axillary, internal mammary or supraclavicular lymph nodes
- *Distant recurrence*, when disease relapses outside the ipsilateral breast, chest wall or regional lymph nodes

*Epidemiology*. In the past, most of the series published had reported that approximately 10–20 % of patients with stage I/II invasive BC can develop an IBTR within 10 years of breast-conserving surgery and radiation therapy [6, 7]. In approximately 60–90 % of cases, IBRT occurs in the same quadrant where the original primary tumour was located, and 60–85 % of recurrences show the same histologic subtype of the primary tumour.

However, nowadays a very low incidence of local recurrences has been shown, with a cumulative incidence of 1.1 % at 5 years [8]. This important result highlights the unequivocal improvement of the conservative approach achieved in the last few years, as well as the significantly prolonged median interval after adjuvant systemic therapy. In addition local recurrence should not be considered as a failure of conservative approach or responsible for systemic progression by itself: previous randomised trials have shown that groups of patients with a high incidence of local recurrences have the same overall survival as that of patients with a low rate of local recurrence [1, 2]. A plausible interpretation is that local recurrence is a marker of tumour aggressiveness and an indicator of an increased likelihood of distant metastases [3–5].

*Risk Factors*. Several investigators have proposed combining multiple factors responsible of local recurrence. These comprise tumour size, nodal status, oestrogen receptor status, molecular subtype, young age, positive microscopic margins, extensive intraductal component, higher grading, vessel invasion multifocality and lymphovascular invasion. Multivariate analysis stratified by treatment showed that young age was an independent prognostic factor for increased local recurrence.

Moreover, the clinical features of recurrent BC together with their therapeutic implications could be highly influenced by some previous treatments as:

- In BCS, the use of neoadjuvant therapy to downsize the primary tumour
- In mastectomy, the radiation therapy for women at risk of chest wall recurrence
- In SLNB, the possible presence of missed involved residual nodes
- In oncoplastic surgery, the structural modification of the area targeted by the radiation boost

### 20.1.2 Clinical Presentations

*Ipsilateral breast recurrences*. Approximately one fourth to one half of local recurrences after initial treatment of invasive cancers with BCT are detected solely by routine mammography. This variability in detecting local recurrences emphasises

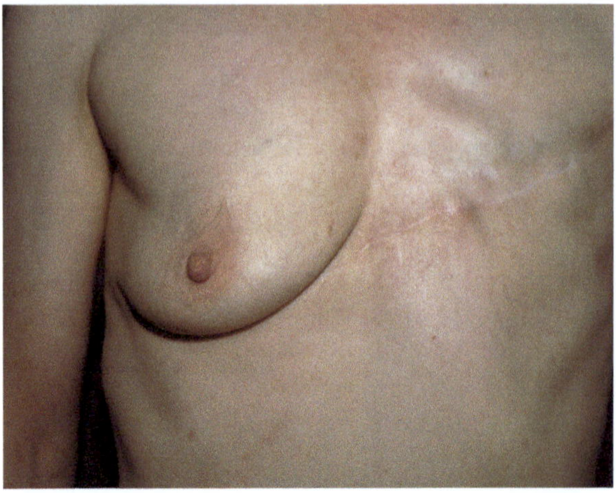

**Fig. 20.1** Solitary nodular chest wall recurrence 3 years after a mastectomy

the need for following patients with both mammography and physical examination. In general, the clinical and radiologic characteristics of recurrent lesions are similar to those of the initially presenting tumours, so that tumours initially presenting as masses or distortions without calcifications usually recurred as masses or distortions and tumours initially presenting with calcifications recurred with calcifications.

The physical examination following breast-conservation treatment often shows only mild thickening without a mass effect. Changes in the physical examination that occur more than 1–2 years following the completion of radiation treatment must be viewed as suspicious. Either surgery or radiation treatment may cause a change in physical examination, such as a mass-like region of fibrosis that may occasionally be difficult clinically to distinguish from a local recurrence. The findings associated with a local recurrence may be subtle, especially when the primary tumour was infiltrating lobular carcinoma. Recurrences of these lesions can produce only minimal thickening or retraction at the biopsy site without a mass [9], while nodular appearances are rare, usually due to a more aggressive disease.

*Chest wall recurrence* after a mastectomy may appear as one (single spot) or more (multiple spots) painless nodules, located either on or under the skin, or as an area of skin thickening along or close to the mastectomy scar. Solitary nodules (Fig. 20.1) are observed in more than half of patients with chest-wall-only recurrences while the remainder have more than one nodule or diffuse chest wall disease. A widespread skin and soft tissue involvement is rare, and it is generally associated with inflammatory changes. The majority of these recurrences involves the chest wall alone, while they rarely occur simultaneously with regional nodal failure.

In the presence of postirradiation fibrosis, early diagnosis of local recurrence may be challenging. Recurrences appear as macular erythema, pruritic or no pruritic, or small papules, or hyperpigmented superficial plaques with surrounding areas of erythema (Fig. 20.2). If the skin lesions had appeared 1 month earlier and

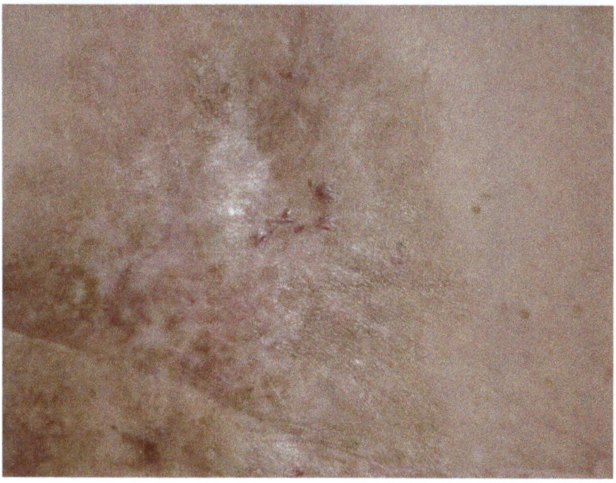

**Fig. 20.2** Hyperpigmented superficial plaques with surrounding erythema, a kind of biopsy-proven recurrence appeared about 1 year after a mastectomy followed by radiation therapy

had not improved with over-the-counter topical preparations applied by the patient, biopsy is mandatory.

*Loco-regional failures* may include lump or swelling of lymph nodes in the axilla or in the supraclavicular fossa. The presence of a palpable mass in the axilla or in the supraclavicular fossa should be considered a tumour recurrence until otherwise proven. In some cases, patients may present with a suddenly occurred lymphoedema, pain in the arm and shoulder or increasing sensory or motor loss in the arm or hand. These latter symptoms are often the result of brachial plexus involvement.

Internal mammary recurrences are rare and often present with a deep, fixed mass in an intercostal space next to the ipsilateral sternal border. These recurrences often first present with pain and tenderness, without noticeable mass, and it may be difficult to differentiate them from sternal metastases.

*Differential diagnosis*. The clinical significance of distinction between an IBTR as a recurrence of the initial tumour and a new primary tumour arising in the breast remains uncertain and in many cases misleading. The differential diagnosis is generally made on clinical grounds, such as the distance of new tumour from the site of the initial tumour, and on disease-free interval. Several series have found that survival decreased with local failures in the same location as the initial tumour (compared to elsewhere in the breast), but others have not. However, this may be related to the longer interval to failure for the recurrences elsewhere in the breast rather than the location itself.

Clinical differential diagnosis should be made with postradiation or postoperative change, foreign body cyst around suture material, cellulitis, severe inflammation of dermal and subcutaneous layers of the skin, fat necrosis from trauma or lipofilling, bony nodule on a rib or costal cartilage from surgical trauma. In patients who had postoperative radiation therapy, a radiation-induced angiosarcoma could be rarely observed, typically late with a median interval of 10 years posttreatment.

### 20.1.3 Role of Imaging

*Mammography*. The role of mammography after BCT is close surveillance of the treated breast for clinically occult recurrent BC as well as screening of the contralateral breast. Patients typically undergo their first posttreatment mammogram 6–12 months after completion of radiation treatment. The degree of oedema and distortion that is seen on the mammogram can vary significantly from one patient to another. At the time of the baseline mammogram after completion of treatment, some patients will have extensive oedema, trabecular thickening and architectural distortion, while other patients will have minimal mammographic changes. These posttreatment changes tend to be maximal at about 6 months after treatment and may pose a challenge to the breast imager in detecting recurrent disease. On subsequent mammograms, the posttreatment changes may remain stable but usually decrease in prominence over time. Therefore, any new or worsening finding on subsequent screening mammography, such as new calcifications, new mass or increasing architectural distortion, needs to be viewed cautiously and evaluated carefully for recurrent disease [10].

*Ultrasound*. For the evaluation of new or suspicious mammographic masses as well as clinically palpable findings, breast ultrasound is an essential tool that plays a complementary role to mammography and physical examination. In the evaluation of palpable breast masses, sonography is particularly helpful, since the mammographic evaluation can be limited due to the posttreatment changes. In patients presenting with palpable breast masses, prospective and retrospective studies have reported the negative predictive value of combined mammography and sonography to be very high, approaching 100 %. In addition, if a lesion is visible on ultrasound, a minimally invasive core-needle biopsy or fine-needle aspiration can be performed under sonographic guidance [11].

*Breast MRI* is well known to detect mammographically occult BC. Unlike mammography and sonography, MRI dynamically evaluates the breast tissue. In addition to assessing the morphology of the breast lesions, the vascularity of any lesions may be evaluated after intravenous contrast enhancement (see Sect. 5.3). Lesion enhancement is based on the number and the permeability of the blood vessels.

There is, however, some overlap in enhancement characteristics seen in benign and malignant lesions. In women with equivocal mammographic findings after breast-conservation treatment, the enhancement pattern on contrast-enhanced MRI can be helpful in differentiating posttreatment scar from recurrent cancer. Breast MRI can also detect mammographically occult local recurrence in the breast BCT [12, 13].

### 20.1.4 Workup

Since local or regional recurrence is a marker of increased aggressiveness, all patients experiencing a relapse, both local and regional, have to undergo proper systemic workup to rule out the presence of synchronous distant metastases. In addition to a complete history and physical exam, patients should have a CT of the chest/abdomen/pelvis and a bone scan. On the other hand, CT should be considered in any patient with new onset pain, paralysis, paraesthesia or lymphoedema, even in the absence of palpable disease. PET scans are used in uncertain situations or when the results of the CT or bone scan are equivocal.

For a woman, learning that she has a recurrent BC may be harder than dealing with the initial diagnosis. An appropriate intervention, including psycho-education, is needed for patients diagnosed with first recurrence in order to detect and manage psychological distress.

## 20.2 Treatment of Isolated Local or Regional Recurrence

**Clinical Practice Points**

- In a patient previously treated for an invasive BC, local recurrence presents a unique challenge to the oncologist because there is a paucity of randomised studies to guide in choosing the optimal combination and sequence of therapies.
- The management of each patient requires a multidisciplinary approach that depends not only on factors specific to the recurrence itself but also on factors related to the original treatment.
- Durable local salvage is important in preventing the consequences of uncontrolled loco-regional disease.
- Wide local excision of all gross disease is recommended with the purpose of both maximising subsequent local control and moderating the required dose of chest wall irradiation.
- Chemotherapy significantly increases overall and disease-free survival, particularly in receptor-negative patients.

### 20.2.1 Local Treatment

*Local recurrence after mastectomy.* Patients with isolated chest wall recurrence after mastectomy should be treated with wide local excision of the relapse after complete local and systemic workup. This is also recommended for multiple nodules amenable to resection with negative margins.

Postoperative loco-regional radiotherapy is added for those patients who did not receive it after primary treatment. For isolated chest wall recurrences, the supraclavicular nodes should be electively treated concurrently with the entire chest wall because of the increased risk of subsequent relapse without radiation. Elective irradiation of a clinically uninvolved axillary or internal mammary node region is not necessary [14].

*Ipsilateral breast tumour recurrence (IBTR).* Up to now, IBTR after BCS has been almost exclusively treated by mastectomy even in patients with small and late recurrences [15, 16]. The number of published studies reporting the outcome of patients treated with conservative surgery alone is limited. There are only retrospective small series, which compared repeat lumpectomy and mastectomy.

Kurtz et al. [17] reported a series of 50 patients with stage I or II BC treated with breast-conserving surgery and radiation who subsequently underwent wide local excision for a clinically isolated IBTR, with or without axillary recurrence. Of the recurrences, 80 % were less than 2 cm in size, 62 % were in the vicinity of the original tumour, and all were without skin involvement. The second local failure rate in the salvaged breast was 38 % at 5 years, with a 5- and 10-year survival of 67 and 42 %, respectively. The only significant factors for local control on multivariate analysis were a disease-free interval greater than 5 years (92 % vs 49 %) and negative resection margins (73 % vs 36 %).

Salvadori et al. [18] reported that the risk of further local recurrence after BCS was higher compared with mastectomy (19 % vs 4 %). While the most published studies recommend a second conservative approach only in selected groups with small and late recurrences, a large observational analysis published by Chen and Martinez [19] discouraged the use of lumpectomy for all patients with ipsilateral breast recurrence. In fact the author found that the group of patients undergoing BCS had significantly worse overall survival compared to the mastectomy group (67 % vs 78 %).

Despite this data subsequent and current studies have shown encouraging results with the use of lumpectomy alone. The largest and most recent series has been published by Gentilini et al. [20]. This retrospective study evaluated 161 patients who underwent second BCS in an attempt to identify the best candidates for BCS. The 5-year OS was 84 % and 5-year cumulative incidence for a further local recurrence was 29 %. Tumour size and time to breast recurrence <48 months increased significantly the risk of second local relapse.

A repeat BCT demands tumour-free margins and an interstitial brachytherapy. Despite that, the indication for second lumpectomy is restricted for suited patients (small size, low risk). As data from prospective randomised clinical trials are missing, an impaired regional tumour control (without disadvantages for overall survival) cannot be ruled out completely. Systemic therapy after resected local recurrence (re-adjuvant) is associated with improved disease-free and overall survival.

Endocrine treatment in hormone-sensitive tumours improves disease-free survival. The impact on overall survival is still debatable. Repeat irradiation breast for recurrent BC is feasible. If no prior radiotherapy has performed after BCS, whole-breast radiation should be performed.

There has been limited experience with repeating radiation therapy for an IBTR following breast-conserving surgery and whole-breast radiotherapy. Deutsch [21] reported on 39 patients who received initial radiation doses of 45–50 Gy to the breast (with or without a boost) and who were treated for local recurrence with repeat lumpectomy and re-irradiation. The prescribed re-irradiation dose was 50 Gy in 25 fractions using electrons. The rate of second local recurrence was 29 % (8/39). Overall cosmetic outcome was excellent or good for 75 % (27/36) of the evaluable patients. Trombetta et al. [22] reported on 21 patients treated for local recurrence using excision plus interstitial brachytherapy to a dose of 45–50 Gy. The rate of second local recurrence was 5 % (1/21), and 10 % (2/21) of the patients developed metastatic disease.

The GEC-ESTRO group [23] published a multricentric retrospective study on the clinical outcome of 217 women who presented IBTR and who had previously undergone BCS and radiation therapy. These women underwent repeat lumpectomy plus re-irradiation using multi-catheter brachytherapy. After a median follow-up of 3.9 years, 5- and 10-year local recurrence rates were, respectively, 5.7 and 7.6 %.

*Loco-regional recurrence.* If there is no evidence of distant metastasis and the axillary recurrence is surgically resectable, surgery should be the initial approach. If the loco-regional recurrence seems difficult to resect, or unresectable (chest wall involvement, brachial plexus involvement), preoperative therapy should be considered to improve the likelihood of complete resection.

For patients who were previously submitted to SLN biopsy only, resection should include a complete ALND. For patients who had a previous ALND, resection is still recommended although the surgical procedure in these cases might be more technically challenging. In most of such cases reported on in the literature, it becomes clear that an incomplete clearance or level I dissection was performed, while in these cases a formal level I and II dissection should be performed.

Radiation therapy in most cases is the only local treatment for supraclavicular recurrence and should target chest wall and infraclavicular and supraclavicular basins. Surgery generally is not indicated in patients with supraclavicular recurrences, unless a coincidence of favourable factors could suggest removing some nodes in order to reduce the tumour mass for the radiation therapy.

## 20.2.2 Systemic Therapy

There are few data on the role of systemic therapy after local recurrence. Adjuvant systemic therapy is now commonly used following initial diagnosis of the primary tumour. Therefore, for many patients who suffer local recurrence, questions of drug resistance and tolerance to further systemic treatment must be considered. The ESMO guidelines [24] published in 2012 tried to target adjuvant therapy categories on the basis of biological characteristics of the tumour.

Systemic therapy alone, without surgery or radiation, is of questionable long-term efficacy. Some individuals with chest wall fixation may respond sufficiently to chemotherapy or hormonal therapy to allow subsequent surgery. However, systemic therapy alone is not effective in obtaining permanent local control of inoperable disease.

Because of the scarcity of existing data and lack of a recognised standard for the optimal systemic treatment after local-regional relapse, participation in ongoing multicentre clinical trials should be encouraged. CALOR trial [25], a multicentric randomised trial, enrolled 162 patients from worldwide institutions and tried to establish whether adjuvant chemotherapy improves the outcome of such patients.

Eligible patients were women of any age with histologically proven and completely excised first isolated recurrence after unilateral BC who had undergone a mastectomy or lumpectomy with clear surgical margins. Patients were randomly allocated to either chemotherapy or no chemotherapy. Radiotherapy was recommended for all patients but was required for those with microscopically involved surgical margins, using at least 50 Gy.

Endocrine therapy was recommended for all patients with receptor-positive recurrent tumours. In patients randomly assigned to receive chemotherapy, choice of chemotherapy, dose adjustments and supportive therapies were left to the discretion of the investigators.

The protocol recommended at least two cytotoxic drugs for 3–6 months (docetaxel, capecitabine, cyclophosphamide, methotrexate, fluorouracil, gemcitabine). Five-year disease-free survival was 69 % (95 % CI 56–79) in the chemotherapy group compared with 57 % (44–67) in the no-chemotherapy group (HR 0.59 [95 % CI 0.35–0.99]; $p=0.046$). Overall survival was also significantly longer in the chemotherapy group; 5-year overall survival was 88 % (95 % CI 77–94) in the chemotherapy group and 76 % (63–85) in the no-chemotherapy group (HR 0.41 [95 % CI 0.19–0.89]; $p=0.024$).

Patients assigned to chemotherapy for receptor-negative LRR had a greater chance of disease-free survival than did those assigned to no chemotherapy (HR 0.32 [95 % CI 0.14–0.73]). Five-year disease-free survival was 67 % (95 % CI 44–82) in the chemotherapy group versus 35 % (18–53) in the no-chemotherapy group.

The results of this trial showed that chemotherapy significantly increased overall and disease-free survival in these patients, particularly those with an oestrogen receptor-negative loco-regional recurrence reducing the relative risk of further relapses by about two-thirds. These findings provide strong evidence that isolated BC recurrences are a marker of concurrent occult systemic disease and that a second adjuvant course of chemotherapy should be recommended in this population of patients.

### 20.2.3 Prognosis

Broadly speaking, the interval to local recurrence is the most generic but significant prognostic factor following either mastectomy or BCT. In most cases, local failure within 2 years is a marker of more aggressive disease and simultaneous distant micrometastases. In contrast, the prognosis improves for the favourable subgroups of patients with chronological late local failures.

Wapnir et al. in 2006 [3] have recognised which are the most important prognostic factors involved in loco-regional recurrence. They confirmed results from NSABP protocol B-06 and concluded that IBTR emerged as an independent predictor of distant disease, conferring a 3.41-fold increased risk. Five years after an IBTR, only 51.4 % of patients were free of distant disease. The average annual death and distant disease rates in the first 5 years after IBTR were 10.2 and 14.9 %, respectively.

The time to IBTR has been proposed as an additional prognostic factor of survival. Among patients with recurrences in the breast within 5 years of initial therapy, the 5-year OS rate was 65 % and the 5-year distant-recurrence-free survival rate was 61 %. In contrast, the 5-year OS rate was 81 % and the 5-year distant-recurrence-free survival rate was 80 % in patients who developed IBTR 5 or more years after diagnosis. This finding suggests that a higher proportion of late IBTRs represents metachronous second primaries in the breast rather than recurrence of the index lesion.

In addition they found that nodal status was not a significant predictor of IBTR whereas is a highly significant predictor for LRR, along with age and hormone receptor status. Higher local recurrence rates in premenopausal versus postmenopausal women have also been reported.

Panet-Raymond et al. [26] have investigated in their study the role of clinicopathologic characteristics of the recurrent tumour in determining survival. They evaluated the impact on disease-free survival and overall survival of lymphovascular invasion, ER status, grade and margin status. Close or positive margins after resection of the recurrence were associated with poor outcome on multivariate analysis.

The negative prognostic impact of a close or positive margin was equally applicable to patients who underwent secondary breast conservation and those who underwent salvage mastectomies. OS at 10 years was most favourable for patients treated with salvage mastectomy compared with those who underwent secondary BCS or biopsy alone. These results underscore the importance of achieving local control at time of recurrence and suggest that secondary breast conservation be used with caution.

Lymphovascular invasion has been a frequently described as a prognostic factor at the time of initial BC diagnosis but has been an under-evaluated factor in the recurrent specimen. ER status at time of recurrence is a significant independent variable associated with OS. It is increasingly recognised that ER status at initial presentation cannot be used as a surrogate for ER status at time of recurrence, because IBTRs may represent an independent new primary within the breast with its own unique histopathological features.

## References


1. Fisher B, Anderson S, Bryant J, et al. Twenty-year follow-up of a randomized trial comparing total mastectomy, lumpectomy, and lumpectomy plus irradiation for the treatment of invasive breast cancer. N Engl J Med. 2002;347:1233–41.
2. Veronesi U, Cascinelli N, Mariani L, et al. Twenty-year follow-up of a randomized study comparing breast-conserving surgery with radical mastectomy for early breast cancer. N Engl J Med. 2002;347:1227–32.
3. Wapnir IL, Anderson SJ, Mamounas EP, et al. Prognosis after ipsilateral breast tumor recurrence and locoregional recurrences in five National Surgical Adjuvant Breast and Bowel Project node-positive adjuvant breast cancer trials. J Clin Oncol. 2006;24:2028–37.
4. Punglia RS, Morrow M, Winer EP, Harris JR. Local therapy and survival in breast cancer. N Engl J Med. 2007;356:2399–405.
5. Anderson SJ, Wapnir I, Dignam JJ, et al. Prognosis after ipsilateral breast tumor recurrence and locoregional recurrences in patients treated by breast-conserving therapy in five National

Surgical Adjuvant Breast and Bowel Project protocols of node-negative breast cancer. J Clin Oncol. 2009;27(15):2466–73.

6. van Dongen J, Voogd AC, Fentiman IS, et al. Long-term results of a randomized trial comparing breast-conserving therapy with mastectomy: European Organization for Research and Treatment of Cancer 10801 trial. J Natl Cancer Inst. 2000;92:1143–50.
7. Fisher B, Anderson S, Redmond CK, et al. Reanalysis and results after 12 years of follow-up in a randomized clinical trial comparing total mastectomy with lumpectomy, with or without irradiation, in the treatment of breast cancer. N Engl J Med. 1995;333:1456–61.
8. Botteri E, Bagnardi V, Rotmensz N, et al. Analysis of local and regional recurrences in breast cancer after conservative surgery. Ann Oncol. 2010;21:723–8.
9. Voogd AC, van Tienhoven G, Peterse HL, et al. Local recurrence after breast conservation therapy for early stage breast carcinoma: detection, treatment and outcome in 266 patients. Dutch Study Group on Local Recurrence after Breast Conservation (BORST). Cancer. 1999;85:437–46.
10. Weinstein SP, Orel SG, Pinnamaneni P, et al. Mammographic appearance of recurrent breast cancer after breast conservation therapy. Acad Radiol. 2008;15:240–4.
11. Moy L, Slanetz PJ, Moore R, et al. Specificity of mammography and US in the evaluation of a palpable abnormality: retrospective review. Radiology. 2002;225:176–81.
12. Lehman CD, Blume JD, Thickman D, et al. Added cancer yield of MRI in screening the contralateral breast of women recently diagnosed with breast cancer: results from the International Breast Magnetic Resonance Consortium (IBMC) trial. J Surg Oncol. 2005;92:9–15.
13. Morris EA, Liberman L, Ballon DJ, et al. MRI of occult breast carcinoma in a high-risk population. AJR Am J Roentgenol. 2003;181:619–26.
14. Halverson KJ, Perez CA, Kuske RR, et al. Isolated locoregional recurrence of breast cancer following mastectomy: radiotherapeutic management. Int J Radiat Oncol Biol Phys. 1990;19:851–8.
15. Burger AE, Pain SJ, Peley G. Treatment of recurrent breast cancer following breast conserving surgery. Breast J. 2013;19:310–8.
16. Hannoun-Levi JM, et al. Local treatments options for ipsilateral breast tumor recurrence. Cancer Treat Rev. 2013;39:737–41.
17. Kurtz JM, Jacquemier J, Amalric R, et al. Is breast conservation after local recurrence feasible? Eur J Cancer. 1991;27:240–4.
18. Salvadori B, Marubini E, Miceli R, et al. Reoperation for locally recurrent breast cancer in patients previously treated with conservative surgery. Br J Surg. 1999;86:84–7.
19. Chen SL, Martinez SR. The survival impact of the choice of surgical procedure after ipsilateral breast cancer recurrence. Am J Surg. 2008;196:495–9.
20. Gentilini O, Botteri E, Veronesi P, et al. Repeating conservative surgery after ipsilateral breast tumor reappearance: criteria for selecting the best candidates. Ann Surg Oncol. 2012;19: 3771–6.
21. Deutsch M. Repeat high-dose external beam radiation for in-breast tumor recurrence after previous lumpectomy and whole breast irradiation. Int J Radiat Oncol Biol Phys. 2002;53:687–91.
22. Trombetta M, Julian T, Bhandari T, et al. Breast conservation surgery and interstitial brachytherapy in the management of locally recurrent carcinoma of the breast: the Allegheny General Hospital experience. Brachytherapy. 2008;7:29–36.
23. Hannoun-Levi JM, Resch A, Gal J, and on behalf of the GEC-ESTRO Breast Cancer Working Group. Accelerated partial breast irradiation with interstitial brachytherapy as second conservative treatment for ipsilateral breast tumour recurrence: multicentric study of the GEC-ESTRO Breast Cancer Working Group. Radiother Oncol. 2013;108:226–31.
24. Cardoso F, Harbeck N, Fallowfield L, Kyriakides S, Senkus E, and on behalf of the ESMO Guidelines Working Group. Locally recurrent or metastatic breast cancer: ESMO Clinical Practice Guidelines for diagnosis, treatment and follow-up. Ann Oncol. 2012;23(Suppl 7): vii11–vii19.

25. Aebi S, Gelber S, Anderson SJ, et al. Chemotherapy for isolated locoregional recurrence of breast cancer (CALOR): a randomised trial. Lancet Oncol. 2014;15:156–63.
26. Panet-Raymond V, Truong PT, Alexander C, Lesperance M, McDonald RE, Watson PH. Clinicopathologic factors of the recurrent tumor predict outcome in patients with ipsilateral breast tumor recurrence. Cancer. 2011;117:20135–43.

## Further Reading

Aebi S, Gelber S, Anderson SJ, et al. Chemotherapy for isolated locoregional recurrence of breast cancer (CALOR): a randomised trial. Lancet Oncol. 2014;15:156–63.

Freedman GM, Fowble BL. Local recurrence after mastectomy or breast-conserving surgery and radiation. Oncology. 2000;14:1561–81.

Taras AR, Thorpe JD, Morris AD, et al. Irradiation effect after mastectomy on breast cancer recurrence in patients presenting with locally advanced disease. Am J Surg. 2011;201:605–10.

# Follow-Up

# 21

Giorgio Macellari and Alfonso M. Pluchinotta

## Contents




G. Macellari (✉)
Surgical Breast Clinic, Hospital "Guglielmo da Saliceto", Piacenza, Italy
e-mail: g.macellari@ausl.pc.it

A.M. Pluchinotta
Breast Surgery, Policlinic of Abano Terme, Padova, Italy
e-mail: pluchinotta.alfonso@gmail.com







A.M. Pluchinotta (ed.), *The Outpatient Breast Clinic: Aiming at Best Practice*,
DOI 10.1007/978-3-319-15907-2_21

**Abstract**

• Follow-up should not be seen exclusively from the physical perspective as women often have increased levels of anxiety after treatment completion, when close contact with the treatment team decreases. • Issues involving work, family and sexuality are often not closely addressed during follow-up, resulting in women not being able to cope effectively. • Depression and intense fatigue may occur in the months following the end of adjuvant chemotherapy and/or RT. Different set of challenges and realities should be addressed to encompass the physical and psychosocial needs of these women. • The role of a specialised breast nurse throughout the individual experience of cancer (*cancer journey*) is extremely important for the patient. In consideration of the huge number of BC survivors all over the world, the magnitude of an extensive follow-up could require a very costly monitoring, probably impossible to be met.

*Future Directions.* As the prevalence of BC rises, a dramatic increase in the number of BC survivors will place clinical and financial demands on the long-term surveillance system. Despite these challenges, evidence is mounting to suggest that disease relapse may be curable if diagnosed and treated early. *One size fits all* prescription has led to an increase in resource utilisation and expensive workups of false-positive tests. Moving forward, developing testing models relevant to a risk stratification system for individualised care may help better elicit the clinical benefit of early detection.

## 21.1 Follow-Up Care Plan

**Clinical Practice Points**

- There is a lack of noticeable evidence for what constitute best practices in follow-up for patients with a history of BC.
- Follow-up should be stratified according to the risk of disease. For early stage BC, a minimalist regimen, based on periodic physical examination and mammography, seems a reasonable option.
- Patients should be given information regarding their personal care plan comprised of clinical and imaging follow-up.
- There is no agreement about the professional who should best be charged with follow-up (GP, gynaecologist, oncologist, surgeon, radiation oncologist, breast nurse).
- Patients with early stage BC (tumour up to 5 cm and less than four positive nodes) who wish to be followed exclusively by a GP may be transferred to them approximately 1 year after the end of BC therapies.
- Many patients expect routine follow-up from their physicians because of unrealistic expectations: they should be properly educated about the very limited value of routine investigations for distant metastases and about the great importance of self-reporting symptoms.
- Patients with early stage BC may present in the months following the end of adjuvant chemotherapy and/or RT. Different set of challenges and realities should be addressed to encompass their physical and psychosocial needs.

### 21.1.1 Introduction

Any person who has or has had cancer, starting from the moment of diagnosis, during treatment and without any evidence of disease, is defined *cancer survivor*. There is far from universal agreement among those who have had cancer about the term cancer survivor. Some object to it, saying they are cured. Others say they are living with cancer. And still others prefer to put cancer behind them and argue that being called a cancer survivor stigmatises them. However, nowadays there is no term that is considered widely accepted.

Patients who are living for decades beyond cancer experience the normal issues of ageing, which are often compounded by the long-term effects of having had cancer and cancer therapy. These patients are at risk for a BC recurrence (which is most common in the first 5 years but may occur even decades following treatment), a new primary BC, other cancers and short-term and long-term adverse effects of treatment.

Essential elements of management for BC survivors who have completed active treatment and have no evidence of disease are cancer surveillance, encouragement of adherence with ongoing treatment and lifestyle recommendations, treatment of medical and psychosocial consequences of cancer and its therapy and care coordination between specialists and primary care providers.

Additional issues for BC patients are related to genetic counselling if indicated, reproductive function if a pregnancy is desired and functional outcome following surgery, sometimes with social and employment concerns. Most of these issues are not easy to deal with, but anyway they need to be identified, focused on and coped with.

*Aims of follow-up* are here listed:

- Early detection and early treatment of recurrent disease, either local or metastatic. Recurrences are concentrated in the first 3 years then having a stable 1–2 % yearly incidence.
- Surveillance of the (ipsilateral and/or contralateral) breast with a five times higher risk of developing a metachronous cancer which may have an independent impact on prognosis.
- Improvement of quality of life by reassuring the patient.
- Monitoring and preventing negative side effects of treatment (e.g. endometrial cancer in tamoxifen users or osteoporosis in premenopausal women undergoing hormone deprivation).

Each of these aims has been the object of discussion over time, based on several conflicting experiences. No definitive evidence is available thus far that early detection and treatment of recurrence may have a favourable impact on prognosis (this subject is addressed in Chap. 20). It is well known that earlier detection is associated with less extensive recurrence and that limited recurrent tumour burden is associated with prolonged survival, but this is not sufficient to demonstrate a real benefit, as improved survival might be simply due to diagnostic anticipation (lead time) with no improvement of overall survival.

### 21.1.2 Follow-Up Regimens

Follow-up of BC patients is standard practice all over the world. Unfortunately, the investigation of distant metastases aimed at early detection and treatment seem to have no prognostic impact, for the present state of the art of diagnosis and treatment. However, taking into account that treatment are changed with the introduction of new agents (as monoclonal antibodies or synthetic oestrogen receptor antagonist), new therapeutic strategies may be validated as favourably influencing overall survival.

Conversely, the evidence of long-term cure of limited as compared to extensive local recurrences suggests a possible favourable prognostic impact of early detection of these events, particularly as regards recurrences in the axilla and in the surgical scar or conserved breast. Such events are likely to become more frequent with the adoption of conservative therapeutic options as tumourectomy and sentinel node technique. Although no definitive evidence of a favourable prognostic impact of early detection of local recurrences is available, the presumed benefit and the fact that early detection in the asymptomatic phase is achieved by palpation and mammography, which are included in a minimalist follow-up approach, justify such a current practice.

In intermediate or intensive regimens, patients should be seen every 4–6 months during the first 2–3 years after primary therapy, every 6–12 months for the next 2 years and then annually, consistent with American Society of Clinical Oncology (ASCO) 2012 guidelines. However, this schedule is arbitrary; no studies have evaluated the benefit of less frequent clinical visits in patients with low-risk disease or more frequent visits in those with higher-risk disease. Some indicative follow-up regimens in relation to the risk and in the absence of associated diseases are set out below.

**Low (*Minimalist*) Regimen**
- Breast self-examination
- Semi-annual or annual physical control (by GP, primary care; by surgeon, secondary care; or both, shared care)
- Annual mammography
- Other instrumental tests in relation to any symptoms

**Intermediate Regimen**
- Breast self-examination
- Semi-annual oncological control
- Annual surgical control (twice a year in the absence of oncological control)
- Annual mammography
- Semi-annual laboratory test including marker
- Other instrumental tests in relation to any symptoms

**Intensive Regimen**
- Breast self-examination
- Oncological control every 4 months for 2 years and then every 6 months for 5 years

- Annual surgical control
- Semi-annual laboratory test including markers
- Annual chest X-ray, liver ultrasound and bone scintigraphy
- Other investigations (CT, MRI) based on the symptoms

**Additional Investigation in Long-Term Medications**

- In case of tamoxifen (TAM) medication: transvaginal ultrasound at baseline and then only in presence of vaginal discharge
- In case of aromatase inhibitors (AIs) medication: bone densitometry annual or biennial

### 21.1.3 Care Plan Coordination

Patients treated for BC should have an agreed, written care plan, which should be recorded by a named healthcare professional (or professionals); a copy should be sent to the GP and a personal copy given to the patient.

This plan should include:

- Designated named healthcare professionals
- Dates for review of any adjuvant therapy
- Details of surveillance mammography
- Signs and symptoms to look for and seek advice on, contact details for immediate referral to specialist care
- Contact details for support services, for example, support for patients with lymphoedema

Whatever the follow-up protocol and the frequency of visits, every visit should include history taking, eliciting of symptoms and physical examination.

Guidelines from the American Society of Clinical Oncology (ASCO) suggest that patients with early stage BC (tumour <5 cm and fewer than four positive nodes) may follow-up exclusively with a general practitioner (GP); for patients and clinicians who agree with this plan, care may be transferred approximately 1 or 2 years after ending the therapies [1]. If care is transferred to a GP (primary care), both the GP and the patient should be informed of the appropriate follow-up and management strategy.

A variety of clinicians may adequately follow women after their primary therapy for BC. Clinicians should be experienced in the surveillance of these patients, the complications that may arise from treatment, and in breast examination, including the examination of irradiated breasts. A shared care model that integrates both specialists and primary care providers on ongoing follow-up care may provide the best adherence to guidelines for recommended care; but communication and coordination of care is required.

In patient with advanced BC, physical controls should be carried out by oncologist (secondary care) or annually by the oncologist and semi-annually by the GP (shared care).

Last but not least, the emotional aspects of BC should always be taken into account. Focus on tests and treatments should not prevent from considering a Women's emotional, psychological, and spiritual health as well. Once treatment ends, almost all women find themselves overwhelmed by emotions. They still think about the possibility of their own death or the effect of cancer on their family, friends, and career, but may also re-evaluate their relationship with spouse or partner. A major concern is, for instance, how to be healthier and have fewer doctor visits, though seeing the health care team less often is a source of anxiety for some.

This is an ideal time to suggest emotional and social support. Almost everyone who has been through cancer can benefit from getting some type of support, though what is best for a patient depends on their own situation and personality. Some people feel safe in peer-support groups or education groups. Others would rather talk in an informal setting, such as spiritual groups. Others may feel more at ease talking one-on-one with a trusted friend or counsellor, or visiting online support communities (see Appendix). Whatever the source of strength or comfort, women should have a place to go with their concerns. The cancer journey can feel very lonely, and it is not necessary or realistic to go through it all on one's own. Friends and family should not feel shut out even if the woman decides not to include them.

## 21.2 Clinical and Instrumental Follow-Up

**Clinical Practice Points**

- Physical exam may be crucial in the identification of local recurrences and regional pathologic lymph nodes.
- Although the evidence is limited, surveillance mammography appears to be associated with a reduction in mortality.
- In asymptomatic patients, radiologic imaging to screen for distant metastasis is of little value and should not be performed.
- As some imaging test, laboratory tests used for surveillance have significant false-positive and false-negative rates.
- A strong body of evidence shows that the optimal follow-up requires very little testing and could be performed by an interested, motivated and well-informed caregiver.

### 21.2.1 Clinical Examination

*HISTORY.* In addition to the general components of a medical history, the BC patient should be screened for symptoms of local recurrence as well as metastatic disease. The history should include any interval changes in the patient's health and social environment (including family history, which may be important to discussions regarding genetic counselling) that may have arisen since the end of treatment.

A review of systems should not only screen for metastatic disease but also may identify issues related to prior treatment. The review of systems should include the following:

- Constitutional symptoms, as anorexia, weight gain, malaise, fatigue, insomnia
- Bone pain, if current, and its characteristics (i.e. location, character, chronic or intermittent, associated symptoms, exacerbating factors and what provides relief)
- Pulmonary symptoms, as persistent cough or dyspnoea (at rest or with exertion)
- Neurologic symptoms, as headache, nausea, vomiting, confusion, weakness, numbness or tingling
- Gastrointestinal symptoms, as right upper quadrant pain, change in bowel habits, presence of bloody or tarry stools
- Genitourinary symptoms, as vaginal bleeding, pelvic pain, difficulty urinating
- Psychological symptoms, as depression, anxiety
- Reproductive/endocrine symptoms, as hot flashes, dyspareunia, vaginal dryness, sexual dysfunction, fertility concerns (in women with intact ovarian function)

*SPECIFIC QUESTIONS RELATED TO THE TREATMENT* (see Sect. 18.2.3): *Tamoxifen or Toremifene*. If a woman is taking tamoxifen or toremifene, doctor should inquire about any abnormal vaginal bleeding, such as vaginal bleeding or spotting after menopause, bleeding or spotting between periods, or a change in the periods. Although these symptoms are usually caused by a non-cancerous condition, they should be investigated, especially in women who have gone through menopause. It is always advisable to regularly undergo a gynaecological visit with gynaecological ultrasound and smear test at least every two years.

*AROMATASE INHIBITORS (AIS)*. In case of treatment with aromatase inhibitors the risk of bone fractures is increased. For this reason, it is advisable to evaluate the bone condition by basal bone densitometry. In case of osteopenia/osteoporosis, specific treatment and periodic checks are advisable. It is also very useful to advise women on their lifestyle, suggesting walking as a physical activity and a healthy diet. If a woman is taking AIS her risk of hypercholesterolemia is increased. It is advisable, therefor, an annual check of cholesterol and triglycerides, besides advising her on maintaining a healthy diet.

*GnRH ANALOGUES*. The most common side effects are hot flashes, increased sweating, night sweats, tiredness, vaginal discomfort and reduced sexual interest. See Sect. 21.3.2 for a proper evaluation and available measures.

*BREAST SELF-EXAMINATION*. About 40 % of locoregional recurrences are detected outside routine follow-up, mainly because patients report themselves signs or symptoms. This leads to recommend self breast examination. This should be performed every 3 or 4 months, either after mastectomy or breast-conserving surgery, provided the patient agrees and can be properly educated.

*PHYSICAL EXAMINATION: Examination of the Breast and Axilla*. Thorough examination should be performed of the preserved and/or contralateral breast, the bilateral axillary regions and the supraclavicular fossae. Evidence of local recurrence includes newly discovered lumps (on the skin, within the breast or the nodal regions). Other worrisome findings may include skin changes in the breast. For women who have undergone mastectomy with or without breast reconstruction, the incision site and surrounding skin of the chest wall should be examined visually and palpated for abnormalities.

*Lymphoedema* requires examination of the arms that should include circumferential measurement of the upper extremities bilaterally.

*In addition*, palpation of the spine, sternum, ribs and pelvis for bone tenderness should be routinely performed. Lungs should be evaluated for breath sounds and percussion changes, right upper abdominal quadrant for tenderness and/or hepatomegaly and so on.

For patients receiving adjuvant hormonal therapy, informed decisions regarding long-term options may necessitate periodic referral for oncology assessment since treatment strategies are evolving over time. Furthermore, input from an oncology specialist is warranted if there is suspicion or evidence of disease recurrence or if questions arise regarding the safety of certain interventions (e.g. vaginal oestrogen in a patient who has severe atrophic vaginitis).

### 21.2.2 Imaging

*IMAGING OF THE BREAST.* Although the evidence is limited, surveillance mammography appears to be associated with a reduction in mortality. Mammography should be performed yearly after completion of locoregional therapy. Women treated with breast-conserving therapy should have their first posttreatment mammogram no earlier than 6 months after definitive radiation therapy.

The purpose of mammographic surveillance is to detect ipsilateral local recurrences after breast-conserving therapy (BCT), which develops in up to 4 % of women treated for early BC. In addition, mammography is performed as surveillance for a contralateral BC. There is a lack of high-quality evidence to inform the optimal timing and survival benefit of mammographic surveillance for detecting ipsilateral recurrence or a contralateral BC. For women in long-term follow-up, mammographic surveillance should be performed annually.

*Detection of local recurrence.* There are no prospective trials that address the utility of mammography in the detection of local recurrence. Data from retrospective series suggest that mammography detects earlier lesions with a more favourable prognosis and that survival is improved in women whose lesions are detected by mammography as compared with those detected by other means. However, other data suggest that mammographic screening in women with a personal history of BC performs less well (lower sensitivity and slightly lower specificity) than in women without such a history. Moreover, women with a personal history of BC had a higher rate of interval cancers compared with women without a history of BC.

*Contralateral BC.* There are no randomised trials that address the role of mammography or its impact on survival in detecting contralateral BCs. However, recommendations for mammographic surveillance are based upon the benefits seen in the general population without a history of BC. In general, BC survivors are higher-risk women than the general population, and it would seem reasonable to assume that they get as much or even more benefit from mammography of the contralateral breast.

There is indirect evidence from retrospective series that supports a beneficial impact for mammography of the contralateral breast. As shown by several controlled studies of screening by mammography, contralateral tumours are more often smaller than 10 mm or in situ, so that their early detection may reduce BC mortality. There is no reason why this should not occur also for contralateral metachronous BC, although the magnitude of such an impact is certainly reduced for the concurrent prognostic effect of first BC.

A recent report has shown a higher risk of BC death for subjects developing a symptomatic rather than an asymptomatic metachronous contralateral BC detected by periodic mammography. Periodic mammography with a higher frequency (as compared to screening of healthy subjects) is currently performed even in a minimalist follow-up approach.

*Surveillance of reconstructed breasts.* For women who have undergone mastectomy, surveillance is usually performed by physical examination. Routine mammographic imaging is technically limited in patients who have prosthetic implants and is generally not advocated. However, mammography is technically feasible following autogenous myocutaneous flap reconstruction. Anyway, since the only place where cancer can occur is either right below the skin in the subcutaneous tissue or just over the pectoral muscle, physical examination remains the cornerstone of detection of recurrent BC after reconstruction.

*Breast MRI.* Breast MRI is not routinely recommended for BC survivors because of a lack of evidence to inform of its role in this population. However, breast MRI can be useful for patients suspected of a BC recurrence when mammography (with or without breast ultrasound) is inconclusive.

Breast MRI is indicated in the follow-up of women at high risk for recurrent disease based on a known BRCA mutation or strongly positive family history. However, this practice is extrapolated from the indications for breast MRI as a screening tool in high-risk women.

*Ultrasound.* Routine use of breast ultrasound as part of surveillance is not widely recommended. Compared with mammography alone, ultrasound plus mammography increased the diagnostic yield but also increased the rate of false-positive results and therefore lowered the positive predictive value.

However, although locoregional recurrence infrequently occurs after mastectomy for BC, screening US enables detection of non-palpable cancer before it can be detected by clinical examination. This is particularly true for recurrent cancers at the mastectomy site located in subcutaneous fat and deep muscle layers. Moreover, the false-negative rate of physical examinations of axillae has been reported to be as high as 39 %.

*IMAGING TO SCREEN DISTANT DISEASE.* In asymptomatic patients, there are no data to indicate that other imaging tests (e.g. bone scans, liver ultrasound exams, CT) can produce a survival benefit. In a 1994 study [2], intensive follow-up [chest X-ray, liver echography, radionuclide bone scan, mammography and physical examinations every 6 or 12 months] showed no effect on mortality at 5 and 10 years, when compared with minimal follow-up (mammography and physical examinations only).

However, the available studies were performed in an era where treatment for advanced disease, both systemic and locoregional, was less efficacious. Nowadays a small percentage of patients with limited metastatic disease (e.g. isolated pulmonary or liver metastases) may be treated with a multimodality approach. Whether such patients are best identified by intensive posttreatment surveillance is unknown, and new trials are needed to reassess this question to new therapeutic option, especially in some specific subgroups of patients.

Until now, for the present state of the art, chest X-rays, bone scans, ultrasound of the abdomen, CT scanning and FDG-PET scanning are not recommended for routine surveillance of patients with early stage BC. However, for some women additional considerations need to be made.

*Evaluation of bone density*. Women with a history of BC may be at increased risk of osteoporosis as a result of prior cancer treatment. Therefore, ASCO guidelines include performing a baseline screening evaluation (typically with dual-energy X-ray absorptiometry) in the following patients:

- Women over 65 years
- Women aged 60–64 years in the presence of any of the following: a family history of osteoporosis, body weight <70 kg, a history of a non-traumatic fracture or other risk factors for osteoporosis (e.g. smoking, a sedentary lifestyle, alcohol use)
- Postmenopausal women taking an aromatase inhibitor (AI), including those in whom an AI has been recommended but not yet initiated
- Premenopausal women who develop treatment-related premature menopause

It is not clear what role vitamin D supplementation should play in women treated for BC or whether or not levels should be checked routinely. In the absence of prospective data to inform of the benefits specifically in these patients, the assessment of vitamin D levels and the role of vitamin D supplementation for women with low vitamin D levels should follow similar guidance as for women without a prior history of BC.

*Bone scan and serum alkaline phosphatase*. There is no evidence that early detection of bone metastases changes the clinical course of the disease. Metastases to bone are almost always diagnosed by symptoms, even when patients undergo routine surveillance with bone scans.

*Abdominopelvic imaging*. Neither liver ultrasound nor abdominopelvic CT scan is recommended as a routine component of posttreatment surveillance. In one large series of over 2,400 patients that included 6,628 pelvic CT scans performed over a 9-year period, pelvic metastases were the only site of metastatic disease in 0.5 % of cases. However, the findings led to over 200 additional radiographic and 50 surgical procedures, which were negative (benign results) in 84 % of the cases.

Regular gynaecologic follow-up is recommended for all women. Patients who receive tamoxifen therapy are at increased risk for developing endometrial cancer and should be advised to report any vaginal bleeding to their physician.

*PET scanning*. There is no role for positron emission tomography (PET) scans in posttreatment follow-up. In retrospective cohort studies and a meta-analysis of 16 studies, PET scanning has been consistently more sensitive than conventional imaging and serum tumour markers for early diagnosis of recurrent disease. However, the impact on survival and quality of life has not been addressed, and it seems unlikely that this approach would provide a survival or quality of life benefit.

### 21.2.3 Laboratory Testing

Laboratory testing, as many imaging tests, used for surveillance have significant false-positive and false-negative rates. The unnecessary additional testing generated by a false-positive result and the misleading reassurance generated by a false-negative test can adversely affect the BC survivor. Therefore, automated chemistry studies are not recommended for routine surveillance in asymptomatic BC patients.

*Liver function tests*. Routine liver function tests are falsely elevated in up to 80 % of women without liver metastases.

*Serum tumour markers*. A number of serum markers that can detect early BC recurrence are available, including CA 15–3, CEA and CA 27.29. These biochemical markers of BC increase in conjunction with advancing primary disease stage and reflect the total body burden of disease. However, they are neither sensitive nor specific for BC relapse. Therefore, measurement of serum tumour markers should only be used to monitor treatment response of patients with metastatic BC, in the absence of readily measurable advanced disease.

At the moment most of the International Societies recommend against or do not recommend the use of routine tumour markers in the surveillance of patients with early stage BC as there is good evidence not to include blood work (as well as diagnostic imaging) as part of screening for distant disease.

## 21.3 Rehabilitative Follow-Up

**Clinical Practice Points**

- People who have many lymph nodes removed during surgery may be at great risk of developing lymphoedema. Complete decongestive therapy remains the initial treatment of choice for lymphoedema. Pharmacological and surgical therapies are investigational.
- Cancer treatment may affect many aspects of sexuality, and BC survivors should be routinely questioned about concerns related to sexual health and counselled or referred as needed.
- Doctors should apply criteria for establishing anxiety and depressive states and promote disclosure of psychological problems.
- Fatigue is one of the most distressing and underestimated side effects of cancer treatment.

### 21.3.1 Lymphoedema and Postsurgical Complications

*Lymphoedema* is an increasingly common and recognised comorbidity of cancer therapy affecting nearly half of all patients who self-report symptoms following ALND and XRT, with incidence ranging from 4 to 17 % following SNLB and RT [3]. Subjective complaints routinely precede the onset of clinically apparent swelling, implying a need to screen all surgical candidates before and after surgical intervention to detect changes, assess risk levels and develop a strategy for early intervention when indicated. Although breast surgeons cannot prevent lymphoedema with current cancer management techniques, understanding the risk levels, early signs and availability of specialised resources can lead to interruption of this chronic, dreaded disease process.

Incidence of postsurgical lymphoedema usually develops within 6 months after surgery, but may be delayed much longer. The oedema is related to several constitutional, technical and managerial factors. People who have had clearance of the axilla are at risk of developing lymphoedema in 10–30 % of cases. After axillary sampling alone lymphoedema is less common, roughly from 5 up to 10 % of cases. After SNB lymphoedema is quite rare. The incidence is increased in patients who receive postoperative RT. Lymphoedema usually develops gradually over time and the swelling can be mild, moderate or severe.

Lymphoedema is assessed by measuring both arms at the same site in the mid biceps region, the antecubital fossa, the mid forearm and the wrist. The measurements are made with the arm straightened in a recumbent position. Care is taken not to pinch the skin when measuring the circumference at the different sites. Hand swelling is rated as none, minimal, moderate or severe in relation to increase on the limb volume (Table 21.1).

*Preventive and therapeutic measures* for the treatment of lymphoedema are listed below [3]:

**Table 21.1** Staging of lymphoedema according to the International Society of Lymphology and grade of severity based on limb volume [4, mod]

| Stage | Description | Severity |
|---|---|---|
| 0 | Lymphostasis: a subclinical condition where swelling isn't evident despite impaired lymph transport. It may exist for months or years before oedema occurs | *None* |
| I | An early accumulation of fluid relatively high in protein content. Oedema decreases with elevation. Pitting may occur. It may take up to a few hours of rest and elevation to reverse | *Minimal* (<20 % increase) |
| II | Pitting occurs, and the oedema is not appreciably reduced with elevation of the affected limb. In late Stage II, the tissue hardens and becomes fibrotic, and pitting no longer occurs | *Moderate* (20–40 % increase) |
| III | This stage is also referred to as elephantiasis. Pitting is absent. Skin changes like acanthosis, fat deposits and warty overgrowths may develop. Fluid may ooze from the skin due to high pressure in the lymphatic and venous vessels. It most commonly occurs in the legs and results from long-standing, inadequately treated or untreated lymphoedema | *Severe* (>40 % increase) |

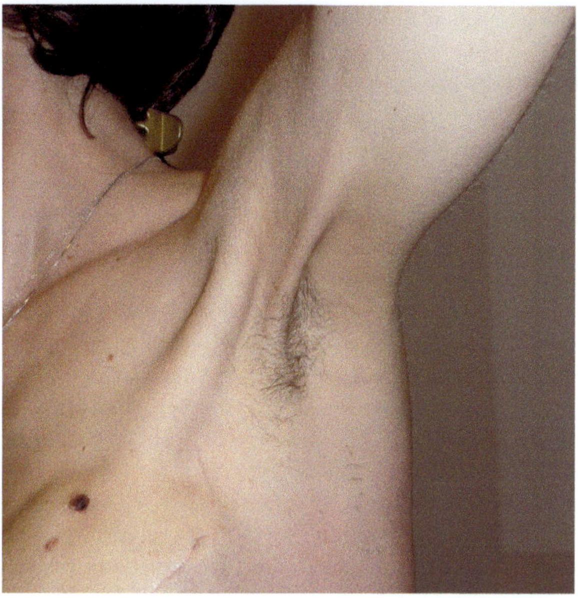

**Fig. 21.1** The ropelike appearance of lymphatic cording (axillary web syndrome) visible under the left axilla of a 48-year-old woman, 2 months after she underwent lumpectomy and axillary dissection

- Skin care is required to maintain good skin hydration and tropism and reduce the risk of infection.
- Exercise promotes lymph flow and maintains good limb function.
- Manual lymphatic drainage is a gentle skin massage that encourages lymph flow and is carried out by a trained therapist.
- Support/compression with multilayer bandaging is applied to reduce the size and improve the condition of the limb to allow fitting of elastic compression garments, which when fitted correctly control swelling and encourage lymph flow. Compression garments should be worn while the patient is exercising to reduce lymphatic filtration.
- Maintaining an adequate weight helps to prevent lymphoedema development, so dietary advice is important in all patients, but particularly in those who are overweight.

*Lymphoedema of the arm without pain* (lymphostasis) may be also due to massive axillary lymph node involvement, to scar tissue that cause blockages in lymph flow and make the enlargement of new lymphatic pathways harder and (rarely) to steroids used in some chemotherapy regimens that can cause fluid retention, usually temporary until the end of treatment.

*Lymphoedema of the arm with pain or paraesthesia* occurring several months after surgery may reflect recurrent tumour. This event is rare and the cancer is often not clinically discernible because it resides high in the apex of the axilla or lung and involves the brachial plexus. Patients may complain of tingling or pain in the hands and progressive weakness and atrophy of the hand and arm muscles. If sufficient time passes, a tumour mass becomes palpable in the axilla or supraclavicular fossa, but the patient is usually left with a paralysed hand unresponsive to therapy. These patients may receive RT to the axilla and supraclavicular fossa, if radiation has not previously been delivered to this region. The recurrence to the brachial plexus may not be easily seen on MRI or CT scanning. PET scanning may be useful in this circumstance. Occasionally, the pain of this nerve involvement is so severe that nerve blocks by a pain management specialist are necessary.

*Range restriction of movement* is assessed by the surgeon as active ranging at the shoulder joint, which was scored as equal to or decreased relative to the non-operated side.

*Numbness and paraesthesia* are evaluated by standard questions asked to each patient regarding the location and severity of the symptoms at the time of evaluation and compared with those in the postoperative period (unchanged, improved, significantly improved or completely resolved). Zones of persistent numbness, due to intercostobrachial nerve damage or section, should be outlined by the examining physician and confirmed by the patient.

*Lymphatic cording*, or *axillary web syndrome*, refers to one or more ropelike structures (more axillary *strings* characterise the *web* appearance) that develop mainly under the axilla (Fig. 21.1) but can extend to involve the medial aspect of the ipsilateral arm down to the antecubital fossa [5]. The syndrome usually appears after ALND, rarely after SLNB, 1–2 months after surgery of the axilla.

Lymphatic cording is associated with pain and limitation of shoulder movement. Symptoms resolve in all patients usually in 2–3 months. The duration of symptoms did not appear to be shortened by nonsteroidal anti-inflammatory drugs, physiotherapy or active range of motion exercises. Physiotherapy is anyway recommended and usually involves a combination of gentle stretching of the cord, exercises and manual lymph drainage.

*Chronic pain after breast surgery.* Some women have problems with neuropathic pain in the chest wall, armpit, and/or arm after surgery that doesn't subside over time. This is called post-mastectomy pain syndrome (PMPS) because it was first described in women who had mastectomies, but it can also happen after BCT. Studies have shown that about 20 % of women develop symptoms of PMPS after surgery. The classic symptoms of PMPS are pain and tingling in the chest wall, armpit, and/or arm. Pain may also be felt in the shoulder or surgical scar. Other common complaints include numbness, shooting or pricking pain, or unbearable itching.

PMPS is thought to be linked to damage done to the nerves in the armpit and chest wall during surgery, but the true causes are still unknown. Women who are younger, had an ALND, or who were treated with radiation after surgery are more likely to have problems with PMPS. PMPS can limit the use of the arm so that over time the woman could lose the ability to use it normally. Most women with PMPS say their symptoms are not severe. Severe PMPS (about 1 to 5 %) can be treated. Drugs commonly used to treat pain don't always work well for nerve pain, but some new available narcotic-like medications, as pregabalin and tramadol, are effective and not as addictive as narcotics.

### 21.3.2 Gynaecological, Sexual and Reproductive Issues

Treatment may affect many aspects of sexuality, and BC survivors should be routinely questioned about concerns related to sexual health and counselled or referred as needed. Menopausal symptoms that result from chemotherapy (in premenopausal women) and hormonal therapy (regardless of menopausal status) may make sexual activity less enjoyable and even painful.

The psychological sequelae of a BC diagnosis can include strains on relationships and changes in body image, both of which can be detrimental to sexual functioning. Sexual dysfunction is associated with depression in BC survivors. It is important for physicians to routinely ask BC survivors about their sexual functioning. Referral to a sexual health and/or mental health expert may be helpful, and this issue is above all an investigational subject. Five questions facilitating discussion are the following.

- Are you bound to be upset?
- Is inability to relax persistent for more than half of the time?
- Often women feel some change in their intimate relationship after BC diagnosis. How has this been for you?
- People frequently feel some change sexually during this time. What have you noticed?
- Speaking to a counsellor for a few sessions is often helpful because of the impact of BC diagnosis and its treatment on sexuality. Would you like a list of local counsellors?

Interventions for women who report dyspareunia or difficulty reaching orgasm may benefit from one or more of the following: local hormonal therapy, lubricants and counselling.

*Local oestrogen therapy*. Local oestrogen therapy comes in the form of creams and tablets, and it may provide relief of symptoms, but its use is controversial, particularly among women with a history of hormone receptor-positive BC. Although one study demonstrated that vaginal oestrogen results in a detectable increase in circulating oestradiol levels among women taking an aromatase inhibitor, another study suggests that vaginal oestrogen therapy does not result in an increased risk of recurrence in women taking endocrine therapy.

One study evaluating the impact of vaginal oestrogen on recurrence risk reported a low (less than 3 %) proportion of patients who used vaginal oestrogen (predominantly women taking TAM) and the finding that the use of vaginal oestrogen was not associated with an increased risk of recurrence. In light of this low-quality evidence, a decision to use vaginal oestrogens must be individualised, taking into account tumour characteristics, current symptoms and the risks and potential benefits of therapy, with input from both the primary oncologist and GP.

*Topical lidocaine*. For women with dyspareunia that appears to be isolated to tenderness at the vulvar vestibule, data from a prospective, randomised, double-blind trial suggest that topical lidocaine may provide relief. Treatment with topical aqueous 4 % lidocaine resulted in significant reduction in their worst pain score with intercourse and in no tenderness with speculum placement in almost all cases. Therefore, the data suggest that this intervention may be specific to women who have pain with penetration localised to the vulvar vestibule.

*Vaginal dehydroepiandrosterone.* Dehydroepiandrosterone (DHEA) is a steroid hormone produced by the adrenal glands. It is an indirect precursor to both oestrogen and testosterone, and levels decline with age. Vaginal DHEA preparations have been reported to improve vaginal health and sexual function in postmenopausal women. However, their safety and effectiveness in women treated for BC has not been cleared. A randomised multicentre trial examining the efficacy of adding dehydroepiandrosterone (DHEA) to a vaginal bioadhesive moisturiser in postmenopausal survivors of BC has found that daily rather than as-needed use of such a moisturiser significantly relieves symptoms of vaginal atrophy in these women and that when DHEA is added, survivors report significant improvements in sexual desire, arousal, pain and overall sexual function.

At 12 weeks, women treated reported improvements in sexual function and symptoms associated with vaginal atrophy. In addition, DHEA was associated with statistically significant improvements in sexual satisfaction as measured using standardised questionnaires. Compared with placebo, vaginal DHEA (at the 6.5 mg dose level) was associated with a higher incidence of voice changes and headaches, but well tolerated otherwise [6]. Although oestradiol levels were slightly increased by the vaginal DHEA in the study overall, this was not true in women receiving aromatase inhibitors. Although other studies are needed, current data support the use of vaginal DHEA as an option for postmenopausal BC survivors who suffer substantial vaginal complaints.

*Ospemifene* (Osphena®) is an oral selective oestrogen receptor modulator (SERM) acting similarly to an oestrogen on the vaginal epithelium, indicated for the treatment of dyspareunia. The FDA approved the medication in February 2013, but additional research addressing the expanded use of ospemifene in breast cancer patients is needed.

*Fertility and pregnancy after BC.* Young BC survivors may experience infertility after BC due to chemotherapy-related gonadotoxicity and the delay in childbearing required when women are taking the recommended 5 years of hormonal therapy.

For women with a history of BC, a subsequent pregnancy does not appear to compromise survival in patients with positive receptor status. A recent meta-analysis of 14 case–control studies that evaluated the impact of pregnancy on the overall survival of women with BC showed that BC patients who became pregnant had a 40 % reduction in the risk of death, compared with those who did not get pregnant. This outcome is likely explained by a selection bias known as the healthy mother effect, such that only healthy BC survivors were able to conceive and carry a pregnancy. However, other studies confirm pregnancy after BC is safe regardless of receptor status.

While some experts recommend that patients wait 2 years after completing adjuvant therapy before attempting conception in order to avoid pregnancy during the time of highest relapse risk, limited data suggest that pregnancy sooner is safe.

Encouragingly, prior BC treatments do not appear to increase the risk of congenital malformation.

*Contraception after BC.* While women with a history of BC may wish to preserve fertility, they may not have an imminent desire to become pregnant. The safety and efficacy of hormonal contraception has not been well studied in women with BC, as these women have traditionally been excluded from studies of hormonal contraceptives. The levonorgestrel-releasing intrauterine device (LNG-IUD) has been evaluated in women with a history of BC, although primarily as a method of endometrial protection from the effects of TAM rather than as a contraceptive modality. Data are limited and inconclusive, but suggest an increased risk of cancer recurrence, although the difference was not statistically significant, despite a low rate of systemic hormone absorption.

World Health Organization guidelines for medical eligibility for contraceptive use suggest avoiding hormonal contraception in women with a current or past history of BC, particularly in those with hormone receptor-positive disease. Clinicians should discuss the use of a nonhormonal contraceptive method (condom, diaphragm, copper IUD) and help the woman choose the method most consistent with her lifestyle and beliefs.

### 21.3.3 Psychological and Relational Issues

Up to 30 % of women with BC develop an anxiety state or depressive illness within a year of diagnosis, which is three to four times the expected rate in matched community samples. After mastectomy without reconstruction, 20–30 % of patients develop persisting problems with body image and sexual difficulties. Breast-conserving surgery reduces problems with body image, but this may be offset by increased fears of recurrence.

After reconstruction some patients are predominantly worried about the satisfaction of their own needs and poorly sensitive to the attitudes and the reactions of the others. On the contrary, women with a strong personality face reconstruction as the conclusive symbolic action to overcome the illness and to repair the mutilation.

The same with regard to communication. A more practical division of psychological types is the Miller Behavioural Style Scale, where patients are divided into *monitors* or *blunters*. The former group of patients request much information, while the latter avoid asking questions. Yet, although some patients may demand information, they do not wish to be burdened with responsibility for any final decisions on treatment. Other patients express little interest in obtaining information about their disease or appear unreceptive to any information that is offered, either in verbal or written form.

Doctors can promote disclosure of such problems by asking questions and clarifying the responses about patients' perceptions of the nature of their illness, their reactions to it and about their experience of losing a breast or having radiotherapy or chemotherapy. By being empathic, making educated guesses about how a patient is feeling and summarising what has been disclosed, doctors promote disclosure and expression of related feelings.

When there is any hint of *anxiety or depression* (Table 21.2), clinicians should inquire about key symptoms by asking open directive questions (*What changes have you noticed while you have been depressed? How have you been sleeping?*). Patients with problems with their *body image* should be asked how much they avoid looking at their chest wall and how they react if they catch sight of it. In patients with *sexual difficulties*, doctors should check whether they represent a new problem and explore the reactions of patients and their partners.

Patients who have a core mood change but too few symptoms to justify a clinical diagnosis usually respond to basic emotional support and do not merit psychiatric referral, especially given the stigma perceived to be associated with such a referral.

*Markers of risk for affective disorders* may be listed as below:

**Table 21.2** Basic criteria for establishing anxiety or depressive state [7, mod.]

| |
|---|
| *Criteria for anxiety state* |
| Persistent anxiety, tension or inability to relax |
| Present for more than half of the time for 4 weeks |
| Cannot pull self out of it or be distracted by others |
| Substantial departure from normal mood |
| *Plus at least four of the following:* |
| Initial insomnia |
| Irritability |
| Impaired concentration |
| Intolerance of noise |
| Panic attacks |
| Somatic manifestations |
| *Criteria for depressive state* |
| Persistent low mood, tension or inability to relax |
| Present for more than half of the time for 4 weeks |
| Cannot be distracted out of it by self or others |
| Qualitatively or quantitatively significantly different from normal mood |
| Inability to enjoy oneself |
| *Plus at least four of the following:* |
| Diurnal variation of mood |
| Repeated or early waking |
| Impaired concentration or indecisiveness |
| Feeling hopeless or suicidal |
| Feelings of guilt, self-blame, being a burden or worthlessness |
| Irritability and anger for no reason |
| Loss of interest |
| Retardation or agitation |
| No confiding tie |
| Low self-esteem |
| Unresolved concerns |

- Past psychiatric illness
- Toxicity as a result of radiotherapy or chemotherapy
- Lymphoedema or pain
- Problems with body image

The diagnosis of BC and its aftermath undoubtedly lead to major life changes for most patients, but these changes are not always negative. The way in which a person who has a diagnosis of BC copes is likely to be consistent with their normal functioning style or personality traits. Coping skills that are characterised by an active and optimistic approach, such as a *fighting spirit*, tend to lead to better outcomes in psychological terms.

*Denial* of the experience of cancer tends to lead to higher distress and maladaptive adjustment, although denial in a pure sense is an unusual response. At present, significant psychological distress in women with BC continues to be underestimated and therefore undertreated. Referral to specialist services should be considered for those patients who are recognised and experiencing adjustment disorders or depression, especially if some markers of risk for affective disorders are present.

### 21.3.4 Family and Social Issues

BC may affect not only the patient but her family too. Even if most of cases of BC are sporadic, a genetic inheritance should be considered.

*Genetic Counselling.* BRCA testing should be strongly considered for men and for women diagnosed under the age of 40 or with Ashkenazi heritage and/or a strong family history of breast or ovarian cancer. Prior to testing, it is important that patients be counselled about the potential ramifications of test results for themselves and their families, both medically and psychosocially (see Sect. 2.3).

Genetic testing of the BC survivor is important, particularly in order to facilitate testing in other family members. Once a particular mutation has been identified, testing other family members is technically straightforward. While it is possible to begin the genetic testing process in an unaffected individual, there is a greater chance that these results will be inconclusive. Therefore, the BC survivor should be tested, particularly if her own children and first-degree relatives are also interested in their personal genetic susceptibility.

*Fatigue.* Fatigue, one of the relatively common side effects of cancer and its treatment, blemishes relational wealth in the family and working environment. Fatigue, in contrast to common tiredness, is a daily lack of energy, an unusual or excessive whole-body tiredness not relieved by sleep. Usually, it comes on suddenly, does not result from activity or exertion and is not relieved by rest or sleep. It often is described as *paralysing*.

Fatigue can prevent a person from functioning normally and impacts the individual quality of life and relational wealth. Our human welfare depends on both material and relational wealth. Relational wealth, in contrast with material wealth made up of commodities, emanates from our interconnections with other human beings. It gives us inner strength and emotional security and defines our quality of life.

The exact reason of fatigue is unknown. It is not predictable by tumour type, treatment or stage of illness. Radiation therapy and any chemotherapy drug may cause fatigue. Patients frequently experience fatigue after several weeks of chemotherapy, but this varies among patients. It may continue even after treatment is complete and can be acute (lasting a month or less) or chronic (lasting from 1 to 6 months or longer).

After having excluded other causes (among the most common: anaemia, hypothyroidism, stress, depression, malnutrition, side effect of medicaments, etc.), the patient should be advised to take some specific measures as:

- Keep a positive attitude and be assertive instead of aggressive.
- Eat well-balanced meals.
- Choose activities which promote mental activation (it is essential that they plan, schedule and take ownership of their own time); undertake daily physical activities (e.g. walking).
- Seek opportunity to be listened to and talk about their own symptoms.

In any case, a patient who experiences fatigue should not be told that symptoms are *part of the disease*.

## 21.4 Educational Follow-Up

**Clinical Practice Points**

- Outpatient breast clinics should take the chance to foster health and well-being messages. Many helpful websites are also available for patient education.
- Lifestyle modification can empower and boost physical and mental health in BC survivors and seems to improve outcomes.
- After menopause most of a woman's oestrogen comes from fat tissue; therefore, women who are overweight should be offered dietary advice and counselling.
- Multiple studies have shown that exercise improves quality of life in BC survivors.

### 21.4.1 Recommended Actions to Improve Quality of Life

Quality of life is a multidimensional construct that takes into account the physical, mental, social, economic and spiritual aspects of life. Limited data suggest that patients treated for BC have good quality of life, particularly as they move beyond the treatment period. However, they may continue to have some lingering concerns.

Patients often ask what they can do to improve their overall outcome from BC. Lifestyle modification can be an empowering and effective way to boost physical and mental health in BC survivors and seems to improve outcomes. Observational data suggest that exercise, avoidance of obesity and minimisation of alcohol intake are associated with a decreased risk of BC recurrence and death in survivors.

*Diet, physical activity and body weight* are collectively considered energy balance factors because they describe the relationship between energy consumed (diet), energy expended (physical activity) and energy stored (adiposity). They have each been linked to cancer outcomes, particularly in survivors of BC.

*BODY WEIGHT.* It is known that being overweight or obese after menopause increases recurrence risk. After menopause most of a woman's oestrogen comes from fat tissue. Having more fat tissue after menopause can increase chance of recurrences by raising oestrogen levels. Also, as said before (see Sect. 2.1), women who are overweight tend to have higher blood insulin levels. Higher insulin levels have also been linked to some cancers, including BC. However, the connection between weight and BC risk is complex. For example, the risk appears to be increased for women who gained weight as an adult but may not be increased among those who have been overweight since childhood. Also, excess fat in the waist area may affect risk more than the same amount of fat in the hips and thighs. Researchers believe that fat cells in various parts of the body have subtle differences that may explain this.

*DIETARY FACTOR.* Western lifestyle, characterised by reduced physical activity and a diet rich in fat, refined carbohydrates and animal protein, is associated with high prevalence of excessive weight, metabolic syndrome, insulin resistance and high plasma levels of several growth factors and sex hormones. Most of these factors are associated with risk and, in BC patients, with increased risk of recurrences. Recent trials have proven that such a metabolic and endocrine imbalance can be favourably modified through comprehensive dietary modification, shifting from Western to Mediterranean and macrobiotic diet.

At present, recommendations for BC patients include the following measures:

- Reduce calorie intake, through the preferred consumption of highly satiating foods, such as unrefined cereals, legumes and vegetables.
- Reduce high glycaemic index and high insulinaemic index food, such as refined flours, potatoes, white rice, corn flakes, sugar and milk, using instead whole grain cereals (unrefined rice, barley, millet, oat, buckwheat, spelt), legumes (any type, including soy products) and vegetables (any type, except potatoes).
- Reduce sources of saturated fat (red and processed meat, milk and dairy products), preferring instead unrefined vegetable fats, such as olive oil, nuts and oleaginous seeds.
- Reduce protein intake, mainly animal proteins (except fish).

*Fats*. Research is still mixed on the role that fats, and which specific types of fats, play in BC risk and prevention. According to results from the Women's Health Initiative study of dietary fat and BC, there is no definite evidence that a low-fat diet will help prevent BC. However, a low-fat or non-fat dairy products are a healthier choice than high-fat ones.

*Fruits and Vegetables* are important sources of antioxidants, which may help protect against the tissue damage linked to increased cancer risk. Antioxidants include vitamin C, vitamin E and carotenoids such as beta-carotene and lycopene. Richly coloured fruits and vegetables – not supplements – are the best sources for these nutrients. These fibre-rich foods are an essential part of a healthy diet. However, it is not clear whether fruits and vegetables can specifically prevent BC development or recurrence.

*Soy*. The American Cancer Society recommends that women with BC eat only moderate amounts of soy foods and avoid taking dietary supplements that contain high amounts of isoflavones, a type of phytoestrogen. Although there is no convincing evidence that soy affects the risk of recurrence, the theoretical risk that phytoestrogens could stimulate the growth of hormonally sensitive cancers raises the concern that high soy intake could be dangerous. Similarly, the safety and efficacy of many other complementary therapies including mistletoe, high doses of vitamins and trace elements like selenium, zinc and copper remains uncertain.

*Alcohol intake*. Even if there is likelihood that alcohol increases the risk of BC (see Sect. 2.1), this evidence in recurrence is limited. However, overweight and postmenopausal women seemed to experience the greatest harm from alcohol intake as measured by BC recurrence risk.

*PHYSICAL ACTIVITY*. Epidemiological studies consistently showed that a sedentary lifestyle is associated with increased risk of BC, both before and after menopause. Women who practice regularly at least some physical activity decrease their risk by 30 % or more. There is evidence that physical activity may also protect against cancer recurrence. Daily physical activity corresponding to about 30 min of brisk walking may reduce recurrences by 50 %. More intense activity does not seem to add any benefit.

In short, sedentary lifestyle and excessive weight are associated with insulin resistance and increased androgenic activity. Physical activity improves insulin sensitivity and decreases testosterone levels and, in the long term, IGF-I levels. Moreover, exercise can help reduce body fat, which in turn lowers levels of cancer-promoting hormones such as oestrogen. The American Cancer Society recommends engaging in 45–60 min of physical activity at least 5 days a week.

Even if evidence is not clearly proven, many studies indicate that both aerobic and weight training exercises benefit the body and the mind and improve quality of life for BC survivors. Physical activity contributes to health by reducing the heart rate, decreasing the risk for cardiovascular disease and reducing the amount of bone loss that is associated with age and osteoporosis. Physical activity also helps the body use calories more efficiently, thereby helping in weight loss and maintenance. It can increase basal metabolic rate, reduces appetite and helps in the reduction of body fat.

Multiple studies have shown that exercise improves quality of life in BC survivors. Therefore, patients should be encouraged to adopt a physically active lifestyle following treatment for BC.

### 21.4.2 Complementary and Alternative Medicine Treatments (CAMs)

The growing interest in complementary and alternative medicine (CAM) has been particularly marked in patients diagnosed with cancer. As known, *complementary* generally refers to using a non-mainstream approach together with conventional medicine, while *alternative* refers to using a non-mainstream approach *in place of* conventional medicine. CAM is defined by the National Institutes of Health (NIH) as incorporating four separate domains: mind–body medicine (patient support groups, cognitive–behavioural therapy, meditation, prayer), biologically based practices (herbs, dietary supplements, vitamins), manipulative/body-based practices (osteopathic manipulation, massage) and energy medicine (qi gong, electromagnetic field therapies). In addition, a separate domain that includes whole systems of practice has been defined (homoeopathic medicine, naturopathic medicine, traditional Chinese medicine).

The widespread use of CAM has to be acknowledged and the reasons for this understood [8]. Deficiencies in the practice of conventional medicine that lead to the adoption of CAM need to be addressed. The goal of complementary medicine is to balance the whole person physically, mentally and emotionally. For many people diagnosed with BC, complementary medicine may help to relieve symptoms, relieves treatment side effects and improves quality of life. From this standpoint, the boundaries between complementary and conventional medicine may overlap and change with time. For example, acupuncture and guided imagery, both once considered complementary or alternative, are now used in some hospitals to help with pain management.

In almost all cases a consensual rather than an integrative approach may be reached. Medical and paramedical practitioners are working in good faith towards the same direction to improve the length and quality of life. The way forward is to build bridges between the culture based on the guidelines and the culture based on a non-mainstream approach.

### 21.4.3 Support Services

*CANCER COUNSELLING CENTRES.* Knowledge is power not only for the physician. The more educated the patients are about their disease process, the more opportunities they have to learn about available therapeutic and supporting options. Assistance in social care differs from country to country. In some countries, such as Germany, special state-sponsored cancer counselling centres are available to the public. In France nearly all hospitals employ highly qualified social workers that are responsible for securing outside social care. In other countries, charity institutions, self-help organisations and support groups take charge of the social and legal aspects of outpatient patient care.

The social services of most clinics, as well as counselling services of the national cancer organisations and self- help groups, provide the patient, the family or the physician responsible for further outpatient care of address list. It is important that such lists are made available to patients who request them. The number of patients asking for this kind of information might be higher than expected. Doctors must not, at the same time, undervalue the importance of certain aspects such as the fact that:

- About 10 % of patients need a customised psycho-oncological support.
- About one third of patients have a clinical and individual situation not requiring a specific assistance.
- Counselling centres are visited more frequently by higher-educated women and by patients with advanced disease, less frequently by lower class people and older survivors.
- Some patients are afraid of facing their own fears and the distress caused by what they experienced.
- Some members of the patient's family may need supporting services.
- Sometimes members of the family may hinder the decisional process, and their advice, which may be given with good intent, may not ultimately be in the patient's best interest.
- Counselling centres strive to inform patients and family members and to soothe the fears and the prejudices, but attendance of some distrustful patients can lead to an outcome conflicting with that they actually pursue.

With the explosion of the Internet, many cancer centres and hospitals, non-profit foundations, women's coalitions and pharmaceutical companies have built solid websites on which various topics are featured (see Appendix). Among the organisations that provide services to cancer patients, most notable are the services offered by the different national cancer societies (usually dot *org* or dot *gov* domains). Most organisations not only provide written material for cancer patients but also have helplines for patients to call. Doctors must take into account that the creation of interactive online support is becoming a reality.

Occasionally, patients can feel overwhelmed with the information that they can be exposed to, if such information is gathered *before* the decision-making process. It would be preferable that patients waited until *after* they processed the more personal information obtained by their physicians regarding their treatment.

*PSYCHO-ONCOLOGICAL CARE.* In some contextual and individual cases, a diagnosis of BC can significantly impact the psychological and emotional well-being of patients and their families. For some women having to face cancer is probably one of the most stressful situations they will ever be likely to experience. Challenges include adjusting to the illness; the stresses of medical treatment; emotional needs; depression, anxiety, relationship and caregiving strains; coping with pain, insomnia and other symptoms; and much more. Some patients (and sometimes their caregivers) may require a short- or longer-term support to help them address these emotional difficulties and mental health problems. There is no right or wrong way to cope, but only a right way for every individual. Patients need time to adapt to their change without expecting too much too soon, but having realistic expectations; therefore, it is important that patients be aware of all of available support services.

Patients admitted in a clinic for the treatments can benefit from an inpatient service. A psychological multidisciplinary team should include a psychiatrist, a counsellor, a psychotherapist and a specialist nurse and should provide the psycho-oncology service working closely with other staff. However, for some women this may result in an additional reliance with the clinic, so they rather prefer outside operating venues.

Outpatient cancer counselling centre models should include psycho-oncologists who usually are better employed to actively approach patient groups. In some cases, even if everything is nicely arranged, attendance will be no longer satisfactory. It is important to keep in mind that the not-use of these services not necessarily means that patients do not need help but that other factors may represent barriers to psychological care access when patients have to actively seek help.

The most onerous task is to address those who are unable, cannot or do not want call for help. Every local GP, oncologist, surgeon or oncology nurse specialist should refer to a psychological support centre for any patient they think may benefit from these services. For a doctor, referring a patient to a support centre is far from being a sign of incompetence, and well for a patient, it is not a sign of failure asking for help or to feeling unable to cope relying only on her own strengths.

*HEALTH INSURANCE.* The limited ability to obtain credit poses a particularly large problem for cancer patients, who would like to arrange an independent existence and require financial coverage in order to do so, taking out health insurance. Most life insurance providers only accommodate potentially curatively treated cancer patients who show no signs of tumour activity. In general, they accept the clinical findings that were obtained in the framework of the aftercare examinations when concluding the contract.

On top of that, life insurance companies make a distinction between various risk classes, based primarily on life expectancy. These risk classes result in different waiting periods. This means that the insurance sum is only paid out following a specific waiting period, the length of which is dependent on the prognostic criteria.

Even when the carcinoma is in an early stage and exhibits a good prognosis, life insurance companies require a postponement of payment for 2 years beginning at the inception of therapy. In case of a poor prognosis, insurance companies generally decline life insurance. This is very disheartening.

*PREJUDICES AND DISCRIMINATIONS.* Finally, some cancer patients suffer discrimination in their own family and in society. At work some patients are denied taking time off for medical appointments; others are overtaken for promotion. Some patients feel abused by their colleagues, who may give them unfair or demeaning tasks, or fail to make reasonable changes to enable them to do their job. Despite the recent introduction of the Equality Act, which should protect workers with cancer, some patients feel so harassed that they quit their jobs.

Cancer patients can experience damaging prejudices inside their own families, friends or be victim of their own prejudices. In the *Illness as Metaphor* the writer Susan Sontag, a cancer patient, challenged the *blame the victim* mentality behind the language society when used to describe diseases as cancer or AIDS. Some diseases are associated with personal psychological traits, and the metaphor used to describe it leads to an association between repressed passions and the physical disease itself. Especially in the past, wrapping diseases in metaphors discourages, silences and shames patients, while the clearest and most truthful way of thinking about disease is to remain realistic. Prejudices, unfortunately, still persist, as do the consequences inherent to them. It is not our place to deal with them, but only to help to recognise them. In an outpatient breast clinic, alongside a greatly animated work, anything unusual may occur, and it is important to remember that it is not always required to open doors leading to secret places, unless we are able to close them safely.

## References

1. Khatcheressian JL, Hurley P, Bantug E, et al. Breast cancer follow-up and management after primary treatment: American Society of Clinical Oncology clinical practice guideline update. J Clin Oncol. 2013;31:961–5.
2. Rosselli Del Turco M, Palli D, Cariddi A, Ciatto S, Pacini P, Distante V. Intensive diagnostic follow-up after treatment of primary breast cancer. A randomized trial. National Research Council Project on Breast Cancer follow-up. JAMA. 1994;271:1593–7.
3. Chagpar AB. The axilla: current management including sentinel node and lymphoedema. In: Dixon JM, editor. Breast surgery. London: Elsevier; 2014.
4. Sabel MS. Regional management of breast cancer. In: Sabel MS, editor. Essentials of breast surgery. Philadelphia: Mosby; 2009.
5. Moskovitz AH, Anderson BO, Yeung RS, et al. Axillary web syndrome with subcutaneous nodules following axillary surgery. Am J Surg. 2001;181:434–9.
6. Archer DF. Dehydroepiandrosterone intravaginal administration for the management of post-menopausal vulvovaginal atrophy. J Steroid Biochem Mol Biol. 2015;145:139–43.
7. Hacking B. Psychological impact of breast cancer. In: Dixon JM, editor. ABC of breast diseases. 4th ed. Oxford: Wiley-Blackwell; 2012.
8. Baum M, Ernst E, Lejeune S, Horneber M. Role of complementary and alternative medicine in the care of patients with breast cancer. Report on the European Society of Mastology (EUSOMA) Workshop, Florence, Italy, December 2004. Eur J Cancer. 2006;42:1702–10.

## Further Reading

Eyles C, Leydon GM, Hoffman CJ, et al. Mindfulness for the self-management of fatigue, anxiety, and depression in women with metastatic breast cancer: a mixed methods feasibility study. Integr Cancer Ther. 2015;14:42–56.

Ghose A, Kundu R, Toumeh A, Hornbeck C, Mohamed I. A review of obesity, insulin resistance, and the role of exercise in breast cancer patients. Nutr Cancer. 2015;27:1–6.

Grunfeld E, Levine MN, Julian JA, et al. Randomized trial of long-term follow-up for early-stage breast cancer: a comparison of family physician versus specialist care. J Clin Oncol. 2006;24:848–55.

Hayes DF. Clinical practice. Follow-up of patients with early breast cancer. N Engl J Med. 2007;356:2505–13.

Kushi LH, Doyle C, McCullough M, et al. American Cancer Society guidelines on nutrition and physical activity for cancer prevention: reducing the risk of cancer with healthy food choices and physical activity. CA Cancer J Clin. 2012;62:30–67.

Patricolo GE, Armstrong K, Riutta J, Lanni T. Lymphedema care for the breast cancer patient: an integrative approach. Breast. 2015;24:82–5.

Puglisi F, Fontanella C, Numico G, et al. Follow-up of patients with early breast cancer: is it time to rewrite the story? Crit Rev Oncol Hematol. 2014;91:130–41.

Shahpar H, Atieh A, Maryam A, et al. Risk factors of lymph edema in breast cancer patients. Int J Breast Cancer. 2013. doi:10.1155/2013/641818.

Taib NA. Recognizing pitfalls in breast cancer follow-up: a necessity reply. World J Surg. 2015;39:548–9.

van Hezewijk M, Smit DJF, Bastiaannet E, et al. Feasibility of tailored follow-up for patients with early breast cancer. Breast. 2014;23:852–8.

**Websites in Appendix**: *Complimentary and Alternative Medicine*, A-4.7; *Lymphedema*, A-4.12; *Quality of Life/Nutrition/Exercises*, A-4.18.

# Appendix

## A. Breast Diseases in the Net

A wise use of the information that can be found online can be an opportunity for growth, not just from a professional point of view, but because it serves as a spur for a variety of actions. The right words for a correct communication can be found online, together with the questionnaires and the technical sheets, and, moreover, all the recommendations by the biggest institutions, and the possibility of reading about clinical trials that could be beneficial to some patients who have specific needs. This personal selection of the most reliable websites (updated 30 January 2015) is meant to provide the users with some useful coordinates that will help them hold the helm steady in order to follow the right course.

### A.1 Main Websites Including Professional and Supporting Information

- *Bestcancersites* (www.bestcancersites.com) is a very comprehensive summary of the best websites, though there is much to discover in the links of the following sites.
- The *American Cancer Society* (*ACS*) (www.cancer.org) is one of the most comprehensive websites that provides in-depth information on all cancer topics on the net. http://www.cancer.org/cancer/breastcancer/index.
- The *National Cancer Institute* (*NCI*) (www.cancer.gov) is another very good source of information presented in an easily understandable way. http://www.cancer.gov/cancertopics/types/breast.
- The *National Library of Medicine* (*NLM*) and The *National Institute of Health* (*NIH*) (www.medlineplus.gov) develops a well-designed site at www.nlm.nih.gov/medlineplus/breastcancer.html.
- The *National Comprehensive Cancer Network* (*NCCN*) is an alliance of 21 of the world's leading cancer centres and updates a complete library of clinical practice guidelines. Guidelines *for physicians* are at www.nccn.org/professionals/



A.M. Pluchinotta (ed.), *The Outpatient Breast Clinic: Aiming at Best Practice*,
DOI 10.1007/978-3-319-15907-2

physician_gls/default.asp, while guidelines *for patients* are at www.nccn.com/patient-guidelines.html.

- *Cancer Research UK* focuses on diagnosis, treatment, and also clinical trials. http://www.cancerresearchuk.org/about-cancer/type/breast-cancer/.
- *Breast Cancer Org* (www.breastcancer.org) is one of the best sites specifically devoted to BC, covering a wide range of matters with many articles easy to understand.
- *Breast Cancer Care* (www.breastcancercare.org.uk) is the UK's leading provider of information, practical assistance, and emotional support.
- *WebMD, Breast Cancer Health Center* (http://www.webmd.com/breast-cancer/default.htm) offers the latest in news and technology on BC.
- *MedLine Plus* is the National Institutes of Health web portal which also covers BC. http://vsearch.nlm.nih.gov/vivisimo/cgi-bin/query-meta?v%3Aproject=medlineplus&query=breast+cancer.

## A.2 Main Websites Addressed to Patients, Families, and Caregivers

- *ACS, Caregivers*. www.cancer.org/treatment/caregivers/index.
- *NCI, For Caregivers, Family, and Friends*. www.cancer.gov/cancertopics/coping/familyfriends.
- *Susan G. Komen* (http://www.komen.org) is the largest source of non-profit funds dedicated to the fight against BC in the world, also well-known for its Komen Race for the Cure events. Site includes excellent questionnaire sheets that the patient can use when speaking with her care providers.
- *Breast Cancer Support* (www.bcsupport.org) is a worthwhile online support group.
- The *Nancy's list* (www.nancyslist.org) is filled of up-to-date information.
- *Living Beyond Breast Cancer* connects people with trusted BC information and gets support. www.lbbc.org.
- *Maggie's Cancer Caring Centres* is popular in UK. http://www.maggiescentres.org.
- *ABCD after breast cancer diagnosis* offers a one-to-one support customized support for patients and family members. http://www.abcdbreastcancersupport.org/.
- *Macmillan Cancer Support* (www.macmillan.org.uk) is a very popular UK's cancer information site.
- *Breakthrough Breast Cancer* (www.breakthrough.org.uk) is another UK's well-known provider.
- *Cancer Care* (www.cancercare.org) is a large USA-based organisation that provides information resources, but also advice on matters such as financial assistance, and counselling.
- *Rethink Breast Cancer* (http://rethinkbreastcancer.com) helps patients understand the different forms of BC.

## A.3 Breast Cancer Coalitions for Advocacy

- *Europa Donna* (www.europadonna.org/) with its 46 member countries is the most widespread European Breast Cancer Coalition, and represents the interests of women regarding BC to local and national authorities as well as to institutions of the European Union.
- *National Breast Cancer Coalition* (*NBCC*) is committed to knowing how to end BC by 2020. To do this *Breast Cancer Deadline 2002 project* takes actions to disrupt the *status quo* of BC for positive social change. www.breastcancerdeadline2020.org/get-involved/training/online-center-for-advocacy-training/.

## A.4 Websites Addressed to Specific Issues

### A.4.1 Advanced BC

- *Advanced BC* (www.advancedbc.org) helps patients with advanced BC to make good treatment decisions based on the latest clinical research.
- *Medhelp* (medhelp.org) runs a *Breast Cancer Stage 3 & 4* forum.

### A.4.2 Adjuvant Systemic Therapy/Adjuvant Radiotherapy

- *Adjuvanonline*! (www.adjuvantonline.com) is addressed to professionals and provides information about the risk of the cancer recurrence within the following 10 years and what benefits might be expected from hormone therapy and/or chemotherapy.
- *Mayo Clinic* (www.mayoclinic.org) is addressed to patients and helps to evaluate the benefits of adjuvant therapy. www.mayoclinic.org/diseases-conditions/cancer/in-depth/adjuvant-therapy/art-20046687.
- *Chemocare* provides the latest information about chemotherapy to patients and their families, caregivers, and friends. www.chemocare.com.
- *NCI*, *Radiation Therapy and You*: *Support for People With Cancer* (book). www.cancer.gov/cancertopics/coping/radiation-therapy-and-you.

### A.4.3 Benign Conditions/Breast Pain

- *Breast Cancer Care*, *Benign Breast Conditions*. www.breastcancercare.org.uk/breast-cancer-breast-health/diagnosis/benign/.
- *ACS*, *Non-Cancerous Breast Conditions*. www.cancer.org/docroot/CRI/content/CRI_2_6X_Non_Cancerous_Breast_Conditions_59.asp.
- *WebMD*, *Breast Pain* (*Mastalgia*) – *Topic Overview*. www.webmd.com/women/tc/breast-pain-mastalgia-topic-overview.
- *Society of Obstetricians and Gynaecologists of Canada* (*SOGC*), *Clinical Practice Guideline*. http://sogc.org/wp-content/uploads/2013/01/170E-CPG-January20061.pdf.

### A.4.4 Breast Forms/Implants

- *Breast Cancer Care*, *Prosthesis*. www.breastcancercare.org.uk/search/site/prosthesis.
- *Breast Cancer Org*, *Prosthetics*: *An Alternative to Reconstruction*. www.breastcancer.org/treatment/surgery/reconstruction/prosthetics.

- *ACS-Reach to Recovery* program, *Prostheses*. www.cancer.org/treatment/treatmentsandsideeffects/physicalsideeffects/dealingwithsymptomsathome/caring-for-the-patient-with-cancer-at-home-prostheses.
- *Food and Drug Administration* (*FDA*), *Risk of Breast Implants*. www.fda.gov/MedicalDevices/ProductsandMedicalProcedures/ImplantsandProsthetics/BreastImplants/ucm064106.htm.

### A.4.5 Breast Self-Examination

- *Breast Cancer Org* is a reliable website that explains how to do a breast self-exam. www.breastcancer.org/symptoms/testing/types/self_exam/.
- The *AJC* provides a detailed guide at www.cancer.org/cancer/breastcancer/detailedguide/breast-cancer-detection?sitearea=.

### A.4.6 Clinical Trials

- *NCI*, *Clinical Trials*. www.cancer.gov/clinicaltrials/ or also http://www.clinical-trials.gov.
- *ACS*, *Emerging Med Clinical Trials Matching Service*. http://clinicaltrials.cancer.org.

### A.4.7 Complementary and Alternative Therapies

- *Quackwatch*, *A Special Message for Cancer Patients Seeking "Alternative" Treatments*. www.quackwatch.org/00AboutQuackwatch/altseek.html.
- *ACS*, *Complementary and Alternative Therapies*. www.cancer.org/Treatment/TreatmentsandSideEffects/ComplementaryandAlternativeMedicine/index.
- *National Center for Complementary and Alternative Medicine*. www.nccam.nih.gov.

### A.4.8 Fatigue

- *Breast Cancer Org*, *Managing Fatigue*. www.breastcancer.org/tips/fatigue.
- *AJC*, *Fatigue*. www.cancer.org/treatment/treatmentsandsideeffects/physicalsideeffects/fatigue/index.
- *NCI*, *Fatigue*. www.cancer.gov/cancertopics/pdq/supportivecare/fatigue/patient.
- *WebMD*, *Cancer-Related Fatigue*. www.webmd.com/breast-cancer/guide/combating-fatigue-breast-cancer.

### A.4.9 Fertility

- *Best Cancer Sites* (www.bestcancersites.com/fertility) provides links to websites with information and support on fertility issues.
- *Young Survival Coalition* (www.youngsurvival.org), *Can I preserve my fertility*? http://www.youngsurvival.org/breast-cancer-in-young-women/faq/can-i-preserve-my-fertility
- *German Breast Group*, *BC in Pregnancy* (http://www.germanbreastgroup.de/en/trials/adjuvantpreventive/pregnancy.html) or *Brustkrebs in der Schwangerschaft* (http://www.germanbreastgroup.de/studien/adjuvant/brustkrebs-in-der-schwangerschaft.html).
- *Oncofertility Consortium* (www.myoncofertility.org).

### A.4.10 Guidelines/Treatment Options (See Also Sects. A.1, A.4.17, and A.4.20)

- The *NCI* (www.cancer.gov) and the (*NCCN*) (www.nccn.org) are good sources of information and guidelines (see Sect. A.1).
- The *American Society of Clinical Oncology* (*ASCO*) publishes online guidelines/recommendations for unusual clinical conditions. http://www.instituteforquality.org/practice-guidelines.
- *Canadian Medical Association Journal* (CMAJ), *Clinical Practice Guidelines for the Care and Treatment of Breast Cancer*. http://www.cmaj.ca/content/158/3/suppl/DC1#physicians.
- *World Health Organisation* (*WHO*), *Guidelines for management of breast cancer*. http://applications.emro.who.int/dsaf/dsa697.pdf.

### A.4.11 Imaging/Screening

- *Radiopaedia*, the online collaborative radiology resource, at http://radiopaedia.org.
- *U.S. Preventive Services Task Force*, *Breast Cancer: Screening*. http://www.uspreventiveservicestaskforce.org/uspstf/uspsbrca.htm.
- *NCI*, *Screening and Testing to Detect Cancer: Breast Cancer*. http://www.cancer.gov/cancertopics/screening/Breast.
- *American College of Physicians*, *Screening Mammography for Women 40–49 Years of Age: a Clinical Practice Guideline*. http://annals.org/article.aspx?articleid=733957.

### A.4.12 Inflammatory Breast Cancer

- *Breast Cancer Org*, *Inflammatory Breast Cancer*. www.breastcancer.org/symptoms/types/inflammatory/.
- *IBC Support* (by Breast Cancer Research Foundation), *Inflammatory breast cancer help and support*. www.ibcsupport.org.
- *Inflammatory Breast Cancer Research Foundation* is another site that includes a list of misleading symptoms of IBC. www.ibcresearch.org.
- *Inflammatory Breast Cancer*. www.theibcnetwork.org.
- *ACS*, *Inflammatory Breast Cancer*. www.cancer.org/Cancer/BreastCancer/MoreInformation/InflammatoryBreastCancer/index.
- *NCI*, *Inflammatory Breast Cancer*. www.cancer.gov/cancertopics/factsheet/Sites-Types/IBC.

### A.4.13 Lymphedema

- *Best Cancer Sites*, *Best Lymphedema Websites*. www.bestcancersites.com/lymphedema.
- *Breast Cancer Org*, *Lymphedema*. www.breastcancer.org/treatment/lymphedema.
- *ACS*, *Lymphedema: What Every Woman with Breast Cancer Should Know*. http://www.cancer.org/acs/groups/cid/documents/webcontent/002876-pdf.pdf.

### A.4.14 Male BC

- *NCI*, *Male Breast Cancer Treatment*. www.cancer.gov/cancertopics/pdq/treatment/malebreast/.

- *MedlinePlus* is a major source of information with a wide range of topics related to BC in men at http://www.nlm.nih.gov/medlineplus/malebreastcancer.html.
- The *ACS* provides a detailed guide to links about male BC (http://www.cancer.org/cancer/breastcancerinmen/detailedguide/breast-cancer-in-men-additional) and has a *What are the risk factors for breast cancer in men*? Page at http://www.cancer.org/cancer/breastcancerinmen/detailedguide/breast-cancer-in-men-risk-factors.
- *Facing Our Risk of Cancer Empowered* (*FORCE*), *Men with Mutation* at http://www.facingourrisk.org/understanding-brca-and-hboc/information/previvors-survivors/men/. See also Sect. A.4.19.

### A.4.15 Non-English Languages

Links in many other languages are provided by *DMOZ* (www.dmoz.org). Moreover, *External Links* can be easily found in most topics of *Wikipedia* selected according to the language of the country.

#### German Language

- *Instituts für Qualität und Wirtschaftlichkeit im Gesundheitswesen, Brustkrebs*. http://www.gesundheitsinformation.de/brustkrebs.2276.de.html.
- *Krebsinformationsdienst des Deutschen Krebsforschungszentrums* (*DKFZ*), *Brustkrebs*. https://www.krebsinformationsdienst.de/tumorarten/brustkrebs/.
- *Deutch Krebsgeselleschaft* (www.krebsgesellschaft.de). *Onko Internetportal der Deutschen Krebsgesellschaft, Patienteninformationen zu Brustkrebs*. http://www.krebsgesellschaft.de/onko-internetportal/basis-informationen-krebs/krebsarten/brustkrebs-definition-und-haeufigkeit.html.
- *Breast Cancer Action* (www.bcaction.de). *Nationale, europäische und internationale Leitlinien zu Brustkrebs* (*Linkliste*). http://www.bcaction.de/bcaction/nationale-europaeische-und-internationale-leitlinien-zu-brustkrebs/#section-3.

#### French Language

- *Le Cancer du Sein, Parlons-en*! (www.cancerdusein.org).
- *Fédération Nationale des Centres de Lutte contre le Cancer* (*FNCLCC*), at www.unicancer.f
- *Groupe de recherche en cancer du sein* (*GRCS*), at http://www.grcs-crchum.ca/.
- *Radio Curie* (http://radio.curie.fr/), is a web broadcast for women with BC and their families.

#### Italian Language

- *Associazione Italiana Ricerca sul Cancro* (*AIRC*), http://www.airc.it/tumori/tumore-al-seno.
- *Associazione Italiana di Oncologia Medica* (*AIOM*) (www.aiom.it) provides also Italian Guidelines (http://www.aiom.it/area+pubblica/area+medica/prodotti+scientifici/linee+guida/1%2C333%2C1%2C).
- *Seno Salvo* (www.senosalvo.com) is the most popular Italian website dealing with breast diseases, both benign and malignant.

### Spanish Language

- The *ACS* proposes many texts in Spanish. http://www.cancer.org/espanol/cancer/cancerdeseno/.
- The *NIC* too offers information in Spanish. http://www.cancer.gov/espanol/tipos/seno.
- *ABCD after breast cancer diagnosis*, one-to-one support also in Spanish. http://www.abcdbreastcancersupport.org/espanol/.
- *Grup d'Ajuda Mama i Salut* (*GAMIS*). http://www.gamisassociacio.org/esp/index_esp.php.
- *Association de Mujeres afectadas por càncer de mama* (*AMACMEC*). http://www.amacmec.org/.

### Other Languages

- *Dutch*, *Borstkanker*. https://www.dmoz.org/World/Nederlands/Gezondheid/Aandoeningen_en_Ziekten/Kanker/Borstkanker;
- *Danish*, *Landsforeninngen mod Brystkraeft*. http://www.brystkraeftforeningen.dk/;
- *Swedish*, *Bröstcancer*. http://www.cancerfonden.se/brostcancer.

## A.4.16 Paget Disease

- *NCI*, *Paget Disease of the Breast*. www.cancer.gov/cancertopics/factsheet/Sites-Types/pagets-breast.
- *Macmillan*, *Paget's disease of the breast*. http://www.macmillan.org.uk/Cancerinformation/Cancertypes/Breast/Aboutbreastcancer/Typesandrelatedconditions/Pagetsdisease.aspx.

## A.4.17 Predictive Markers

- The *Triple Negative Breast Cancer Foundation* (www.tnbcfoundation.org) is dedicated to the advancement of research for triple negative BC.
- The *Her2 Support Group* (www.her2support.org) gives information and support to patients who are HER2 positive.
- The *ASCO* publishes online guidelines/recommendations for assays and predictive markers. http://www.instituteforquality.org/practice-guidelines.

## A.4.18 Quality of Life/Nutrition/Exercises

- *Macmillan*, *Adjusting to life after cancer*, provides information about post-treatment challenges and ways to minimize difficulties. www.macmillan.org.uk/Cancerinformation/Livingwithandaftercancer/Lifeaftercancer/.
- *Reach to Recovery*. http://ww w.cancer.org/treatment/supportprogramsservices/reach-to-recovery
- *NCI*, *Facing Forward: Life after Cancer Treatment*. www.cancer.gov/cancertopics/coping/life-after-treatment/.
- *Susan G. Komen*, *Quality of Life* (ww5.komen.org/BreastCancer/QualityofLife.html) and *Healthy Weight and Diet* (http://ww5.komen.org/BreastCancer/HealthyWeightampDiet.html).

- *ACS, ACS Guidelines on Nutrition and Physical Activity for Cancer Prevention.* (http://www.cancer.org/healthy/eathealthygetactive/acsguidelinesonnutrition-physicalactivityforcancerprevention/index), and *Exercise after Breast Surgery* (http://www.cancer.org/cancer/breastcancer/moreinformation/exercises-after-breast-surgery).
- *Breast Cancer Org, Nutrition.* www.breastcancer.org/nutr_intro.html.
- *Australian Cancer Institute, Guidelines on Diet, Physical Activity and Weight for Cancer Prevention.* http://www.cancerinstitute.org.au/publications/guidelines-on-diet,-physical-activity-and-weight-for-cancer-prevention.
- *American Council of Exercise (ACE), Exercise for Breast Cancer Survivors.* http://www.acefitness.org/acefit/healthy_living_fit_facts_content.aspx?itemid=3320.

### A.4.19 Risk Assessment Models/Genetics

- *Breast Cancer Org, Breast Cancer Risk Factors.* www.breastcancer.org/risk/factors/genetics.jsp.
- *Breast Cancer Research, Breast cancer risk-assessment models.* http://breast-cancer-research.com/content/9/5/213.
- *ACS, Causes, Risk Factors, and Prevention Topics*, at http:/www.cancer.org/cancer/breastcancer/detailedguide/breast-cancer-risk-factors.
- *NCI, Breast Cancer: Prevention, Genetics, Causes* (www.cancer.gov/cancertopics/prevention-genetics-causes/breast), and *Cancer Genetics* (www.cancer.gov/cancertopics/prevention-genetics-causes/genetics).
- *FORCE* (www.facingourrisk.org) is an organization devoted to hereditary breast and ovarian cancer. Its mission includes support, research, and advocacy for anyone with a BRCA mutation or a family history of cancer. *Hereditary Breast and Ovarian Cancer Information and Advocacy.* http://www.facingourrisk.org/index.php.
- *Myriad Pro, Hereditary Breast and Ovarian Cance*r (HBOC). Although this is trademark, the site shows a wide source of information data for professionals. https://www.myriadpro.com/hereditary-cancer-testing/hereditary-breast-and-ovarian-cancer-hboc-syndrome/hboc-cancer-risks/.

### A.4.20 Second Opinion

- The *Johns Hopkins Hospital Breast Center* (www.hopkinsmedicine.org/breast-center), *Ask the Expert.* http://www.hopkinsbreastcenter.org/services/ask_expert/.
- *ACS, Talking with your doctor getting a second opinion.*
- www.cancer.org/Treatment/UnderstandingYourDiagnosis/TalkingaboutCancer/TalkingWithYourDoctor/talking-with-your-doctor-getting-a-second-opinion.
- *Breast Cancer Org, Asking for a Second Opinion.* www.breastcancer.org/treatment/second_opinion/asking.jsp.

### A.4.21 Surgery

- *Breast Cancer Org, Biopsy.* http://www.breastcancer.org/symptoms/testing/types/biopsy.

- *WebMD, Breast Biopsy* (http://www.webmd.com/women/guide/breast-biopsy) and other topics as *Types of Mastectomy* and *Breast Reconstruction.*
- *eMedicine Health, Mastectomy* (http://www.emedicinehealth.com/mastectomy/article_em.htm) and other topics as *Lumpectomy, Sentinel Node Biopsy, Breast Reconstruction.*
- *American Society of Plastic Surgeons (ASPS), 2012 Post-Mastectomy Fat Graft/Fat Transfer ASPS Guiding Principles*, at http://www.plasticsurgery.org/Documents/medical-professionals/health-policy/guiding-principles/2012Post-MastectomyFatGraft-FatTransferASPSGuidingPrinciples.pdf.
- *British Assoc. of Plastic, Reconstructive and Aesthetic Surgeons (BAPRAS), Lipomodelling Guidelines for Breast Surgery.* http://www.bapras.org.uk/docs/default-source/commissioning-and-policy/2012-august-lipomodelling-guidelines-for-breast-surgery.pdf.
- *Options for Breast Reconstruction.* http://www.optionsforbreastreconstruction.com.
- *Breast Free* (www.breastfree.org) offer information about alternatives to reconstruction and support for women who have already decided against it.

### A.4.22 Trials for Special Situations

- *Your Treatment Choices* makes easy to find and connect with a clinical research trial in Europe. https://yourtreatmentchoices.com/.
- *UK Clinical Trials Gateway* provides information about clinical trials running in the UK. http://www.ukctg.nihr.ac.uk/default.aspx.
- *MARIBS (Magnetic Resonance Imaging for Breast Screening) study*, coordinated by the Institute of Cancer Research, compares regular mammographic screening and regular magnetic resonance imaging (MRI) for women with a high risk of carrying gene BRCA1/2. http://www.icr.ac.uk/news-archive/magnetic-resonance-imaging-more-sensitive-than-mammograms-in-detecting-breast-cancer-in-high-risk-under-50%27s.
- *Sister study* (www.sisterstudy.org) has enrolled 50,000 women who have sisters with BC. This study will follow these women for at least 10 years and collect information about genes, lifestyle, and environmental factors. An offshoot of the Sister Study, the Two Sister Study, contributes to learn about genetic and environmental causes of young-onset BC (see also Sect. A.4.19).

### A.4.23 Young Women

- The *Young Survival Coalition* (www.youngsurvival.org) is an international network of BC survivors and supporters dedicated to the concerns and issues that are unique to young women (under age 41).
- *Macmillan* has a section *Cancer info for teens and young adults* at www.click4tic.org.uk.
- *Rethink Breast Cancer* (www.rethinkbreastcancer.com) helps young women facing BC, inter alia, making sure that they have timely access to prevention surgery and reconstruction.

- The *I'm Too Young For This! Cancer Foundation* is a support and research organization working exclusively on behalf of survivors under the age of 40 and their care providers. *Stupid Cancer* (www.stupidcancer.org) is one of the sections with comprehensive list of other cancer-related net resources for adolescents-teens and young adults.
- *How Can We Help You* [Resource Directories] provides links to a wide variety of resources relevant to young adults with cancer. In the link there are forums (http://forums.stupidcancer.org), and also a weekly radio broadcast (http://www.blogtalkradio.com/stupidcancershow).
- *Planet Cancer* (http://planetcancer.org) has launched a social networking section of their website for very young adults with cancer, at http://myplanet.planetcancer.org.

# Epilogue

During the drafting of this handbook, memories of friendly conversations with *Uccio* Querci della Rovere accompanied me: memories of the time and the words that physicians needed in order to think; the time and the words that patients needed more than some drugs; the time and the words, but music too (especially by the Beatles); the good reads; and the loves with which it was important to fill our lives and which made us feel more genuine and credible. Among so many, some of the exchanges *Uccio* and I had had a deep impact on me and I felt the need to share them, in the body of the text and in these last lines. Although *Uccio* is not with us anymore, his legacy continues to speak.

- *The eye sees only what the mind is prepared to comprehend* is a quote of Henry Bergson. At risk of appearing self-conceited, we hope to have helped you to *know and hold* in mind in order to *recognise* the many aspects of breast diseases.
- *It takes a vocation to art of observation, as with all the other arts* is a quote of Jean-Baptiste Bouillaud about the *esprit d'observation*, which must be constantly cultivated, but primarily in those cases where a mistake was made.
- *A rolling stone gathers no moss* is an old English proverb that means that a person who is always changing ideas and methods is unable to retain something of his background. Retaining means not to be confused by the large array of concepts, but still make wise choices and establish good habits.
- *Use technology to confirm your diagnostic impression, not to rule it out*, a statement of Barry B. Lowitz that emphasises the value of intuition, especially when based on a solid experience.
- *The good teacher explains, the superior teacher demonstrates, but the great teacher inspires* is a quote of William Arthur Ward. Look at *inspiration* as a long-term goal that never really has an ending. Be inspired and aim to inspire.
- *The anatomical types of the breast cancer are so numerous, the variations in clinical course so wide, the paths of dissemination so diverse, the difficulty of determining the actual conditions so complex... as to render impossible in the majority of cases a reasonably accurate adjustment of means to ends.* This James Ewing's statement is one of the quotes of the past that have kept intact its great value over time.



A.M. Pluchinotta (ed.), *The Outpatient Breast Clinic: Aiming at Best Practice*,
DOI 10.1007/978-3-319-15907-2

- *The female breast is the chest elevated to the status of a mystery – the moralized chest,* writes Novalis who adds: *such elevation to the status of a mystery expresses the very relationship of soul, spirit and matter in the cosmos.* That says a lot about the several symbolisms of the breast and its importance in our culture.
- Women should *have a finger in every pie* is an idiomatic expression meaning to be involved in and have influence in decision-making process. Ultimately, women should *have a finger in their own destiny*, as wrote Rose Kushner, an American journalist and pioneering advocate for breast cancer patients.
- *Anything that changes your values changes your behaviour* is a teaching quote of George Sheehan. Also in medical practice the biggest challenge for concordance comes from a change in beliefs and values, as much, and probably more than, from information and logic.
- *When a woman feels uncomfortable in her skin it is of little use to put something else in her breasts, no surgeon is able to give her charm or to modify a glance.* This statement of Dominique Gros may be questionable, but still has value in some cases.
- *A bad workman blames his tools* is an idiom suitable for both (few) radiologists and surgeons in certain (rare) situations.
- *The devil is in the detail* is another idiom, which refers to a catch or mysterious element hidden in the details and derives from the earlier phrase *God is in the detail* expressing the idea that whatever one does should be done thoroughly; i.e. details are important and should never be disregarded.
- *The decision of one is more useful than the opinion of many* describes, for the surgeon, the moment when they find themselves alone facing difficult choices, none of which seems to be a definite solution.
- *The long and winding road* was the last single released by the Beatles. Same as long and winding is the road *across the universe* (another line by the Beatles) of the breast identity.

The Editor

MIX
Papier aus verantwortungsvollen Quellen
Paper from responsible sources
FSC® C105338

If you have any concerns about our products,
you can contact us on
**ProductSafety@springernature.com**

In case Publisher is established outside the EU,
the EU authorized representative is:
**Springer Nature Customer Service Center GmbH**
**Europaplatz 3, 69115 Heidelberg, Germany**

Printed by Libri Plureos GmbH
in Hamburg, Germany